MOTOR NEURON DISEASE

'The tongues of dying men enforce attention like deep harmony'

John of Gaunt in Richard III,
Shakespeare

MOTOR NEURON DISEASE

EDITED BY

A.C. WILLIAMS

Professor of Clinical Neurology and
Head of the University Department of Neurology,
University of Birmingham, UK

CHAPMAN & HALL MEDICAL
London · Glasgow · New York · Tokyo · Melbourne · Madras

Published by Chapman & Hall, 2–6 Boundary Row, London SE1 8HN, UK

Chapman & Hall, 2–6 Boundary Row, London SE1 8HN, UK
Blackie Academic & Professional, Wester Cleddens Road, Bishopbriggs, Glasgow G64 2NZ, UK
Chapman & Hall Inc., One Penn Plaza, 41st Floor, New York NY 10119, USA
Chapman & Hall Japan, Thomson Publishing Japan, Hirakawacho Nemoto Building, 6F, 1–7–11 Hirakawa-cho, Chiyoda-ku, Tokyo 102, Japan
Chapman & Hall Australia, Thomas Nelson Australia, 102 Dodds Street, South Melbourne, Victoria 3205, Australia
Chapman & Hall India, R. Seshadri, 32 Second Main Road, CIT East, Madras 600 035, India

First edition 1994

Typeset in 10/12 Palatino by Photoprint, Torquay, Devon
Printed in Great Britain by the University Press, Cambridge

ISBN 0 412 54780 5

A catalogue record for this book is available from the British Library

Library of Congress Cataloging-in-Publication data available

∞ Printed on acid-free text paper, manufactured in accordance with ANSI/NISO Z39.48–1992

Contents

Contents

Contents

Contributors

S.P. ALLISON
Queen's Medical Centre, Department of Medicine, Ward C54, University Hospital, Nottingham NG7 2UH, UK

STANLEY H. APPEL
Department of Neurology, Baylor College of Medicine, One Baylor Plaza, Texas Medical Center, Houston, Texas, USA

DARYN BELDEN
University of Wisconsin-Madison Medical School, Department of Neurology, Madison, Wisconsin, USA

BENJAMIN RIX BROOKS
University of Wisconsin Hospital, ALS Clinical Research Center, CSC H6–558, Madison, Wisconsin 53792–0001, USA

PETER CARDY
Motor Neurone Disease Association, PO Box 246, Northampton NN1 2PR, UK

MARINOS C. DALAKAS
Neuromuscular Diseases Section, NINDS, National Institutes of Health, Building 10, Room 4N248, Bethesda, Maryland 20892, USA

JACQUELINE DE BELLAROCHE
Department of Biochemistry, Neurosciences Research Group, Charing Cross & Westminster Medical School, Fulham Palace Road, London W6 8RF, UK

ROXANNE DEPAUL
University of Wisconsin-Madison Medical School, Department of Neurology, Madison, Wisconsin, USA

YAN DE TAN
University of Wisconsin-Madison Medical School, Department of Neurology, Madison, Wisconsin, USA

Contributors

VICTOR DUBOWITZ
Royal Postgraduate Medical School, Hammersmith Hospital, Du Cane Road, London W12 0NN, UK

FELIX P. ECKENSTEIN
School of Medicine, Department of Cell Biology, Oregon Health Sciences University, 3181 S W Sam Jackson Park Road, Portland, Oregon 97201–3098, USA

JOZSEF I. ENGELHARDT
Department of Neurology and Psychiatry, Albert-szent-Gyorgyi University, Szeged, Hungary

ROBERT J. FALLAT
ALS and Neuromuscular Research Foundation, 2351 Clay Street, RM 416, San Francisco, CA 94115, USA

DENISE A. FIGLEWICZ
Neuromuscular Disease Center, University of Rochester Medical Center, 601 Elmwood Avenue, Box 673, Rochester, New York 14642, USA

JAMES GAFFNEY
University of Wisconsin-Madison Medical School, Department of Neurology, Madison, Wisconsin, USA

SALLY J. GIBSON
Department of Histochemistry, Royal Postgraduate Medical School, Hammersmith Hospital, Du Cane Road, London W12 0NN, UK

HISHAM HAKIM
University of Wisconsin-Madison Medical School, Department of Neurology, Madison, Wisconsin, USA

SARAH HARPER
Department of Experimental Pathology, Medical School, Guy's Hospital, London Bridge, London SE1 9RT, UK

TOM HEAFIELD
Department of Clinical Neurology, Queen Elizabeth Hospital, Edgbaston, Birmingham, B15 2TH, UK

PAUL JOLICOEUR
Laboratory of Molecular Biology, IRCM 110 avenue des Pins Quest, Montreal, Quebec, Canada H2W 1R7

Contributors

BURK JUBELT
Department of Neurology, College of Medicine, State University of New York, 750 East Adams Street, Syracuse, NY 13210, USA

DOROTHY C. KELLEY-GERAGHTY
Department of Neurology, College of Medicine, State University of New York, 750 East Adams Street, Syracuse, NY 13210, USA

LEONARD KURLAND
Senior Consultant and Professor of Epidemiology, Mayo Clinic, Rochester, Minnesota 55905, USA

P.N. LEIGH
Institute of Psychiatry, De Crespigny Park, Denmark Hill, London SE5 8AF, UK

DAVID LEWIS
University of Wisconsin-Madison Medical School, Department of Neurology, Madison, Wisconsin, USA

CHRISTOPHER N. MARTYN
MRC Environmental Epidemiology Unit, University of Southampton, Southampton General Hospital, Southampton SO9 4XV, UK

JOSEPH E. MAZURKIEWICZ
Department of Anatomy, Cell Biology and Neurobiology, A–135, Albany Medical College, 47 New Scotland Avenue, Albany, New York 12281, USA

N.M.F. MURRAY
The National Hospital for Neurology & Neurosurgery, Queen Square, London WC1N 3BG, UK

RAE NISHI
School of Medicine, Department of Cell Biology, Oregon Health Sciences University, 3181 S W Sam Jackson Park Road, Portland, Oregon 97201–3098, USA

FORBES H. NORRIS
ALS and Neuromuscular Research Foundation, 2351 Clay Street, RM 416, San Francisco, CA 94115, USA

PETER B. NUNN
Kings College London, Division of Molecular Sciences, Department of Biochemistry, Strand, London WC2R 2LS, UK

DAVID OLIVER
Medway Health Authority, The Wisdom Hospice, St William's Way, Rochester, Kent ME1 2NU, UK

Contributors

HARDEV S. PALL
University Department of Clinical Neurology, Queen Elizabeth Hospital, Edgbaston, Birmingham B15 2TH, UK

BERNARD M. PATTEN
Bayor College of Medicine, Department of Neurology, One Baylor Plaza, Houston, Texas 77030, USA

ROSALIND PEGG
Clevedon, Avon, UK

JULIA M. POLAK
Department of Histochemistry, Royal Postgraduate Medical School, Hammersmith Hospital, Du Cane Road, London W12 0NN, UK

AMANDA POWELL
Department of Clinical Neurology, Queen Elizabeth Hospital, Edgbaston, Birmingham B15 2TH, UK

KURUPATH RADHAKRISHNAN
Section of Clinical Epidemiology, Department of Health Sciences Research, Mayo Clinic, Rochester, Minnesota 55905, USA

JON RAWLING
University of Wisconsin-Madison Medical School, Department of Neurology, Madison, Wisconsin, USA

J.K. RAWLINGS
Queen's Medical Centre, Department of Medicine Ward C54, University Hospital, Nottingham, NG7 2UH, UK

MARCO ROSSI
The Midland Centre for Neurosurgery & Neurology, Holly Lane, Smethwick, Warley, West Midlands B67 7JX, UK

GUY A. ROULEAU
Centre for Research in Neurosciences, McGill University, The Montreal General Hospital Research Institute, 1650 Cedar Avenue, Montreal PQ H3G 1A4, Canada

MOHAMMED SANJAK
University of Wisconsin-Madison Medical School, Department of Neurology, Madison, Wisconsin, USA

R. GLENN SMITH
Department of Neurology, Baylor College of Medicine, One Baylor Plaza, Texas Medical Center, Houston, Texas 77030, USA

RICHARD SMITH
ALS and Neuromuscular Research Foundation, 2351 Clay Street, RM 416, San Francisco, CA 94115, USA

ENRICO STEFANI
Department of Molecular Physiology and Biophysics, Baylor College of Medicine, One Baylor Plaza, Texas Medical Center, Houston, Texas, USA

T.J. STEINER
Academic Unit of Neuroscience, Charing Cross and Westminster Medical School, The Reynolds Bld, St Dunstan's Road, London W6 8RP, UK

ROBERT SUFIT
University of Wisconsin-Madison Medical School, Department of Neurology, Madison, Wisconsin, USA

RUP TANDAN
Department of Neurology, University Health Center, One South Prospect Street, Burlington, Vermont 05401, USA

NEIL H. THOMAS
Royal Postgraduate Medical School, Hammersmith Hospital, Du Cane Road, London W12 0NN, UK

P. K. THOMAS
Royal Free Hospital, Rowland Hill Street, London NW3 2PF, UK

JIM UNSWORTH
Director of Rehabilitation, Selly Oak Hospital, Raddlebarn Road, Selly Oak, Birmingham B29, UK

LISA VIRGO
Department of Biochemistry, Charing Cross and Westminster Medical School, Fulham Palace Road, London, UK

FRANK WALSH
Department of Experimental Pathology, Medical School, Guy's Hospital, London Bridge, London SE1 9RT, UK

ROSEMARY WARING
School of Biochemistry, University of Birmingham, Edgbaston, Birmingham B15 2TT, UK

STEPHEN C. WARING
Section of Clinical Epidemiology, Department of Health Sciences Research, Mayo Clinic, Rochester, Minnesota 55905, USA

Contributors

DANNY F. WATSON
Department of Neurology, Wayne State University, 421 East Canfield Avenue, 3124 Elliman Building, Detroit, Michigan 48201, USA

ADRIAN WILLIAMS
University Department & Regional Centre for Neurology, Queen Elizabeth Hospital, Edgbaston, Birmingham B15 2TH, UK

DAVID B. WILLIAMS
Senior Consultant and Professor of Epidemiology, Mayo Clinic, Rochester, Minnesota 55905, USA

H.J. WILLISON
Royal Free Hospital, Rowland Hill Street, London NW3 2PF, UK

Preface

My first recollection of a discussion on research in motor neurone disease (MND) was when some 15 years ago a distinguished professor of neurology said that if someone gave him a million pounds to work on the cause and cure of motor neurone disease he would not know where to start. How encouraging that times have changed such that there are now several different approaches, though no single approach, that will lead, no doubt by a tortuous route and with much attendant serendipity, towards understanding the pathogenesis. In turn, though unpredictable whether it arrives early or late in this process, treatment for this thoroughly unpleasant disease will emerge. As an illness that rarely runs in families and where epidemics do not occur we are looking at a multifactorial process presumably with a genetically determined Achilles heel, leading to individual susceptibility to environmentally derived perturbations. The genetic elements may be most easily unravelled in familial cases with the hope that they also relate to susceptibility factors in the sporadic case, and advances being made in this arena are described herein. We have no MPTP story equivalent for motor neurone disease, which is unfortunate as that discovery has been so stimulating in the parallel world of Parkinson's disease, but not surprising as the MPTP miniepidemic was a fluke event. Nevertheless, clues as to the environmental triggers from the situation on Guam and other speculations, whether viral or chemical toxins, are included. Biochemical mechanisms involved in the life and death of a motor neurone are clearly important in understanding the selective neuronal involvement and current knowledge outlined in several chapters, though differentiating predisposing factors from the terminal process will not be easy. Either way, understanding the biochemical chain of events could lead to therapeutic loopholes, as will be mentioned, together with the design of trials to test such hypotheses.

The management of the patient with MND is demanding and requires input from quite a range of medical and paramedical specialties at all stages of the illness. Another trend over the last decade has been towards more effort from physicians in helping with the management of

Preface

this and other incurable diseases. Welcome though this is, there are major deficiencies in most parts of the world at many levels in the delivery of good and humane health care to patients with motor neurone disease. Many agencies, including the voluntary organizations, need to get their act together; I know that this is not easy, but expense, the usual excuse, is only one of the problems, as there also needs to be a change of attitude. Many of these aspects are discussed by various authors and, though it is not always easy to prove how bad services are, anecdotal reports from patients give no room for complacency, particularly when such reports often give a catalogue of poor management rather than isolated events.

I have encouraged authors to use the format of this volume to be outspoken and controversial if they wish and have not edited out contradictions and hope this compilation is a lively overview of where the action is in motor neurone disease circles.

A. C. Williams
Birmingham

PART ONE

1 Clinical features and differential diagnosis of classical motor neuron disease

RUP TANDAN

1.1 INTRODUCTION

The progressive neurodegenerative disorder of adults resulting from variable combined degeneration of the lower motor neurons (LMN) and upper motor neurons (UMN) is referred to as motor neuron disease (MND) in the UK and some European countries, as amyotrophic lateral sclerosis (ALS) in the USA and as Charcot's disease in France. The first clinical and pathological descriptions of MND were given by Charcot in several publications in the second half of the nineteenth century (Charcot and Joffroy, 1869; Charcot, 1873). At least three types of the disease are recognized: classical sporadic disease (Tandan and Bradley, 1985a; Mitsumoto, Hanson and Chad, 1988; Williams and Windebank, 1991), familial and usually dominantly inherited disease (Mulder *et al.*, 1986), and the type seen in the high-incidence foci in the western Pacific Ocean (Guam, Kii Peninsula of Japan and West New Guinea) (Lavine *et al.*, 1991). Although the precise etiology of the motor neuron degeneration in this disease is not yet known (Tandan and Bradley, 1985b; Mitsumoto, Hanson and Chad, 1988; Williams and Windebank, 1991), several authors have recently reported motor neuron disorders in association with immunological abnormalities that are potentially treatable (Sadiq *et al.*, 1990; Pestronk, 1991), while others have described the clinical and genetic characteristics of the disease seen as part of a widespread systems degeneration in association with deficiency of the lysosomal hydrolase N-acetyl-β-hexosaminidase (β-hex) (Johnson *et al.*, 1982; Specola *et al.*, 1990). Increased awareness, early diagnosis and more aggressive supportive management have led to increased life expectancy in this disease (Caroscio *et al.*, 1987).

1.2 TRENDS IN THE EPIDEMIOLOGY OF CLASSICAL MOTOR NEURON DISEASE

The annual incidence rate of classical sporadic MND has varied between 0.5 and 2.4 per 100 000 population, and the annual prevalence rate between 2.5 and 7 per 100 000 population worldwide in different studies (Kurtzke, 1991). The annual average death rate from the disease is about 1 per 100 000 population. There are no significant racial differences in the incidence, prevalence or death rate of the disease, and it is believed that the low incidence rates reported from Eastern Europe, Russia and Mexico probably reflect incomplete case ascertainment. Recent reports from the USA, England, Scotland, Canada, Israel, France, Finland and Japan suggest that the annual incidence rate and average annual death rate may be rising, especially amongst the Caucasian population, and most notably in females older than 60 years (Durrleman and Alpero-vitch, 1989). A detailed description of the epidemiology of the disease is provided in Chapter 18.

1.3 CRITERIA FOR THE DIAGNOSIS OF MOTOR NEURON DISEASE

The heterogeneity of clinical involvement early in the course of the disease makes diagnosis difficult and adversely affects the inclusion of patients in clinical research trials and molecular genetics studies. In order to achieve a consensus on the diagnostic criteria of the disease, the World Federation of Neurology Subcommittee on Motor Neuron Disease convened a meeting of esteemed clinicians and researchers at El Escorial, Spain, in May 1990. The clinical criteria for the diagnosis are listed in Table 1.1. For the diagnosis of MND to be suggested, a careful history and physical and neurological examinations must demonstrate clinical evidence of LMN and UMN signs in the bulbar, cervical, thoracic and lumbosacral regions (Table 1.2). The topography of UMN and LMN signs in these four regions determines the certainty of the diagnosis (definite, probable, possible or suspected MND, Table 1.1). The accuracy, sensitivity and specificity of these clinical diagnostic criteria have been validated in a recent clinicopathological study (Gaffney *et al.*, 1992).

1.4 CLINICAL VARIANTS OF MOTOR NEURON DISEASE

There is good consensus amongst investigators that the clinical variant forms of classical MND probably result from early and predominant degeneration of the LMN and UMN in certain anatomical locales. Thus, degeneration of the LMN of the limb muscles produces the progressive muscular atrophy (PMA) variant, and degeneration of the cranial motor neurons subserving bulbar muscles causes progressive bulbar palsy (PBP). Further, striking degeneration of the UMN controlling the limb muscles produces the rare clinical and probably distinct disorder, primary lateral sclerosis (PLS), while significant degeneration of the corticobulbar system underlies progressive pseudobulbar palsy (PPP). Nevertheless, these clinical variant forms of classical MND can often

Table 1.1 Clinical criteria for the diagnosis and degree of diagnostic certainty in classical motor neuron disease

---

Diagnostic criteria for motor neuron disease
   Criteria *required* for the diagnosis:
   (i)   Lower motor neuron signs
   (ii) Upper motor neuron signs and
   (iii) Progression
   Criteria *supportive* of the diagnosis:
   (i)   Fasciculations in one or more regions
   (ii)   Isokinetic/isometric strength abnormalities
   (iii) Pulmonary function abnormalities
   (iv) Speech abnormalities
   (v)   Swallowing dysfunction
   (vi) Muscle biopsy evidence of denervation–reinnervation
   (vii) Normal nerve biopsy
   Criteria *inconsistent* with the diagnosis:
   (i)   Sensory loss
   (ii)   Sphincter dysfunction
   (iii) Movement disorder
   (iv) Dementia
   (v)   Anterior visual system abnormalities
   (vi) Other causes of MND-like syndromes
Clinical diagnostic certainty in motor neuron disease
   Definite: LMN and UMN signs in three regions (brainstem, cervical, thoracic, lumbosacral), e.g. classical Charcot-type MND
   Probable: LMN and UMN signs in two different regions and UMN signs rostral to the LMN signs, e.g. UMN bulbar, LMN spinal; UMN and LMN bulbar, LMN spinal; etc.
   Possible: LMN and UMN signs in one region or UMN signs in two or three regions, e.g. monomelic MND; progressive bulbar palsy
   Suspected: LMN signs in two or three regions, e.g. progressive muscular atrophy, or cases not meeting requirements for possible MND

---

only be distinguished early in the course of the disease, because with the typical progression most patients usually develop clinical features of combined LMN and UMN involvement that can be verified at autopsy (Swank and Putnam, 1943; Lawyer and Netsky, 1953; Brownell, Oppenheimer and Hughes, 1970; Bonduelle, 1975; Norris, 1991).

1.5 CLINICAL FEATURES OF CLASSICAL MOTOR NEURON DISEASE

1.5.1 Classical motor neuron disease

Degeneration of the LMN typically produces focal or multifocal and often asymmetric muscle weakness and atrophy, cramps, prominent

Clinical features and differential diagnosis

Table 1.2 Lower and upper motor neuron signs in the four regions in classical motor neuron disease

	Bulbar	*Cervical*	*Thoracic*	*Lumbosacral*
LMN signs	Tongue, larynx, palate, lips, jaw	Neck, arm, hand, diaphragm	Back, abdomen	Back, abdomen, leg, foot
UMN signs	Clonic jaw reflex, brisk, gag reflex, exaggerated snout reflex, pseudobulbar features	Pathologically brisk or clonic tendon reflexes, Hoffmann reflex, spread of reflexes, spasticity	Loss of superficial abdominal reflexes	Pathologically brisk or clonic tendon reflexes, spasticity, extensor plantar response

fasciculations, fatigue, dysarthria and dysphagia (Table 1.2). Clinical involvement from UMN degeneration results in spasticity, pathological hyperreflexia, Babinski sign, brisk jaw jerk and emotional lability (Table 1.2). By the time of presentation, however, features of combined LMN and UMN degeneration are seen in the majority of classical MND patients, in various combinations (Table 1.3), occurring in about two-thirds of such patients (Table 1.4).

Muscle weakness is universal, and muscle atrophy with fasciculations is seen in most patients except in the very overweight, in whom they are difficult to discern. Muscle cramps are reported by over 50% of all patients, particularly after mild exertion or stretching. Motor involvement is frequently asymmetrical, and at onset is more common in the hands and arms than in the legs and bulbar muscles (Table 1.5). With eventual progression of the disease, bulbar weakness develops in almost 50% of patients, and respiratory muscle weakness occurs almost universally. Spasticity is seen in 50–75% of all patients. Only 30–50% of all patients with classical MND show a Babinski sign, even though other features of UMN involvement such as spasticity and pathological hyperreflexia might be present (Table 1.3).

1.5.2 Progressive bulbar palsy and pseudobulbar palsy

In different series reported in the literature, about 15–40% of patients with classical MND show prominent dysarthria and dysphagia at onset,

Table 1.3 Distribution of signs in some series of patients with motor neuron disease

Reference	No. of patients	Lower motor neuron involvement				Upper motor neuron involvement				
		Weakness	Atrophy	Cramps	Fasciculations	Spasticity	Babinski sign	Emotional lability	Sphincter dysfunction	Sensory abnormalities
Swank and Putnam, 1943	151	80	80	30	30	69	40	6	25	0
Friedman and Freedman, 1950	111	98	98	?	>90	75	?	27	15	10
Lawyer and Netsky, 1953	53	75	?	8	100	?	?	20	15	12
Mackay, 1963	70	83	83	?	?	67	?	?	?	20
Bonduelle, 1975	125	75	84	16	?	?	19	?	?	?
Gubbay et al., 1985	318	100	100	9	73	47	?	2	5	12
Caroscio et al., 1987	397	100	>90	50	>90	47	50	?	?	?

All values denote percentage of patients.

Table 1.4 Clinical characteristics and survival profiles in some series of patients with motor neuron disease

Reference	No. of patients	Mean age of onset (years)	Male-Female ratio	Clinical variants (percentage of patients)			Mean disease duration (months)				Survival (%)		Remarks
				Classical MND	PMA	PBP	Classical MND	PMA	PBP	All	5-year	10-year	
Mackay, 1963	70	52.5	2.5 : 1	71	11	16	36	33	17	?	?	?	Exceptionally survival 5–20 years
Boman and Meurman, 1967	140	47.3 (spinal) 54.7 (bulbar)	1.3 : 1	75	75	25	56	56	30	34	28	15	Bulbar-onset patients older, poorer prognosis
Veijajiiva, Foster and Miller, 1967	51	52.7	1.8 : 1	53	27	20	36	42	22	36	8	2	
Osuntokun, Adeuja and Bademosi, 1974	92	35.6	3 : 1	36	21	43	73	66	66	?	54	29	Relatively benign disease
Bonduelle, 1975	125	56.5	1.2 : 1	56	16	28	35	32	20	32	8	?	Bulbar disease more common in females
Kristensen and Mulgaard, 1977	118	57.2	1.9 : 1	83	10	7	36	36	24	30	19	8	Bulbar-onset patients older

Study													Comments
Rosati et al., 1977	86	57.0	2.1 : 1	66	14	20	29	40[a]	30	31	?	?	Bulbar disease more common in females Longer survival in younger cases
Forsgren et al., 1983	128	59.5	1.1 : 1	63	19	18	32	70	30	34	28	15	Bulbar-onset patients older. 5/10 year survival 23%/14% in classical and 64%/31% in PMA cases
Caroscio, 1987	397	57.0	1.5 : 1	82	7	9	52	182	48	49	38	30	
Schiffer et al., 1987	520	53.2	2.4 : 1	64	32	4	19	152	17	24	33	?	
Jablecki, Berry and Leach, 1989	194	59.0	1.4 : 1	73	0	27	–	–	?	37[b]	38	20	Bulbar-onset patients older
Christensen, Hojer-Petersen and Jensen, 1990	186	63.5	1.4 : 1	89	2	9	?	–	–	23[b]	26	7	Survival shorter in bulbar-onset and older patients

[a] Pseudopolyneuritic type.
[b] Median values.

Clinical features and differential diagnosis

Table 1.5 Site of onset in some series of patients with motor neuron disease

Reference	No. of patients	Upper extremities[a]	Lower extremities[a]	Bulbar[a]	Mixed[a]	Axial[a]
Friedman and Freedman, 1950	111	31	38	21	10	0
Lawyer and Netksy, 1953	53	26	46	26	0	2
Vejjajiva, Foster and Miller, 1967	51	40	25	25	10	0
Brownell, Oppenheimer and Hughes, 1970	45	29	40	31	16	0
Kristensen and Mulgaard, 1977	118	46	20	34	0	0
Rosen, 1978	668	41	40	19	0	0
Gubbay et al., 1985	318	29	49	22	?	?
Munsat et al., 1988	50	48	32	20	0	0
Jablecki, Berry and Leach, 1989	194	34	36	27	?	3

[a] All values represent percentage of patients.

with variable and at times no involvement of the limbs (Table 1.4). These patients typically show fasciculations and atrophy of the tongue due to loss of intrinsic muscles, decreased mobility of the tongue and pharyngeal muscle weakness. With disease progression, anarthria and aphagia ultimately ensue, leading to a verbally non-communicative state, and a propensity for repeated episodes of aspiration, choking, and aspiration pneumonitis. Early features in some patients may include spasticity of the tongue, diminished voluntary control over emotions, particularly with inappropriate crying; brisk jaw, gag and facial reflexes; and presence of primitive reflexes. These patients exhibit the entity of pseudobulbar palsy (Gallagher, 1989). In almost 90–100% of patients with a bulbar presentation, limb involvement eventually develops.

Table 1.6 Clinical characteristics and speech parameters in non-dysarthric and dysarthric MND patients at presentation

Clinical features	Non-dysarthric	Dysarthric
Number	12	13
Male–female	7:6	4:8
Age (years)	57.6 ± 10.9	59.6 ± 6.2
Duration (months)	13.4 ± 8.0	25.4 ± 16.0
Mode of onset		
Spinal	13	8
Bulbar	0	4
Norris score	81.2 ± 7.8	73.9 ± 11.9
Forced vital capacity (l)	3.1 ± 0.6	2.2 ± 0.7
Speech parameters		
Intelligibility (%)	98.3 ± 1.4	94.0 ± 4.5
Frenchay dysarthria assessment (%)	97.1 ± 4.1	81.5 ± 16.7
Tongue	96.8 ± 8.4	75.3 ± 23.5
Larynx	95.2 ± 9.5	75.6 ± 17.6
Palate	96.8 ± 5.4	81.9 ± 21.2
Lips	97.6 ± 3.3	86.2 ± 14.3
Jaw	100.0	100.0
Diadochokinetic rate	11.8 ± 2.2	8.5 ± 2.4
Maximum phonation time for /a/ (s)	21.0 ± 7.7	15.9 ± 5.5

In patients with bulbar involvement, measurement of maximum forces generated using sensitive transducers has shown that weakness is greatest in the tongue, followed by that in the jaw and lip muscles (DePaul *et al.*, 1988). This predilection is also suggested by results of the Frenchay dysarthria assessment, which shows most significant decline of lingual function (Enderby, 1980; Table 1.6), and is substantiated by several pathological studies that reveal profound loss of hypoglossal motor neurons (Lawyer and Netsky, 1953; Bonduelle, 1975). Weakness of the tongue, jaw and lip muscles is also seen, although to a lesser extent, in non-dysarthric MND patients with involvement confined to the limbs (DePaul *et al.*, 1988; Rosenfield *et al.*, 1991); compensatory movements of the jaw and the less involved extrinsic lingual muscles probably account for preserved speech function in these patients (DePaul and Abbs, 1987).

Several studies of swallowing have improved the understanding of this complex function in MND. In patients with bulbar presentation, swallowing and speech are usually simultaneously affected, and often accompanied by chewing difficulty (Robbins, 1987). There is generally no correlation between the presence or extent of swallowing difficulty and the absence or briskness of the jaw reflex or the gag reflex. Choking and coughing with solids and liquids reflect decreased force or coordination of the tongue; aspiration, particularly of liquids, results from decreased function of the vagus-innervated pharyngeal structures that protect the airway (true and false vocal folds); and problems in chewing, as evidenced by increased eating time, are the result of jaw muscle involvement. Video fluoroscopic recordings of swallowing have shown increased oral transit time, delay in elevation of the larynx and vallecular pooling that is more pronounced with liquids than with semisolids, especially in patients with bulbar involvement. Patients with bulbar dysfunction also demonstrate repetitive swallows of the same bolus, repetitive lingual pumping and use of compensatory strategies (e.g. head tilting) to facilitate swallowing.

The dysarthria in MND is associated with decreased range, rate and strength of articulatory movements of the tongue and oropharyngeal musculature; it results in progressively decreased intelligibility of speech (Kent *et al.*, 1990). Subjective abnormalities of perceptual speech in dysarthric patients relate to LMN and UMN dysfunction in the bulbar distribution, with perhaps UMN involvement being a better predictor of speech difficulty than LMN dysfunction (Rosenfield *et al.*, 1991). Perceptual abnormalities reported include temporal disruption, prolongation of segments, imprecise articulation of consonants, inappropriate pause times, hypernasality, vocal harshness, breathiness and voice tremor (Carpenter, McDonald and Howard, 1978).

Single-word intelligibility, Frenchay dysarthria assessment, maximum diadochokinetic rate for a series of three syllables (/pataka/) and maximum phonation duration for production of /a/ are all bedside clinical tests that differentiate dysarthric and non-dysarthric patients reliably (Table 1.6), and can be used to follow disease progression (Mulligan *et al.*, in press).

The imprecision and lack of objectivity associated with perceptual measures of speech categorization have prompted a few investigators, including the author's own group, to examine the acoustic characteristics of speech in intelligible MND patients (Kent *et al.*, 1989; Mulligan *et al.*, in press). These studies, using spectrograms of target words embedded in carrier phrases, have shown slow rate of speech, increased stop-gap and vowel duration, the occurrence of spirantization and changes in the second-format trajectories with increased duration and decreased slope and extent. The most vulnerable phonetic features involved in MND with progressive dysarthria are those associated with lingual–alveolar and velopharyngeal function and laryngeal configuration, and result from slowness of tongue movements and laryngeal gestures.

1.5.3 Progressive muscular atrophy

In reported series about 10–20% of patients present with a pure LMN disorder (Table 1.4). PMA accounted for 17 out of 761 cases (2.2%) of motor neuron diseases in northern California, with a calculated annual incidence of 0.02 per 100 000 population (Norris, 1991). The annual death rate from the disorder between 1950 and 1960 was reportedly 0.4 per 100 000 population. Most authorities believe that the majority of PMA cases evolve into classical MND clinically and pathologically over time. PMA occurs at an earlier age than classical MND, has a more striking male predilection, typically shows no bulbar involvement or only mild and late bulbar dysfunction and lacks UMN features.

Nevertheless, it is well recognized that the absence of UMN clinical signs predicts corticospinal tract involvement inaccurately, as in several series patients that appeared to have pure PMA on clinical grounds showed corticospinal tract degeneration pathologically (Friedman and Freedman, 1950; Lawyer and Netsky, 1953; Brownell, Oppenheimer and Hughes, 1970; Norris, 1991).

Asymmetrical distal upper extremity weakness and atrophy precedes distal lower extremity and proximal involvement. Symptoms can be exacerbated by exposure to cold. In general, muscle fasciculations and cramps are less frequent than in classical MND, although contraction fasciculations can be seen. The disease course is long-lasting, often extending from 10 to 15 years (Chio et al., 1985).

1.5.4 Primary lateral sclerosis

This chronic and perhaps distinct sporadic motor disorder, which is about twice as common in males as in females, usually begins after the age of 50 years (Younger et al., 1988). The presentation includes slowly progressive prominent spastic paraparesis or quadriparesis over many years, pathological hyperreflexia with clonus and minimal associated weakness in the lower extremities. Bilateral Babinski signs and decreased or absent abdominal reflexes are usually seen. In some patients the sequence of emotional lability, dysarthria, dysphagia and spastic tetraparesis more appropriately classifies them as having chronic progressive spinobulbar spasticity, probably a subtype of PLS (Gastaut, Michel and Figarella-Branger, 1988). Anterior horn cell involvement is not seen in PLS, based on clinical, electrophysiological and histological evidence. The disorder has to be differentiated from isolated instances of hereditary spastic paraplegia, chronic progressive myelopathy of multiple sclerosis, adrenomyeloneuropathy, human T-lymphotrophic virus

Clinical features and differential diagnosis

type I-associated myelopathy and structural lesions of the foramen magnum or cervical cord (Younger *et al.*, 1988).

1.5.5 Respiratory muscle involvement in classical motor neuron disease

Impairment of respiratory muscle function as determined by objective measures is common at presentation in classical MND (Fallat *et al.*, 1979; Ioli *et al.*, 1987; Schiffman and Belsh, 1989). However, early involvement of the diaphragm and external intercostal muscles (the major inspiratory muscles), and the abdominal wall and internal intercostal muscles (the principal expiratory muscles), is usually clinically asymptomatic. Nevertheless, with progressive disease patients successively report dyspnea on exertion and dyspnea at rest or during speaking, chewing or swallowing. Significant diaphragmatic involvement is suggested by greater breathing difficulty in the recumbent than sitting or upright positions. Symptomatic respiratory muscle involvement is more likely in patients with bulbar weakness, and in those with atrophy of the deltoids and trapezii. Rapid loss of pulmonary function usually occurs in the years preceding death, and terminal respiratory failure, which is the most common cause of death, is precipitous (Fallat *et al.*, 1979).

Studies of pulmonary function undertaken in several series of classical MND patients have shown a decrease in maximum voluntary ventilation (MVV), inspiratory pressure (IP) and expiratory pressure (EP) of 20–60% of predicted values, and increase in residual volume (RV) of 10–30% of predicted values, even in asymptomatic patients (Fallat *et al.*, 1979). Although most studies describe increasing abnormality of MVV, IP, EP and RV with disease progression, decline in forced vital capacity (FVC) generally lags behind, and may not occur until 1–3 years from onset. Deterioration in respiratory parameters occurred faster in patients followed until death than in those still alive at a mean interval of 20 months in one series (Fallat *et al.*, 1979). An FVC of less than 50% of predicted increases the chances of respiratory failure developing in patients, as do intercurrent infection, respiratory muscle fatigue, debility, aspiration and heart failure. Although the rate of decline of FVC is quite variable among patients (Munsat *et al.*, 1988), it is usually rapid just before death.

1.5.6 Classical MND and dementia

Clinically detectable dementia can accompany about 5% of otherwise typical patients with classical MND, being slightly more prevalent in bulbar-onset and familial cases (Hudson, 1981; Wikstrom *et al.*, 1982;

14

Horoupian *et al.*, 1984). The clinical features in some reviews and reports are given in Table 1.7. Overall, the demographic characteristics are not very different from those seen in classical MND without dementia. In about 50% of patients clinical dementia precedes the classical symptoms and signs of MND, while in 25% each it either follows motor involvement or is uncovered simultaneously. In one review of 231 patients with MND and dementia from the USA, UMN involvement was identified in 80%, bulbar abnormalities in 45%, myoclonus in 15% and cerebellar dysfunction in 6% of patients (Salazar *et al.*, 1983). Although patients with these features were previously reported under the heading of 'amyotrophic' Creutzfeldt–Jakob disease (CJD), none fulfilled other clinical or electroencephalographic criteria of CJD, and in none studied was the disease transmitted to laboratory animals (including non-human primates). The current consensus is that in these patients the disease is more closely related to classical MND than to transmissible CJD (Hudson, 1981; Salazar *et al.*, 1983).

Detailed neuropsychological testing undertaken by several investigators (including in some series in clinically non-demented patients) has defined abnormalities of attention, learning, confrontation naming, insight, judgement and calculations in a significant proportion of patients with classical MND (Neary *et al.*, 1990; Peavy *et al.*, 1992). However, memory deficits recorded by some observers in classical MND may really be the result of poor attention or difficulty in initiating behavior secondary to frontal lobe dysfunction, rather than true memory impairment (Peavy *et al.*, 1992).

1.5.7 Classical MND and parkinsonism

Although pathological degeneration of the substantia nigra is often reported in classical MND patients (Lawyer and Netsky, 1953; Brownell, Oppenheimer and Hughes, 1970; Bonduelle, 1975), clinical parkinsonism is rarely encountered (Hudson, 1981). When parkinsonism does occur in patients with MND, it is usually accompanied by dementia (Table 1.8). Parkinsonism can precede, accompany or follow the signs of MND; its features are no different from those seen elsewhere (Salazar *et al.*, 1983).

1.6 UNUSUAL CLINICAL MANIFESTATIONS IN CLASSICAL MND

1.6.1 Classical MND and oculomotor function

Although the usual teaching has been that oculomotor function is generally spared in classical MND (Bonduelle, 1975), several reports in

Table 1.7 Classical motor neuron disease and dementia

Reference	No. of patients	Male–female ratio	Mean age of onset (years)		Mode of onset			Mean duration of disease (years)		Remarks
			MND	Dementia	MND first	Dementia first	Simul-taneously	MND	Dementia	
Hudson, 1981	26	2 : 1	52.4	52.8	5	9	12	1.9	2.1	Duration till death
Wikstrom et al., 1982	3	0 : 3	71.3	70.7	1	2	0	1.7	2.3	Bulbar onset in all; duration till death
Salazar et al., 1983	37	2 : 1	56.0[a]		? 13/34	21/34	?	2.5[a]		Positive family history in 18%
Horoupian et al., 1984	2	1 : 1	45,52	45,50	0	1	1	7,2	7,4	Bulbar onset in both patients
Peavy et al., 1992	2	0 : 2	66.5,69	65,59	0	2	0	2,2	2.5,11	Bulbar onset in majority
	13 (prior reports)	5 : 8	54.1	53.2	0	8[b]	4[b]	1.1 (bulbar) 1.5 (limb)	2.3	

[a] Data for all patients with motor neuron disease and dementia.
[b] Data not clear from history in one patient.

Table 1.8 Classical motor neuron disease Parkinsonism and dementia

	Parkinsonism Hudson, 1981	MND–parkinsonism–dementia	
		Hudson, 1981	Salazar et al., 1983
Number of patients	8	8	26
Male–female ratio	7:1	3:1	2.8:1
Mean age of onset (years)			
MND	58.3	51.6	57.9[a]
Parkinsonism	54.8	53.1	?
Dementia	N/A	52.1	?
Mode of onset			
MND before parkinsonism or dementia	1/8	5/8	?11/26
Dementia before MND or parkinsonism	N/A	2/8	15/26
Parkinsonism before MND	5/8	0/8	?
Simultaneously	2/8	1/8	?
Mean duration of disease (years)			
MND	2.7	2.1	2.3[a]
Parkinsonism	6.2	0.9	
Dementia	N/A	1.9	

[a] Data for patients with MND, parkinsonism and dementia.

the last 15 years have noted abnormalities in a significant proportion of patients, particularly in those with bulbar involvement (Hayashi *et al.*, 1987; Esteban, De Andres and Giminez-Roldan, 1978). Clinically evident cog-wheeling of pursuit eye movements has been confirmed by electro-oculography (EOG). Other abnormalities reported, usually on the basis of EOG, include presence of frequent square-wave jerks and interruption saccades, reduced saccade velocity, mild conjugate gaze defects, asymmetry of optikokinetic nystagmus, spontaneous nystagmus with eyes closed and impaired visual scanning. One series described oculomotor paralysis in MND patients on respirators, that developed only after involvement of muscles of the lower face, pharynx, neck, tongue, lips and jaw (Hayashi *et al.*, 1987). These authors also reported the successive occurrence of abnormal Bell's phenomenon, slow ocular and eyelid movements, impersistent eyelid closure and dissociated movements of eyeballs and eyelids during corneal stimulation, an order of impairment that is the reverse of the normal ontogenetic sequence of these functions. Despite the above reports, a recent study reiterates the idea of oculomotor sparing in MND (Gizzi *et al.*, 1992), arguing that unrecognized coexistent parkinsonism could have accounted for the oculomotor abnormalities in some earlier series, a notion that seems less plausible from the evidence available.

1.6.2 Classical MND and sensory abnormalities

It has long been known that about 15–20% of patients with classical MND may either volunteer or admit to experiencing sensory symptoms. Careful bedside clinical examination can often reveal sensory abnormalities, while quantitative computerized sensory testing, as employed by some investigators, has shown abnormal thresholds, particularly for vibration and touch–pressure sensations (Mulder *et al.*, 1983; Jamal *et al.*, 1985). These observations are in keeping with loss of myelinated nerve fibers in the sensory superficial peroneal and sural nerves, and the pathological demonstration of degeneration of the posterior columns, spinocerebellar tracts, dorsal root ganglia and large myelinated nerve fibers in the dorsal roots in patients with classical MND (Kawamura *et al.*, 1981; Hamida *et al.*, 1987). They are also consistent with abnormalities of near-field (sural nerve) and far-field (after median nerve stimulation) responses seen in up to 50% of patients with classical MND (Shefner, Tyler and Krarup, 1991).

1.6.3 Classical MND and autonomic nervous system involvement

Traditional teaching, with support from clinical and pathological studies (Mannen *et al.*, 1982; Sung, 1982), has maintained that bladder and bowel dysfunction does not occur in classical MND. However, some investigators have noted dysautonomia as evidenced by resting tachycardia, decreased variability of the R–R cardiac interval, postural abnormalities of heart rate and blood pressure, and deranged gastroesophageal motility in a few patients with classical MND (Nogues and Stalberg, 1989).

1.7 TOPOGRAPHY OF ONSET AND MODE OF SPREAD OF DISEASE IN CLASSICAL MND

Several large series of patients with MND have indicated that, overall, about 65% of patients present with combined LMN and UMN involvement (classical MND or ALS), 25% with bulbar features (PBP) and 10% with LMN degeneration (PMA) (Table 1.4). Pseudobulbar palsy and PLS are rare presentations. When onset and spread of symptoms from LMN degeneration were recorded in 702 patients with classical MND followed up to 7 years, onset was characterized as being in one leg in 174 (25%), in one arm in 213 (30%) and in the bulbar region in 96 (14%) (Brooks, 1991). Spread of disease in unilateral limb-onset cases occurred successively to the contralateral limb, the homolateral limb and the bulbar area. Similar patterns of progression have been found in 150 classical MND patients followed over 5 years (Pajeau *et al.*, in preparation). Three years after onset, spread to bulbar muscles had occurred in 62% and 52% of arm- and leg-onset cases respectively, and spread to arm and leg muscles had occurred in 76% and 66%, respectively, of bulbar-onset cases (Brooks, 1991). In examining sex effects, spread to other regions after leg onset was faster in females, and to arms after bulbar onset was faster in males. These studies provide information on the sequence of spread of LMN degeneration, and corroborate non-random regional involvement of motor neurons.

1.8 CLINICAL COURSE AND PROGNOSIS OF CLASSICAL MND AND ITS VARIANTS

Several earlier clinical studies and semiquantitative analyses of motor function have shown a progressive decline of parameters in almost all patients. Quantitative tests of isometric muscle strength, activities of daily living, timed tasks, and respiratory parameters usually show a variable decrease of function of up to 20–50% per year (Andres *et al.*, 1988; Appel *et al.*, 1988; Munsat *et al.*, 1988; Jablecki, Berry and Leach, 1989). Deterioration is usually linear, with considerable difference in the rate of decline between patients (up to 20- to 40-fold), although in a given patient variability of loss of function between regions is less. In 40 patients with classical MND followed for 6 months, a 10–40% decrease from baseline values in a series of ordinal and quantitative measures of clinical, isometric muscle strength, activities of daily living, pulmonary function and electrophysiological parameters was found (Table 1.9). In another study of 50 MND patients followed monthly for a mean duration of 20 months, progressively increasing rates of deterioration were recorded for bulbar, leg strength, arm strength, pulmonary and timed hand functions (Munsat *et al.*, 1988). The natural history of the disease is discussed in detail in Chapter 6.

Although the overall median survival in classical MND is usually about 3 years from onset of the disease, early diagnosis and more aggressive management have led to increased survival in recent years, including in variants traditionally known to show poorer prognosis (Caroscio *et al.*, 1987). Two major factors that determine length of survival in classical MND are age of onset and clinical variant of the disease present. It is generally agreed that, independent of the clinical

Clinical features and differential diagnosis

Table 1.9 Change in some parameters over a 6-month period in 40 patients with classical motor neuron disease

Parameter	Baseline value Mean	SD	Percentage change at 6 months
Norris score[a]	74.93	10.09	−10.20
Grip strength, right (kg)	22.25	22.59	−39.15
Grip strength, left (kg)	19.64	23.47	−39.79
Activities of daily living (arms)[b]	54.97	11.21	−10.03
Activities of daily living (legs)[b]	47.34	12.23	−17.11
Forced vital capacity (l)	2.64	0.92	−23.99
Maximum isometric torque, biceps (ft lb)	21.00	12.06	−24.56
Surface macro compound muscle action potential amplitude, biceps (μV)	9281.05	4679.49	−17.93
Fiber density, biceps	2.79	1.19	10.83
Number of motor units, biceps	216.24	200.98	−28.80

[a] Normal = 100 (Norris *et al.*, 1974).
[b] Normal = 70 for arms and 63 for legs (Fillyaw *et al.*, 1989).

variant of MND present, survival is greater in patients with onset of symptoms before the age of 50 years than after. Survival is usually longest in the PMA variant, shortest in PBP and intermediate in patients with classical disease (ALS) (Table 1.4). Since bulbar disease is more common in older individuals, some researchers believe that the relatively poorer survival in PBP may be due to late age of onset in these patients rather than to the site of involvement. As shown in Table 1.4, overall 5-year survival ranges between 8 and 38%, and 10-year survival between 7 and 30%. Rarely, classical MND can be reversible, with either spontaneous improvement (Tucker *et al.*, 1991) or complete resolution after appropriate therapy, just as has been described for MND in association with intoxication due to lead (Boothby, de Jesus and Rowland, 1974) and mercury (Adams, Ziegler and Lynn, 1983), lymphoma (Younger *et al.*, 1991), dysproteinemia (Parry *et al.*, 1986) and cancer (Evans *et al.*, 1990).

1.9 DIFFERENTIAL DIAGNOSIS OF CLASSICAL MND

In view of the lack of a specific biochemical marker for the disease, the diagnosis of MND is purely clinical along with support from laboratory data. It can, however, be difficult to diagnose the disease early, and this

Table 1.10 Disorders that can produce a motor neuron disease-like syndrome

Inherited	
Enzymopathy	Hexosaminidase deficiency
Degenerative	Familial spastic paraplegia
Acquired	
Traumatic	Post-traumatic syringomyelia
Inflammatory	Myopathy, chronic demyelinating polyneuropathy
Immune-mediated	Motor neuropathy, radiculopathy or neuropathy associated with paraproteins or anti-GM1 antibody
Degenerative	Cervical myeloradiculopathy and multiple lumbosacral radiculopathy
Post-infectious	Post-polio syndrome
Endocrine	Thyroid and parathyroid disorders, diabetic 'amyotrophy'
Exogenous toxins	Lead, mercury
Tumors	Lymphoma, cancer
Post-radiation	Lumbar motor neuron degeneration
Miscellaneous	Cramp–fasciculation syndrome, cervical or foramen magnum region tumors

has to be based upon exclusion of conditions that produce an MND-like disorder (reviewed in Tandan, 1993). There is no doubt that classical MND has probably been underdiagnosed and misdiagnosed in the past (Caroscio *et al.*, 1987), especially in the elderly, in whom clinical features of the disease are often ascribed to debility of old age. Electrophysiological studies help to confirm the clinical diagnosis (see Chapter 7). Peripheral nerve conduction studies are usually normal and can serve to distinguish some disorders that may present similarly (Table 1.10), particularly chronic inflammatory demyelinating polyneuropathy (Barohn *et al.*, 1989) and multifocal motor neuropathy with conduction block seen in association with serum anti-GM1 antibodies (Pestronk, 1991). Cerebrospinal fluid examination and routine blood and urine studies are usually normal. A muscle or nerve biopsy may be necessary in selected cases to confirm denervation–reinnervation, and exclude inflammatory conditions that can produce an MND-like disorder (Table 1.10). Radiologic studies of the cervical and lumbar regions might be necessary, in appropriate cases, to exclude structural abnormalities in posterior fosa, foramen magnum region, cervical area or lumbosacral region.

Amongst other diseases or conditions that can produce a clinical syndrome resembling MND are endocrine disorders (thyroid, parathyroid and pancreas), the post-polio syndrome (Chapter 4), motor neuropathies (Chapter 3), the spinal muscular atrophies (Chapter 2), post-

Clinical features and differential diagnosis

radiation lumbar motor neuron degeneration, segmental spinal muscular atrophy confined to one limb (Oryema, Ashby and Spiegel, 1990; Riggs, Schochet and Gutmann, 1984) or both arms (Tandan *et al.*, 1990), and the cramp–fasciculation syndrome (Tahmoush *et al.*, 1991). These can be differentiated from classical MND, albeit at times with some difficulty, by appropriate history, clinical course, laboratory testing and electrophysiological studies.

1.10 CONCLUSION

The development of strict diagnostic criteria for MND and increased awareness will not only allow early diagnosis, but also facilitate research in the clinical, pathological and molecular areas of the disease. The incidence of the disease is probably rising, and with a more aggressive treatment approach leading to longer survival the prevalence of the disease is likely to increase. Several research groups have elegantly begun to chart the overall clinical course of the disease in different anatomical regions, as a prelude to understanding heterogeneity and defining the natural history of the disease. Finally, better understanding of immunological, pathological and genetic features of the disease has taken us closer to unravelling the mystery behind the cause of this enigmatic disease.

ACKNOWLEDGMENTS

The author is supported by grants from the Food and Drug Administration, Muscular Dystrophy Association, General Clinical Research Center Division of the National Institutes of Health, and Tyson & Associates, Inc., Santa Monica, CA. The author is grateful to Judy Gilmour for secretarial help in the preparation of this manuscript.

REFERENCES

Adams, C.R., Ziegler, D.K. and Lynn, J.T. (1983) Mercury intoxication simulating amyotrophic lateral sclerosis. *J. Am. Med. Assoc.*, **250**, 642–3.

Andres, P.L., Finison, L.J., Conlon, T. *et al.* (1988) Use of composite scores (megascores) to measure deficit in amyotrophic lateral sclerosis. *Neurology*, **38**, 405–8.

Appel, S.H., Stewart, S.S., Appel, V. *et al.* (1988) A double-blind study of the effectiveness of cyclosporine in amyotrophic lateral sclerosis. *Arch. Neurol.*, **45**, 381–6.

Barohn, R.J., Kissel, J.T., Warmolts, J.R. and Mendell, J.R. (1989) Chronic inflammatory demyelinating polyradiculoneuropathy: clinical characteristics, course, and recommendations for diagnostic criteria. *Arch. Neurol.*, **46**, 878–84.

Bonduelle, M. (1975) Amyotrophic lateral sclerosis, in *Handbook of Clinical Neurology*, Vol. 22 (eds P.J. Vinken, G.W. Bruyn and J.M. DeJong), New York, Elsevier, pp. 281–338.

Boman, K. and Meurman, T. (1967) Prognosis of amyotrophic lateral sclerosis. *Acta Neurol. Scand.*, **56**, 299–308.

Boothby, J.A., deJesus, P.V. and Rowland, L.P. (1974) Reversible forms of motor neuron disease: lead 'neuritis'. *Arch. Neurol.*, **31**, 18–23.

Brooks, B.R. (1991) The role of axonal transport in neurodegenerative disease: a meta-analysis of experimental and clinical poliomyelitis compared with amyotrophic lateral sclerosis. *Can. J. Neurol. Sci.*, **18**, 435–8.

Brownell, B., Oppenheimer, D.R. and Hughes, J. (1970) The central nervous system in motor neuron disease. *J. Neurol. Neurosurg. Psychiatry*, **33**, 338–57.

Caroscio, J.T., Mulvihill, M.N., Sterling, R. and Abrams, B. (1987) Amyotrophic lateral sclerosis. Its natural history. *Neurol. Clin.*, **5**, 1–8.

Carpenter, R.J., McDonald, T.J. and Howard, F.M. (1978) The otolaryngotic presentation of amyotrophic lateral sclerosis. *Otolaryngology*, **86**, 33–44.

Charcot, J.-M. (1873) Lecons sur les maladies du systeme nerveux. IInd Series, collected by Bourneville Paris, Delahaye, pp. 192–242. (English translation by G. Sigerson, New Sydenham Society, London, 1881; reprinted by the New York Academy of Medicine, Hafner, 1962, pp. 163–204.)

Charcot, J.M. and Joffroy, A. (1869) Deux cas d'atrophie musculaire progressive. *Arch. Physiol. Norm. Pathol.*, **2**, 354–67 and 629–490.

Chio, A., Brignolio, F., Leone, M. *et al.* (1985) A survival analysis of 155 cases of progressive muscular atrophy. *Acta Neurol. Scand.*, **72**, 407–13.

Christensen, P.B., Hojer-Pedersen, E. and Jensen, N.B. (1990) Survival of patients with amyotrophic lateral sclerosis in 2 Danish counties. *Neurology*, **40**, 600–4.

DePaul, R. and Abbs, J.H. (1987) Manifestations of ALS in the cranial motor nerves. Dynametric, neuropathologic and speech motor data. *Neurol. Clin.*, **5**, 231–50.

DePaul, R., Abbs, J.H., Caligiuri, M. *et al.* (1988) Hypoglossal, trigeminal, and facial motoneuron involvement in amyotrophic lateral sclerosis. *Neurology*, **38**, 281–3.

Durrleman, S. and Alperovitch, A. (1989) Increasing trend of ALS in France and elsewhere: are the changes real? *Neurology*, **39**, 768–73.

Enderby, P.M. (1980) Frenchay dysarthria assessment. *Br. J. Disord. Commun.*, **15**, 165–73.

Esteban, A., DeAndres, C. and Gimenez-Roldan, S. (1978) Abnormalities of Bell's phenomenon in amyotrophic lateral sclerosis: a clinical and electrophysiological evaluation. *J. Neurol. Neurosurg. Psychiatry*, **41**, 690–8.

Evans, B.K., Fagan, C., Arnold, T. *et al.* (1990) Paraneoplastic motor neuron disease and renal cell carcinoma: improvement after nephrectomy. *Neurology*, **40**, 960–2.

Clinical features and differential diagnosis

Fallat, R.J., Jewitt, B, Bass, M. *et al.* (1979) Spirometry in amyotrophic lateral sclerosis. *Arch. Neurol.*, **36**, 74–80.

Fillyaw, M., Tandan, R., Bradley, W.G. *et al.* (1989) Quantitative measures of neurological function in chronic neuromuscular disease. *J. Neurol. Sci.*, **92**, 17–36.

Forsgren, L., Almay, B.G.L., Holmgren, G. and Wall, S. (1983) Epidemiology of motor neuron disease in northern Sweden. *Acta Neurol. Scand.*, **68**, 20–9.

Friedman, A.P. and Freedman, D. (1950) Amyotrophic lateral sclerosis. *J. Nerv. Ment. Dis.*, **111**, 1–18.

Gaffney, J.S., Sufit, R.L, Hartmann, H. *et al.* (1992) Clinical diagnosis of amyotrophic lateral sclerosis (ALS): a clinicopathologic study of 'El Escorial' Working Group criteria in 36 autopsied patients (abstract). *Neurology*, **42**, 455.

Gallagher, J.P. (1989) Pathologic laughter and crying in ALS: a search for their origin. *Acta Neurol. Scand.*, **80**, 114–17.

Gastaut, J.L., Michel, B., Figarella-Branger, D. and Somma-Mauvais, H. (1988) Chronic progressive spinobulbar spasticity. A rare form of primary lateral sclerosis. *Arch. Neurol.*, **45**, 509–513.

Gizzi, M., DiRocco, A., Sivak, M. and Cohen B. (1992) Ocular motor function in motor disease. *Neurology*, **42**, 1037–46.

Gubbay, S.S., Kahana, E., Zilber, N. *et al.* (1985) Amyotrophic lateral sclerosis: a study of its presentation and prognosis. *J. Neurol.*, **232**, 295–300.

Hamida, M.B., Letaief, F., Hentati, F. and Hamida, C.B. (1987) Morphometric study of the sensory nerve in classical (or Charcot disease) and juvenile amyotrophic lateral sclerosis. *J. Neurol. Sci.*, **78**, 313–29.

Hayashi, H., Kato, S., Kawada, T. and Tsubaki, T. (1987) Amyotrophic lateral sclerosis: oculomotor function in patients on respirators. *Neurology*, **37**, 1431–2.

Horoupian, D.S., Thal, L., Katzman, R. *et al.* (1984) Dementia and motor neuron disease: morphometric, biochemical and Golgi studies. *Ann. Neurol.*, **16**, 305–13.

Hudson, A.J. (1981) Amyotrophic lateral sclerosis and its association with dementia, parkinsonism and other neurological disorders: a review. *Brain*, **104**, 217–47.

Ioli, F., DiLorenzo, G., Donner, C.F. *et al.* (1987) Some remarks on lung function in amyotrophic lateral sclerosis. *Adv. Exp. Med. Biol.*, **209**, 139–42.

Jablecki, C.K., Berry, C. and Leach, J. (1989) Survival prediction in amyotrophic lateral sclerosis. *Muscle Nerve*, **12**, 833–41.

Jamal, G.A., Weir, A.I., Hansen, S. and Ballantyne, J.P. (1985) Sensory involvement in motor neuron disease: further evidence from automated thermal threshold determination. *J. Neurol. Neurosurg. Psychiatry*, **48**, 906–10.

Johnson, W.G., Wigger, H., Karp, H.R. *et al.* (1982) Juvenile spinal muscular atrophy: a new hexosaminadase phenotype. *Ann. Neurol.*, **11**, 11–16.

Kawamura, Y., Dyck, P.J., Shimono, M. *et al.* (1981) Morphometric comparison of the vulnerability of peripheral motor and sensory neurons in amyotrophic lateral sclerosis. *J. Neuropath. Exp. Neurol.*, **40**, 667–75.

Kent, R.D., Weismer, G., Kent, J.F. *et al.* (1989) Relationships between speech intelligibility and the slope of second-format transitions in amyotrophic lateral sclerosis. *Clin. Linguist. Phonet.*, **3**, 347–58.

Kent, R.D., Kent, J.F., Weismer, G. *et al.* (1990) Impairment of speech intelligibility in men with amyotrophic lateral sclerosis. *J. Speech Hearing Dis.*, **55**, 721–8.

Kristensen, O. and Melgaard, B. (1977) Motor neuron disease. Prognosis and epidemiology. *Acta Neurol. Scand.*, **56**, 299–308.

Kurtzke, J.F. (1991) Risk factors in amyotrophic lateral sclerosis. *Adv. Neurol.*, **56**, 245–70.

Lavine, L., Steele, J.C., Wolfe, N. *et al.* (1991) Amyotrophic lateral sclerosis/ Parkinsonism–dementia complex in Southern Guam: is it disappearing? *Adv. Neurol.*, **56**, 271–85.

Lawyer, T. and Netsky, M.G. (1953) Amyotrophic lateral sclerosis: a clinico-anatomic study of fifty-three cases. *Arch. Neurol. Psychiat.*, **69**, 171–92.

Mackay, R.P. (1963) Course and prognosis in amyotrophic lateral sclerosis. *Arch. Neurol.*, **8**, 117–27.

Mannen, T., Iwata, M., Toyokura, Y. and Nagashima, K. (1982) The Onuf's nucleus and the external anal sphincter muscles in amyotrophic lateral sclerosis and Shy–Drager syndrome. *Acta Neuropathol.*, **58**, 255–60.

Mitsumoto, H., Hanson, M.R. and Chad, D.A. (1988) Amyotrophic lateral sclerosis. Recent advances in pathogenesis and therapeutic trials. *Arch. Neurol.*, **45**, 189–202.

Mulder, D.W., Bushek, W., Spring, E. *et al.* (1983) Motor neuron disease (ALS): evaluation of detection thresholds of cutaneous sensations. *Neurology*, **33**, 1625–7.

Mulder, D.W., Kurland, L.T., Offord, K.P. and Beard, C.M. (1986) Familial adult motor neuron disease: amyotrophic lateral sclerosis. *Neurology*, **36**, 511–17.

Mulligan, M., Riddle, J., Delaney, M. *et al.* Longitudinal study of intelligibility and the acoustic characteristics of speech in amyotrophic lateral sclerosis. *J. Speech Hearing Dis.* (in press).

Munsat, T.L., Andres, P.L., Finison, L. *et al.* (1988) The natural history of motoneuron loss in amyotrophic lateral sclerosis. *Neurology*, **38**, 409–13.

Neary, D., Snowden, J.S., Mann, D.M.A. *et al.* (1990) Frontal lobe dementia and motor neuron disease. *J. Neurol. Neurosurg. Psychiatry*, **53**, 23–32.

Nogues, M.A. and Stalberg, E.V. (1989) Automatic analysis of heart rate variation. II. Findings in patients attending an EMG laboratory. *Muscle Nerve*, **12**, 1001–8.

Norris, F.H. (1991) Adult progressive muscular atrophy and hereditary spinal muscular atrophies, in *Handbook of Clinical Neurology*, Vol. 59 (eds P.J. Vinken, G.W. Bruyn, H.L. Klawans and J.M.B.V DeJong), Elsevier, New York, pp. 13–34.

Clinical features and differential diagnosis

Norris, F.H., Colanchini, P.R., Fallat, R.J. *et al.* (1974) Administration of guanidine in amyotrophic lateral scleroris. *Neurology*, **24**, 721–8.

Oryema, J., Ashby, P. and Spiegel, S. (1990) Monomelic atrophy. *Can. J. Neurol. Sci.*, **17**, 124–30.

Osuntokun, B.O., Adeuja, A.O.G. and Bademosi, O. (1974) The prognosis of motor neuron disease in Nigerian Africans. *Brain*, **97**, 385–94.

Pajeau, A., Badger, G., Kruinski, P. and Tandan, R. Onset and spread of motor neuron loss in amyotrophic lateral sclerosis. In preparation.

Parry, G.J., Holtz, S.J., Benn-Zeev, D. and Drori, J.B. (1986) Gammopathy with proximal motor axonopathy simulating motor neuron disease. *Neurology*, **36**, 273–6.

Peavy, G.M., Herzog, A.G., Rubin, N.P. and Mesulam, M.-M. (1992) Neuropsychological aspects of dementia of motor neuron disease: a report of two cases. *Neurology*, **42**, 1004–8.

Pestronk, A. (1991) Motor neuropathies, motor neuron disorders, and antiglycolipid antibodies. *Muscle Nerve*, **14**, 927–36.

Riggs, J.E., Schochet, S.S. and Gutmann, L. (1984) Benign focal amyotrophy. Variant of chronic spinal muscular atrophy. *Arch. Neurol.*, **41**, 678–9.

Robbins, J. (1987) Swallowing in ALS and motor neuron disorders. *Neurol. Clin.*, **5**, 213–29.

Rosati, G., Pinna, L., Granieri, E. *et al.* (1977) Studies on epidemiological, clinical and etiological aspects of ALS disease in Sardinia, southern Italy. *Acta Neurol. Scand.*, **55**, 231–44.

Rosen, A.D. (1978) Amyotrophic lateral sclerosis. Clinical features and prognosis. *Arch. Neurol.*, **35**, 638–42.

Rosenfield, D.B., Viswanath, N., Herbrich, K.E. and Nudelman, H.B. (1991) Evaluation of the speech motor control system in amyotrophic lateral sclerosis. *J. Voice*, **5**, 224–30.

Sadiq, S.A., Thomas, F.P., Kilidireas, K. *et al.* (1990) The spectrum of neurologic disease associated with anti-GM1 antibodies. *Neurology*, **40**, 1067–72.

Salazar, A.M., Masters, C.L., Gajdusek, D.C. and Gibbs, C.J. (1983) Syndromes of amyotrophic lateral sclerosis and dementia: relation to transmissible Creutzfeldt–Jakob disease. *Ann. Neurol.*, **14**, 17–26.

Schiffer, D., Briguolio, F., Chio, A. *et al.* (1987) A study of prognostic factors in motor neuron disease. *Adv. Exp. Med. Biol.*, **209**, 255–63.

Schiffman, P.L. and Belsh, J.M. (1989) Effect of inspiratory resistance and theophylline on respiratory muscle strength in patients with amyotrophic lateral sclerosis. *Annu. Rev. Respir. Dis.*, **139**, 1418–23.

Shefner, J.M., Tyler, H.R. and Krarup, C. (1991) Abnormalities in the sensory action potential in patients with amyotrophic lateral sclerosis. *Muscle Nerve*, **14**, 1242–6.

Specola, N., Vanier, M.T., Goutieres, F. *et al.* (1990) The juvenile and chronic forms of GM2 gangliosidosis. Clinical and enzymatic heterogeneity. *Neurology*, **40**, 145–50.

Sung, J.H. (1982) Autonomic neurons of the sacral spinal cord in amyotrophic lateral sclerosis, anterior poliomyelitis and 'neuronal intranuclear hyaline inclusion disease': distribution of sacral autonomic neurons. *Acta Neuropathol.*, **56**, 233–7.

Swank, R.L. and Putnam, T.J. (1943) Amyotrophic lateral sclerosis and related conditions: Clinical analysis. *Arch. Neurol. Psychiat.*, **49**, 151–77.

Tahmoush, A.J., Alonso, R.J., Tahmoush, G.P. and Heiman-Patterson, T.D. (1991) Cramp-fasciculation syndrome: a treatable hyperexcitable peripheral nerve disorder. *Neurology*, **41**, 1021–4.

Tandan, R. (1993) ALS-like syndromes and ALS-variants, in *ALS: Diagnosis and Management for the Clinician* (eds J. Belsh and P. Schiffman), Futura Publishing, New York.

Tandan, R. and Bradley, W.G. (1985a) Amyotrophic lateral sclerosis. 1. Clinical features, pathology and ethical issues in management. *Ann. Neurol.*, **18**, 271–80.

Tandan, R. and Bradley, W.G. (1985b) Amyotrophic lateral sclerosis. 2. Etiopathogenesis. *Ann. Neurol.*, **18**, 419–31.

Tandan, R., Sharma, K.R., Bradley, W.G. *et al.* (1990) Chronic segmental spinal muscular atrophy of upper extremities in identical twins. *Neurology*, **40**, 236–9.

Tucker, T., Layzer, R.B., Miller, R.G. and Chad, D. (1991) Subacute, reversible motor neuron disease. *Neurology*, **41**, 1541–4.

Vejjajiva, A., Foster, J.B. and Miller, H. (1967) Motor neuron disease. A clinical study. *J. Neurol. Sci.*, **4**, 299–314.

Williams, D.B. and Windebank, A.J. (1991) Motor neuron disease (Amyotrophic lateral sclerosis). *Mayo Clin. Proc.*, **66**, 54–82.

Wikstrom, J., Paetau, A., Palo, J. *et al.* (1982) Classic amyotrophic lateral sclerosis with dementia. *Arch. Neurol.*, **39**, 681–3.

Younger, D.S., Chou, S., Hays, A.P. *et al.* (1988) Primary lateral sclerosis. A clinical diagnosis re-emerges. *Arch. Neurol.*, **45**, 1304–7.

Younger, D.S., Rowland, L.P., Latov, N. *et al.* (1991) Lymphoma, motor neuron diseases, and amyotrophic lateral sclerosis. *Ann. Neurol.*, **29**, 78–86.

2 *Spinal muscular atrophies*

NEIL H. THOMAS and VICTOR DUBOWITZ

2.1 INTRODUCTION

The spinal muscular atrophies (SMA) are a genetically heterogeneous group of inherited conditions that are characterized by degeneration of anterior horn cells or cranial nerve motor nuclei and resultant wasting and weakness affecting voluntary muscles. The commonest and best-defined group is that which comprises the childhood autosomal recessive spinal muscular atrophies: these will be discussed in detail in this chapter. There are, however, both autosomal dominant and X-linked forms, and the clinical features of SMA may be associated with other neurological abnormalities.

The childhood autosomal recessive spinal muscular atrophies are characterized by symmetrical weakness and wasting affecting the proximal muscles with relative sparing of the cranial motor nuclei. The major determinant of both morbidity and mortality in these conditions is the degree of respiratory muscle weakness, which in the severe form leads to death within the first few years of life. Intellect is unimpaired and the mild form is compatible with an almost normal lifespan.

The recognition of forms of SMA of varying severity is a phenomenon that has become more clearly defined over the last 20 years, although in the earliest reports of Werdnig and Hoffmann, prolonged survival was already described.

2.2 HISTORICAL REVIEW

Neurological wasting conditions in children were not discussed at any length in literature prior to the nineteenth century. Pearn (1984), in an excellent review of the evolution of the classification of childhood neuromuscular disease, points out that a combination of short survival and social ostracism due to deformity ensured that such children were not readily available for study.

29

Spinal muscular atrophies

Neuroanatomical and neurophysiological developments from the middle of the nineteenth century were important in forming a classification of disease in this area. Claude Bernard (1858) pointed out the difference between neural and muscular forms of paralysis, and Luys (1860) and Charcot (1869) demonstrated the relationship between anterior horn cell degeneration and progressive muscular atrophy (i.e. motor neurone disease). Duchenne (1861) described the X-linked muscular dystrophy that now bears his name, but also pointed out that progressive childhood paralysis might be caused by different diseases. He described one female patient who was thin, wasted and of advanced intelligence; examination of her muscle biopsy suggests a neurogenic atrophy.

Numerous publications from this time describe cases that fit the phenotype of spinal muscular atrophy: Bennett (1883) discussed 'chronic atrophic spinal paralysis in children': one case is clearly severe spinal muscular atrophy, although not recognized as such.

Two important points become evident at this time: firstly, the genetic nature of these conditions became a concern, with Gowers (1892) writing specifically on this, and secondly, the splitters of differential diagnosis such as Erb (1884) were opposed by the lumpers, who considered infantile paralyses as a single clinical condition. An attempt to consider neuromuscular conditions separate from more generalized neurological disorders in which hypotonia and weakness occurred with mental retardation and other neurological features became apparent at this time.

Then, in 1891, Guido Werdnig published his classical paper 'Two hereditary cases of progressive muscular atrophy in early infancy presenting as muscular dystrophy, but on a neural basis'. He described two brothers who developed a progressive proximal weakness affecting the legs; tremor was noted in their arms, and one child died of pertussis aged 3 years. Autopsy, which did not include the brain, showed bilateral symmetrical loss of anterior horn cells.

A further report from Werdnig in 1894 described six children, and commented on the variability of severity. Hoffmann in 1900 reported six cases in four families, and suggested that there were 21 other affected relatives in these families. It is perhaps worth mentioning that the children described by both Werdnig and Hoffmann would not fall into the category of severity now associated with the eponym 'Werdnig–Hoffmann disease'.

Attention was drawn to the milder forms of SMA by the description by Kugelberg and Welander in 1956 of 12 cases with onset between 2 and 17 years and survival into adult life, with continued ambulation. Subsequent publications in the 1960s served to highlight the fact that there were milder forms of SMA that did not have the uniformly fatal prognosis of Werdnig–Hoffmann disease. However, the variety of views expressed in such publications has caused some confusion in the nomenclature associated with the various forms of childhood spinal muscular atrophy, a situation that causes difficulty in efforts to coordinate international projects to locate the gene for SMA.

2.3 CLASSIFICATION

The classification of the childhood forms of SMA arose out of the realization that there were individuals who survived beyond the few years that is normally the span of infants with what has become known as Werdnig–Hoffmann disease. As has been mentioned, numerous authors of the first half of the century made reference to prolonged survival in SMA, but the recognition of the less severe forms of SMA was promoted in a series of publications from 1950 onwards.

Brandt (1950) described 112 patients from 69 families in Denmark, including a small number of patients with later onset and prolonged survival. Kugelberg and Welander (1956) described 12 patients who developed clinical signs between 2 and 17 years, in whom walking was not lost and in whom there was prolonged survival. The later onset patients with spinal muscular atrophy in whom walking is preserved have subsequently continued to be described as having Kugelberg–Welander disease.

In 1964, Dubowitz described a further 12 patients with spinal muscular atrophy with prolonged survival. Only one child achieved the ability to walk, but all the others could sit unsupported. Onset was between 9 and 16 months. At least two of these patients are still alive at the time of writing, being now aged 46 and 44 years respectively. One family had previously lost a boy to the more severe (Werdnig–Hoffmann disease) form of the condition, highlighting the possibility of variability in clinical severity within a family. Dubowitz pointed out that, while this group of patients appeared to be a distinct and clearly defined clinical subgroup, there was difficulty in drawing a distinct division between this intermediate group and the severe infantile form on the one hand and the mild adolescent/adult form on the other, and that there appeared to be a continuum of clinical severity, from the severest form involving antenatal onset and birth with extreme weakness to the milder forms compatible with continued ambulation and prolonged survival. In expounding this view, Dubowitz also favoured genetic homogeneity in SMA with allelic genes accounting for variation in severity.

Spinal muscular atrophies

This view was supported by Munsat *et al.* (1969), who pointed out that there are families in which severe and milder forms coexist within the same sibship, and that clinical, electrophysiological and pathological features are the same in patients regardless of the length of survival.

However, Emery (1971) suggested that the spinal muscular atrophies could be divided into four types, infantile, intermediate, juvenile and adult. Fried and Emery (1971) also felt that the childhood disease could be divided into three clinically and genetically distinct groups, on the basis of age of onset and length of survival: type I (Werdnig–Hoffmann disease), characterized by onset at birth or the first few months of life, and death usually before the age of 2 years; type II (intermediate form) with onset between 3 and 15 months and survival beyond 4 years; and type III (Kugelberg–Welander disease) with onset after 24 months and with prolonged survival. There would, however, be children who would fall outside this classification.

The picture had become more complex when Hausmanowa-Petrusewicz *et al.* (1968) subdivided their cases into a severe infantile form (Ia) with onset at birth and death within 2–4 years, a less severe infantile form with inability to walk but longer survival (Ib), an intermediate form or late infantile form (type II) with onset after 2 years, subsequent immobilization and prolonged survival, and a type III with later onset, mildly progressive course and prolonged survival. Type Ia corresponds broadly to Werdnig–Hoffmann disease, Ib and II to the intermediate type and III to Kugelberg–Welander disease.

Pearn, Carter and Wilson (1973) used sib–sib analysis in looking at a large cohort of familial cases and felt able to define what they termed acute generalized SMA (Werdnig–Hoffmann disease): this condition was fatal by 3 years and led to delayed motor milestones, evident by 3 and at latest 6 months. All other cases were termed chronic. Pearn and Wilson (1973a,b) amplified this description in later publications, but pointed out that there was overlap between the groups on the basis of length of survival.

The clinical classification of the spinal muscular atrophies is not easy. This is partly because there is overlap between the different clinical subgroups in terms of their measurable parameters such as age of onset or age of milestones. Classification is important, however, in terms of prognosis and management. It has been the practice at Hammersmith Hospital, London, to classify SMA into severe, intermediate and mild forms on the basis of the ability to sit and walk unaided (Dubowitz, 1989), an approach that has the advantage of simplicity and is of use in focusing management to specific problems and determining prognosis. It is this scheme that is used below.

2.4 PHENOTYPE

2.4.1 Proximal childhood-onset spinal muscular atrophies

This group of patients is characterized by symmetrical muscle wasting and weakness that is due to anterior horn cell degeneration. The weakness is greater proximally and affects legs more than arms. Autosomal recessive inheritance is usual, although a small number of cases may be sporadic (Pearn, 1980). In general, there is little variation in severity within a sibship, but there are reports of children with Werdnig–Hoffmann disease and the milder forms within one sibship, a situation difficult to explain on the basis of a single allelic gene.

SEVERE SPINAL MUSCULAR ATROPHY

This is also known as Werdnig–Hoffmann disease or acute SMA; patients are never able even to sit unaided. The onset of weakness is *in utero* or in the first few months of life. Pearn (1973a) estimated that a history of reduced fetal movements was present in approximately one-third of patients with Werdnig–Hoffmann disease, a frequency similar to our own clinical experience. Hypotonia, weakness and respiratory or swallowing difficulties are the main presenting symptoms. On examination, the infants are found to be markedly hypotonic, to have severe limb and trunk weakness and to have poor head control. A mixture of diaphragmatic breathing and intercostal recession leads to a bell-shaped chest and the arms are held internally rotated. Facial movements are normal, and the infants have a bright interested expression. Tongue fasciculation is present. Tendon reflexes are absent. Intellectual development is normal.

Although the weakness is severe, it appears to be non-progressive, but the tendency to respiratory infections means that the prognosis is poor with the majority of infants with severe SMA dying of pneumonia within the first few years. Management is supportive, and no specific curative treatment is available.

INTERMEDIATE SPINAL MUSCULAR ATROPHY

This group of patients is characterized by the ability to sit unaided, but not to stand. The onset is somewhat later, between 6 and 12 months, and presentation is usually with failure to stand or walk unaided or with weak legs. Once again the weakness is symmetrical and proximal and affects the legs more than the arms. Fasciculation of the tongue is present in the majority of children, there is tremor of the hands and tendon jerks are diminished or absent. Hypotonia and joint laxity may be a feature, and there may be a progressive scoliosis. Intellect is normal or even advanced.

The weakness is usually non-progressive, although there may be a slow decline in motor abilities over a long period. There may be deterioration, too, associated with periods of rapid growth and weight gain.

Long-term prognosis depends entirely on respiratory function, which may be compromised by both intercostal muscle weakness and the development of restrictive lung disease secondary to the scoliosis. Diagnosis may be confirmed by electromyography and muscle biopsy (see below, section 2.5). Creatine kinase is usually normal, while an electrocardiogram is also normal but shows a characteristic baseline tremor.

The management of children with intermediate SMA includes prevention or treatment of scoliosis by spinal bracing. It may be necessary to resort to surgical fixation of the spine as the scoliosis may be progressive despite use of a spinal brace. By the use of standing frame or callipers, it may be possible to achieve a standing posture, and ambulation in orthoses may be achieved by children with disease at the milder end of this spectrum.

MILD SPINAL MUSCULAR ATROPHY

Mild SMA, also known as Kugelberg–Welander disease, is characterized by the ability to walk unaided. The onset is later again, usually becoming manifest in the second year of life onwards. Children with this condition present with difficulty in walking, running or jumping. They have an abnormal, waddling gait and may exhibit Gowers' sign in having difficulty in rising from the floor. Tongue fasciculation may be present, and tendon reflexes may be absent, diminished or present. Joints once more are hypermobile. Investigations are as above for intermediate SMA.

The weakness is relatively static although deterioration may occur during growth spurts (e.g. puberty). The outlook for long-term survival is good, and depends on respiratory function. Management includes encouraging mobility, rehabilitation in callipers if walking is lost and vigorous treatment of respiratory infections.

2.4.2 Autosomal dominant spinal muscular atrophy

As mentioned above, autosomal dominant inheritance is recognized in proximal spinal muscular atrophy. It has been suggested that there are two major forms of autosomal dominant SMA (Pearn, 1978). One is a childhood-onset (0–8 years) form, which runs a mild course. This form is not limited to proximal muscles, and the gene appears to exhibit complete penetrance. It is estimated to account for 2% of all childhood spinal muscular atrophy. A second dominant gene appears to result in an adult-onset form; median age of onset was 37 years in Pearn's study, the gene was fully penetrant, but the clinical course was perhaps more rapid than the childhood form. Thirty per cent of adult cases appear to be of autosomal dominant inheritance. These genes appear unrelated to that involved in childhood-onset proximal SMA (Kausch *et al.*, 1991).

2.4.3 Distal spinal muscular atrophy

Hereditary distal spinal muscular atrophy constitutes one cause of the clinical syndrome of peroneal muscular atrophy (Harding and Thomas, 1980). These authors reviewed 34 patients who were identified from a larger study. They suggested that the condition resembled hereditary motor and sensory neuropathy types I and II, but differed in showing less upper limb weakness, relative preservation of the tendon reflexes and normal sensory function tested both clinically and electrophysiologically. Motor nerve conduction velocity was normal and there was electromyographic evidence of denervation. Nearly all patients developed symptoms before 20 years, most in the first decade. Weakness affected the legs and in one-quarter the arms. Reflexes are preserved in the majority of cases.

Young and Harper (1980) have also reported a family affected by hereditary distal SMA in which an additional potentially hazardous feature was vocal cord paralysis. Presentation is usually in the teens. A more recent report (Pridmore *et al.*, 1992) of a new family with this syndrome confirms autosomal dominant inheritance.

2.4.4 Atypical spinal muscular atrophy

Various forms of neurogenic muscle atrophy occur in association with other neurological abnormalities or in a particular distribution. Their place in a scheme of classification of the spinal muscular atrophies is uncertain, as is their relationship to the more clearly defined childhood-onset forms of SMA.

SPINAL MUSCULAR ATROPHY WITH SPECIAL DISTRIBUTION

There have been a number of reports of individuals with symmetrical neurogenic muscle wasting and weakness affecting localized areas of the

Spinal muscular atrophies

body. Progressive bulbar palsy due to depletion of the neurones in the cranial motor nuclei with subsequent loss of anterior horn cells in the upper cervical cord is a rare variant of SMA. Sometimes known as Fazio–Londe disease, this condition is seen in children between 1 and 12 years, presenting with stridor, palatal palsy, facial weakness and dysphagia. Ophthalmoplegia may also occur. Some cases appear to be inherited in a recessive fashion (Gomez, Clermont and Bernstein, 1962). Death results from aspiration in most cases, although survival into adult life has been reported.

A genetically distinct form of progressive bulbar palsy is the Vialetto–van Laere syndrome, which combines cranial nerve palsies with sensorineural deafness. Presentation is usually between 10 and 20 years, and the bulbar weakness, which is progressive, may be associated with limb weakness and respiratory difficulties. The inheritance in familial cases appears to be recessive. It has been suggested that the disease is more severe in males. The prognosis is variable: in the report from Gallai (Gallai *et al.*, 1981), one sibling had died at 2 years, while another was still alive at 15 years.

Goutières, Bogicevic and Aicardi (1991) recently reported five cases of a predominantly cervical form of spinal muscular atrophy. Two were brothers born to normal consanguineous parents. These children presented with poor head control between the ages of 3 and 6 months and were found to have atrophic weak neck muscles. Initially the limbs were affected only mildly, but over a period of 1–2 years, the legs were affected. In this caudal progression, the intercostal muscles may become weak, and three children died from respiratory complications. Electromyography performed on neck muscles confirmed a neurogenic abnormality, and muscle biopsy of quadriceps or deltoid showed neurogenic fascicular atrophy.

SPINAL MUSCULAR ATROPHY ASSOCIATED WITH OTHER ABNORMALITIES

Anterior horn cell disease has been reported in association with a number of other abnormalities. Goutières, Aicardi and Farkas (1977) reported three sibs with severe mental retardation, cortical blindness and extensive peripheral paralysis of the lower motor neurone type. Spinal cord necropsy findings were indistinguishable from those of Werdnig–Hoffmann disease; in addition there was hypoplasia and atrophy of the cerebellum, and atrophy of the ventral surface of the pons. Other authors have reported similar cases, but their relationship to classical forms of SMA is unclear and may be clarified when the gene for childhood-onset spinal muscular atrophy is characterized.

Arthrogryposis is a feature of some forms of anterior horn cell disease, although it is a specific exclusion from the criteria of classical autosomal recessive spinal muscular atrophy agreed at a recent International SMA Workshop (Munsat, 1991). There appear to be neuropathological differences in the alpha motor neurones affected in Werdnig–Hoffmann disease and those in arthrogryposis (Clarren and Hall, 1983). Fleury and Hageman (1985) have reported an autosomal dominant form of lower motor neurone disorder that presents with arthrogryposis.

SPINAL MUSCULAR ATROPHY ASSOCIATED WITH
HEXOSAMINIDASE DEFICIENCY

Deficiency of the isoenzymes of the lysosomal enzyme N-acetyl-β-hexosaminidase results in a number of neurological disorders, the best characterized being deficiency of hexosaminidase A, resulting in Tay–Sachs disease. However, deficiency of hexosaminidase A has also been described to result in a phenotype similar to that of Kugelberg–Welander disease (Johnson et al., 1982). There has also been a report of a progressive motor neurone syndrome associated with deficiency of hexosaminidase B: this individual exhibited dysarthria, muscle wasting, fasciculation and pyramidal tract dysfunction, the last being a feature not seen in spinal muscular atrophy (Cashman et al., 1986). This report was of interest when the gene for childhood-onset SMA was localized to chromosome 5q as the gene for the hexosaminidase β subunit was in the same region. The SMA gene has now been shown to be separate from that of hexosaminidase B (Daniels et al., 1992).

2.5 DIAGNOSIS

2.5.1 Clinical

The clinical phenotype of anterior horn cell disease is wide, and it has proved necessary to establish diagnostic criteria to achieve a degree of international uniformity in running genetic projects investigating spinal muscular atrophy. A recent international SMA collaborative workshop came to a consensus view as to the definitive criteria in order to diagnose SMA (Munsat, 1991). These were broad criteria to achieve consensus, and it has been pointed out that certain patients will not fit exactly any of the categories.

The clinical features for inclusion agreed were as follows: the weakness is symmetrical, is more proximal than distal and affects legs more than arms. The trunk is also affected. There is evidence of denervation, either clinically or by EMG or muscle biopsy (see below).

Spinal muscular atrophies

Specific exclusions include associated CNS dysfunction, arthrogryposis, involvement of other neurological systems or other organs, sensory loss, eye muscle weakness and marked facial weakness.

A classification of the childhood-onset autosomal recessive SMA agreed defined three broad groups on the basis of clinical severity, augmented by age at death.

2.5.2 Electrophysiology

Electromyography will usually confirm denervation. The EMG shows discrete voluntary motor unit potentials of large amplitude that are often unstable. Fibrillation, positive sharp waves and complex repetitive discharges may be present (Payan, 1991). Spinal muscular atrophy with onset before 2 years has been shown to be associated with motor units discharging in relaxed muscles. This phenomenon is not present in mild SMA. Hausmanowa-Petrusewicz and Karwanska (1986) confirmed that the EMG findings vary in the different forms of childhood SMA; their conclusions were that recording of increased numbers of large, long potentials was a feature of more chronic forms with a better prognosis, this feature being due to reinnervation.

Peripheral nerve studies show normal motor nerve conduction velocity (Moosa and Dubowitz, 1976), although slowing can occur in the face of motor unit fall-out. The compound muscle action potential is reduced in amplitude, while the mixed-nerve action potential is normal.

2.5.3 Ultrasound examination of muscle

Ultrasound examination is also fairly distinctive, showing increased echo within the affected muscle plus atrophy of the muscle with reduction in bulk (Heckmatt and Dubowitz, 1984). In experienced hands, ultrasound examination may reduce the need for invasive electrophysiological examination.

2.5.4 Histopathology – muscle

The severe and intermediate forms have similar histological appearances. Atrophic fibres are seen in all biopsies, having a circular outline (Dubowitz, 1985). Large groups of atrophic fibres are interspersed with fascicles containing hypertrophied fibres. The large fibres are usually type 1.

Variation in the extent of atrophy is seen throughout the muscle, and thus the severity of disease is not easy to determine from a particular biopsy. In addition, in early severe SMA, the characteristic large reinnervated fibres may not be present, the biopsy consisting mainly of small fibres, and diagnosis is therefore difficult.

2.6 GENETICS

2.6.1 Population genetics

Estimation of the incidence of forms of the spinal muscular atrophies is complicated by the difficulties of establishing their mode of inheritance in all cases. An international collaboration in the 1970s, which included mainly chronic cases, concluded that the majority were inherited in an autosomal recessive fashion, with the incidence of dominant forms being relatively low (Emery *et al.*, 1976).

Pearn, Carter and Wilson (1973), in the course of studies in the 1970s, were able to estimate the prevalence and gene frequency of forms of spinal muscular atrophy. For severe SMA, they suggested a gene frequency of between 1 in 60 and 1 in 90 on the basis of the cases presenting to the Hospital for Sick Children over a 10-year period. They acknowledge the difficulties of complete case ascertainment for a given population. Pearn was able to refine this figure in a population study of the disease in north-east England. He found a prevalence of 1 in 25 708 live births for the severe form, which gave a gene frequency of 1 in 80 (Pearn, 1973b). There have been reports of culturally or geographically isolated populations with a much higher prevalence than this: for example, the prevalence in the Karaite community in Israel may be one or two orders of magnitude greater than that in western populations (Fried and Mundel, 1977).

For the more chronic forms (intermediate and mild SMA), Pearn (1978) found a prevalence of 1 in 24 100 live births, which gave a gene frequency of between 1 in 76 and 1 in 111, with a working frequency of 1 in 90 for genetic counselling purposes. The variability of this figure relates to the incidence of new dominant mutations (phenocopies), which is difficult to determine with accuracy. It is of interest too that there have been reports of an excess of males in the milder forms of childhood-onset SMA (Hausmanowa-Petrusewicz *et al.*, 1976).

2.6.2 Molecular genetics

Childhood-onset autosomal recessive SMA has not been shown to be associated with a specific chromosomal deletion: it was therefore necessary to apply linkage analysis techniques in a random search within the genome to try to locate the gene. A concerted international collaboration involving researchers from the USA, UK, Finland and

Spinal muscular atrophies

Germany has recently resulted in the identification of the gene on chromosome 5q (Brzustowicz *et al.*, 1990), a location that has been confirmed by a French group working on a similar project (Melki *et al.*, 1990a). Both these groups have confirmed that there is genetic homogeneity between the severe (acute) forms and more chronic forms (Gilliam *et al.*, 1990; Melki *et al.*, 1990b).

Initially, results in the linkage analysis suggested that there was genetic heterogeneity, but careful clinical evaluation of the apparently unlinked families suggested that their clinical features were not typical of classical SMA (Munsat *et al.*, 1990). Recent publication of extended linkage analysis studies has confirmed genetic homogeneity (Sheth *et al.*, 1992; Daniels *et al.*, 1992a). It remains to be seen, however, whether the single allelic gene or multiple gene theory to account for clinical heterogeneity is correct. The gene for autosomal dominant forms of the condition appears not be linked to chromosome 5q markers (Kausch *et al.*, 1991).

The location of the gene to chromosome 5q and the existence of tightly linked polymorphic markers have created the possibility of offering prenatal diagnosis to families who have previously had an affected child (Daniels *et al.*, 1992b; Melki *et al.*, 1992). There remain a number of issues that complicate the provision of genetic advice for families in this situation. Firstly, SMA may show variable severity within a sibship. In addition, while segregation ratios in severe SMA are 0.25, supporting the hypothesis that this is an autosomal recessive disorder, this ratio is significantly less than 0.25 in intermediate and mild SMA, suggesting a more complex genetic model.

2.7 RELATIONSHIP TO OTHER MOTOR NEURONE DISEASES

Various authors have considered the spinal muscular atrophies under the umbrella of motor neuropathies, but there appears to be no apparent genetic link between phenotypically similar forms of spinal muscular atrophy such as, for example, the childhood-onset autosomal recessive form and the adult-onset autosomal dominant forms. The genetic origins of other motor neuropathies remain undefined.

The hereditary motor and sensory neuropathies (HMSN) are both clinically and genetically distinct from the spinal muscular atrophies. These disorders are characterized by distal wasting and weakness affecting arms and legs, and exist in different forms, classified on the basis of neuronal pathology (demyelination or axonal degeneration) and pattern of inheritance. The genes for demyelinating forms of HMSN have been located to chromosomes 1 and 17.

2.8 CONCLUSION

The spinal muscular atrophies are an important cause of inherited morbidity and mortality in childhood and later life. Their clinical phenotype is wide, and the overall classification of these disorders is still incomplete. As with many areas of medicine, it is hoped that advances in molecular genetics may illuminate our understanding of the relationships between the different forms of the condition, and that understanding the basic gene defect will allow the development of a treatment for conditions that at present are amenable only to supportive therapy.

ACKNOWLEDGEMENT

NHT has been supported as a clinical research fellow at the Royal Postgraduate Medical School by a clinical research grant from the Muscular Dystrophy Group of Great Britain.

REFERENCES

Bennett, A.H. (1883) On chronic atrophic spinal paralysis in children. *Brain*, **6**, 289–301.

Bernard, C. (1858) Leçons sur la Physiologie et la Pathologie du Systeme Nerveux. *Lecon*, **11**, 205.

Brandt, S. (1950) *Werdnig-Hoffmann's Infantile Progressive Muscular Atrophy: Clinical Aspects, Pathology, Heredity and Relation to Oppenheim's Amyotonia Congenita and Other Morbid Conditions with Laxity of Joints or Muscles in Infants.* Ejnar Munksgaard Forlag, Copenhagen.

Brzustowicz, L.M., Lehner, T., Castilla, L.H. *et al.* (1990) Genetic mapping of chronic childhood-onset spinal muscular atrophy to chromosome 5q11.2–13.3. *Nature*, **344**, 540–1.

Cashman, N.R., Antel, J.P., Hancock, L.W. *et al.* (1986) N-acetyl-β-hexosaminidase β locus defect and juvenile motor neuron disease: a case study. *Ann. Neurol.*, **19**, 568–72.

Charcot, J.M. (1869) Deux cas d'atrophie musculaire progressive avec lésions de la substance grise et des faisceaux antéro-lateraux de la moelle épiniere. *Arch. Physiol. Norm. Path.*, **2**, 744–60.

Clarren, S.K. and Hall, J.G. (1983) Neuropathological findings in the spinal cords of 10 infants with arthrogryposis. *J. Neurol. Sci.*, **58**, 89–102.

Daniels, R.J., Thomas, N.H., MacKinnon, R.N. *et al.* (1992a) Linkage analysis of spinal muscular atrophy. *Genomics*, **12**, 335–9.

Daniels, R.J., Suthers, G.K., Morrison, K.E. *et al.* (1992b) Prenatal prediction of spinal muscular atrophy. *J. Med. Genet.*, **29**, 165–70.

Dubowitz, V. (1964) Infantile muscular atrophy. A prospective study with particular reference to a slowly progressive variety. *Brain*, **87**, 707–18.

Spinal muscular atrophies

Dubowitz, V. (1985) *Muscle Biopsy: A Practical Approach*, 2nd edn, Bailliere Tindall, London.

Dubowitz, V. (1989) *A Colour Atlas of Muscle Disorders in Childhood*. Wolfe Medical Publications, London, p. 66.

Duchenne, G.-B. (1861) *De L'Electrisation Localisée et son Application a la Pathologie et a la Therapeutique*. J.-B. Bailliere et Fils, Paris, p. 275.

Emery, A.E.H. (1971) The nosology of the spinal muscular atrophies. *J. Med. Genet.*, **8**, 481–95.

Emery, A.E.H., Davie, A.M., Holloway, S. and Skinner, R. (1976) International collaborative study of the spinal muscular atrophies. 2. Analysis of genetic data. *J. Neurol. Sci.*, **30**, 375–84.

Erb, W. (1884) On chronic atrophic spinal paralysis in the child; and on a rare modification of the reaction of degeneration. *Brain*, **6**, 7–19.

Fleury, P. and Hageman, G. (1985) A dominantly inherited lower motor neuron disorder presenting at birth with associated arthrogryposis. *J. Neurol. Neurosurg. Psychiat.*, **48**, 1037–48.

Fried, K. and Emery, A.E.H. (1971) Spinal muscular atrophy type II. A separate genetic and clinical entity from type I (Werdnig–Hoffmann disease) and type III (Kugelberg–Welander disease). *Clin. Genet.*, **2**, 203–9.

Fried, K. and Mundel, G. (1977) High incidence of spinal muscular atrophy type 1 (Werdnig–Hoffmann disease) in the Karaite community in Israel. *Clin. Genet.*, **12**, 250–1.

Gallai, V., Hockaday, J.M., Hughes, J.T. *et al.* (1981) Ponto-bulbar palsy with deafness (Brown–Vialetto–van Laere syndrome). *J. Neurol. Sci.*, **50**, 259–75.

Gilliam, T.C., Brzustowicz, L.M., Castilla, I..H. *et al.* (1990) Genetic homogeneity between acute and chronic forms of spinal muscular atrophy. *Nature*, **345**, 823–5.

Gomez, M.R., Clermont, V. and Bernstein, J. (1962) Progressive bulbar paralysis in childhood (Fazio–Londe's disease). *Arch. Neurol.*, **6**, 317–23.

Goutières, F., Aicardi, J. and Farkas, E. (1977) Anterior horn cell disease associated with pontocerebellar hypoplasia in infants. *J. Neurol. Neurosurg. Psychiat.*, **40**, 370–8.

Goutières, F., Bogicevic, D. and Aicardi, J. (1991) A predominantly cervical form of spinal muscular atrophy. *J. Neurol. Neurosurg. Psychiat.*, **54**, 223–5.

Gowers, W.R. (1892) Acute atrophic paralysis, in: *A Manual of Diseases of the Nervous System*, Vol. 1, 2nd edn. Blakiston, Philadelphia, pp. 352–78.

Harding, A.E. and Thomas, P.K. (1980) Hereditary distal spinal muscular atrophy. *J. Neurol. Sci.*, **45**, 337–48.

Hausmanowa-Petrusewicz, I. and Karwanska, A. (1986) Electromyographic findings in different forms of infantile and juvenile spinal muscular atrophy. *Muscle and Nerve*, **9**, 37–46.

Hausmanowa-Petrusewicz, I., Askanas, V., Badurska, B. *et al.* (1968) Infantile and juvenile spinal muscular atrophy. *J. Neurol. Sci.*, **6**, 269–87.

Hausmanowa-Petrusewicz, I., Zaremba, J., Borkowska, J. and Prot, J. (1976) Genetic investigations on chronic forms of infantile and juvenile spinal muscular atrophy. *J. Neurol.*, **213**, 335–46.

References

Heckmatt, J.Z. and Dubowitz, V. (1984) Diagnosis of spinal muscular atrophy with pulse echo ultrasound imaging, in: *Progressive Spinal Muscular Atrophies* (eds I. Gamstorp and H.B. Sarnat) Raven Press, New York, pp. 141–52.

Hoffmann, J. (1900) Uber die hereditaire progressive spinale Muskelatrophie im Kindesalter. *Muenchen Med. Wschr.*, **47**, 1649–51.

Johnson, W.G., Wigger, H.J., Karp, H.R. *et al.* (1982) Juvenile spinal muscular atrophy: a new hexosaminidase deficiency phenotype. *Ann. Neurol.*, **11**, 11–16.

Krausch, K., Muller, C.R., Grimm, T. *et al.* (1991) No evidence for linkage of autosomal dominant proximal spinal muscular atrophies to chromosome 5q markers. *Hum. Genet.*, **86**, 317–18.

Kugelberg, E. and Welander, L. (1956) Heredo-familial juvenile muscular atrophy simulating muscular dystrophy. *Arch. Neurol. Psychiat.*, **75**, 500–9.

Luys, J.B. (1860) Lesions histologiques de la substance grise de la moelle epinierie. *Gaz. Med. Paris*, **15**, 505.

Melki, J., Abdelhak, S., Sheth, P. *et al.* (1990a) Gene for chronic proximal spinal muscular atrophies maps to chromosome 5q. *Nature*, **344**, 767–8.

Melki, J., Sheth, P., Abdelhak, S. *et al.* (1990b) Mapping of acute (type I) spinal muscular atrophy to chromosome 5q12–q14. *Lancet*, **336**, 271–3.

Melki, J., Abdelhak, S., Burlet, P. *et al.* (1992) Prenatal prediction of Werdnig-Hoffmann disease using linked polymorphic DNA probes. *J. Med. Genet.*, **29**, 171–4.

Moosa, A. and Dubowitz, V. (1976) Motor nerve conduction velocity in spinal muscular atrophy of childhood. *Arch. Dis. Childh.*, **51**, 974–7.

Munsat, T.L. (1991) Workshop Report. International SMA Collaboration. *Neuromuscular Disorders*, **1**, 81.

Munsat, T.L., Woods, R., Fowler, W. and Pearson, C.M. (1969) Neurogenic muscular atrophy of infancy with prolonged survival. *Brain*, **92**, 9–24.

Munsat, T.L., Skerry, L., Korf, B. *et al.* (1990) Phenotypic heterogeneity of spinal muscular atrophy mapping to chromosome 5q11.2–13.3 (SMA 5q). *Neurology*, **40**, 1831–6.

Payan, J. (1991) Clinical electromyography in infancy and childhood, in *Paediatric Neurology*, 2nd edn (ed E. Brett), Churchill Livingston, Edinburgh, pp. 816–18.

Pearn, J.H. (1973a) Fetal movements and Werdnig–Hoffmann disease. *J. Neurol. Sci.*, **18**, 373–9.

Pearn, J.H. (1973b) The gene frequency of acute Werdnig-Hoffmann disease (SMA type 1). A total population survey in North-East England. *J. Med. Genet.*, **10**, 260–5.

Pearn, J.H. (1978) Incidence, prevalence, and gene frequency studies of chronic childhood spinal muscular atrophy. *J. Med. Genet.*, **15**, 409–13.

Pearn, J. (1980) Classification of spinal muscular atrophies. *Lancet*, **i**, 919–22.

Pearn, J. (1984) The discovery of neuronopathy and neuropathy as a cause of progressive paralysis in childhood. *J. Neurol. Sci.*, **64**, 99–107.

Pearn, J.H. and Wilson, J. (1973a) Acute Werdnig–Hoffmann disease. *Arch. Dis. Childh.*, **48**, 425–9.

Spinal muscular atrophies

Pearn, J.H. and Wilson, J. (1973b) Chronic generalized spinal muscular atrophy of infancy and childhood. *Arch. Dis. Childh.*, **48**, 768–74.

Pearn, J.H., Carter, C.O. and Wilson, J. (1973) The genetic identity of acute infantile spinal muscular atrophy. *Brain*, **96**, 463–70.

Pridmore, C., Baraitser, M., Brett, E.M. and Harding, A.E. (1992) Distal spinal muscular atrophy with vocal cord paralysis. *J. Med. Genet.*, **29**, 197–9.

Sheth, P., Abdelhak, S., Bachelot, M.F. *et al.* (1992) Linkage analysis in spinal muscular atrophy, by six closely flanking markers on chromosome 5. *Am. J. Hum. Genet.*, **8**, 764–8.

Werdnig, G. (1891) Zwei fruhinfantile hereditare Falle von progressiver Muskelatrophie unter dem Bilde der Dystrophie, aber auf neurotischer Grundlage. *Arch. Psychiat.*, **22**, 437–81.

Werdnig, G. (1894) Die fruhinfantile progressive spinale Amyotrophie. *Arch. Psychiat.*, **26**, 706–44.

Young, I.D. and Harper, P.S. (1980) Hereditary distal spinal muscular atrophy. *J. Neurol. Neurosurg. Psychiat.*, **43**, 413–18.

3 Motor neuropathies

P.K. THOMAS and H.J. WILLISON

The terminology used to identify motor neuropathies is confused (Thomas, 1991). In pathological terms **motor neuronopathies** comprise conditions in which there is a loss of the lower motor neurone *in toto*, whereas in **motor neuropathies** the parent cell bodies, in general, survive, but there is either a selective degeneration of motor axons (**motor axonopathy**) or a primary demyelinating disorder (**demyelinating motor neuropathy**). Clinically it is difficult to distinguish between motor neuronopathies and axonopathies. The term 'spinal muscular atrophy', dating back to Hoffmann (1893), is equivalent to a motor neuronopathy, although its use is not always appropriate as brainstem motor neurones are often also affected. This chapter will consider a range of disorders usually included within the category of neuropathies in which involvement of the lower motor neurones is a salient feature of the clinical picture. A number, by virtue of their clinical course or other features, are not confused with motor neurone disease (amyotrophic lateral sclerosis), whereas in others the clinical differentiation is not always easy. Emphasis will be placed on the latter. Motor neuropathies of acute onset will not be included, or neuropathies in which there is substantial sensory or autonomic involvement.

3.1 INHERITED MOTOR NEUROPATHIES AND NEURONOPATHIES

3.1.1 The peroneal muscular atrophy syndrome (Charcot–Marie–Tooth disease)

Patients with an inherited distal and approximately symmetric denervating disorder, usually with lower limb predominance, were separated from those with other progressive lower motor neurone disorders by Charcot and Marie (1886) and Tooth (1886). It is now evident that the syndrome of peroneal muscular atrophy that they delineated is subdivisible into an increasingly large number of genetic entities. A

45

Motor neuropathies

major advance was achieved by Dyck and Lambert (1968a,b) on the basis of combined clinical, genetic, electrophysiological and nerve biopsy findings. They were able to separate patients with pure lower motor neurone involvement, which they designated the spinal form of Charcot–Marie–Tooth (CMT) disease. Such patients are now usually said to have a distal spinal muscular atrophy (Harding and Thomas, 1980a). The second category comprised patients in whom there is accompanying involvement of the primary sensory neurones. These were designated as hereditary motor and sensory polyneuropathy by Thomas, Calne and Stewart (1974), abbreviated to hereditary motor and sensory neuropathy (HMSN) by Dyck (1975). 'Motor' was placed before 'sensory' to emphasize the greater severity of motor involvement. Dyck and Lambert showed that some of these patients had a demyelinating neuropathy (HMSN type I) and others an axonopathy (HMSN type II). Their genetic distinction was established by intrafamilial correlation of nerve conduction velocity (Thomas, Calne and Stewart, 1974; Harding and Thomas, 1980b). Dyck and Lambert also defined a further type of HMSN in which hypomyelination was shown to be a distinctive feature (HMSN III). X-linked families were identified later. Complex forms of HMSN also exist in which there are additional features associated with the peroneal muscular atrophy syndrome.

HEREDITARY DISTAL SPINAL MUSCULAR ATROPHY

Instances of hereditary spinal muscular atrophy (SMA) constituted 34 out of 262 patients with the peroneal muscular atrophy syndrome reported by Harding and Thomas (1980a). Pearn and Hudgson (1979) found that examples of distal SMA made up 10% of all cases with SMA in a population survey in north-east England. Such patients are genetically heterogeneous. At least two forms with autosomal dominant and three with autosomal recessive inheritance have probably been identified (Harding, 1993). No X-linked families have been reported.

Symptoms in the more common autosomal dominant form usually appear before the age of 20 years and most often in the first decade (Davis *et al.*, 1978; Harding and Thomas, 1980a), but dominantly inherited families in which the onset is delayed until the third or fourth decades are recognized (Nelson and Amick, 1966; McLeod and Prineas, 1971). The condition usually begins with distal wasting and weakness in the legs, especially of the anterolateral compartment lower leg muscles. Foot deformity is often pronounced in cases of early onset. Tendon reflex loss may be confined to the ankle jerks. Progression is slow but extension to distal upper limb muscles occurs later in the disease.

Families with an autosomal dominant inheritance in which affected members have weakness that predominantly affects (Meadows *et al.*,

Inherited motor neuropathies and neuronopathies

1969; Harding and Thomas, 1980a) or is confined to (Lander *et al.*, 1976) distal upper limb muscles are on record. Onset has been in the first or second decades, again with slow progression. A large family in which distal spinal muscular atrophy of autosomal dominant inheritance was combined with vocal cord paresis has been described in South Wales (Young and Harper, 1980). Silver (1966) described a kinship in which hereditary spastic paraplegia was consistently associated with wasting of the small hand muscles.

Cases of distal spinal muscular atrophy with autosomal recessive inheritance tend to have a less favourable prognosis with a greater tendency to spread to proximal muscle and a more rapid evolution. There is a severe infantile form of distal SMA with probable autosomal recessive inheritance in which diaphragmatic paralysis and respiratory failure are an early feature and death usually occurs before the age of 12 months (Bertini *et al.*, 1989).

TYPE I HEREDITARY MOTOR AND SENSORY NEUROPATHY

This is the commonest variant of HMSN in the UK and North America. The onset is usually in the first decade, not infrequently in the second, and only rarely later than this. It may be apparent in infancy. The initial symptoms are usually difficulty in walking because of distal lower limb weakness leading to bilateral foot drop, or foot deformity. The foot deformity usually consists of clawing of the toes, often associated with an equinovarus deformity of the foot and shortening of the calf muscles. Distal upper limb muscle wasting and weakness follow. An upper limb postural tremor was present in 89% in the series reported by Harding and Thomas (1980b). It resembles essential tremor and may be pronounced (Roussy–Lévy syndrome). There is widespread loss of tendon reflexes. Sensory loss is often not detectable clinically in the earlier stages, but a variable degree of distal sensory loss for all modalities is usually detectable in established cases. Scoliosis develops in a proportion of patients. The peripheral nerves are palpably or visibly thickened in about a third (Harding and Thomas, 1980b). In patients with severe limb weakness, diaphragmatic involvement may occur, leading to dyspnoea on recumbency. Progression is slow. Occasionally patients deteriorate very shortly after adolescence. Rapid deterioration raises the possibility of a superimposed chronic inflammatory demyelinating polyneuropathy (Dyck *et al.*, 1982).

Most families with HMSN I show autosomal dominant inheritance, and in the majority the disease has been shown to be linked to the short arm of chromosome 17 (Vance *et al.*, 1989; Timmerman *et al.*, 1990). This type has been designated HMSN Ia (or CMT Ia) and was linked to 17p12

47

Motor neuropathies

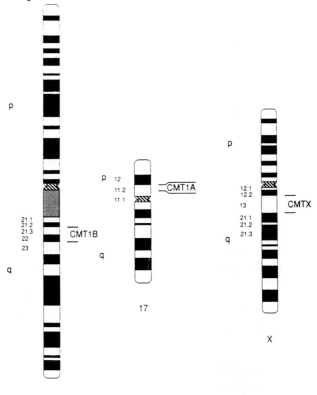

Figure 3.1 Diagrams showing localization of HMSN Ib (CMT Ib), HMSN Ia (CMT Ia) and X-linked HMSN (CMT XI) on chromosomes 1 and 17 and the X chromosome respectively. (Reproduced with permission of Dr R.V. Lebo.)

by Chance *et al.* (1990) (Figure 3.1). Most cases have been shown to have a segmental chromosome duplication in band 17p11.2 (Lupski *et al.*, 1991; Raeymakers *et al.*, 1991) (Figure 3.2). The mechanism of the production of the duplication, which constitutes a partial trisomy, is probably unequal crossing over at meiosis. A high proportion of sporadic cases of HMSN I are found to display this duplication (Hoogendijk *et al.*, 1992), which is therefore a valuable asset in genetic counselling. In occasional families a point mutation at this site is present. In a small number of families with HMSN I, the disorder has shown linkage to markers on chromosome 1 (Bird *et al.*, 1982; Guiloff *et al.*, 1982; Lebo *et al.*, 1992) with a localization on the long arm in the region of the Duffy blood group and Fcγ or Fcγ RII gene loci (Figure 3.1). This form has been designated HMSN Ib (or CMT Ib). In other families linkage to markers on both chromosomes 1 and 17 appears to have been excluded,

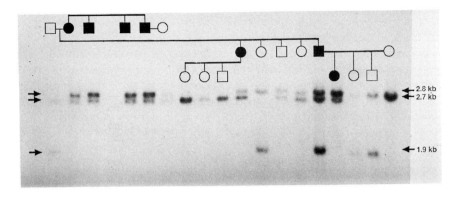

Figure 3.2 In the upper part of the figure is the pedigree for a family with HMSN Ia. Symbols: circles, female; squares, male. Filled symbols indicate affected individuals. In the lower part of the figure are autoradiographs of a Southern blot, using a probe that hybridizes to a DNA sequence in 17 p11.2. This detects three alleles with sizes 2.8, 2.7 and 1.9 kb. Normal individuals either display two of these alleles or are homozygous for one of them. Affected individuals show increased hybridization density of one of two alleles (e.g. the 2.8-kb fragment in the four affected siblings in the top left of the figure) or all three (affected male, second generation). (Figure kindly provided by Dr S. Malcolm.)

indicating further genetic heterogeneity. At present it is not known whether there are clinical differences between the different forms.

Motor nerve conduction velocity is severely reduced, usually to the range between 20 and 40 m/s in the median nerve (Harding and Thomas, 1980b), although values as low as 10 m/s can be encountered. Sensory action potentials are depressed or unrecordable. Nerve biopsy shows myelinated fibre loss, usually with prominent hypertrophic changes with concentric Schwann cell proliferation ('onion bulbs') and evidence of widespread segmental demyelination in teased fibre preparations. Myelin thickness may be reduced relative to axon diameter in remyelinating fibres but is also increased in some fibres. This has led to the proposal that the disease produces axonal atrophy and secondary demyelination (Nukada *et al.*, 1983). It now seems more likely to involve myelin or Schwann cell function directly, at least for HMSN Ia, as a disturbance affecting PMP22 (peripheral myelin protein 22) is probably implicated (see Thomas and Harding, 1993).

Rare patients with type I HMSN with autosomal recessive inheritance have been described (Harding and Thomas, 1980c). They tend to be more severely affected than patients with autosomal dominant inheritance and motor nerve conduction velocity is somewhat slower. Nerve biopsy shows hypertrophic changes similar to those of autosomal dominant HMSN I. In contrast to HMSN III, myelin sheaths of normal or relatively increased thickness are present. As has been pointed out by A.A.W.M. Gabreëls-Festen (personal communication, 1992) the Schwann cell processes in the onion bulbs may be extremely attenuated, often with approximation of their two cell membranes so that they resemble single myelin lamellae. A second type of autosomal recessive HMSN I that appears to be genetically distinct is characterized by highly irregular myelin sheaths with multiple outpouchings (Ohnishi et al., 1989; Gabreëls-Festen et al., 1990).

TYPE II HEREDITARY MOTOR AND SENSORY NEUROPATHY

Type II HMSN is also usually of autosomal dominant inheritance. The responsible gene(s) has not yet been localized. The onset is later than for HMSN I. In most patients the condition becomes manifest during the second decade but the onset is often delayed, sometimes as late as the seventh decade (Harding and Thomas, 1980b). It again usually begins with distal muscle wasting and weakness in the lower limbs but, in contradistinction to HMSN I, the calf muscles are often quite markedly affected in addition to the anterolateral lower leg muscles. Tendon reflex depression or loss tends to be less, as does the degree of sensory loss and upper limb motor involvement. Postural tremor in the arms may occur but is usually not obtrusive and the peripheral nerves are not thickened. Progression is slow.

Autosomal recessive HMSN II is occasionally encountered in the UK (Harding and Thomas, 1980c) and is the commonest variant in Algeria (Tazir, Attal and Ait-Kaci-Ahmed, 1992). Such patients tend to be more severely affected. A variant with onset in childhood with probable autosomal recessive inheritance and a considerably more aggressive course has been reported by Ouvrier et al. (1981) and Gabreëls-Festen et al. (1991).

TYPE III HEREDITARY MOTOR AND SENSORY NEUROPATHY

This disorder was originally defined by Dyck and Lambert (1968a) as a mixed motor and sensory neuropathy of autosomal recessive inheritance with an onset in early childhood and more severe involvement than HMSN I. Nerve conduction velocity was severely reduced to less than 10 m/s. Histologically there was a hypertrophic 'onion bulb' neuropathy characterized by severe hypomyelination, i.e. the myelin sheaths were consistently reduced in thickness on fibres of all diameters. It was equated with Dejerine–Sottas disease. A further study was undertaken by Ouvrier, McLeod and Conchin (1987).

It is now apparent that HMSN III is genetically heterogeneous. It encompasses at least three disorders. The first has the features already described. In the second, the onion bulbs differ from those of HMSN I in that they are frequently composed not of concentric layers of Schwann cells but of multiple double layers of basal laminae (Lyon, 1969; Guzzetta, Ferrière and Lyon, 1982). These presumably originally encased Schwann cell processes that disappeared. The third form of HMSN III is a congenital disorder in which there is amyelination of peripheral nerve fibres. Affected children have a limited life expectancy (Karch and Urich, 1975; Kennedy, Sung and Berry, 1977; Guzzetta, Ferrière and Lyon, 1982).

X-LINKED HEREDITARY MOTOR AND SENSORY NEUROPATHY

Several families with X-linked dominant HMSN have been identified (Rozear et al., 1987; de Weerdt et al., 1978; Hahn et al., 1990). In this pattern of inheritance, males are more severely affected than females and there is no male-to-male transmission. The disorder is designated HMSN X1 (CMT X1). The clinical features in affected males resemble those of type 1 HMSN. Heterozygote females are either asymptomatic or are mildly affected. Nerve biopsy studies have suggested a primary axonopathy with secondary demyelination (Hahn et al., 1990). The gene for the disorder has been localized to the Xq13 region (Beckett et al., 1986) (Figure 3.1).

An X-linked recessive variety of HMSN (HMSN X2) (CMT X2) has also been described, associated with mental retardation and deafness with linkage to a marker on the proximal long arm of the X chromosome (Fischbeck et al., 1985). The condition was considered to be an axonopathy.

3.1.2 X-linked bulbospinal neuronopathy

This syndrome was first clearly identified by Kennedy et al. (1968), although cases can be picked out in earlier series in which its characteristic features were not appreciated. It is frequently misdiagnosed as motor neurone disease. The onset is usually in the third or fourth decade, but it can range from 15 to 60 years. Muscle cramps and an upper limb postural tremor resembling essential tremor may antedate the development of weakness by many years. The weakness, accompanied by muscle wasting and fasciculation, generally begins proximally in the lower and then in the upper limbs, slowly spreading over 10–20 years to distal limb muscles. At this stage bulbar involvement is added, with dysarthria and dysphagia and a wasted fasciculating tongue.

Motor neuropathies

Prominent contraction fasciculation of the face is a particularly characteristic feature, rarely being encountered in other disorders.

Although the syndrome was initially considered to be a purely motor
disorder, Harding et al. (1982) found that sensory action potentials are
regularly reduced in amplitude or absent. Minor degrees of sensory loss
may be found (Sobue et al., 1989). Electromyography reveals the usual
features of chronic partial denervation. Motor nerve conduction velocity
is preserved or slightly reduced. Muscle biopsy shows chronic partial
denervation with evidence of collateral reinnervation and secondary
myopathic changes. The latter may account for the elevated serum
creatine kinase level, which may be up to five times the upper limit of
normal.

Autopsy studies (Sobue et al., 1989) have shown a distally accentuated loss of motor and sensory fibres in the peripheral nerves and a
rostrally accentuated loss of fibres in the gracile fasciculi. There is also
loss of bulbar and spinal motor neurones and, to a lesser extent, of
dorsal root ganglion cells. The condition therefore appears to involve a
distal axonopathy leading to loss of lower motor and sensory neurones
in toto.

An additional manifestation of some interest is the presence of
gynaecomastia in about 50% of cases. Secondary sexual characteristics
are normal but affected individuals may have reduced fertility. Diabetes
mellitus can also be associated.

The disorder has been localized to the proximal long arm of the X
chromosome (Fischbeck et al., 1986). Recently it has been shown that the
defect is an abnormally long repeated sequence in the androgen receptor
gene, leading to an increase in the size of a polyglutamine tract in the
receptor (La Spada et al., 1991). How this leads to the neurological
syndrome is so far uncertain, but it may be of relevance that androgen
receptors are present on anterior horn cells.

3.1.3 Hereditary proximal spinal muscular atrophy

These disorders are of greater clinical importance during the first two
decades of life. The childhood and juvenile spinal muscular atrophies
are considered in Chapter 2. This section will therefore be restricted to
hereditary proximal spinal muscular atrophies with onset in adult life.
These are so far rather poorly characterized and the loci for the
responsible genes have not been established. There is evidence for the
existence of both autosomal dominant and autosomal recessive forms,
which are genetically distinct from those with an onset below the age of
15 years (Harding, 1993). The onset of symptoms in the recessive form
(Pearn, Hudgson and Walton, 1978) is between 15 and 60 years

with a mean of 35 years. Progression is slow, distal limb muscles becoming involved later. Bulbar involvement is rare and reported isolated male patients or brothers in which this has been present may have been examples of X-linked bulbospinal neuronopathy. Distinction from motor neurone disease may be difficult in the early stages, particularly as the weakness may be asymmetric (Pearn, Hudgson and Walton, 1978). The possibility of hexosaminidase deficiency (see later) has to be borne in mind.

The existence of an autosomal dominant form of hereditary proximal spinal muscular atrophy, although it is rare, seems firmly established (Bundey and Lovelace, 1975; Pearn, 1978). The age of onset is usually in the third or fourth decades, but it may range from 25 to 65 years. Pearn (1978) found a mean age of 37 years in three families. Progress is gradual and the mean life expectancy from onset of symptoms is about 20 years (Pearn, 1978). Involvement of distal limb and bulbar muscles occurs as the disease advances. It can be confused with familial motor neurone disease in the earlier stages, but progression in that condition is more rapid, involvement is often asymmetric and pyramidal signs usually appear even if not present at first.

3.1.4 Hereditary motor neuronopathies with complex distributions

It is difficult to be certain of the nature of the cases of 'scapuloperoneal amyotrophy' described by Davidenkow (1939) as they were reported before the introduction of electromyography and nerve conduction studies. Some had distal sensory loss and can be accepted as an inherited neuropathy (Davidenkow's syndrome). Myopathic disorders with this distribution are now well documented. The possibility of the existence of an autosomal dominant motor neuronopathy with this distribution mainly dates to the report by Kaeser (1965), but the distribution of muscle weakness in some members of his family was not of scapuloperoneal pattern, and some findings suggested a myopathy. More acceptable cases have been recorded by Serratrice *et al.* (1976). In two patients with neuronopathies observed by the author, both with a scapuloperoneal distribution and both sporadic, investigations that included electromyography, nerve conduction studies and muscle biopsy initially suggested a motor neuronopathy or neuropathy. Serial sensory conduction studies later showed evidence of involvement of the primary sensory neurones. Neither had clinically detectable sensory loss. The existence of an autosomal dominant form of scapuloperoneal motor neuronopathy must therefore be considered to be provisional. A point of some interest is that in patients with the scapuloperoneal syndrome, it is notoriously difficult to establish by electromyography whether the disorder is neurogenic or myopathic and the interpretation of muscle biopsies can also present problems.

A hereditary motor neuronopathy of facioscapulohumeral distribution has been reported on a few occasions (Fenichel, Emery and Hunt, 1967; Cao et al., 1976; Furukawa and Toyokura, 1976). Inheritance has been of autosomal dominant pattern with onset in the second decade and slow progression. There is a single report of a Japanese family with a motor neuronopathy that combined distal limb and oculopharyngeal involvement (Matsunaga et al., 1973). Onset was in the fourth decade. Although the disease affected two generations, inheritance was uncertain because of consanguinity. Either an autosomal dominant or autosomal recessive pattern was possible.

3.1.5 Hexosaminidase deficiency

The GM2 gangliosidoses are the consequence of a deficiency either of the hexosaminidase enzyme that hydrolyses the terminal N-acetylgalactosamine from GM2 ganglioside or of the activator protein for the enzyme. There are two major hexosaminidase isoenzymes, A and B (hex A and hex B). Hex A is made up of α- and β-subunits coded for on chromosomes 15 and 5 respectively, whereas hex B is composed only of β-subunits. A mutation of the α-locus thus gives rise to a deficiency of hex A, the usual manifestation of which is Tay–Sachs disease. A β-locus mutation produces a deficiency of hex A and hex B and leads to Sandhoff disease. These disorders are of autosomal recessive inheritance. In recent years examples of both hex A and combined hex A and B deficiency presenting during adolescence or early adult life as a chronic spinal muscular atrophy have been described (Jellinger et al., 1982; Dale, Engel and Rudd, 1982; Barbeau et al., 1984; Mitsumoto et al., 1985; Parnes et al., 1985; Johnson, Wigger and Karp, 1982; Karni, Navon and Sadeh, 1988; Thomas, Young and King, 1989). Most often this has been associated with involvement of other systems, including cognitive impairment, ataxia and pyramidal signs, but some cases can present with a virtually pure proximal spinal muscular atrophy resembling Kugelberg–Welander disease. Progression is slow.

3.2 SEGMENTAL MOTOR NEURONOPATHIES

3.2.1 Chronic asymmetric spinal muscular atrophy (CASMA)

This is a relatively common condition, although reports as to its prevalence are not available. Descriptions of cases have been given by Meadows, Marsden and Harriman (1969), and Harding, Bradbury and

Murray (1983). The designation given above was introduced by the latter authors and seems to be the most satisfactory. Weakness and muscle wasting, often with fasciculation, usually begin in one limb, either lower or upper, and then extend to other limbs. Initially these patients may be exceedingly difficult to distinguish from those with motor neurone disease. Progression is slow and spontaneous arrest can occur. Pyramidal signs do not develop and bulbar involvement did not occur in the 18 patients reported by Harding, Bradbury and Murray (1983). It is intriguing that two of these patients had first-degree relatives with acute infantile spinal muscular atrophy (Werdnig-Hoffmann disease), raising the possibility that CASMA could be a heterozygote manifestation of this condition.

3.2.2 Other segmental motor neuronopathies

A distinctive disorder that develops during adolescence or early in the third decade and which is virtually confined to males appears to be particularly common in Japan (Sobue et al., 1978), although reports of similar cases have appeared from India (Singh, Sachdev and Susheela, 1980) and Australia (O'Sullivan and McLeod, 1978). The authors have also observed such patients in the UK. Muscle weakness and wasting that affect the small hand and forearm muscles unilaterally or occasionally bilaterally progress quite rapidly initially and then slow or arrest. Recovery does not occur. Electromyography and nerve conduction studies suggest anterior horn cell disease. The condition is sporadic except in the case of a father and son who were both affected in the series of 71 patients reported by Sobue et al. (1978).

Cases of benign monomelic lower limb spinal muscular atrophy ('wasted leg syndrome') have been reported from India (Gourie-Devi, Suresh and Shankar, 1984).

3.3 METABOLIC NEUROPATHIES

3.3.1 Diabetes mellitus

The commonest peripheral neuropathy that is associated with diabetes mellitus is a distal sensory/autonomic neuropathy. 'Diabetic amyotrophy' constitutes a predominantly motor syndrome. It seems possible that this can be separated into two forms. One consists of an asymmetric lower limb proximal motor neuropathy that mainly affects the thigh muscles and the iliopsoas. It is often of relatively acute or subacute onset and therefore will not be discussed further. It may well be ischaemic in origin (Raff, Sangalang and Asbury, 1968). The second form is a relatively symmetric proximal lower limb motor neuropathy of insidious onset. It is more likely to be associated with the distal sensory neuropathy than the asymmetric form (Subramony and Wilbourn, 1982) and has been considered to be likely to have a metabolic rather than an ischaemic basis (Asbury, 1977).

3.3.2 Other conditions

Chronic renal failure may give rise to a peripheral neuropathy. This is usually a distal length-related sensorimotor neuropathy. Rarely a pure motor syndrome is encountered (Thomas *et al.*, 1971). Amyloidosis (primary or inherited) may also be responsible for a peripheral neuropathy. Most commonly this is initially of 'small fibre' type with predominant loss of pain and temperature sensation and autonomic involvement. Occasional patients present with a slowly progressive distal predominantly motor involvement, as in a patient encountered by the authors, who was initially considered to have type II HMSN.

3.4 TOXIC NEUROPATHIES

Of the neuropathies related to environmental toxins, that caused by lead characteristically produces predominantly motor involvement. The older literature described focal weakness as a common presentation with five distinct patterns. In order of frequency of occurrence these were wrist and finger extensors, shoulder girdle muscles, intrinsic hand muscles, the peronei and the laryngeal muscles. It was considered that the particular distribution was related to habitual use of the affected muscles. Lead neuropathy is now rare, as are such focal patterns of weakness (Boothby, DeJesus and Rowland, 1974). More usually, progressive generalized weakness occurs, with loss of tendon reflexes and mild distal wasting, sometimes with fasciculation. In children, lower limb involvement tends to predominate. Electromyography reveals signs of denervation. Motor nerve conduction velocity is preserved, sensory action potentials being diminished in amplitude (Buchthal and Behse, 1979).

Distinction from motor neurone disease can be difficult. Associated anaemia with basophilic stippling of erythrocytes and alimentary symptoms (anorexia, vomiting, abdominal pain), if present, will suggest the diagnosis. Confirmation can be obtained by the finding of an elevated blood level or, if this is equivocal, by the examination of urine levels following a chelation challenge. Improvement occurs following removal from exposure and treatment with chelating agents.

Although vincristine neuropathy usually begins with sensory symptoms in the limbs, it is predominantly a motor neuropathy. Weakness tends to begin in the upper limbs with finger and wrist drop and then extends to affected distal lower limb muscles. The tendon reflexes are depressed or lost. Sensory loss remains mild and affects the distal limbs and sometimes the trigeminal territory. Nerve conduction studies demonstrate an axonopathy. The neuropathy is dose related and may be a result of binding to axonal microtubules with consequent impairment of fast axonal transport. Slow recovery occurs on withdrawal of the drug.

3.5 INFLAMMATORY NEUROPATHIES

3.5 Chronic inflammatory demyelinating polyneuropathy (CIDP)

The presentations of this condition are extremely varied. Although an ataxic sensory form occurs, this is uncommon. In most cases the involvement is predominantly motor and ranges from a diffuse symmetric polyneuropathy, through multifocal motor neuropathies, to focal brachial plexus or limb presentations.

The symmetric polyneuropathy is the commonest variant. This can display a relapsing and remitting or a chronic progressive course. It can develop at any age from childhood to late life. The mean age of onset for the relapsing cases is appreciably lower than for the chronic progressive cases (McCombe, Pollard and McLeod, 1985). This distribution of weakness may be proximal, distal or generalized. Not infrequently there is an upper limb postural tremor resembling essential tremor. The tendon reflexes are depressed or absent. Sensory loss, when present, is usually relatively mild, is distal in distribution and affects mainly large-fibre modalities. The peripheral nerves may be thickened. Motor nerve conduction velocity is moderately or severely reduced and sensory action potentials can be depressed or absent, or sometimes fully preserved. Conduction block in motor fibres is often demonstrable, although strict criteria must be fullfilled before this can be accepted (see Cornblath *et al.*, 1991).

Over the past decade a syndrome has been defined characterized by a multifocal demyelinating neuropathy with conduction block that can persist at one site for prolonged periods (Lewis *et al.*, 1982; Parry and Clarke, 1985; Van Den Bergh, Logigan and Kelly, 1989). If accompanied by sensory changes, initially it can mimic entrapment syndromes (Lewis *et al.*, 1982) or motor neurone disease if sensory changes are absent (Parry and Clarke, 1985). Some patients with a clinically similar syndrome have been shown to have high titres of anti-GM1 or GD1b ganglioside antibodies (Pestronk *et al.*, 1988a). These are discussed later.

Motor neuropathies

The first instance of focal hypertrophic neuropathy to be identified was the variant that affects the brachial plexus (Adams, Asbury and Michelson, 1965). This gives rise to upper limb weakness, usually out of proportion to the amount of wasting, which may affect distal or proximal muscles, or both. Sensory loss is usually trivial or absent. The involvement is usually unilateral. Pathologically there is a focal demyelinating hypertrophic neuropathy affecting the brachial plexus (Cusimano, Bilboa and Cohen, 1988). Confusion with motor neurone disease of progressive muscular atrophy form is frequent, as there are electromyographic signs of denervation but motor conduction velocity (and sensory conduction) in the limb itself may be normal. F-wave latencies, on the other hand, are often markedly prolonged. Alternatively, proximal conduction can be shown to be reduced using recording from limb muscles and high-voltage electrical stimulation of spinal roots. Enlargement of the brachial plexus may be shown by magnetic resonance imaging (MRI).

Focal demyelinating neuropathy affecting isolated limb nerves is less common. Again motor changes predominate with disproportionate weakness in relation to the degree of wasting. Fasciculation or myokymia can be a striking manifestation (Mitsumoto et al., 1990). Again, MRI can demonstrate focal nerve enlargement. The condition has to be distinguished from focal lesions that have been described as being hypertrophic but which consist of the formation of multiple small whorls composed of perineurial cells (Bilboa et al., 1984).

3.6 NEUROPATHY ASSOCIATED WITH ANTI-GM1 GANGLIOSIDE ANTIBODIES

Much evidence has recently accumulated to suggest an important role for antibodies directed against carbohydrate residues present on glycolipids and gangliosides in the pathogenesis of autoimmune neuropathies (Quarles, Ilyas and Willison, 1986; Latov, 1990). Of particular relevance are the many recent reports of anti-GM1 antibodies in the serum of patients with different patterns of motor neuropathy and neuronopathy, including typical motor neurone disease (MND). This section will review the background and current status of this rapidly evolving field.

3.6.1 Ganglioside structure and function

Gangliosides are ubiquitous components of many cell membranes highly concentrated in the nervous system. Structurally they comprise

Table 3.1 Structure of GM1 and related gangliosides

Compound	Carbohydrate sequence
GM1	Gal (β1–3) GalNAc (β1–4) Gal (β1–4) Glc (β1–1) Ceramide (α2–3) NeuAc
GD1b	Gal (β1–3) GalNAc (β1–4) Gal (β1–4) Glc (β1–1) Ceramide (α2–3) NeuAc (α2–8) NeuAc
GD1a	Gal (β1–3) GalNAc (β1–4) Gal (β1–4) Glc (β1–1) Ceramide (α2–3) (α2–3) NeuAc NeuAc
GM2	GalNAc (β1–4) Gal (β1–4) Glc (β1–1) Ceramide (α2–3) NeuAc
Asialo-GM1	Gal (β1–3) GalNAc (β1–4) Gal (β1–4) Glc (β1–1) Ceramide

the hydrophobic, ceramide portion of the molecule, which is inserted into the lipid membrane bilayer. The extracellular component comprises a chain of at least two carbohydrate residues linked to variable amounts of sialic acid (see Table 3.1). It is the presence of sialic acid that defines the molecule as a ganglioside.

The major species of brain ganglioside are GM1, GD1a, GD1b and GT1b, the most abundant being GM1, which is present in both neural membranes and myelin. GM1 is also present to a lesser extent in the peripheral nervous system (PNS), where cholera toxin-binding studies have shown it to be concentrated at nodes of Ranvier and nerve terminals (Hanson, Holmgren and Svennerholm, 1977; Ganser, Kirschner and Willinger, 1983). Many details of ganglioside function are unknown. They are the natural ligands for a variety of toxins, including tetanus, botulinum and cholera toxins. They are also able to modulate a wide range of cellular processes in both normal and pathological states, such as neurite outgrowth (Leeden, 1989; Barletta, Bremer and Culp, 1991).

3.6.2 Clinical features of anti-GM1 ganglioside antibody-associated diseases

Although there has been considerable recent emphasis on the association of anti-GM1 antibodies with motor system diseases, the clinical spectrum of nerve disease described in association with anti-GM1

Motor neuropathies

antibodies is very varied and includes patients with clear sensory nerve involvement. In addition to neuropathies and neuronopathies, significant titres of anti-GM1 antibodies, including those associated with monoclonal immunoglobulins (mIgs) (Marcus et al., 1989a), have also been found in a wide variety of normal people (Marcus et al., 1989b) and in those with other diseases, including multiple sclerosis, brain injury, stroke, systemic lupus erythematosis (Endo et al., 1984) and Alzheimer's disease (Chapman et al., 1988). Identical clinical syndromes frequently occur in the absence of anti-GM1 antibodies. It is thus important to realize that many factors other than simply the presence of anti-GM1 antibodies need to be identified in order to unravel the pathogenetic factors in the complex array of motor neurone syndromes.

The first evidence to link antibodies to GM1 ganglioside with motor system diseases appeared in 1986 when Freddo et al. (1986) described a patient with a purely lower motor neurone disease comprising progressive weakness with fasciculations and areflexia in all four limbs, widespread denervation on EMG examination and normal motor and sensory conduction studies. Cerebrospinal fluid (CSF) examination was normal. The patient's serum contained an IgM lambda mIg reactive with GM1, asialo-GM1 and GD1b, which all share a terminal Gal (β1–3) GalNAc moiety. Despite immunosuppressive treatment with plasma exchange, chlorambucil and prednisolone, her symptoms progressed and she died 2 years after onset of her illness (Latov et al., 1988). A further case with an identical serological specificity was reported in 1988 (Latov et al., 1988). This patient had progressive upper limb wasting with weakness and mild sensory symptoms with less marked abnormalities in the legs. He was areflexic. Nerve conduction studies were normal and EMG examination revealed widespread denervation with fasciculation and fibrillation. The CSF had an elevated protein content at 1.1 g/l and 10 lymphocytes/mm^3. The patient responded well to treatment with immunosuppressive therapy with chlorambucil and plasma exchange. In this patient sensory features were present and CSF examination was abnormal, which would argue strongly against MND as the primary diagnosis. Nardelli et al. (1988) reported another patient with a lower motor neurone syndrome and an IgM mIg with anti-GM1, GD1b and asialo-GM1 antibody activity.

At the same time three further patients were described with mixed sensorimotor neuropathies and IgM monoclonal antibodies reactive with GM1 (llyas et al., 1988). The first of these was initially diagnosed as having a lower motor neurone form of MND, but 3 years later developed sensory symptoms and on re-evaluation was found to have antibodies to GM1 also reactive with GD1b and asialo-GM1. Interestingly, the other two patients had anti-GM1 antibodies cross-reactive with GM2 and also had a second IgM mIg reactive with the myelin-associated glycoprotein (MAG); both these patients had more prominent sensory symptoms.

A report from Pestronk *et al.* (1988a) identified two patients with polyclonal anti-GM1 antibodies and a multifocal motor syndrome in which conduction block was present along many motor nerves. Minor sensory features were also present. Both of these patients responded to treatment with cyclophosphamide. Although 'multifocal motor neuropathy' (MMN) with demyelinating conduction block had been previously recognized as a clinical entity (Lewis *et al.*, 1982), this was the first description of it occurring in the context of anti-GM1 antibodies.

Since this original description many investigators have described further patients with a similar clinical pattern (Pestronk, 1991). These patients thus typically have an asymmetric syndrome of weakness with wasting and fasciculation, often starting distally in the upper limbs and spreading to involve other sites. Sensory symptoms and signs are mild or absent. Onset in middle age is usual and slow progression may occur over many years. Men are more frequently affected than women. Although many of these patients have anti-GM1 antibodies, this is not invariable (Pestronk, 1991; Lange *et al.*, 1992). Conduction block is present on motor nerves, which may need to be extensively and carefully sampled in order to detect this. The difficulties associated with distinguishing conduction block from conduction delay with abnormal temporal dispersion in this context have been recently discussed in detail (Cornblath *et al.*, 1991). Many of these patients respond to treatment with immunosuppressive agents, particularly cyclophosphamide (Feldman *et al.*, 1991), although again this is variable.

Whether this clinical pattern of MMN constitutes a distinct entity or whether it is part of the increasingly wide spectrum of CIDP remains an issue for discussion. However, we and many others have seen patients who fit remarkably closely the MMN pattern as described by Pestronk and colleagues (Pestronk *et al.*, 1988a; Pestronk, 1991). Current evidence favours the existence of a fairly uniform but uncommon clinical entity comprising MMN with conduction block and often with anti-GM1 antibodies (Adams *et al.*, 1991; Pestronk, 1991; Lange *et al.*, 1992). The precise characterization of such cases must await further studies to establish the nature of the underlying pathology and to determine the significance of these antibodies.

Since the early descriptions of cases of anti-GM1 antibody-associated motor neurone syndromes, many screening studies for anti-GM1 antibodies on larger groups of patients with typical MND and other neuromuscular diseases have been performed (Pestronk *et al.*, 1989; Nobile-Orazio *et al.*, 1990; Sadiq *et al.*, 1990; Salazas-Grueso *et al.*, 1990; Adams *et al.*, 1991; Gregson, Jones and Willison, 1991; Lamb and

Motor neuropathies

Patten, 1990). These studies have produced conflicting information as a result of two major problems: the lack of a standardized anti-ganglioside antibody assay procedure and differences in the diagnostic categorization and selection criteria for patients and appropriate controls.

Although incompletely resolved, some unifying patterns have now emerged. First, many early reports suggested that anti-GM1 antibodies are found significantly more frequently in MND patients (50–60%) than in controls (<25%) (Pestronk et al., 1988b, 1989; Shy et al., 1989). Other studies (Latov et al., 1988; Salasaz-Grueso et al., 1990) found a similar frequency (10–20%) in MND patients and controls. A recent community based series of 82 MND patients and age/sex-matched controls by Chancellor et al. (1992) again showed similar frequencies (20–25% positive) between the two groups. It thus seems that, despite early claims to the contrary, there is no significant increase in anti-GM1 antibodies in classical MND.

Secondly, most neurological patients with high titres of anti-GM1 antibodies (variably defined, but at least > 1:350) have either a lower motor neuronopathy, motor neuropathy or CIDP with little sensory involvement (Lamb et al., 1991; Pestronk, 1991; Sadiq et al., 1990); anti-GM1 antibodies have not been found in sensory neuropathies alone, although this is not true for anti-GD1b antibodies (Daune et al., 1992). Apart from MMN with demyelinating conduction block, in which the prevalence of anti-GM1 antibodies is higher than 50%, these antibody-positive patients still represent a small proportion (10–20%) of the total number of patients in these groups. In addition to chronic neuropathies, many patients with acute Guillain–Barré syndrome (GBS) who have high-titre anti-GM1 IgM and/or IgG antibodies are now being identified (Oomes et al., 1990; Yuki et al., 1990; Gregson et al., 1991; Ilyas et al., 1992; Nobile-Orazio et al., 1992). These patients also tend to have prominent or pure motor involvement, often with severe axonal involvement. Again, the anti-GM1 antibody-positive GBS patients account for less than 20% of the total. As can be seen, the clinical spectrum of disease associated with anti-GM1 antibodies is large and uneven but clearly warrants further study in order that these issues can be clarified.

3.6.3 Characteristics of anti-GM1 antibodies

All the anti-GM1 antibodies that have been referred to above are of the IgM class with the exception of some anti-GM1 IgG antibodies that have recently been identified in the sera of GBS patients. The affinities of human anti-GM1 antibodies have not been measured to date since no cloned antibody-producing cell lines have yet been described. Likewise, the immunoglobulin variable-region gene usage of anti-GM1 antibodies has yet to be delineated. Since anti-GM1 antibodies can frequently be detected in normal serum, including umbilical cord blood, it has been postulated that they form part of the naturally occurring autoantibody repertoire (Latov, 1990). These autoantibodies are generally regarded as non-pathogenic under normal circumstances: they are polyreactive low-affinity IgM class antibodies produced by T-cell independent mechanisms (Casali and Notkins, 1989). However, pathological circumstances such as the loss of idiotypic regulation, B-cell transformation or exposure to cross-reactive foreign antigen on microbial polysaccharides may result in an increase in antibody concentration or affinity that could render them pathogenic.

Scrutiny of the basic ganglioside structure (see Table 3.1) shows that there is considerable potential for sharing of epitopes between different gangliosides. All the human antibodies described in relation to neurological disease react with the carbohydrate and/or sialic acid portion of gangliosides. However, the influence of auxiliary lipids and variations in the orientation of the carbohydrate and ceramide portions of the molecule under different physical conditions may have profound influences on antibody binding. For example, it has been shown that antibodies reactive with GM1 in a liposome environment containing lecithin and cholesterol may not react with purified GM1 in a solid-phase assay system (Endo et al., 1984). We have recently examined two monoclonal antibodies developed by Inglis et al. (1987) that react strongly with the Gal (β1–3) GalNAc moiety when synthetically conjugated to albumin but fail to react with GM1, GD1b or asialo-GM1, which share the same terminal Gal (β1–3) GalNAc structure. The converse is also true: antibodies reactive with GM1, GD1b and asialo-GM1 may not react with Gal (β1–3) GalNAc–albumin (Pestronk, 1991). Thus, despite the apparent potential for antibody reactivity with glycolipids in a natural lipid membrane-like environment and for cross-reactivity with glycoconjugates that share similar carbohydrate structures, this may not necessarily occur. It is important to bear these considerations in mind when selecting a screening system for antibodies or considering disease models.

With these cautions in mind, three main patterns of anti-GM1 antibody specificity have been identified. First, antibodies may react with the terminal Gal (β1–3) GalNAc structure and will therefore cross-react with GD1b and asialo-GM1 (Baba et al., 1989; Pestronk, 1991). Secondly, antibodies may react with GM1 and GM2 (Ilyas et al., 1988; Baba et al., 1989), presumably via shared internal sialylated sugar moieties. Thirdly, some antibodies react with GM1 alone (Latov et al., 1988; Pestronk, 1991). Effort has been made by some authors to correlate

A   B

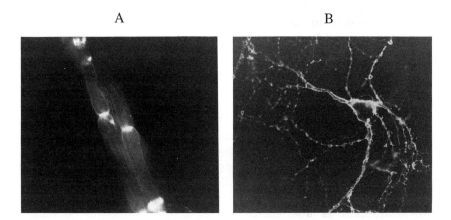

Figure 3.3 (A) Immunostaining of teased rat cauda equina with serum diluted 1:50, from a patient with acute motor neuropathy containing anti-GM1 IgG and IgM antibodies, followed by FITC anti-human IgG. Magnification ×216. (B) Immunostaining of rat primary cortical culture with the same serum as A, followed by FITC anti-human IgM. Magnification ×360. (Courtesy of Dr N. Gregson.) (Reproduced with permission from Gregson *et al.*, 1991.)

these variations in fine specificity with clinical subgroups (Pestronk *et al.*, 1989, 1990; Sadiq *et al.*, 1990). Although this approach is clearly important, no convincing unifying patterns have yet emerged.

3.6.4 Pathogenetic mechanisms

Several different mechanisms have been proposed to explain the possible pathogenic effects of anti-GM1 antibodies: it is most likely that they induce a pathological effect through binding to the extracellular carbohydrate moieties of GM1 and thereby either activate complement and other proinflammatory pathways or create a functional block of GM1-modulated processes. Since the major site of GM1 localization in the PNS is at nodes of Ranvier, conduction block would seem to be a reasonable consequence of this. Direct immunofluorescence studies on peripheral nerve from a patient with MMN (Santoro *et al.*, 1990) have demonstrated immunoglobulin deposits at nodes of Ranvier. However, this was found for sensory fibres in the sural nerve, whereas the patient had a motor neuropathy. Nevertheless, serum from this patient bound to nodes of Ranvier when injected into rat sciatic nerve, which also was considered to develop conduction block. Similar localization of antibody has been found by other researchers (Gregson *et al.*, 1991; see Figure 3.3). The other site at which GM1 is found in the PNS is at motor nerve terminals; binding of antibody at this site may induce local pathological changes or result in uptake of immunoglobulin with retrograde transport to the cell body and subsequent functional disruption. This concept has been studied in detail with antibodies of other specificities by several workers using autoimmune models of MND (Fabian, 1990; Fabian and Ritchie, 1986; Engelhardt and Appel, 1990). GM1 is found in many sites in the central nervous system (CNS) including spinal motor neurones (Gregson et al., 1991; Thomas et al., 1990) and other cortical neurones (Figure 3.3) to which antibodies could presumably bind if they had free access. However, the protection offered by the blood–brain barrier and local factors influencing exposure of antigenic determinants presumably prevent this from occurring in vivo. It is interesting to note that the main site of nerve injury in the neuropathy associated with anti-MAG antibodies is also in the PNS, despite the fact that the concentration of MAG is likewise much higher in the CNS (Latov, 1990; Quarles, Ilyas and Willison, 1986). It is not yet firmly established, however, that MAG is the relevant myelin protein. The identification of MAG as the culprit could reflect a cross-reaction. Many antibodies that bind to GM1 cross-react with other glycolipids and glycoproteins that may have the potential to mediate the pathological events (Thomas et al., 1989), although examples of this have yet to be identified.

3.6.5 Summary

Many studies have indicated that anti-GM1 antibodies are associated with different patterns of motor neurone diseases. Despite incomplete and often contradictory evidence, the main body of opinion suggests that identifying the pathogenetic mechanisms of antibodies to GM1 and related antigens in inducing disease is an important goal for the future. This may conceivably throw light on the mechanisms operating in classical MND. In addition, since autoimmune motor neurone syndromes are potentially treatable, it is particularly important to identify the subgroup of patients with these conditions so that they receive appropriate therapy.

3.7 PARANEOPLASTIC NEUROPATHY

Paraneoplastic diseases are remote effects of cancer unrelated to direct infiltration of tissue by tumour. Many paraneoplastic syndromes have been recognized that involve peripheral nerve, producing different patterns of motor, sensory and sensorimotor neuropathy. In particular, a subacute sensory neuropathy originally described by Denny-Brown (1948) is associated with carcinoma. It should be stated at the outset that,

Motor neuropathies

although many examples of paraneoplastic motor neurone diseases have been described, they are extremely rare. The relative frequency of both cancer and motor neuropathies/motor neurone diseases will ensure that many patients will be found with both conditions coincidentally. The evidence that the two conditions are related in some patients will be briefly reviewed here.

3.7.1 Epidemiological studies

Several large series of patients and national epidemiological surveys have studied the association between malignancy and MND. These surveys were initiated by several early reports of a biased link between the two conditions. For example, a high incidence was reported by Norris and Engel (1965), who found that 10% (13/130) of an unselected group of MND patients had cancer. Many subsequent population-based surveys failed to confirm these early reports. A subsequent survey of 834 ALS patients found a prevalence of cancer of 2.6%, which was not significantly different from the general population (Norris *et al.*, 1989). The overall conclusion from many studies reviewing thousands of patients is that there is no evidence to indicate a general association between the two conditions (Rosenfeld and Posner, 1991). There are, however, a sufficient number of unusual manifestations of MND-like syndromes in cancer patients to indicate that there may be important disease subgroups that warrant further scrutiny. These are described below.

3.7.2 Subacute motor neuronopathy associated with lymphoma

Many references have been made to subacute motor neuronopathy as a distinct clinical syndrome usually occurring with lymphoma. The term was coined by Schold *et al.* (1978), who described 10 patients with this condition. Other authors have reported similar cases (reviewed by Younger *et al.*, 1991). The clinical features comprise an asymmetric lower motor neurone pattern of weakness with wasting and fasciculation, depressed reflexes and normal sensation. Nerve conduction studies are normal, with EMG evidence of denervation. The CSF is acellular but the protein content may be elevated. The course may be chronic and is occasionally modified by treatment of the malignancy. Pathologically, loss of anterior horn cells and demyelination in anterior nerve roots may occur. Inflammatory changes in nerve roots, anterior horns or spinal cord are variably present. The evidence thus indicates that both the nerve root and cell body may be affected.

Younger *et al.* (1991) recently showed that, of their nine patients with lymphoma and a motor neurone syndrome, the majority also had upper motor neurone signs, confirmed in autopsy examination of two cases. They also identified motor nerve conduction block in two patients. In addition, three of their nine patients had mIgs, six had an increased CSF protein concentration and three had oligoclonal CSF IgG bands. These data provide further evidence for dysimmunity in the pathogenesis of paraneoplastic motor neurone diseases.

3.7.3   Other paraneoplastic motor neurone syndromes

Motor neurone involvement occurs in about half the patients with paraneoplastic encephalomyelitis, a well-documented syndrome that can involve all levels of the neuraxis. All these patients have the anti-Hu autoantibody in their serum, which binds to neuronal nuclei throughout the nervous system (Anderson *et al.*, 1988; Szabo *et al.*, 1991); this antibody is not found in patients with purely motor syndromes. Two other case reports have described patients with motor neurone syndromes and cancer in whom immunofluorescence studies with the patient's serum have demonstrated reactivity with motor neurones although the antigens involved have not been characterized further (Dhib-Jalbut and Liwnicz, 1986; Wong *et al.*, 1987).

3.7.4   Summary

Although there is no association between motor neuropathies or motor system diseases and cancer in large population studies, a sufficient number of atypical cases occur to warrant attention to the association at both the clinical and experimental level. The most important relevant overlap is between motor neuronopathies and lymphomas. This in turn converges with paraproteins and dysimmunity, which are frequent associations within this subgroup; it is thus likely that autoimmune factors are pathogenetically significant in the situations when the two conditions are causally rather than coincidentally related.

3.8   PARAPROTEINAEMIC NEUROPATHY

Abnormalities of plasma cell proliferation resulting in the production of monoclonal serum immunoglobulin (mIg, also termed monoclonal gammopathy or paraproteinaemia) have been widely described in association with peripheral neuropathy and motor neurone diseases. The association with neuropathy was first recognized over 20 years ago and since then research in this field has progressed considerably. The structural and pathogenic properties of many mIgs of different isotypes, affinities and antigenic specificities have been studied in considerable detail; however, the pathogenetic relationship between mIgs and neuropathies remains a complicated and contentious field that has yet to be fully elucidated (Quarles, Ilyas and Willison, 1986; Latov, 1990; Gosselin, Kyle and Dyck, 1991; Yeung *et al.*, 1991).

An important issue concerns the definition of mIgs and the value of classifying mIg-associated disease as a separate entity. The presence or absence of a mIg depends upon the sensitivity of the technique used to detect it; now that highly sensitive methods such as isoelectric focusing and immunoblotting are available, the threshold for detecting mIgs has been reduced considerably. Since all antibodies are by nature monoclonal, describing them as such is a matter of degree. Monoclonal or oligoclonal immunoglobulins may occur in normal serum in response to antigen stimulation, where they may be transitory. Benign monoclonal gammopathy occurs when no detectable B-cell disorder is evident. Several different patterns of frank lymphoproliferative disease may produce mIgs, including solitary plasmacytoma, multiple myeloma and B-cell lymphoma. Pathogenetic antibodies of a similar specificity and affinity may be present in serum in insufficient amount to be identifiable as a monoclonal band but produce the same clinical effect (McGinnis *et al.*, 1988), indicating that this distinction may be unhelpful in terms of identifying individual cases or gaining insights into disease pathogenesis.

The clinical patterns of neuropathy that have been encountered in paraproteinaemia are varied and encompass axonopathies, neuronopathies and demyelinating neuropathies affecting the motor and sensory systems to different degrees in symmetric or multifocal patterns (Gosselin, Kyle and Dyck, 1991; Yeung *et al.*, 1991). In general, paraproteinaemic neuropathies are demyelinating and affect sensory fibres more severely than motor fibres. Although very uncommon, purely motor paraproteinaemic neuropathies have been described and are being increasingly identified in association with anti-GM1 antibodies. In addition there are many reports of mIgs associated with otherwise typical MND or MND with unusual features, as discussed below. For the purposes of this section, mIg-associated motor neuropathies that clinically resemble MND in the broadest sense will be included.

3.8.1 Paraproteins in motor neuropathies

Many reports have described individuals or small numbers of patients with motor system disease and mIgs with very variable clinical and pathological features. Some of these reports clearly describe motor neuropathies, others describe typical MND/ALS and in others ambiguity exists. For example, Rowland *et al.* (1982) described a 48-year-old man with an IgM kappa mIg and a diffuse lower motor neurone syndrome that was considered to simulate MND. The patient showed muscle wasting with weakness, widespread fasciculation and tendon areflexia. Sensation was normal. There was EMG evidence of denervation, motor conduction was slowed and there was an elevated CSF protein content at 2.65 g/l. He failed to respond to immunosuppressive treatment and died 14 months after onset. At autopsy there was severe axonal degeneration and demyelination in the ventral roots with milder but definite changes in the dorsal roots. Anterior horn cell morphology was normal with the exception of central chromatolysis and the brain and spinal cord were otherwise normal. It was partly the presence of widespread fasciculation that initially suggested anterior horn cell disease. It is insufficiently recognized that fasciculation may be a prominent manifestation of demyelination of peripheral nerve fibres. The tendon areflexia, slow motor nerve conduction velocity and elevated CSF protein concentration strongly favoured a demyelinating neuropathy in this patient, and the autopsy findings confirmed a polyradiculopathy. Although the sensory system was clinically and electrophysiologically spared, pathological changes were present in the dorsal roots. The specificity of the mIg was not determined and there was no mention of mIg deposition within the nerve roots.

Parry *et al.* (1986) described a 38-year-old man with a subacute proximal motor axonopathy evolving over 4 months which rendered him tetraparetic. Apart from early paraesthesiae, the sensory system was again clinically spared. He responded to immunosuppressive therapy but died from pulmonary embolism. The main pathological findings were focal axonal swellings and lymphocytic infiltration of the ventral roots. Occasional degenerating neurones were seen in the dorsal root ganglia. Although the serum IgM was elevated to twice normal, there was no evidence of a mIg, although the term gammopathy was used by the authors.

A report by Rudnicki *et al.* (1987) documented a more chronic pattern of evolution. They described a 69-year-old man with distal limb wasting with weakness and widespread denervation evolving over 8 years. Initial investigation showed a polyclonal increase in serum IgM, but further evaluation 5 years after onset demonstrated an IgM kappa mIg, and 2 years later an IgA mIg was also identified. The patient responded partially to immunosuppressive therapy and remained clinically stable. The clinical and electrophysiological studies were considered to be indicative more of a chronic spinal muscular atrophy than a proximal motor axonopathy. However, as indicated earlier in this chapter, the distinction between an axonopathy and a neuronopathy may not be possible in the absence of autopsy studies. In addition, a mIg evolved out of an apparent polyclonal increase in serum IgM, thereby reinforcing the view that this distinction is also a relative one.

In the series of 25 patients with peripheral neuropathy and IgM paraproteinaemia described by Dellagi *et al.* (1983), two had a purely motor syndrome, although further details of these cases were not recorded. Other case reports describe patients in whom the dominant lesion appears to be a motor neuropathy, although no pathological proof is provided.

3.8.2 Paraproteins in motor neurone disease

There are many case descriptions in which the clinical and pathological diagnosis is clearly that of MND rather than motor neuropathy. For example, in the same paper as referred to above, Rudnicki *et al.* (1987) described a 69-year-old man with an IgG lambda mIg and progressive limb and bulbar weakness who died within a year of onset of symptoms despite immunosuppressive therapy. Post-mortem demonstrated typical features of ALS with widespread severe cortical motor neurone, corticospinal tract and anterior horn cell degeneration. In another example, Kreiger and Melmed (1982) described a 63-year-old man with an IgG kappa mIg and progressive lower motor neurone weakness with fasciculation, bilateral pyramidal signs and bulbar palsy who died 2 years after the onset of symptoms. The pathology was again typical of ALS. In neither of these cases were detailed immunopathological studies undertaken, making the association with the mIg circumstantial.

Apart from the cases associated with anti-GM1 antibodies (see above), there is only one example to date of an individual case of MND in which the specificity of the mIg has been determined and appears to be relevant to the clinical syndrome. Hays *et al.* (1990) have reported a patient who died with ALS and an IgA mIg in whom IgA was deposited in the cell bodies and processes of surviving anterior horn cells in the lumbar cord. On Western blots the IgA reacted with the 200-kDa neurofilament protein and also reacted with an as yet uncharacterized 65-kDa protein found in spinal cord. Interestingly, Inuzuka *et al.* (1989) reported two patients with MND whose serum also reacted on Western blots with a 65-kDa protein present in spinal cord, although these antibodies were not mIgs.

In a large retrospective series of 206 patients with MND reported by Shy *et al.* (1986), 10 patients were identified as having mIg, giving a prevalence of 4.9%. The addition of selected patients allowed them to identify a total of 21 cases of mIg-associated MND. IgG and IgM mIgs were equally represented and one patient had an IgA mIg. The clinical features of these patients were not unusual, either in terms of the pattern of upper (UMN) or lower motor neurone (LMN) involvement or the disease duration. Only one patient had an autopsy, again without atypical features. They noted that, in general, MND patients with IgM paraproteins tended to have more prominent LMN involvement and often had a mildly elevated CSF protein. IgG paraproteins occurred with mixed UMN and LMN disease and normal CSF protein. However, these were not absolute findings. Treatment with immunosuppressive therapy was largely disappointing, with the exception of one patient with an IgG paraprotein, who clearly responded to combination chemotherapy.

In another large series reported by Younger et al. (1990), mIgs were detected in 9% of 120 MND patients by conventional immunofixation. No particular trends in disease pattern were identified, most patients having mixed UMN and LMN signs. IgG, IgM and IgA mIgs were found, an elevation of CSF protein content was observed frequently (36% compared with 1% in the MND cases without mIg) and three gammopathy patients also had lymphoma. Another study by Younger et al. (1991) has again noted this association between MND and lymphoma with or without mIg.

Duarte et al. (1991) have used a very sensitive Western blotting technique capable of detecting mIgs in concentrations as low as 25 ng/ml, to perform a prospective survey of 30 MND cases with matched controls. They found a 60% incidence of mIg in their MND group as compared with 13% in the control group. The mIg isotype was IgG in 73% and IgM in the remainder. No clinical subgroup correlations were identified and the antigenic specificity of the mIgs remains unknown.

A more recent study by Chancellor et al. (1992) comprising 82 MND patients and carefully matched controls failed to show any difference in mIg frequencies between the two groups, using either standard high-resolution agarose electrophoresis or a very sensitive isoelectric focusing and immunoblotting method.

3.8.3 Summary

Epidemiological observations on the frequency of mIgs in motor neurone syndromes and appropriate controls are hampered by the relative rarity of the cases and the lack of straightforward diagnostic criteria, particularly in distinguishing pure neuropathy cases from lower motor neurone forms of MND. In carefully defined MND comprising UMN and LMN signs there may be an increased incidence of mIgs, although a recent extensive study (Chancellor *et al.*, 1992) has failed to confirm this. It is thus our view that paraproteinaemia is not associated with the generality of MND, but may be relevant in rare cases. Paraproteinaemic neuropathy is now a well-recognized clinical entity, although only a very small proportion of cases are purely motor. It is equally clear that a great number of clinically indistinguishable cases of motor neurone syndromes exist in whom mIgs are not found. When present, the mIg isotypes that have been described include IgG, IgM and IgA with both kappa and lambda light-chain types. With few exceptions, the specificity of the mIgs remains unknown. Deposition of the mIg within nerve or evidence of complement activation or cellular infiltration has infrequently been observed. There is thus very little direct evidence that can be extracted from the majority of clinicopathological case reports to support a central role for the mIg in mediating disease pathogenesis. However, exceptions such as the case described by Hays *et al.* (1990) may support a primary role for antibody in mediating disease in some cases: this highlights the importance of careful analysis of individual cases in providing directions for future research initiatives. Considerable effort is needed to define these relationships in further detail.

REFERENCES

Adams, D., Kuntzer, T., Burger, D. *et al.* (1991) Predictive value of anti-GM1 antibodies in neuromuscular diseases: a study of 180 sera. *J. Neuroimmunol.*, **32**, 223–30.

Adams, R.D., Asbury, A.K. and Michelson, J.J. (1965) Multifocal pseudohypertrophic neuropathy. *Trans. Am. Neurol. Assoc.*, **90**, 30.

Anderson, N.E., Rosenblum, M.K., Graus, F. *et al.* (1988) Autoantibodies in paraneoplastic syndromes associated with small cell lung cancer. *Neurology*, **38**, 1391–8.

Asbury, A.K. (1977) Proximal diabetic neuropathy. *Ann. Neurol.*, **2**, 179–80.

Baba, H., Daune, G.C., Ilyas, A.A. *et al.* (1989) Anti-GM1 ganglioside antibodies with differing fine specificities in patients with multifocal motor neuropathy. *J. Neuroimmunol.*, **25**, 143–50.

Barbeau, A., Plasse, L., Cloutier, T. *et al.* (1984) Lysosomal enzymes in ataxia: discovery of two cases of late onset hexosaminidase A and B deficiency (adult Sandhoff disease) in French Canadians. *Can. J. Neurol. Sci.*, **11**, 601–6.

Barletta, E., Bremer, E.G. and Culp L.A. (1991) Neurite outgrowth in dorsal root neuronal hybrid clones modulated by ganglioside GM1 and disintegrins. *Exp. Cell Res.*, **193**, 101–11.

Beckett, J., Holden, J.J.A., Simpson, N.E. *et al.* (1986) Localization of X-linked dominant Charcot–Marie–Tooth disease (CMT 2) to Xq13. *J. Neurogenet.*, **3**, 225–31.

Bertini, E., Gadisseux, J.L., Palmieri, G. *et al.* (1989) Distal infantile spinal muscular atrophy associated with paralysis of the diaphragm: a variant of spinal muscular atrophy. *Am. J. Med. Genet.*, **33**, 328–34.

Bilboa, J.M., Khoury, N.J.S., Hudson, A.R. and Briggs, S.J. (1984) Perineuroma (localized hypertrophic neuropathy). *Arch. Pathol. Lab. Med.*, **108**, 557–62.

Bird, T.D., Ott, J. and Giblett, E.R. (1982) Evidence for linkage of Charcot–Marie–Tooth neuropathy to the Duffy locus on chromosome 1. *Am. J. Hum. Genet.*, **34**, 388–94.

Boothby, J.A., DeJesus, P.V. and Rowland, L.P. (1974) Reversible forms of motor neuron disease. *Arch. Neurol.*, **31**, 18–29.

Buchthal, F. and Behse, F. (1979) Electrophysiology and nerve biopsy in men exposed to lead. *Br. J. Indust. Med.*, **36**, 135–42.

Bundey, S. and Lovelace, R.E. (1975) A clinical and genetic study of chronic spinal muscular atrophy. *Brain*, **98**, 455–72.

Cao, A., Cianchetti, C., Calisti, L. and Tangheroni, W. (1976) A family of juvenile proximal spinal muscular atrophy with dominant inheritance. *J. Med. Genet.*, **13**, 131–45.

Casali, P. and Notkins, A.L. (1989) CD5+ B lymphocytes, polyreactive antibodies and the human B cell repertoire. *Immunol. Today*, **9**, 364–8.

Chance, P.F., Bird, T.D., O'Connell, P. *et al.* (1990) Genetic linkage and heterogeneity in type I Charcot–Marie–Tooth disease (hereditary motor and sensory neuropathy type I). *Am. J. Hum. Genet.*, **47**, 915–25.

Chancellor, A.M., Willison, H.J., Paterson, G. *et al.* (1992) The frequency of anti-GM1 antibodies and paraproteins in MND: a population based control study. *J. Neurol.*, **239** (Suppl. 2), S100.

Chapman, J., Sela, B.A., Wertman, E. *et al.* (1988) Antibodies to ganglioside GM1 in patients with Alzheimer's disease. *Neurosci. Lett.*, **86**, 235–40.

Charcot, J.M. and Marie, P. (1886) Sur une forme particulière d'atrophie musculaire progressive, souvent familial débutant, par les pieds et les jambes et atteignant plus tard les mains. *Rev. Méd.*, **6**, 97–138.

Cornblath, D.R., Sumner, A.J., Daube, J. *et al.* (1991) Issues and opinions: conduction block in clinical practice. *Muscle Nerve*, **14**, 869–71.

Cusimano, M.D., Bilboa, J.M. and Cohen, S.M. (1988) Hypertrophic brachial plexus neuritis: a pathological study of two cases. *Ann. Neurol.*, **24**, 615–22.

Dale, A.J.D., Engel, A.G. and Rudd, N.L. (1982) Familial hexosaminidase deficiency with Kugelberg–Welander phenotype and mental change. *Ann. Neurol.*, **14**, 109.

Daune, G.C., Farrer, R.G., Dalakas, M.C. and Quarles, R.H. (1992) Sensory neuropathy associated with monoclonal immunoglobulin M to GD1b ganglioside. *Ann. Neurol.*, **31**, 683–5.

Davidenkow, S. (1939) Scapuloperoneal amyotrophy. *Arch. Neurol. Psychiatr.*, **41**, 694–8.

Davis, C.J.F., Bradley, W.G. and Madrid, R. (1978) The peroneal muscular atrophy syndrome (clinical, genetic, electrophysiological and nerve biopsy studies). *J. Génet. Hum.*, **26**, 311–49.

Dellagi, K., Dupouey, P., Brouet, J.-C. *et al.* (1983) Waldenström's macroglobulinaemia and peripheral neuropathy: a clinical and immunological study of 25 patients. *Blood*, **62**, 280–5.

Motor neuropathies

Denny-Brown, D. (1948) Primary sensory neuropathy with muscular changes associated with carcinoma. *J. Neurol. Neurosurg. Psychiatr.*, **11**, 73–8.

de Weerdt, C.J. (1978) Charcot–Marie–Tooth disease with sex-linked inheritance: linkage studies and abnormal serum alkaline phosphatase levels. *Eur. Neurol.*, **17**, 336–43.

Dhib-Jalbut, S. and Liwnicz, B.H. (1986) Immunocytochemical binding of serum IgG from a patient with oat cell tumour and motoneuron disease to normal human cerebral cortex and molecular layer of the cerebellum. *Acta Neuropathol. (Berl.)*, **69**, 96–102.

Duarte, F., Binet, S., Lacomblez, L. *et al.* (1991) Quantitative analysis of monoclonal immunoglobulins in serum of patients with amyotrophic lateral sclerosis. *J. Neurol. Sci.*, **104**, 88–91.

Dyck, P.J. and Lambert, E.H. (1968a) Lower motor and primary sensory neuron diseases with peroneal muscular atrophy. I. Neurologic, genetic and electrophysiologic findings in hereditary polyneuropathies. *Arch. Neurol. (Chic.)*, **18**, 603–18.

Dyck, P.J. and Lambert, E.H. (1968b) Lower motor and primary sensory neuron diseases with peroneal muscular atrophy. II. Neurologic, genetic and electrophysiologic findings in various neuronal degenerations. *Arch. Neurol.*, **18**, 619–25.

Dyck, P.J., Low, P.A., Bartelson, J.D. *et al.* (1982) Prednisone responsive hereditary motor and sensory neuropathy. *Mayo Clin. Proc.*, **57**, 239–45.

Endo, T., Scott, D.D., Stewart, S.S. *et al.* (1984) Antibodies to glycosphingolipids in patients with multiple sclerosis and SLE. *J. Immunol.*, **132**, 1793–7.

Engelhardt, J.I. and Appel, S.H. (1990) Motoneuron reactivity of sera from animals with autoimmune models of motoneuron destruction. *J. Neurol. Sci.*, **96**, 333–52.

Fabian, R.H. (1990) Uptake of anti-neuronal IgM by CNS neurons: comparison with anti-neuronal IgG. *Neurology*, **40**, 419–22.

Fabian, R.H. and Ritchie, T.C. (1986) Intraneuronal IgG in the central nervous system. *J. Neurol. Sci.*, **73**, 257–67.

Feldman, E.L., Bromberg, M.B., Albers, J.W. and Pestronk, A. (1991) Immunosuppressive treatment in multifocal motor neuropathy. *Ann. Neurol.*, **30**, 397–401.

Fenichel, G.M., Emery, E.S. and Hunt, P. (1967) Neurogenic atrophy simulating facioscapulohumeral dystrophy. *Arch. Neurol.*, **17**, 257–63.

Fischbeck, K.H., Ar-Rushdi, N., Pericak-Vance, M. *et al.* (1986) X-linked neuropathy: gene localization with DNA probes. *Ann. Neurol.*, **20**, 527–32.

Freddo, L., Yu, R.K., Latov, N. *et al.* (1986) Gangliosides GM1 and GD1b are antigens for M-proteins in a patient with motor neuron disease. *Neurology*, **36**, 454–8.

Furukawa, T. and Toyokura, Y.(1976) Chronic spinal muscular atrophy of facio-scapulohumeral type. *J. Med. Genet.*, **13**, 285–71.

Gabreëls-Festen, A.A.W.M., Joosten, E.M.G., Gabreëls, F.J.M. *et al.* (1990) Congenital demyelinating motor and sensory neuropathy with focally folded myelin sheaths. *Brain*, **113**, 1629–44.

References

Gabreëls-Festen, A.A.W.M., Joosten, E.M.G., Gabreëls, F.J.M. *et al.* (1991) Hereditary motor and sensory neuropathy of neuronal type with onset in early childhood. *Brain*, **114**, 1855–70.

Ganser, A.L., Kirschner, D. and Willinger, L.W. (1983) Ganglioside localisation on myelinated nerve by cholera toxin binding. *J. Neurocytol.*, **12**, 921–38.

Gosselin, S., Kyle, R.A. and Dyck, P.J. (1991) Neuropathy associated with monoclonal gammopathies of undetermined significance. *Ann. Neurol.*, **30**, 54–61.

Gourie-Devi, M., Suresh, T.G. and Shankar, S.K. (1984) Monomelic amyotrophy. *Arch. Neurol.*, **41**, 388–97.

Gregson, N.A., Jones, D. and Willison, H.J. (1991) Antibodies to GM1 ganglioside in motor neuron diseases, in *Recent Advances in MND/ALS Research* (ed. F. Clifford Rose), Butterworths, London.

Gregson, N.A., Jones, D., Thomas, P.K. and Willison, H.J. (1991) Acute motor neuropathy with antibodies to GM1 ganglioside. *Neurology*, **238**, 447–51.

Guiloff, R.J., Thomas, P.K., Contreras, M. *et al.* (1982) Evidence for linkage of type I hereditary motor neuropathy to the Duffy locus on chromosome 1. *Ann. Hum. Genet.*, **46**, 25–7.

Guzzetta, F., Ferrière, G. and Lyon, G. (1982) Congenital hypomyelinating polyneuropathy: pathological findings compared with polyneuropathies starting later in life. *Brain*, **105**, 395–416.

Hahn, A.F., Brown, W.F., Koopman, W.J. *et al.* (1990) X-linked dominant hereditary motor and sensory neuropathy. *Brain*, **113**, 1511–25.

Hanson, H.-A., Holmgren, J. and Svennerholm, L. (1977) Ultrastructural localization of cell membrane GM1 ganglioside by cholera toxin. *Proc. Natl. Acad. Sci. USA*, **704**, 3782–6.

Harding, A.E. (1993) Inherited neuronal atrophy and degeneration predominantly of lower motor neurons, in *Peripheral Neuropathy*, 3rd edn (eds P.J. Dyck, P.K. Thomas *et al.*), W.B. Saunders, Philadelphia, pp. 1051–64.

Harding, A.E. and Thomas, P.K. (1980a) Hereditary distal spinal muscular atrophy: a report on 34 cases and a review of the literature. *J. Neurol. Sci.*, **45**, 337–48.

Harding, A.E. and Thomas, P.K. (1980b) The clinical features of hereditary motor and sensory neuropathy types I and II. *Brain*, **103**, 259–80.

Harding, A.E. and Thomas, P.K. (1980c) Autosomal recessive forms of hereditary motor and sensory neuropathy types I and II. *J. Neurol. Neurosurg. Psychiatr.*, **43**, 669–78.

Harding, A.E., Bradbury, P.G. and Murray, N.M. (1983) Chronic asymmetrical spinal muscular atrophy. *J. Neurol. Sci.*, **59**, 69–83.

Harding, A.E., Thomas, P.K., Baraitser, M. *et al.* (1982) X-linked bulbospinal neuronopathy: a report of ten cases. *J. Neurol. Neurosurg. Psychiatr.*, **45**, 1012–9.

Hays, A.P., Roxas, A., Sadiq, S.A. *et al.* (1990) A monoclonal IgA in a patient with amyotrophic lateral sclerosis reacts with neurofilaments and surface antigen on neuroblastoma cells. *J. Neuropathol. Exp. Neurol.*, **49**, 383–98.

Motor neuropathies

Hoffmann, J. (1893) Über chronische Spinalmuskelatrophie in Kindesalter, auf familiäre Basis. *Deutsch. Z. Nervenheilk.*, **3**, 427.

Hoogendijk, J.E., Hensels, G.W., Gabreëls-Festen, AAWM. *et al.* (1992) De-novo mutation in hereditary motor and sensory neuropathy type 1. *Lancet*, **339**, 1081–2.

Ilyas, A.A., Willison, H.J., Dalakas, M.C. *et al.* (1988) Identification and characterization of gangliosides reacting with IgM paraproteins in three patients with neuropathy associated with biclonal gammopathy. *J. Neurochem.*, **51**, 851–8.

Ilyas, A.A., Mithen, F.A., Dalakas, M.C. *et al.* (1992) Antibodies to acidic glycolipids in Guillain–Barré syndrome and chronic inflammatory demyelinating polyneuropathy. *J. Neurol. Sci.*, **107**, 111–21.

Inglis, G., Fraser, R.H., Mitchell, A.A.B. *et al.* (1987) Serological characterisation of a mouse monoclonal anti-P-like antibody. *Vox Sang.*, **52**, 79–82.

Inuzuka, T., Sato, S., Yanagisawa, K. and Miyatake, M. (1989) Antibodies to human spinal cord proteins in sera from patients with motor neuron disease and other neurological diseases. *Eur. Neurol.*, **29**, 328–32.

Jellinger, K., Anzil, A.P., Seeman, D. and Bernheimer, H. (1982) Adult GM$_2$ gangliosidosis masquerading as slowly progressive muscular atrophy. Motor neuron disease phenotype. *Clin. Neuropathol.*, **1**, 31–44.

Johnson, W., Wigger, H.J. and Karp, H.R. (1982) Juvenile spinal muscular atrophy. A new hexosaminidase deficiency phenotype. *Ann. Neurol.*, **11**, 11–16.

Kaeser, H.E. (1965) Scapuloperoneal muscular atrophy. *Brain*, **88**, 407–18.

Karch, S.B. and Urich, H. (1975) Infantile polyneuropathy with defective myelination: an autopsy study. *Devel. Med. Child Neurol.*, **17**, 504–11.

Karni, A., Navon, R. and Sadeh, M. (1988) Hexosaminidase A deficiency manifesting as spinal muscular atrophy. *Ann. Neurol.*, **24**, 451–3.

Kennedy, W.R., Alter, M. and Sung, J.H. (1968) Progressive proximal spinal and bulbar muscular atrophy of late onset. A sex-linked recessive trait. *Neurology*, **18**, 671–83.

Kennedy, W.R., Sung, J.H. and Berry, J.F. (1977) A case of congenital hypomyelination neuropathy: clinical, morphological, and chemical studies. *Arch. Neurol.*, **34**, 337–45.

Kreiger, C. and Melmed, C. (1982) Amyotrophic lateral sclerosis and paraproteinemia. *Neurology*, **32**, 896–8.

Lamb, N.L. and Patten, B.M. (1991) Clinical correlations of anti-GM1 antibodies in amyotrophic lateral sclerosis and neuropathies. *Muscle Nerve*, **14**, 1021–7.

Lander, C.M., Eadie, M.J and Tyrer, J.H. (1976) Hereditary motor peripheral neuropathy predominantly affecting the arms. *J. Neurol. Sci.*, **28**, 389–94.

Lange, D.J., Trojaborg, W., Latov, N. *et al.* (1992) Multifocal motor neuropathy with conduction block: Is it a distinct clinical entity? *Neurology*, **42**, 497–505.

La Spada, A.R., Wilson, E.M., Lubahn, D.B. *et al.* (1991) Androgen receptor gene mutations in X-linked spinal and bulbar muscular atrophy. *Nature*, **352**, 77–8.

Latov, N. (1990) Antibodies to glycoconjugates in neurological disease. *Clin. Asp. Autoimmun.*, **4**, 18–29.

Latov, N., Hays, A.P., Donofrio, P.D. *et al.* (1988) Monoclonal IgM with unique reactivity to gangliosides GM1 and GD1b and to lacto-N-tetraose in two patients with motor neuron disease. *Neurology*, **38**, 763–8.

Lebo, R.V., Chance, P.F., Dyck, P.J. *et al.* (1992) Chromosome 1 Charcot–Marie–Tooth syndrome (HMSN1B) locus in Fcygamma RII gene region. *Hum. Genet.*, **88**, 1–12.

Ledeen, R.W. (1989) Biosynthesis, metabolism and biological effects of gangliosides, in *Neurobiology of Glycoconjugates* (eds R.U. Margolis and R.K. Margolis), Plenum Press, New York, pp. 43–83.

Lewis, R.A., Sumner, A.J., Brown, M.J. and Asbury, A.K. (1982) Multifocal demyelinating neuropathy with persistent conduction block. *Neurology*, **32**, 958–64.

Lupski, J.R. Montes de Oca-Luna, R., Slaugenhaupt, S. *et al.* (1991) DNA duplication associated with Charcot–Marie–Tooth disease type Ia. *Cell*, **66**, 219–32.

Lyon, G. (1969) Ultrastructural study of a nerve biopsy from a case of early infantile chronic neuropathy. *Acta Neuropathol. (Berl.)*, **13**, 131–42.

McCombe, P.A., Pollard, J.D. and McLeod, J.G. (1985) Chronic inflammatory demyelinating polyradiculoneuropathy. *Brain*, **110**, 1617–30.

McGinnis, S., Kohriyama, T., Yu, R.K. *et al.* (1988) Antibodies to sulfated glucuronic-acid containing glycosphingolipids in neuropathy associated with anti-MAG antibodies and in normal subjects. *J. Neuroimmunol.*, **17**, 119–26.

McLeod, J.G. and Prineas, J.W. (1971) Distal type of chronic spinal muscular atrophy: clinical, electrophysiological and pathological studies. *Brain*, **94**, 703–19.

Marcus, D.M., Perry, L., Gilbert, S. *et al.* (1989a) Human IgM monoclonal proteins that bind 3-fucosyllactosamine, asialo-GM1 and GM1. *J. Immunol.*, **143**, 2929–32.

Marcus, D.M., Latov, N., Hsi, B.P. *et al.* (1989b) Measurement and significance of antibodies against GM1 ganglioside. *J. Neuroimmunol.*, **25**, 255–9.

Matsunaga, M., Inokuchi, T., Ohnishi, A. and Kuroiwa, Y. (1973) Oculopharyngeal involvement in familial neurogenic muscular atrophy. *J. Neurol. Neurosurg. Psychiatry*, **36**, 104–11.

Meadows, J.C., Marsden, C.D. and Harriman, D.G.F. (1969) Chronic spinal muscular atrophy in adults. 2. Other forms. *J. Neurol. Sci.*, **9**, 551–66.

Mitsumoto, H., Sliman, R.J., Schafer, I.A. *et al.* (1985) Motor neuron disease and adult hexosaminidase A deficiency in two families: evidence for multisystem degeneration. *Ann. Neurol.*, **17**, 378–85.

Mitsumoto, H., Levin, K.H., Wilbourn, A.J. and Chou, S.M. (1990) Hypertrophic mononeuritis clinically presenting with painful legs and moving toes. *Muscle Nerve*, **13**, 215–21.

Nardelli, E., Steck, A.J., Barkas, T. *et al.* (1988) Motor neuron disease and monoclonal IgM with antibody activity against GM1 and GD1b ganglio-sides. *Ann. Neurol.*, **23**, 524–8.

Nelson, J.W. and Amick, L.D. (1966) Heterofamilial progressive spinal muscular atrophy: a clinical and electromyographic study of a kinship. *Neurology (Minneap.)*, **16**, 306–17.

Nobile-Orazio, E., Carpo, M., Legname, G. *et al.* (1990) Anti-GM1 antibodies in motor neuron disease and neuropathy. *Neurology*, **40**, 1747–50.

Nobile-Orazio, E., Carpo, M., Meucci, N. *et al.* (1992) Guillain–Barré syndrome associated with high titres of anti-GM1 antibodies. *J. Neurol. Sci.*, **109**, 200–6.

Norris, F.H. and Engel, W.K. (1965) Carcinomatous amyotrophic lateral sclerosis, in *The Remote Effects of Cancer on the Nervous System* (eds W.R. Brain and F.H. Norris), Grune & Stratton, New York, pp. 24–34.

Norris, F.H., Denys, E.H., Sang, K. and Mukai, E. (1989) Population study of amyotrophic lateral sclerosis. *Ann. Neurol.*, **26**, 139–40.

Nukada, H., Dyck, P.J. and Karnes, J.L. (1983) Thin axons relative to myelin spiral length in hereditary motor and sensory neuropathy type I. *Ann. Neurol.*, **4**, 648–55.

Ohnishi, A., Murai, Y, Ikeda, M. *et al.* (1989) Autosomal recessive motor and sensory neuropathy with excessive myelin outfolding. *Muscle Nerve*, **12**, 568–75.

Oomes, P.G., van der Meché, F.G.A., Toyka, K.V. and Kleyweg, R.P. (1990) Antibodies to ganglioside GM1 in Guillain–Barré syndrome. Peripheral Neuropathy Association of America Abstracts, Oxford, UK.

O'Sullivan, D.J. and McLeod, J.G. (1978) Distal chronic spinal muscular atrophy involving the hands. *J. Neurol. Neurosurg. Psychiatr.*, **41**, 653–8.

Ouvrier, R.A., McLeod, J.G. and Conchin, T.E. (1987) The hypertrophic forms of hereditary motor and sensory neuropathy. A study of hypertrophic Charcot–Marie–Tooth disease (HMSN type I) and Dejerine–Sottas disease (HMSN type III) in childhood. *Brain*, **110**, 121–48.

Ouvrier, R.A., McLeod, J.G., Morgan, G.J. *et al.* (1981) Hereditary motor and sensory neuropathy of neuronal type with onset in early childhood. *J. Neurol. Sci.*, **51**, 181–97.

Parnes, S., Karpati, G., Carpentier, S. *et al.* (1985) Hexosaminidase A deficiency presenting as atypical juvenile-onset spinal muscular atrophy. *Arch. Neurol.*, **42**, 1176–80.

Parry, G. and Clarke, S. (1985) Pure motor neuropathy with multifocal conduction block masquerading as motor neuron disease. *Muscle Nerve*, **8**, 617–26.

Parry, G.J., Holtz, S.J., Ben-Zeev, D. and Drori, J.B. (1986) Gammopathy with proximal motor neuropathy simulating motor neuron disease. *Neurology*, **36**, 273–76.

Patten, B.M. (1984) Neuropathy and motor neuron syndromes associated with plasma cell disease. *Acta Neurol. Scand.*, **69**, 47–61.

Pearn, J.H. (1978) Autosomal dominant spinal muscular atrophy. A clinical and genetic study. *J. Neurol. Sci.*, **38**, 263–75.

References

Pearn, J.H. and Hudgson, P. (1979) Distal spinal muscular atrophy – a clinical and genetic study of 8 kindreds. *J. Neurol. Sci.*, **43**, 183–92.

Pearn, J.H., Hudgson, P. and Walton, J.N. (1978) A clinical and genetic study of adult-onset spinal muscular atrophy. The autosomal recessive form as a discrete disease entity. *Brain*, **101**, 591–606.

Pestronk, A. (1991) Invited review: motor neuropathies, motor neuron disorders and anti-glycolipid antibodies. *Muscle Nerve*, **14**, 927–36.

Pestronk, A., Cornblath, D.R., Ilyas, A.A. *et al.* (1988a) A treatable multifocal neuropathy with antibodies to GM1 ganglioside. *Ann. Neurol.*, **24**, 73–8.

Pestronk, A., Adams, R.N., Clawson, L. *et al.* (1988b) Serum antibodies to GM1 ganglioside in amyotrophic lateral sclerosis. *Neurology*, **38**, 1457–61.

Pestronk, A., Adams, R.N., Cornblath, D.R. *et al.* (1989) Patterns of serum antibodies to GM1 and GD1a gangliosides in ALS. *Ann. Neurol.*, **25**, 98–102.

Pestronk, A., Chaudhry, V., Feldman, E.L. *et al.* (1990) Lower motor neuron syndromes defined by patterns of weakness, nerve conduction abnormalities and high titres of antiglycolipid antibodies. *Ann. Neurol.*, **27**, 316–26.

Quarles, R.H., Ilyas, A.A. and Willison, H.J. (1986) Antibodies to glycolipids in demyelinating diseases of the human peripheral nervous system. *Chem. Phys. Lipids*, **42**, 235–48.

Raeymaekers, P., Timmerman, V., Nelis, E. *et al.* (1991) Duplication in chromosome 17p11.2 in Charcot–Marie–Tooth neuropathy type IA (CMT 1A). *Neuromusc. Disord.*, **1**, 93–8.

Raff, M., Sangalang, V. and Asbury, A.K. (1968) Ischemic mononeuropathy multiplex associated with diabetes mellitus. *Arch. Neurol. (Chic.)*, **18**, 487–98.

Rosenfeld, M.R. and Posner, J.B. (1991) Paraneoplastic motor neuron disease, in *Advances in Neurology*, Vol. 56 *Amyotrophic Lateral Sclerosis and Other Motor Neuron Diseases* (ed. L.P. Rowland), Raven Press, New York.

Rowland, L.P., Defendini, R. and Sherman, W. *et al.* (1982) Macroglobulinemia with peripheral neuropathy simulating motor neuron disease. *Ann. Neurol.*, **11**, 532–6.

Rozear, M.P., Pericak-Vance, M.A., Fischbeck, K. *et al.* (1987) Hereditary motor and sensory neuropathy, X-linked: a half century follow up. *Neurology*, **37**, 1460–5.

Rudnicki, S., Chad, D.A., Drachman, D.A. *et al.* (1987) Motor neuron disease and paraproteinemia. *Neurology*, **37**, 335–7.

Sadiq, S.A., Thomas, F.P., Kilidirias, K. *et al.* (1990) The spectrum of neurological disease associated with anti-GM1 antibodies. *Neurology*, **40**, 1067–92.

Salazas-Grueso, E.F., Routbort, M.J., Martin, J. *et al.* (1990) Polyclonal IgM anti-GM1 ganglioside antibody in patients with motor neuron disease and variants. *Ann. Neurol.*, **27**, 558–63.

Santoro, M., Thomas, F.P., Fink, M.E. *et al.* (1990) IgM deposits at nodes of Ranvier in a patient with motor neuropathy, anti-GM1 antibodies and multifocal motor conduction block. *Ann. Neurol.*, **28**, 373–9.

Schold, S.C., Cho, E-S., Somasundaram, M. *et al.* (1978) Subacute motor neuronopathy: a remote effect of lymphoma. *Ann. Neurol.*, **5**, 271–87.

Motor neuropathies

Serratrice, G., Gastaut, J.L., Pellissier, J.F. and Pouget, J. (1976) Amyotrophies scapulo-péronières chroniques de type Stark-Kaeser (à propos de 10 observations). *Rev. Neurol.*, **132**, 823–41.

Shy, M.E., Rowland, L.P., Smith, T. *et al.* (1986) Motor neuron disease and plasma cell dyscrasia. *Neurology*, **36**, 1429–36.

Shy, M.E., Evans, V.A., Dublin, F.D. *et al.* (1989) Antibodies to GM1 and GD1b in patients with motor neuron disease without plasma cell dyscrasia. *Ann. Neurol.*, **25**, 511–13.

Singh, N., Sachdev, K. and Susheela, A.K. (1980) Juvenile muscular atrophy localized to the arms. *Arch. Neurol.*, **37**, 297–305.

Silver, J.R. (1966) Familial spastic paraplegia with amyotrophy of the hands. *J. Neurol. Neurosurg. Psychiatry*, **29**, 135–44.

Sobue, I., Saito, N., Iida, M. and Ando, K. (1978) Juvenile type of distal and segmental muscular atrophy of extremities. *Ann. Neurol.*, **3**, 429–32.

Sobue, G., Hashizume, Y., Mukai, E. *et al.* (1989) X-linked recessive bulbospinal neuronopathy. A clinicopathological study. *Brain*, **122**, 209–32.

Subramony, S.H. and Wilbourn, A.J. (1982) Diabetic proximal neuropathy. Clinical and electromyographic studies. *J. Neurol. Sci.*, **53**, 293–301.

Szabo, A., Dalmau, J., Manly, G. *et al.* (1991) HuD, a paraneoplastic encephalomyelitis antigen, contains RNA-binding domains and is homologous to Elav and Sex-lethal. *Cell*, **67**, 325–33.

Tazir, M., Attal, E. and Ait-Kaci-Ahmed, M. (1992) Hereditary motor and sensory neuropathy: a clinical and genetic study. *J. Neurol.*, **239** (Suppl 2), S93.

Thomas, F.P., Lee, A.M., Romas, S.N. and Latov, N. (1989) Monoclonal IgMs with anti-Gal(α1–3) GalNAc activity in lower motor neuron disease; identification of glycoprotein antigens in neural tissue and cross-reactivity with serum immunoglobulins. *J. Neuroimmunol.*, **23**, 164–74.

Thomas, F.P., Thomas, J.E., Sadiq, S.A. *et al.* (1990) Human monoclonal IgM anti-Gal(α1–3) GalNAc autoantibodies bind to the surface of bovine spinal motorneurons. *J. Neurol. Exp. Neuropathol.*, **49**, 89–95.

Thomas, P.K. (1991) Separating motor neuron diseases from pure motor neuropathies: clinical clues and definitions, in *Amyotrophic Lateral Sclerosis and Other Motor Neuron Diseases, Advances in Neurology*, Vol. 56 (ed. L.P. Rowland), Raven Press, New York, pp. 381–4.

Thomas, P.K. and Harding, A.E. (1993) Inherited neuropathies: the interface between molecular genetics and pathology. *Brain Pathol.*, **3**, 129–33.

Thomas, P.K., Calne, D.B. and Stewart, G. (1974) Hereditary motor and sensory polyneuropathy (peroneal muscular atrophy). *Ann. Hum. Genet.*, **88**, 111–53.

Thomas, P.K., Young, E. and King, R.H.M. (1989) Sandhoff disease mimicking adult-onset bulbospinal neuronopathy. *J. Neurol. Neurosurg. Psychiatry*, **52**, 1103–6.

Thomas, P.K., Hollinrake, K., Lascelles, R.G. *et al.* (1971) The polyneuropathy of chronic renal failure. *Brain*, **94**, 761–80.

Timmerman, V., Raeymaekers, R., De Jonghe, P. *et al.* (1990) Assignment of the

Charcot–Marie–Tooth neuropathy type I (CMT 1a) gene to 17p11.2–p12. *Am. J. Hum. Genet.*, **47**, 680–5.

Tooth, H.H. (1886) *The Peroneal Type of Progressive Muscular Atrophy*. Lewis, London.

Vance, J.M., Nicholson, G.A., Yamaoka, L.H. *et al.* (1989) Linkage of Charcot–Marie–Tooth neuropathy type Ia to chromosome 17. *Exp. Neurol.*, **104**, 186–9.

Van den Bergh, P., Logigan, E.L. and Kelly, J. (1989) Motor neuropathy with multifocal conduction blocks. *Muscle Nerve*, **11**, 26–38.

Wong, M.C.W., Salanga, V.D., Chou, S. *et al.* (1987) Immune-associated paraneoplastic motor neuron disease and limbic encephalopathy. *Muscle Nerve*, **10**, 661–2.

Yeung, K.B., Thomas, P.K., King, R.H.M. *et al.* (1991) The clinical spectrum of peripheral neuropathies associated with benign monoclonal IgM, IgG and IgA paraproteinaemia. *J. Neurol.*, **238**, 383–91.

Young, I.D. and Harper, P.S. (1980) Hereditary distal spinal muscular atrophy with vocal cord paresis. *J. Neurol. Neurosurg. Psychiatry*, **43**, 413–21.

Younger, D.S., Rowland, L.P., Latov, N. *et al.* (1990) Motor neuron disease and amyotrophic lateral sclerosis: relation of high CSF protein content to paraproteinemia and clinical syndromes. *Neurology*, **40**, 595–9.

Younger, D.S., Rowland, L.P., Latov, N. *et al.* (1991) Lymphoma, motor neuron diseases and amyotrophic lateral sclerosis. *Ann. Neurol.*, **29**, 78–86.

Yuki, N., Yoshino, H., Sato, S. and Miyatake, T. (1990) Acute axonal polyneuropathy associated with anti-GM1 antibodies following Campylobacter enteritis. *Neurology*, **40**, 1900–2.

4 Post-polio motor neuron disease

MARINOS C. DALAKAS

4.1 INTRODUCTION

The clinical symptoms, histological signs and electrophysiological findings of post-polio syndrome are directly related to new motor neuron deterioration of previously affected motor neurons and the effectiveness of the remaining motor neuron pool in maintaining large motor units for many years. The neuronal dysfunction in the post-polio state can serve as a paradigm for understanding the involvement of motor neurons in patients with other motor neuron diseases such as amyotrophic lateral sclerosis (ALS), if one considers that ALS is the end-result of motor neuron dysfunction caused by putative viral, toxic, immunological or abiotrophic factors that began slowly and evolved gradually.

Like the other enteroviruses affecting motor neurons (Wadia *et al.*, 1981; Melnick, 1984; Johnson, 1982), the poliomyelitis virus causes, most of the time, a non-paralytic disease that presents as a non-specific acute viral illness. Because paralysis or weakness occurs only when more than 50–60% of the motor neurons in a spinal cord segment are destroyed, damage of fewer motor neurons will not cause clinical signs of muscle weakness. The general implication is that, if infections with such neurotrophic viruses occur repeatedly, the motor neuron pool is gradually depleted until a critical threshold is reached for muscle weakness to develop. Furthermore, motor neurons scarred by such enteroviral or other toxic insults can later in life succumb to the ageing process sooner than the non-affected or intact motor neurons because of an abiotrophic interaction between ageing and previous subclinical neuronal injury (Calne *et al.*, 1986).

4.2 RELEVANT OBSERVATIONS OF MOTOR NEURON LOSS DURING ACUTE PARALYTIC POLIOMYELITIS

To place the pathogenetic mechanisms of the post-polio syndrome and generally the post-polio state in perspective, it is helpful to consider

Post-polio motor neuron disease

some original observations, made by Bodian (1949a, 1949b, 1982, 1984) regarding motor neuron injury during acute poliomyelitis infection. As reviewed by Dalakas (Dalakas and Hallett, 1988; Dalakas, 1990a; Dalakas and Illa, 1991), the following observations are of relevance:

1. during the second or third day of the infection, there is a striking scarcity of normal-appearing neurons even in cases of very mild paralysis;
2. the average proportion of injured neurons that are destroyed, the **'case fatality rate'**, is almost 50%, with a 30% probability that an invaded motor neuron will be destroyed by the poliomyelitis virus;
3. up to 50% of neurons corresponding to paralyzed limbs recover histologically;
4. infected neurons exhibiting only mild degree of diffuse chromatolysis generally survive and can support motor units; in contrast, the loss of function in muscle groups appears to correlate only with severe cytoplasmic and nuclear changes within the neurons;
5. up to 20% of neurons corresponding to normal limbs or to limbs with minimal weakness die; and
6. during the acute stage of the disease the distribution of the destroyed neurons is scattered, sparing at times muscle groups innervated by two to three contiguous levels of the spinal cord, which explains the absence of paralysis of certain muscles in the same limb.

Based on the above observations, it is evident that the poliomyelitis virus is widely disseminated throughout the motor neuron pool, causing variable degrees of neuronal destruction. A patient who has survived an acute paralytic attack is, therefore, left with the following different populations of surviving neurons:

1. **Normal, unaffected neurons, away from the areas of lost neurons.**
2. **Normal, unaffected neurons, next to areas of destroyed neurons.** Such cells, although morphologically normal, are stressed to compensate for their neighboring neurons lost in up to three contiguous spinal cord segments, and maintain larger than normal motor units.
3. **Neurons originally affected but seemingly fully recovered.** The lifespan of such cells may be below normal and, if chronically stressed, their metabolic reserves may be limited.
4. **Neurons moderately affected, which escaped death but have survived as small in size, but normal in appearance**. Such cells may have limited reserves and, in spite of their normal appearance, their capacity to establish and maintain more than the normal number of effective synapses is impaired.
5. **Neurons severely affected but incompletely recovered ('scarred'**

84

neurons). Such cells should have abnormal function and shorter life expectancy.

The post-polio spinal cord, therefore, contains fewer than the normal number of normal neurons and an increased number of abnormal neurons, which may not be able to perform to full capacity and maintain large motor units. Consequently, when a muscle is left with more denervated muscle fibers than could be possibly rescued and reinnervated by the existing neurons, new muscle weakness ensues, as discussed below.

4.3 CLINICAL SIGNS AND SYMPTOMS

4.3.1 Definition

The term post-polio syndrome was initially coined by the patients themselves to describe a variety of unexplained and rather stereotyped new physical and psychosocial difficulties that these patients experienced later in life (Dalakas, 1984, 1987a, 1988a, 1990a,b; Dalakas and Hallett, 1988; Dalakas and Illa, 1991; Dalakas et al., 1984a,b, 1986a; Halstead and Wiechers, 1985; Halstead and Wiechers, 1987). At times, this term has been all inclusive because of the tendency of some investigators to include not only the new neurological symptoms but other medical, orthopedic or psychiatric problems that are indirectly related to the long-term post-polio disability. The post-polio syndrome should be defined as 'the constellation of new muscle weakness, fatigue and myalgia of the skeletal or bulbar muscles, unrelated to any other known disease, that begins 25–30 years after an acute attack of paralytic poliomyelitis'. The diagnosis of post-polio syndrome is considered in a patient who has:

1. history of documented acute paralytic poliomyelitis in childhood or adolescence;
2. partial recovery of motor function and functional stability or recovery for at least 15 years;
3. residual asymmetric muscle atrophy with weakness, areflexia, and normal sensation in at least one limb; and
4. normal sphincteric function.

4.3.2 Clinical symptomatology

Post-polio syndrome is a clinical diagnosis and essentially one requiring the need to exclude any other known medical, neurologic, orthopedic or psychiatric illness that could explain the development of such symp-

Post-polio motor neuron disease

toms. Some of these commonly encountered unrelated problems include radiculopathies, degenerative arthritis and compression neuropathies such as carpal tunnel syndrome, ulnar neuropathies at the wrist or elbow and plexopathies due to compression of the above-mentioned nerves as the result of a long-term use of wheelchairs, crutches, braces or poor posture. In addition, a variety of psychosocial concerns, anxieties, depression or non-specific diffuse pains are not uncommon among post-polio patients (Kohl, 1987). Such symptoms, if mild and proportional to those expected in patients with long-term disability, are not of diagnostic concern. However, if they dominate the clinical picture and overshadow the new somatic symptomatology, secondary or psychogenic causes should be excluded.

The post-polio syndrome includes the combination of:

1. a variety of **musculoskeletal symptoms**; and
2. **the post-poliomyelitis progressive muscular atrophy (PPMA)** (Dalakas, 1986, 1987a,b, 1988a, 1990a,b; Dalakas *et al.*, 1984a,b, 1986a; Dalakas and Illa, 1991).

Musculoskeletal symptoms include diminished endurance, fatigue, joint pain in biomechanically deformed or marginally stable joints, worsening mobility owing to long-standing scoliosis or poor posture, and increasing difficulties due to unnatural or unusual mechanics imposed by tendon transfers or uneven size of limbs and recent increase in body weight that further reduces endurance and increases fatigue. Some of these patients describe their symptoms rather vaguely and often with a frustrating degree of variability. Although they feel 'weak', it is often difficult to determine if they have new muscle weakness because the overwhelming fatigue, diminished endurance, various emotional difficulties, and frequent presence of a fibromyalgic-like syndrome may complicate the clinical picture. Such symptoms have been noticed since 1972 (Anderson, Levine and Gellert, 1972).

Post-poliomyelitis progressive muscular atrophy (PPMA) is a term coined to describe the new slowly progressive muscle weakness with or without muscle pain and atrophy that affects certain muscle groups of post-polio patients. In contrast to the previous group, patients with PPMA have objective signs and symptoms that reflect new low motor neuron deterioration, as noted many years ago by several authors (Campbell, Williams and Pearce, 1969; Hayard and Seaton, 1979; Mulder, Rosenbaum and Layton, 1972). These new symptoms include:

1. **New muscular weakness and atrophy.** This involves either previously affected muscles that have fully or partially recovered or, less

often, muscles clinically unaffected by the original disease. The new weakness is asymmetrical, affecting one or two extremities or certain muscles of one or two limbs, and can be associated with new focal atrophy. The asymmetry and random distribution of new weakness even among muscle groups of the same limb is so striking that post-polio patients need to be examined and followed on a 'muscle-by-muscle basis'. Patients with new weakness have increasing difficulties in daily activities such as walking, standing, climbing stairs, ambulating for the same distances as before, transferring from bed to chair, driving, dressing, combing their hair or shaving (Halstead and Wiechers, 1985; Dalakas, 1988b). Because of the very asymmetric nature of their motor weakness even among muscles of the same limb, disabled post-polio patients have demonstrated an extraordinary ability to maintain for years a high level of performance with an unconventional and improvised use of the remaining healthy muscles in any given limb. For this reason, a new weakness, affecting even a single muscle, if critical for a specific movement, often leads to a disturbance of motor balance with a disproportionate loss of functional skill.

2. **Fatigue**. This is a universal phenomenon in post-polio patients. Although fatigue is difficult to define and often times it means 'different things to different patients', the majority of patients define it as lack of energy and stamina that improves after a brief period of ½–2 h of rest, usually at midday. They feel 'pooped out' after they try to maintain or perform a task they used to do not only with their previously weak extremities but even with their healthier muscles. In contrast to the fatigue of patients with **chronic fatigue syndrome**, the post-polio fatigue is prominent in the early hours of the afternoon, and improves after brief periods of rest. Although frustrating and distressing, post-polio fatigue does not usually keep the highly motivated patients out of work and is not often due to psychogenic or depressive causes.

3. **Myalgia**. This is often mixed with arthralgias, but at times it presents as a peculiar deep ache or as an intrinsic muscle pain often like a muscle cramp similar to the one seen in patients with other neurogenic conditions (Glasberg, Dalakis and Engel, 1978). Although myalgia is a recognizable symptom, it should raise the suspicion of coexisting psychogenic causes if it is disproportionate to the rest of the clinical picture or requires narcotics. In such cases it may not be different from myofascial pain syndrome or fibromyalgia.

4. **Fasciculations**. Although infrequent, these can be seen in all the muscles, stable or weakening, if one waits and watches carefully (Cruz-Martinez, Perez Conde and Ferrer, 1983; Cruz-Martinez, Ferrer

and Perez Conde, 1984; Dalakas *et al.*, 1986a; Cashman *et al.*, 1987; Dalakas and Hallett, 1988; Dalakas, 1990a; Ravits *et al.*, 1990; Dalakas and Illa, 1991). The fasciculations in PPMA are less frequent than those seen in ALS and they are not as fine or rippling, but coarser, giving the impression that more fascicles are involved.

5. **Weakness of bulbar muscles**. New weakness in the bulbar muscles is clinically manifested predominantly in patients who have had residual bulbar muscle weakness. However, subclinical asymmetrical weakness in the pharyngeal constrictor muscles is very frequent in PPMA patients, including those who do not complain of new swallowing difficulties. Of 32 patients examined for clinical or subclinical signs of oropharyngeal dysfunction, 14 had symptoms of new swallowing difficulties and 18 were asymptomatic in this respect (Sonies and Dalakas, 1991; Dalakas, 1991a). Only 12 of them had a history of bulbar involvement during acute poliomyelitis. Swallowing function was assessed objectively by ultrasonography, video fluoroscopy and an oral motor index score for 10 components of oral function. It was found that all but one of the 32 patients, regardless of whether they had new symptoms or previous bulbar involvement, had some abnormality on detailed testing of oropharyngeal function; only two patients had any signs of aspiration. The mean oral motor index score (a quantitative measure of oral sensorimotor function) in the patients was higher than that in age-matched normal subjects ($P < 0.001$). Video fluoroscopy showed abnormalities of varying severity, including unilateral bolus transport through the pharynx, pooling in the valleculae or pyriform sinuses, delayed pharyngeal constriction and impaired tongue movements. On ultrasonography, the mean ($\pm$SD) duration of wet swallows was significantly longer in the symptomatic patients than in the asymptomatic patients (2.67 $\pm$ 0.70 *vs.* 1.65 $\pm$ 0.42 s). These findings indicate that in the bulbar neurons of post-polio patients there is a slowly progressive deterioration similar to that occurring in the muscles of the limbs (Sonies and Dalakas, 1991).

6. **New respiratory difficulties**. These are more likely to occur in patients left with some degree of residual respiratory muscle weakness from the original illness and they are very rare in patients left with adequate or normal respiratory muscle function. The reserves of the respiratory muscles in such patients are already diminished and, as new neuronal dysfunction occurs later in life, additional respiratory muscle weakness develops. At times this can be severe, requiring some mechanical support at night (Fisher, 1984, 1987; Bach *et al.*, 1987; Dalakas and Hallett, 1988; Dalakas and Illa,

1991). The new respiratory difficulties in PPMA patients are related not only to the new muscle weakness of the respiratory muscles, but also to other factors such as increasing scoliosis, pulmonary emphysema, cardiovascular insufficiency and, in wheelchair-bound patients, poor posture (Dalakas and Hallett, 1988). A central component may also coexist since acute bulbar polio often affects the medullary structures, including the reticular formation system and the sleep regulatory centers (Plum, 1959; Guilleminault and Motta, 1978; Lane, Haselman and Nichols, 1974).

7. **Sleep apnea**. This is not an uncommon phenomenon in patients left with residual bulbar dysfunction or severe respiratory compromise (Guilleminault and Motta, 1978; Fisher, 1987). It appears to be due to a combination of: (a) central apnea, probably due to a residual dysfunction of the surviving bulbar reticular neurons, (b) obstructive apnea, due to pharyngeal weakness and increasing musculoskeletal deformities from scoliosis or emphysema and (c) PPMA resulting in diminished muscle strength of the respiratory, intercostal and abdominal muscle groups.

4.4 RISK FACTORS

Well established risk factors responsible for the development of post-polio syndrome are unknown. However, based on repeated clinical observations and epidemiological surveys the following factors appear associated with an **earlier** onset of post-polio syndrome (Halstead and Wiechers, 1987; Dalakas and Hallett, 1988):

- new symptoms appearing first in the weakest limbs and in patients with the most severe residual paralysis;
- earlier bulbar or respiratory difficulties in patients with residual bulbar and respiratory weakness;
- symptoms occurring earlier in the patients who had acute poliomyelitis at an older age.

A common clinical diagnostic dilemma occurs with patients who present with some symptoms of post-polio syndrome and give a history of acute paralytic or non-paralytic illness labeled as poliomyelitis, but who do not demonstrate residual signs of an atrophic or weak limb and do not have any available records to document the cause of the original illness. The suspicion of a polio-like illness in these patients is strengthened if the electromyography and muscle biopsy show signs of diffuse denervation and reinnervation that cannot be explained by another disease process. Although such cases are of special interest for studying the function of previously scarred but fully recovered and well-compensated motor neurons, such patients are not included in my studies.

4.5 PROGRESSION AND OUTCOME

The rate of progression of patients with PPMA and the risk of developing ALS were examined in our original follow-up evaluation of patients followed for an average period of 8.2 years (range 4.5–20) (Dalakas *et al.*, 1986a). The new post-polio symptoms appear to begin after a mean period of 28.8 years (range 15–54) after the original attack of acute paralytic poliomyelitis. The pace of worsening, however, differs from patient to patient, being generally slow and variable even within the same patient. Long periods (up to 10 years) of stability are not uncommon. This is different from the pattern seen in ALS even within a 6-month observation period (Dalakas *et al.*, 1986b). Neither the age of onset of new symptoms, the patient's sex nor the degree and type of physical activities preceding the development of new weakness appears to be a significant factor in contributing to the rate of progression. The progression of the new weakness is overall very slow and difficult to appreciate on a year-to-year basis using the Medical Research Council (MRC) scale. Perhaps more sensitive quantitative measurements of muscle strength could provide an accurate assessment of progression. The impact of the new weakness on the patient's functional capabilities is also variable, but it appears to depend mostly on the residual deficit at the outset of PPMA. The more severe the residual poliomyelitis deficit, the greater the functional impact of PPMA on the patient's neuromuscular functions.

Using objective measurements of bulbar function, the rate of progression in the bulbar symptoms, after a mean follow-up period of 2 years, has also been demonstrated in four patients (Sonies and Dalakas, 1991; Dalakas, 1991a). One patient, who was initially asymptomatic, still reported no symptoms 2 years later in spite of a subtle worsening of the oral motor index score. A second patient, who was initially asymptomatic, became aware 1 year later of mild difficulties with tongue control. This was consistent with the finding of new mild-to-moderate weakness of the tongue and jaw and a worsening of the oral motor index score from 1.35 to 2.00. A third patient, who was also asymptomatic initially, became symptomatic 2 years later. Her clear perception of new difficulties in oropharyngeal function was consistent with progression of the objective measures of dysphagia. Lastly, a fourth patient, who was initially symptomatic and had signs of reduced epiglottal descent without aspiration, reported increased difficulty in swallowing, which was confirmed by worsening of the oropharyngeal signs and the development of aspiration 2 years later.

The incidence and prevalence of new weakness in post-polio patients is unknown. Some preliminary data point to a wide-range rate that varies from 25 to 80% (Codd et al., 1984; Windebank et al., 1987). The only parameter that has been consistent in almost every study is the time of onset of the new symptoms, which is 28–35 years after the acute polio attack. The number of polio survivors is also uncertain, although a recent study from the Center for Health Statistics points to approximately one million survivors in the USA. Although some studies suggest increased incidence of ALS in areas prevalent for acute polio (Martyn, Barker and Osmond, 1988; Zilkha, 1962), there is clearly no evidence to indicate that post-polio patients are at risk of developing ALS. We have not seen any patient with the post-polio syndrome develop ALS among the hundreds of patients whose progress we have followed (Dalakas, unpublished observations).

4.6 ELECTROPHYSIOLOGICAL PRINCIPLES

Electrophysiological studies including single-fiber EMG have failed to show specific findings that distinguish post-polio syndrome from other motor neuron disorders. As discussed below, however, the electrophysiological studies have been informative in: (a) showing continuous denervation/reinnervation even in stable muscles on the basis of widespread increased jitter and blocking; and (b) demonstrating, on the basis of absence of neurogenic jitter, that in PPMA the initial site of the pathophysiological process is at the distal axonal sprouts. In contrast, in ALS, in which neurogenic jitter is often present, the initial lesion is more proximal, at or above the axonal branch point (Table 4.1).

At rest, fibrillations, positive sharp waves and fasciculations can be seen in post-polio patients even in stable muscles (Wiechers and Hubbell, 1981; Cruz-Martinez, Perez Conde and Ferrer, 1983; Cruz-Martinez, Ferrer and Perez Conde, 1984; Cashman et al., 1987; Dalakas et al., 1986a; Wiechers, 1987a, 1988; Dalakas and Hallett, 1988; Ravits et al., 1990). The firing of the spontaneous discharges is much more frequent and the number of sites with abnormal activity is much higher in the muscles of ALS patients than in those with PPMA. However, more meaningful quantitative differences between PPMA and ALS exist in the size of the voluntary motor unit action potentials, the fiber density and the degree of blocking. All three of these variables are increased in ALS patients, but they have reached giant proportions in PPMA (Table 4.1).

Although it is generally believed that fibrillation and positive sharp waves are signs of acute denervation and dissipate after 1 or 2 years

Post-polio motor neuron disease

Table 4.1 Electrophysiological findings in post-polio state and ALS

	Post-polio[a]	ALS
Fibrillations and positive sharp waves	Present (+)	+++
Fasciculations	Frequently present (+)	+++
Giant potentials of long duration, polyphasic	Often above 10 mV in amplitude	Rarely above 10 mV in amplitude
Fiber density	Very high	Increased
Jitter and blocking	Increased, even in 'stable' muscles suggestive of ongoing reinnervation (very unstable in weak muscles)	Increased
Neurogenic jitter	Not yet seen, suggestive of instability of sprouts distal to the axonal branch points	Often found
Macro EMG	Amplitude increased, but drops with progressive weakness	Amplitude increased

[a]No significant differences were found between PPMA and stable post-polio muscles.
Modified from Dalakas (1987b).

(Buchthal and Honke, 1944), more careful review even of the old literature has shown that fibrillation and positive sharp waves may persist several years after nerve injury (Buchthal and Pinelli, 1953; Hertz, Madson and Buchthal, 1954; Stalberg, 1982; Lutschg and Ludin, 1981; Kimura, 1983). Fibrillations might be the result of a continuous process of denervation and reinnervation as part of the normal process of repair after nerve injury. Therefore their presence in post-polio muscles does not appear to have any special implication. The same appears to be true for the fasciculations, which exist without special significance in all types of post-polio muscles regardless of whether they are newly weakened or stable (Dalakas *et al.*, 1986a; Dalakas and Hallett, 1988; Ravits *et al.*, 1990). Their presence does not indicate development of motor neuron disease even if at times they are frequent and associated with muscle cramps (Fetell *et al.*, 1982).

Single-fiber EMG shows increased jitter and blocking in both stable and newly weakening post-polio muscles. These signs are also found in ALS patients which indicates that there is no clear distinction between the two conditions as far as jitter is concerned (Dalakas *et al.*, 1986a). Increased jitter, which represents the excessive variation of the time of transmission at the neuromuscular junction or excessive variation of the time of action potential propagation into the two (or more) branches of an axon at the axonal branching point (Kimura, 1983), is difficult to quantify in post-polio patients because of the high number of clusters, in which the individual components cannot be identified well and triggering is not consistent (Dalakas *et al.*, 1986a). Blocking that is due to failure of impulse propagation at one of the neuromuscular junctions or one of the axonal branch points is also frequent in post-polio patients, as it is in ALS (Dalakas *et al.*, 1986a) (Table 4.1). Increased jitter can persist indefinitely after the acute poliomyelitis infection, suggesting the presence of a continuous denervating/reinnervating process that is unrelated to recent deterioration (Wiechers and Hubbell, 1981; Dalakas *et al.*, 1986a; Wiechers, 1988; Ravits *et al.*, 1990). Although jitter is abnormal in post-polio muscles, there is no 'neurogenic jitter' (Dalakas *et al.*, 1986a), the jitter ascribed to the axonal branch points. Neurogenic jitter is characterized by two or more potentials that move together with respect to a third potential and cannot be due to a process at a single endplate. Neurogenic jitter develops in ALS patients (Stalberg, 1982; Kimura, 1983; Lange, Smith and Lovelace, 1989). This negative observation has been interpreted as suggesting that the abnormality in post-polio muscle involves the individual axonal twigs rather than the whole nerve (Dalakas *et al.*, 1986a; Dalakas and Hallett, 1988).

It has been recently found that within the maximally enlarged motor units related to marked reinnervation the synapses may be less effective (Maselli *et al.*, 1992), resulting in impaired neuromuscular transmission as reflected by increased jitter. However, the functional significance of this interpretation is unclear because the impaired transmission in such post-polio muscles is unrelated to the manifestation of new symptoms of fatigue or weakness.

The motor units in post-polio patients are large in amplitude and often in duration in almost all the muscles, including those that appear to be clinically normal or historically not affected. This is expected when one considers the generalized nature of the acute illness. The size of the voluntary motor unit action potentials, the fiber density and the macro EMG amplitude are dramatically increased in PPMA owing to a very successful reinnervating process that results in giant-size motor units. In contrast, in ALS the motor unit size is only mildly increased because the reinnervation process is limited because of short lifespan or sickness of neurons or impaired ability of the existing neurons to fully reinnervate the already denervated fibers. Of interest is the fact that the amplitude on macro EMG drops as weakness progresses (Lange, Smith and Lovelace, 1989), suggesting loss of muscle fibers in the motor unit with progression of the weakness.

Table 4.2 Differences and characteristics in the muscle biopsies of patients with ALS and PPMA

	PPMA	ALS
1. Fiber type grouping of normal-size fibers	Always present even in asymptomatic muscles (large groups, up to 170 fibers per group)	Found in up to 50% of the patients (groups are much smaller than those noted in PPMA)
2. Scattered angulated fibers	A few are present in PPMA (absent in asymptomatic post-polio)	Many are present
3. Group atrophy	Rare in newly weakening and previously healthy muscles	Always present in the weakening and previously healthy muscles
4. Inflammation	Up to 40% of biopsies	Rare
5. Hypertrophic, moth-eaten and targetoid fibers	Often present owing to long-standing partial denervation	Rare
6. N-CAM-positive fibers	Scattered; rarely in small groups but within the large groups of reinnervated fibers	Scattered or in larger groups; often angulated fibers

Modified from Dalakas (1987b).

Nerve conduction studies and repetitive stimulation studies are normal in post-polio patients and they are not different from those in ALS (Dalakas *et al.*, 1986a; Dalakas and Hallett, 1988; Ravits *et al.*, 1990).

4.7 MUSCLE BIOPSY FINDINGS

The characteristic features of the muscle biopsies in post-polio patients are summarized in Table 4.2. In general, the findings depend on the biopsied muscle (Dalakas, 1984; Dalakas, 1988b, 1990a). Muscles originally affected and partially recovered show a variable degree of neurogenic group atrophy combined with myopathic features characterized by increased connective tissue, occasional necrotic or phagocytosed fibers, variation of fiber size with big and small rounded fibers, fiber splitting and internal nuclei. Muscle biopsy specimens from muscles originally affected but fully recovered show fiber type grouping with a large number (up to 200) of normal-size muscle fibers per group. By contrast, in ALS, although grouping of normal-size fibers is frequent, the groups are much smaller in size, reflecting the shorter lifespan of the motor neurons and impaired ability to fully reinnervate, as previously discussed (Dalakas, 1990b; Dalakas and Illa, 1991).

A histological characteristic of the newly weakened muscles is the presence of small, atrophic, esterase-positive angulated fibers, which are scattered among normal-size fibers and suggest recent denervation. Follow-up muscle biopsies, even from the same muscles that had weakened further, reveal additional angulated fibers that are still scattered, although at times they are contiguous or form tiny groups of three to four. The absence of typical group atrophy in previously healthy and newly weakened post-polio muscles contrasts with the findings in the weakening muscles of patients with ALS, in whom atrophic fibers in groups (group atrophy) resulting from death of whole neurons is a common finding. As PPMA progresses, however, more adjacent fibers may become atrophic, eventually producing small-group atrophy resulting either from degeneration of terminal sprouts and major axonal branches that belong to a large motor unit or death of an entire small motor unit that emanated from a previously scarred neuron that has marginal reserves and limited capacity to reinnervate (Dalakas, 1986, 1987a,b, 1988b, 1990a,b; Dalakas et al., 1986a; Dalakas and Illa, 1991).

With immunocytochemistry, using anti-Leu-19/NKH-I monoclonal antibodies, which identify muscle-specific N-CAM molecules (Covault and Sanes, 1985; Dalakas and Illa, 1991), some workers (Cashman et al., 1987; Illa, Leon-Monzon and Dalakas, 1992) have found evidence of a continuous denervation and reinnervation. This was based on the observation that N-CAM, which is expressed only in the recently denervated fibers (Covault and Sanes, 1985; Illa, Leon-Monzon and Dalakas, 1992), was expressed by normal-size fibers found scattered or in small groups within the larger groups of reinnervated fibers (Figure 4.1). This indicates that in PPMA there are at a given time individual muscle fibers that have just lost their reinnervation and became unstable but have not yet become atrophic. These fibers represent failure of re-reinnervation and can be potentially rescued if the collateral sprouts from the surviving motor neurons (which also have N-CAM) will make contact and form a new effective synapse. Recent evidence suggests that some of the re-reinneverated fibers may not be forming effective synapses (Maselli et al., 1992). These observations supplement the electrophysiological findings of increased jitter and lead to the conclusion that the muscles in post-polio patients remain unstable because at a given time there are more denervated fibers than could possibly be

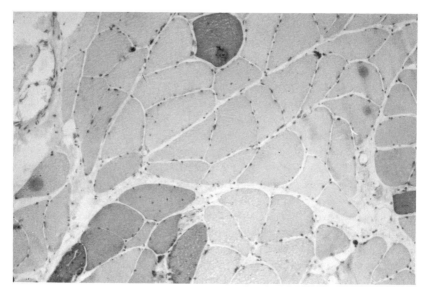

Figure 4.1 Muscle biopsy section from a patient with PPMA immunostained with antibodies to Leu-19 that identify N-CAM-positive fibers indicative of ongoing denervation. Positive muscle fibers are mostly of normal size and they are scattered or in small groups (×375).

reinnervated. If the denervated fibers cannot be rescued and make an effective synapse with a distal sprout, they lose their N-CAM expression and become atrophic.

Another finding in the muscle biopsy of post-polio patients is the presence in up to 40% of PPMA muscles of increased numbers of perivascular or endomysial mononuclear infiltrates (Dalakas, 1986, 1987a,b, 1988b, 1990a; Illa and Dalakas, 1990; Dalakas and Illa, 1991). With immunocytochemistry these cells are CD8[+] or CD4[+] lymphocytes (Figure 4.2) (Illa and Dalakas, 1990; Dalakas and Illa, 1991). A large number of fibers in PPMA muscles also express MHC class I antigen on their surface (Figure 4.3), even in areas remote from the lymphocytic infiltrates, in a pattern analogous to that seen in inflammatory myopathies (Dalakas, 1991a). MHC class II (DR) antigen was seen in rare fibers; we have not observed this even in inflammatory myopathies (Illa and Dalakas, 1990; Dalakas and Illa, 1991). Although the significance of these observations is unclear, the possibility that lymphokines or cytokines released by the previous viral infection can trigger a smoldering, low-grade, immune attack against self antigens cannot be excluded.

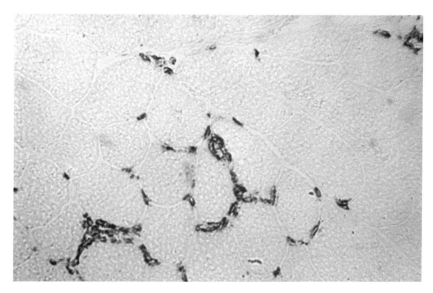

Figure 4.2   Cross-section of a muscle from a patient with PPMA immunostained with antibodies to CD8$^+$ cells shows that the majority of the inflammatory cells surrounding healthy muscle fibers are CD8$^+$ cells ($\times$375).

4.8   SPINAL CORD FINDINGS

A study of spinal cord sections in seven patients with prior polio (three with PPMA and four with stable post-polio but without new symptoms) who died from unrelated causes 9 months to 44 years after the original polio attack revealed mild but definite perivascular inflammation in the parenchyma of the gray matter as well as active gliosis disproportional to the neuronal loss (Pezeshkpour and Dalakas, 1988). Neuronal atrophy and chromatolysis were also noted. In three PPMA patients we found axonal spheroids. Several surviving neurons were present throughout the gray matter, but some of them had abnormal configuration of their somata, consisting of atrophy, accumulation of lipofuscin and loss of Nissl substance (Pezeshkpour and Dalakas, 1988). These findings were unrelated to new weakness or the time of death after the original illness, implying that some degree of activity continues for many years in the post-polio spinal cord, the site of the original viral infection. Although these changes were mild and may be considered non-specific, it is of note that inflammation has been also noted in the post-polio spinal cord by others, 1 year after the original polio attack

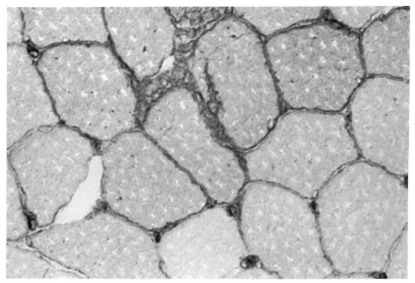

Figure 4.3 Cross-section of a muscle biopsy from a patient with the post-polio syndrome shows strong MHC-I class expression in the muscle fibers.

(Peers, 1943; Plum and Olson, 1973). Similar patterns of inflammation in the spinal cord have been reported in ALS patients (Appel *et al.*, 1990).

4.9 PATHOGENESIS OF PPMA

Based on the above-described clinical, electrophysiological, histological and immunohistochemical findings in the muscle and spinal cords, I have formulated the following hypothesis relating to the function of post-polio motor neurons, as shown diagrammatically in Figure 4.4.

After acute polio, there exist both unimpaired motor neurons that have fully or partially recovered and can resume normal or near-normal function and dying neurons (Figure 4.4). The terminal axons of the surviving motor neurons sprout in an attempt to reinnervate muscle fibers orphaned by the death of their parent motor neurons. During this process, uninvolved or recovered anterior horn cells adopt in their motor unit territories additional muscle fibers that could extend up to four or five new muscle fibers for every muscle fiber innervated originally, increasing the number of muscle fibers innervated by a single motor neuron by four to five times above normal. This process produces large motor units and is so effective that, despite the loss of up to 50% of

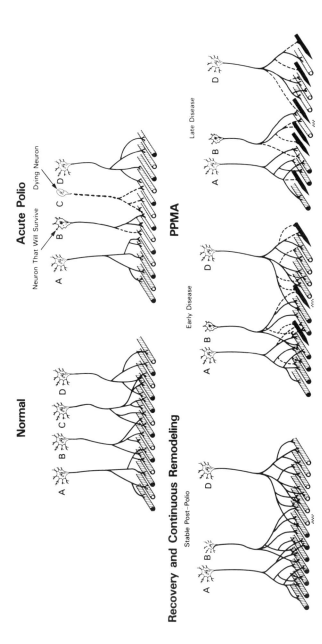

Figure 4.4 Diagrammatic representation of remaining neurons after acute polio and in the chronic post-polio state. In the stable post-polio state, there is continuing remodeling of the motor unit by effective reinnervation of the newly denervated fibers. In early PPMA there are only small scattered angulated fibers (dark) representing disintegration of distal sprouts corresponding to early new muscle weakness. As PPMA progresses, more muscle fibers can become denervated; hence the possible development of atrophic fibers in small groups represented as two contiguous dark fibers. Dots represent the nuclear clumps that remained since the acute polio attack.

the original number of motor neurons, the muscle can retain clinically normal strength (Dalakas and Hallett, 1988; Dalakas, 1990a; Dalakas and Illa, 1991). However, after maximum recovery is achieved the reinnervated motor units have not matured and stabilized as expected. On the contrary, the motor units are unstable because not all of the excessive distal sprouts can form effective synapses, resulting in failure to re-reinnervate all the newly denervated fibers. This ongoing denervating and re-reinnervating process is stressing the neuronal cell bodies, which after a number of years are left with diminished reserves and reduced ability to maintain the metabolic demands of all their sprouts. Consequently, there is slow deterioration of some nerve terminals. As each terminal dies, muscle fibers drop out because they can no longer be reinnervated and weakness progresses slowly. The presence of single, scattered, atrophic, angulated fibers without new group atrophy, along with scattered N-CAM-positive fibers of normal size and the increased jitter with absence of neurogenic jitter, support the notion that in PPMA there is initially denervation of individual fibers, rather than denervation of groups of muscle fibers. As PPMA progresses, however, some adjacent fibers become atrophic, as depicted in Figure 4.4, and eventually small-group atrophy may develop as whole axonal branches that belong to the same or neighboring motor units or whole scarred neurons with minimal muscle reserves disintegrate.

4.10 ETIOLOGY OF THE POST-POLIO SYNDROME AND RELEVANCE TO ALS

The possible etiologic considerations for the above-described pathogenetic mechanisms of the new muscle weakness in patients with old polio include the following:

1. **Normal aging**. Aging alone cannot be the cause of PPMA because motor neuron loss does not occur in people younger than age 60 (Tomlinson and Irving, 1977), and muscle biopsy specimens from normal people younger than 60 years old rarely show small angulated fibers (Hicks, Cutler and Dalakas, 1985) (and M.C. Dalakas, unpublished observations). In addition, the PPMA patients selected for our study were below the age of 60 (average 47 years) to specifically avoid the effect of aging. Epidemiologic data also indicate that it is the length of the interval between onset of acute polio and the appearance of new symptoms that is a determining variable for PPMA and not chronological age (Halstead and Wiechers, 1987).
2. **Attrition and premature neuronal exhaustion or early aging**. This is the theory I favor. PPMA appears to express itself clinically

approximately 30 years after the original polio attack, which suggests that the remaining overstressed post-polio neurons may succumb earlier than normal to the aging process or may even have a shorter lifespan. Motor unit decompensation may be accelerated by normal aging, which has been associated with increased endplate complexity and reduced terminal sprouting (Pestronk, Drachman and Griffin, 1980). These phenomena of normal aging expressed prematurely in a previously affected neuron or facilitated by attrition can explain some of the observations mentioned above.

The phenomenon of attrition of a previously scarred neuron raises an important neurobiological question regarding the lifespan of a healthy or previously scarred (but recovered) motor neuron that has been stressed to oversprout and maintain large motor units. There is no known human model and not enough information from experimental animals regarding the longevity and electrophysiological behavior of such motor neurons. This information is needed to understand not only the post-polio syndrome but also the other motor neuron diseases, especially ALS. Motor neurons subjected for years to various insults (mechanical, viral, other) may have a shorter lifespan. Consequently, a motor neuron disease, such as ALS, may be clinically manifested when the population of the remaining motor neurons crosses a critical threshold during the lifetime of an individual.

3. **Immunopathologic mechanisms**. Although unlikely, as it seems that PPMA is an immune disease, the following primary or secondary immunological abnormalities should be given serious consideration:

- mild inflammation is present in the muscle biopsies consisting of $CD8^+$ and $CD4^+$ cells surrounding healthy muscle fibers that express MHC-I class antigen on their surface, in a pattern similar to that seen in some immune-mediated inflammatory myopathies;
- weak IgG oligoclonal bands are seen in the spinal fluid of some PPMA patients (Dalakas, 1987a, 1990c);
- mild inflammatory changes are present in the spinal cord even up to 44 years after the original polio attack;
- abnormal phenotypic expression of peripheral blood lymphocyte subsets and depletion of naive T cells suggestive of a chronic activation of T cells have been described (Ginsberg et al., 1989);
- an increased association with HLA-DQ 17 haplotype, suggestive of genetic susceptibility to the acute polio infection, has been observed (Dinsmore and Dalakas, 1992).

4. **Chronic persistent poliovirus infection**. Poliovirus is a cytolytic RNA virus and acute poliomyelitis is a monophasic disease. Although

recurrent poliomyelitis is not known to occur, poliovirus can cause a persistent infection in animals or immunosuppressed humans (Miller, 1981). Persistent poliovirus infection has been shown to correlate with a selection of highly mutated viral strains that are capable of producing cytopathic effects in neuroblastoma cell lines even over a 9-month period (Colbere-Garopin et al., 1989). The possibility therefore of residual viral genomes within the remaining motor neurons of post-polio patients, although remote, cannot be ignored. Oligoclonal IgM bands specific for polioviruses were recently detected in the CSF of 21 of 36 patients with post-polio syndrome, and intrathecal synthesis of IgM antibodies against poliovirus was noted among the symptomatic post-polio patients (Sharief, Hentges and Ciardi, 1991). Increased levels of interleukin 2 (IL-2) and soluble IL-2 receptors were also noted in the CSF of these patients. These abnormalities, if confirmed, point towards an intrathecal immune response to the poliovirus unique to symptomatic post-polio patients. High poliovirus IgM antibody titers were seen in 6 of 25 post-polio patients using a sensitive ELISA assay (Leon-Monzon et al., 1991). Although this may imply a response to viral antigens hidden in various tissues, we have not been able to find viral genome in the muscle biopsies or the lymphocytes of these patients using the polymerase chain reaction technique (Leon-Monzon and Dalakas, 1992). We have not yet studied the spinal cord or the gut.

4.11 TREATMENT

There is no specific treatment for the post-polio syndrome. Therapy is entirely symptomatic and includes:

- non-steroidal anti-inflammatory drugs for the pain;
- changes in lifestyle to avoid overexhaustion and to accommodate the fatigue, which sometimes can be disabling if brief periods of rest during the day are not taken;
- healthier diet to avoid gaining weight;
- moderate non-fatiguing exercises, especially swimming; and
- reassurance that there is no evidence of recurrence of poliovirus or that the new symptoms are not life-threatening.

The belief by some that lack of exercise is beneficial because it preserves the neuronal lifespan is not based on experimental data. An active life with activities up 'to tolerance' and a 'commonsense' approach to the amount of physical tasks performed is recommended.

Because of the immunopathological abnormalities noted above, the author's group has been conducting a double-blind placebo-controlled trial with prednisone. Amantadine, a drug used to treat fatigue, is under study in my institution. Mestinon, which enhances acetylcholine release, has been reported to help the fatigue, but controlled studies have not been conducted. In my hands, Mestinon has been ineffective. Guanidine has not been formally tried.

REFERENCES

Anderson, A.D., Levine, S.A. and Gellert, H. (1972) Loss of ambulatory ability in patients with old anterior poliomyelitis. *Lancet*, **ii**, 1061–3.

Appel, S.H., Engelhardt, J.I., Garcia, J. and Stefani, E. (1990) Autoimmunity and ALS: a comparison of animal models of immune-mediated motor neurone destruction and human ALS, in *Advances in Neurology*, vol. 56 (ed. L.P. Rowland) Raven Press, New York, pp. 405–12.

Bach, J.R., Alba, A.S., Bodofsky, E. *et al.* (1987) Glossopharyngeal breathing and non-invasive aids in the management of post-polio respiratory insufficiency, in *Research and Clinical Aspects of the Late Effects of Poliomyelitis*, Vol. 23 (eds L.S. Halstead and D.O. Wiechers) March of Dimes, White Plains NY, pp. 99–113.

Bodian, D. (1949a) Histopathologic basis of clinical findings, in *Poliomyelitis. Am. J. Med.*, **6**, 563–78.

Bodian, D. (1949b) Poliomyelitis: pathologic anatomy, in *Poliomyelitis: Papers and Discussions*. Presented at the First International Poliomyelitis Conference. J.B. Lippincott, Philadelphia, p. 62.

Bodian, D. (1982) Poliomyelitis, in *Pathology of the Nervous System*, Vol. 3 (ed. J. Minckler), McGraw-Hill, New York, pp. 2323–64.

Bodian, D. (1984) Motorneuron disease and recovery in experimental poliomyelitis, in *Late Effects of Poliomyelitis* (eds L.S. Halstead and D.O. Wiechers) Symposia Foundation, Miami, pp. 45–50.

Buchthal, F. and Honke, P. (1944) Electromyographic examination of patients suffering from poliomyelitis. *Acta Med. Scand.*, **116**, 148.

Buchthal, F. and Pinelli, P. (1953) Action potentials in muscular atrophy of neurogenic origin. *Neurology*, **3**, 591–603.

Calne, D.B., Eisen, A., McGeer, E. and Spencer, P. (1986) Alzheimer's disease, Parkinson's disease and motorneurone disease: abiotrophic interaction between aging and environment? *Lancet*, **ii**, 1067–70.

Campbell, A.M.G., Williams, F.R. and Pearce, J. (1969) Late motor neurone degeneration following poliomyelitis. *Neurology*, **19**, 1101–6.

Cashman, N.R., Maselli, R. Wollman, R.L. *et al.* (1987) Late denervation in patients with antecedent paralytic poliomyelitis. *N. Engl. J. Med.*, **317**, 7–12.

Codd, M.B., Mudler, D.W., Kurland, L.T. *et al.* (1984) Poliomyelitis in Rochester Minnesota 1935–1955. Epidemiology and long-term sequelae: a preliminary report, in: *Late Effects of Poliomyelitis* (eds L.S. Halstead and D.O. Wiechers), Symposia Foundation, Miami, pp. 121–34.

Colbere-Garopin, F., Christodoulou, C., Crainic, R. and Pelletier, T. (1989)

Persistent poliovirus infection of human neuroblastoma cells. *Proc. Natl. Acad. Sci. USA*, **86**, 4354–9.

Covault, J. and Sanes, J.R. (1985) Neural cell adhesion molecule (N-CAM) accumulates in denervated and paralyzed skeletal muscles. *Proc. Natl. Acad. Sci. USA*, **82**, 4544–8.

Cruz-Martinez, A., Ferrer, M.T. and Perez Conde, M.C. (1984) Electrophysiological features in patients with non-progressive and late progressive weakness after paralytic poliomyelitis. Conventional EMG, automatic analysis of the electromyogram and single fiber electromyography study. *Electromyogr. Clin. Neurophysiol.*, **24**, 469–79.

Cruz-Martinez, A., Perez Conde, M.C. and Ferrer, M.T. (1983) Chronic partial denervation is more widespread than is suspected clinically in paralytic poliomyelitis: electrophysiological study. *Eur. Neurol.*, **22**, 314–21.

Dalakas, M.C. (1984) Future basic research issues for post-poliomyelitis, in *Late Effects of Poliomyelitis* (eds L.S. Halstead and D.O. Wiechers), Symposia Foundation, Miami, pp. 225–8.

Dalakas, M.C. (1986) New neuromuscular symptoms in patients with old poliomyelitis: a three year follow-up study. *Eur. Neurol.*, **25**, 381–7.

Dalakas M.C. (1987a) New neuromuscular symptoms after polio (the post-polio syndrome): clinical studies and pathogenetic mechanisms, in *Research and Clinical Aspects of the Late Effects of Poliomyelitis*, Vol. 23 (eds L.S. Halstead and D.O. Wiechers), March of Dimes, White Plains NY, pp. 241–64.

Dalakas, M.C. (1987b) ALS and post-polio: differences and similarities, in *Research and Clinical Aspects of the Late Effects of Poliomyelitis*, Vol. 23 (eds L.S. Halstead and D.O. Wiechers), March of Dimes, White Plains NY, pp. 63–81.

Dalakas, M.C. (1988a) Post-polio syndrome, in *Yearbook of Nursing 88*, Springhouse Corporation, pp. 50–4.

Dalakas, M.C. (1988b) Morphological changes in the muscles of patients with post-poliomyelitis neuromuscular symptoms. *Neurology*, **38**, 99–104.

Dalakas, M.C. (1990a) Pathogenesis of post-polio syndrome: clues from muscle and CNS studies, in *The Post-Polio Syndrome* (ed. T. Munsat), Butterworths, Stoneham, pp. 39–65.

Dalakas, M.C. (1990b) Post-poliomyelitis motor neuron disease: what did we learn in reference to amyotrophic lateral sclerosis? in *Amyotrophic Lateral Sclerosis: Concepts in Pathogenesis and Etiology* (ed. A.J. Hudson), pp. 326–56.

Dalakas M. (1990c) Oligoclonal bands in postpoliomyelitis muscular atrophy. *Ann. Neurol.*, **28**, 196–7.

Dalakas, M.C. (1991a) Polymyositis, dermatomyositis and inclusion-body myositis. *N. Engl. J. Med.*, **325**, 1487–98.

Dalakas, M.C. (1991b) Dysphagia in the post-polio syndrome. *N. Engl. J. Med.*, **325**, 1107–9.

Dalakas, M.C. and Hallett, M. (1988) The post-polio syndrome, in *Advances in Contemporary Neurology* (ed. F. Plum), F.A. Davis, Philadelphia, pp. 51–94.

Dalakas, M.C. and Illa, I. (1991) The Post-polio syndrome: concepts in pathogenesis and etiologies, in *Advances in Neurology*, Vol. 56, *Amyotrophic Lateral Sclerosis* (ed. L.P. Rowland), Raven Press, New York, pp. 495–511.

References

Dalakas, M.C., Sever, J.L., Fletcher, M. *et al.* (1984a) Neuromuscular symptoms in patients with old poliomyelitis: clinical, virological, and immunological studies, in *Late Effects of Poliomyelitis* (eds L.S. Halstead and D.O. Wiechers), Symposia Foundation, Miami, pp. 73–90.

Dalakas, M.C., Sever, J.L., Madden, D.L. *et al.* (1984b) Late post-poliomyelitis muscular atrophy: clinical, virological and immunological studies. *Rev. Infect. Dis.*, **6**, S562–7.

Dalakas, M.C., Elder, G., Hallett, M. *et al.* (1986a) A long term follow-up study of patients with postpoliomyelitis neuromuscular symptoms. *N. Engl. J. Med.*, **314**, 959–63.

Dalakas, M.C., Aksamit, A.J., Madden, D.L. and Sever, J.L. (1986b) Recombinant α-2 interferon in a pilot trial of patients with ALS. *Arch. Neurol.*, **43**, 933–5.

Dinsmore, S.T. and Dalakas, M. (1992) Immunogenetic and immunoregulatory factors in patients with the post-polio syndrome (PPS). *Neurology*, **42(S)**, 314.

Fetell, M.R., Smallberg, G., Lewis, L.D. *et al.* (1982) A benign motor neuron disorder: delayed cramps and fasciculation after poliomyelitis or myelitis. *Ann. Neurol.*, **11**, 423–7.

Fisher, D.A. (1984) Poliomyelitis: late pulmonary complications and management, in *Late Effects of Poliomyelitis* (eds L.S. Halstead and D.O. Wiechers), Symposia Foundation, Miami, 185–92.

Fisher, D.A. (1987) Sleep disordered breathing as a late effect of poliomyelitis, in *Research and Clinical Aspects of the Late Effects of Poliomyelitis*, Vol. 23 (eds L.S. Halstead and D.O. Wiechers), March of Dimes, White Plains NY, pp. 115–20.

Ginsberg, A.H., Gale, M.J., Rose, L.M. and Clark, E.A. (1989) T-cell alteration in late post-poliomyelitis. *Arch. Neurol.*, **46**, 497–501.

Glasberg, M., Dalakas, M.C. and Engel, W.K. (1978) Muscle cramps and pains: histochemical analysis of muscle biopsies in 63 patients. *Neurology*, **28**, 387.

Guilleminault, C. and Motta, J. (1978) Sleep apnea syndrome as a long-term sequela of poliomyelitis, in *Sleep Apnea Syndromes*, Vol. 2 (ed C. Guilleminault), Kroc Foundation, New York, pp. 309–15.

Halstead, L.S. and Wiechers, D.O. (eds) (1985) *Late Effects of Poliomyelitis*, Symposia Foundation, Miami.

Halstead, L.S. and Wiechers, D.O. (eds) (1987) *Research and Clinical Aspects of the Late Effects of Poliomyelitis*, Vol. 23, March of Dimes, White Plains NY.

Hayward, S. and Seaton, D. (1979) Late sequelae of paralytic poliomyelitis. A clinical and electromyographic study. *J. Neurol. Neurosurg. Psychiatr.*, **42**, 117–22.

Hertz, H., Madsen, A. and Buchthal, F. (1954) Prognostic implications of electromyography in acute anterior poliomyelitis. *J. Bone Joint Surg.*, **36A**, 902.

Hicks, J.E., Cutler, N.A. and Dalakas, M.C. (1985) Assessment of peripheral nervous system involvement in normal aged and Alzheimer's patients (abstract). *Arch. Phys. Med. Rehabil.*, **16**, 10.

Post-polio motor neuron disease

Illa, I. and Dalakas, M.C. (1990) Immunocytochemical changes in the muscles of patients with post-poliomyelitis muscular atrophy (PPMA): relevance to amyotrophic lateral sclerosis (ALS). *Neurology*, **40(S)**, 429.

Illa, I., Leon-Monzon, M. and Dalakas, M.C. (1992) Regenerating and denervated human muscle fibers and satellite cells express N-CAM recognized by monoclonal antibodies to NK cells. *Ann. Neurol.*, **31**, 46–52.

Johnson, R.T. (1982) *Viral Infections of the Nervous System*, Raven Press, New York.

Katlyar, B.C., Misra, S., Singh, R.B. *et al.* (1983) Adult polio-like syndrome following enterovirus 70 conjunctivitis (natural history of the disease). *Acta Neurol. Scand.*, **67**, 263–72.

Kimura, J. (1983) *Electrodiagnosis in Diseases of Nerve and Muscle*, F.A. Davis, Philadelphia.

Kohl, S.J. (1987) Emotional responses to the late effects of poliomyelitis, in *Research and Clinical Aspects of the Late Effects of Poliomyelitis*, Vol. 23 (eds L.S. Halstead and D.O. Wiechers), March of Dimes, White Plains NY, pp. 135–43.

Lane, D.J., Haselman, B. and Nichols, P.J.R. (1974) Late onset respiratory failure in patients with previous poliomyelitis. *Q. J. Med.*, **43**, 551–68.

Lange, D.J., Smith, T. and Lovelace, R.E. (1989) Postpolio muscular atrophy. Diagnostic utility of macroelectromyography. *Arch. Neurol.*, **46**, 502–6.

Leon-Monzon, M. and Dalakas, M.C. (1992) Absence of persistent infection with enteroviruses in muscles of patients with inflammatory myopathies. *Ann. Neurol.*, **32**, 219–22.

Leon-Monzon, M., Agboatwalla, M., Dinsmore, S. *et al.* (1991) Comparison of antibodies to the poliomyelitis virus in patients with acute paralytic poliomyelitis, post-polio syndrome and ALS. *Ann. Neurol.*, **30**, 301–2.

Lutschg, J. and Ludin, H.P. (1981) Electromyographic findings in patients after recovery from peripheral nerve lesions and poliomyelitis. *J. Neurol.*, **225**, 25–32.

Martyn, C.N., Barker, D.J.P. and Osmond, C. (1988) Motorneuron disease and postpoliomyelitis in England and Wales. *Lancet*, **i**, 1319–22.

Maselli, R.A., Cashman, N.R. and Wallman R.L. *et al.* (1992) Neuromuscular transmission as a function of motor unit size in patients with prior poliomyelitis. *Muscle and Nerve*, **15**, 648–55.

Melnick, J.K. (1984) Enterovirus type 71 infections: a varied clinical pattern sometimes mimicking paralytic poliomyelitis. *Rev. Inf. Dis.*, **6S**, 387–92.

Miller, J.R. (1981) Prolonged intracerebral infection with poliovirus in asymptomatic mice. *Ann. Neurol.*, **9**, 590–6.

Mulder, D.W., Rosenbaum, R.A. and Layton Jr, D.O. (1972) Late progression of poliomyelitis or forme fruste amyotrophic lateral sclerosis. *Mayo Clinic Proc.*, **47**, 756–61.

Peers, J.H. (1943) The pathology of convalescent poliomyelitis. *Am. J. Pathol.*, **19**, 673–96.

Pestronk, A., Drachman, D.B. and Griffin, J.W. (1980) Effects of aging on nerve sprouting and regeneration. *Exp. Neurol.*, **70**, 65–82.

References

Pezeshkpour, G.H. and Dalakas, M.C. (1988) Long term changes in the spinal cord of patients with old poliomyelitis: signs of continuous disease activity. *Arch. Neurol.*, **45**, 505–8.

Plum, F. and Olson, M.E. (1973) Myelitis and Myelopathy, in *Clinical Neurology*, Vol. 3 (eds A.B. Baker and L.H. Baker), Harper & Row, Hagerstown, MD, 1–33.

Plum, F. and Swanson, A.G. (1959) Central neurogenic hypoventilation in man. *Arch. Neurol. Psychiatr.*, **81L**, 531–60.

Ravits, J., Hallet, M., Baker, M. *et al.* (1990) Clinical and electromyographic studies of post-poliomyelitis muscular atrophy. *Muscle Nerve*, **13**, 667–74.

Sharief, M.K., Hentges, R. and Ciardi, M. (1991) Intrathecal immune response in patients with the post-polio syndrome. *N. Engl. J. Med.*, **325**, 748–55.

Sonies, B.C. and Dalakas, M.C. (1991) Dysphagia in patients with the post-polio syndrome. *N. Engl. J. Med.*, **324**, 1162–7.

Stalberg, E. (1982) Electrophysiological studies of reinnervation in amyotrophic lateral sclerosis, in *Human Motor Neuron Disease* (ed. L.P. Rowland), Raven Press, New York, pp. 47–59.

Tomlinson, B.E. and Irving, D. (1977) The numbers of limb motor neurons in the human lumbosacral cord throughout life. *J. Neurol. Sci.*, **34**, 213–19.

Wadia, N.H., Wadia, P.N., Katrak, S.M. and Misra, V.P. (1981) Neurological manifestations of acute hemorrhagic conjunctivitis. *Lancet*, **ii**, 528–32.

Wiechers, D.O. (1987) Reinnervation after acute poliomyelitis, in *Research and Clinical Aspects of the Late Effects of Poliomyelitis*, Vol. 23 (eds L.S. Halstead and D.O. Wiechers), March of Dimes, White Plains, NY, pp. 213–21.

Wiechers, D.O. (1988) New concepts of the reinnervated motor unit revealed by vaccine-associated poliomyelitis. *Muscle Nerve*, **11**, 356–64.

Wiechers, D.O. and Hubbell, S.L. (1981) Late changes in the motor unit after acute poliomyelitis. *Muscle Nerve*, **4**, 524–8.

Windebank, A.J., Daube, J.R., Litchy, W.J. *et al.* (1987) Late sequelae of paralytic poliomyelitis in Olmsted County, Minnesota, in *Research and Clinical Aspects of the Late Effects of Poliomyelitis*, Vol. 23 (eds L.S. Halstead and D.O. Wiechers), March of Dimes, White Plains, NY, pp. 27–38.

Zilkha, K. (1962) Discussion on motor neuron disease. *Proc. R. Soc. Med.*, **55**, 1028–31.

5 Amyotrophic lateral sclerosis–parkinsonism–dementia complex on Guam: epidemiologic and etiological perspectives

LEONARD T. KURLAND,
KURUPATH RADHAKRISHNAN,
DAVID B. WILLIAMS and STEPHEN C. WARING

5.1 INTRODUCTION

Amyotrophic lateral sclerosis (ALS) is a progressive disease whose clinical features are the result of degeneration of upper and lower motor neurons. Dementia, extrapyramidal features or disturbances of ocular movement are not generally present. However, ALS occurs in foci in the Western Pacific islands in combination with dementia and parkinsonism, often with a gaze palsy that resembles progressive supranuclear palsy, and shows widespread Alzheimer-like neurofibrillary tangles pathologically. This has been described in the Chamorro population of the Mariana Islands as amyotrophic lateral sclerosis and parkinsonism–dementia complex (ALS/PDC) (Hirano, Malamud and Kurland, 1961; Kurland *et al.*, 1961). ALS and PDC have also been described in two villages on the Kii Peninsula in Japan (Uebayashi, 1980), and in the Irian Jaya focus of south-west New Guinea, where the disease has also been prevalent but pathological confirmation has not been feasible (Gajdusek and Salazar, 1982).

The small island of Guam in the Mariana Islands of the Western Pacific has been an important focus of research in neurodegenerative diseases (Figure 5.1). For the past 40 years the continued surveillance of ALS and PDC in Guam and other Western Pacific foci has provided insight into the pathogenesis of several neurodegenerative disorders. In this chapter we attempt to reconcile current knowledge of the epidemiologic, clinical and pathologic features of ALS/PDC in the Western Pacific. Primary emphasis will be on the comprehensive studies of ALS/PDC on Guam with reference to similar disease foci in Japan and west New Guinea, relating these studies to reports of other neurodegenerative diseases occurring outside the Western Pacific.

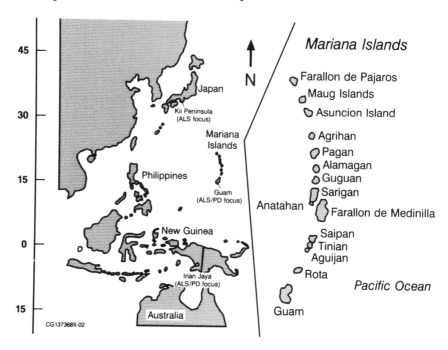

Figure 5.1 Map of the Pacific islands, the Kii Peninsula in Japan, the Mariana Islands and Irian Jaya in western New Guinea.

5.2 THE EPIDEMIOLOGIC DATA FROM GUAM AND THE MARIANA ISLANDS

Although ALS on Guam has been traced through death certificates and church records back to 1815, it is uncertain how long the indigenous Chamorro people have had an abnormally high frequency of neuro-degenerative diseases. An accurate history for both ALS and PDC would be a valuable contribution to understanding the etiology of Guam disease. Padre Diego Luis de Sanvitores led the first Spanish missionaries to Guam in 1668, and in that first year they baptized more than 100 individuals said to be centenarians (Safford, 1903; Haddock, 1973). Early reports describe the Chamorros as 'remarkably free from disease and physical defects' (Safford, 1903).

Guam became a USA possession after the Spanish–American War in 1898. The first recorded diagnosis of amyotrophic lateral sclerosis was made in 1904, on a death certificate written by US Navy personnel (Kurland, 1957). It seems remarkable that in a remote naval outpost in the Western Pacific this diagnosis was confidently made less than 50 years after Charcot had first described and named the disease (Charcot

110

and Joffroy, 1869). ALS was known to the Chamorros as 'lytico', a contraction of the Spanish word 'paralytico'. Early reports by Zimmerman (1945), Koerner (1952), Arnold, Edgren and Palladino (1953) and Tillema and Wynberg (1953) were confirmed in the surveys by Kurland and Mulder (1954), who showed that ALS was 50–100 times more prevalent among the Chamorros of Guam than in the population of the continental USA.

Systematic epidemiological surveillance of ALS and PDC on Guam began 40 years ago with the work of Kurland and Mulder and continued from 1956 through 1983 with the establishment of a Research Center by the National Institute for Neurologic, Communicative Disorders and Stroke (NINCDS). Between 1950 and the early 1980s, ALS and PDC accounted for about 20% of all deaths in Chamorros on Guam in those over age 25 years (Kurland and Mulder, 1954; Kurland *et al.*, 1961; Reed *et al.*, 1966; Brody and Kurland, 1973; Reed and Brody, 1975). An analysis of the NINCDS Research Center Registry, with cases dating from the early 1950s through the early 1980s, indicated that ALS or PDC cases had dramatically declined by the early 1980s (Garruto, Yanagihara and Gajdusek, 1985). During this same time period, the mean age at onset of ALS had increased from 48 to 52 years in men and from 42 to 52 years in women. The mean age at onset for PDC had increased from 55 to 59 years in men and from 51 to 59 years in women (Garruto, Yanagihara and Gajdusek, 1985).

There is, however, uncertainty about the completeness of case ascertainment in the NINCDS Research Center Registry as compared with that attained with the earlier surveys by Kurland and Mulder (1954). This difference is due primarily to the methodologic shortcomings of passive surveillance in the 1970s and 1980s compared with the active (house-to-house) surveillance of Mulder and Kurland (1954).

Geographic differences in the distribution of disease occurrence on Guam have been observed. The highest incidence rates have been noted in the southern villages, while the central and most of the northern villages on the island have had lower rates. ALS/PDC is also prevalent among the Chamorros on the nearby island of Rota (Figure 5.1), but less common among the Chamorros on Saipan. There is some uncertainty about whether an atypical form of motor neuron disease characterized by a slowly progressive paraparesis with fasciculations and minimal muscle atrophy occurs among the Carolinians on Saipan who have partly adopted Chamorro customs. In the Caroline Islands to the south, neither ALS nor PDC has been found (Kurland and Mulder, 1954; Mulder and Kurland, 1954).

Studies of Chamorros from Guam who migrated to California showed that they retain an increased risk of developing ALS and PDC (Torres,

ALS–parkinsonism–dementia complex on Guam

Iriarte and Kurland, 1957; Eldridge *et al.*, 1969; Garruto, Gajdusek and Chen, 1980). Furthermore, ALS and PDC have been reported in Filipino immigrants to Guam, on average two decades after their arrival (Garruto, Gajdusek and Chen, 1981; Chen *et al.*, 1982). It is difficult to determine if exposure of these Filipino migrants to the Guam environment *per se* leads to an increased risk of developing ALS/PDC, since no data are available on the incidence of ALS and PDC in the Philippine Islands (Matsumoto, Yase and Yasui, 1972). Migrants to Guam whose stay is short term, particularly US military personnel and construction workers, are not at increased risk of developing disease (Brody, Edgar and Gillespie, 1978). Thus, the migration studies lend support to the concept that long-term exposure to the environment on Guam may be associated with an increased risk of developing ALS/PDC.

In the other high-incidence foci of ALS/PDC in the Western Pacific, a decline in incidence rates has also been observed. In the Kii Peninsula of Japan, incidence rates have declined from 55 to 14 per 100 000 population in the Hobara subfocus, and no new cases have been observed in the Kosagawa subfocus (Garruto and Yase, 1986). In western New Guinea, with prevalence rates originally reported as high as 1300 per 100 000 population, ALS/PDC has disappeared in at least one village and declined in several other villages coincident with increased westernization and introduction of new foodstuffs (Gajdusek and Salazar, 1982; Gajdusek, 1984).

New patients with ALS/PDC have been identified on Guam as a result of the Micronesian Health Study (MHS), a federally funded project involving Mayo Clinic in Rochester, Minnesota, the University of Guam, and Mount Sinai Medical Center in New York. Surveys conducted from March 1990 through February 1991 among village residents 55 years and older on the islands of Rota and Tinian, and in the village of Yigo on Guam indicate a high prevalence of PDC and dementia on Rota, no definitive cases of ALS or PDC on Tinian and a high prevalence of ALS/PDC in Yigo. Although ALS is less common, the geographic pattern of ALS, PDC and dementia combined was similar to that of ALS and PDC reported in the 1960s, which suggests that the distribution of the presumed etiological agent(s) has not changed significantly in three decades.

Analysis of data from the MHS Registry, which represents patients still alive (or status unknown) in 1983 when the NINCDS Research Center closed, plus newly diagnosed cases through October 1992, indicates a continued upward trend in age at onset as previously reported. Patients with disease onset from 1980 to 1989 had an average age at onset of 53 years for ALS (similar for both males and females) and 63 years for PDC (similar for males and females). Figure 5.2 shows the

112

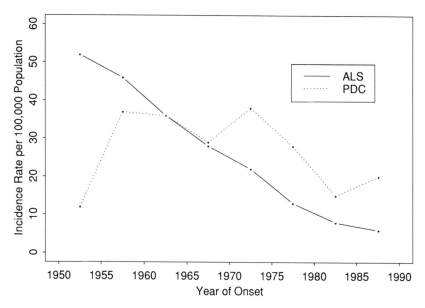

Figure 5.2 Five-year average annual incidence rates of amyotrophic lateral sclerosis (ALS) and parkinsonism–dementia complex (PDC) by year of onset, based on 1950–90 census data for Chamorros on Guam. Rates for the period 1980–84 should be considered underestimates since the numerator included only patients that were still alive at the time of closure of the NINCDS Research Center and, therefore, did not include patients who had disease onset from 1980 to 1983, but died before it closed. (Sources of data: Reed and Brody, 1975; Zhang *et al.*, 1990; NINCDS Registry, unpublished data; Micronesian Health Study Registry, October 1992, unpublished data.)

average annual incidence rates for 5-year intervals from 1950 to 1989, which include data from the previous studies (NINCDS, 1950–79) and the current MHS Registry (1980–89) (S.C. Waring, unpublished data). Although the rates for ALS are consistent with previous reports of a decrease in incidence, recent data do not support the reported dramatic decline in incidence rates for PDC (Garruto, Yanagihara and Gajdusek, 1985).

5.3 CLINICAL FEATURES OF ALS/PDC ON GUAM

Guam ALS, with few exceptions, is clinically indistinguishable from sporadic ALS worldwide. The onset of symptoms is insidious with atrophy, weakness and fasciculations of the skeletal musculature (Rodgers-Johnson, Garruto and Yanagihara, 1986). Muscle weakness and atrophy are progressive and result in flaccid paralysis, often within

113

a year of disease onset; reflexes are usually hyperactive until atrophy is pronounced. PDC, referred to as 'rayput' (slowness) or 'bodig', is a combination of varying degrees of bradykinesia, muscle rigidity, tremor and progressive dementia (Hirano et al., 1961; Chen and Chase, 1986; Rodgers-Johnson, Garruto and Yanagihara, 1986; Zhang et al., 1990). Clinical evidence of anterior horn cell degeneration may develop late in the course of about 20% of PDC patients (Hirano et al., 1961).

In the continental USA, ALS, Parkinson's disease and Alzheimer's disease tend to occur as single disease entities, although as many as one-third of those with Parkinson's disease will develop cognitive impairment. However, on Guam, a combination of two or all three of these disorders (ALS, parkinsonism, and dementia) frequently occurs in the same patient.

In recent years, supranuclear disturbances of ocular motility, usually mild, have been noted in a majority of Guam patients with ALS/PDC (Lepore et al., 1988). These comprise saccadic and pursuit paresis, nystagmus, conjugate gaze limitation, abnormal convergence, opto-kinetic nystagmus and vestibulo-ocular reflex cancellation (Lepore et al., 1988). There is thus the suggestion that the spectrum of neurodegenerative disease on Guam is broader than previously suspected, and includes ALS cases with features of Parkinson's disease, Alzheimer's disease and possibly supranuclear palsy. In a survey conducted in three southern villages on Guam in 1987–88, dementia alone or in association with early parkinsonism was noted predominantly in older women; this may reflect their selective survival (Lavine et al., 1991).

Another recent discovery that is under investigation is a pigmentary retinopathy resembling opthalmomyiasis interna posterior seen in 26 of 49 Chamorros with ALS/PDC as well as in 16% of neurologically asymptomatic individuals aged 50 and over (Cox et al., 1989). In contrast to published case reports of opthalmomyiasis interna posterior (Gass and Lewis, 1976; Syralden, Nitter and Mehl, 1982), the pathologic findings from autopsy of neurological patients from Guam show no evidence of a parasite. This retinopathy can be reliably detected by indirect opthalmoscopy or retinal photography; even when advanced, it may be impossible to confirm this using the direct ophthalmoscope. This retinopathy is characterized by hypopigmented subretinal tracks, which criss-cross in a random fashion and at times form loops. The degree of retinal involvement varies markedly. At autopsy, focal degeneration of the retinal pigmented epithelium has been observed; therefore, it is more accurate to refer to this condition as retinal pigmentary epithelio-pathy (Campbell et al., 1993). We are not aware of a similar pigmentary retinopathy in patients with either ALS or Parkinson's disease in other geographic sites. R.N. Hogan (personal communication) has described the apparent loss of pigment in the cells of the retinal pigmented epithelium in one rhesus monkey following the intracarotid injection of 1-methyl-4-phenyl-1,2,3,6 tetrahydropyridine (MPTP). Pathologically, the cells appeared to be clear except for small aggregations of concentrated pigment or macromelanosomes. Hogan noted similar macromelanosomes in the cases from Guam. However, the cause and pathogenesis of the Guam retinopathy are obscure. Since 1986, more than 100 Guamanian Chamorros with retinal pigmentary epitheliopathy have been identified, but it has been detected in only one non-Chamorro patient, an elderly Filipino who has been a resident of the island for 50 years (Campbell *et al.*, 1993).

The significance of the retinal pigmentary epitheliopathy in ALS/PDC is unclear. Retinal pigmentary epitheliopathy may represent a pre-viously unrecognized pathological manifestation of ALS/PDC, which could mean that ocular involvement in asymptomatic individuals may serve as a marker of subclinical neurological disease or a predictor of future disease. Alternatively, as retinal pigmentary epitheliopathy is asymptomatic and difficult to detect, it may be an endemic disease on Guam that occurs independent of ALS/PDC. Further epidemiologic studies are needed to provide evidence supporting either hypothesis.

Positron emission tomographic studies of Guam PDC have shown marked reduction in striatal [^{18}F]6-fluorodopa uptake. This metabolic abnormality is similar to that found in patients with idiopathic Parkinson's disease. Guam ALS patients have diminished striatal [^{18}F]6-fluorodopa uptake at a level intermediate between controls and indi-viduals with parkinsonism due to PDC (Snow *et al.*, 1990). In addition, two control subjects had diminished [^{18}F]6-fluorodopa uptake, suggest-ing that these clinically normal 'at-risk' subjects may have subclinical disease (Snow *et al.*, 1990).

5.4 NEUROPATHOLOGY OF WESTERN PACIFIC ALS/PDC

The lower and upper motor neuron degeneration in Western Pacific ALS is similar to that of sporadic ALS, with the additional histologic features of an excess of neurofibrillary tangles and intracytoplasmic inclusion (granulovacuolar) bodies, particularly in the nerve cells of the hippo-campus and other subcortical areas (Hirano, Malamud and Kurland, 1961; Malamud, Hirano and Kurland, 1961; Hirano *et al.*, 1966). The specificity of the neurofibrillary tangles in Western Pacific ALS/PDC is unclear because an excess of such tangles has also been found in a large proportion of Chamorros who died apparently free of neurologic symptoms (57% of people aged 40–59 and 95% of people aged ≥60 years) (Chen, 1981).

Ultrastructurally, the neurofibrillary tangles appear as paired helical filaments very similar to those in Alzheimer's disease with single or occasionally triple helical filaments as well (Guiroy et al., 1987, 1990). Paired helical filaments are each composed of two subfilaments 10 nm in diameter with an average crossover periodicity of 180 nm, more than double the crossover periodicity of paired helical filaments observed in Alzheimer's disease (Guiroy et al., 1987). The neurofibrillary tangles occurring in Chamorros, both with and without recognized ALS/PDC, have been shown to be similar to those of Alzheimer's disease by immunocytochemical characterization techniques (Shankar et al., 1989; Ito et al., in press).

Ubiquitin-positive filamentous inclusions are found in the anterior horn cells of all Guam ALS patients and all sporadic ALS cases. In addition, one of six PDC cases had similar abnormalities (Matsumoto, Hirano and Goto, 1990). In Guam PDC, striatal efferent neurons appear normal, but there is histological evidence of severe dopaminergic neuronal loss from both the medial and lateral portions of the substantia nigra (Goto, Hirano and Matsumoto, 1990).

5.5 REPORTS OF ALS ASSOCIATED WITH OTHER NEURODEGENERATIVE DISORDERS FROM OUTSIDE THE WESTERN PACIFIC REGION

Reports of ALS associated with other neurodegenerative diseases outside the Western Pacific have been rare. ALS associated with organic dementia has been recognized in up to 15% of all cases of familial ALS and 2% of cases of sporadic ALS (Burnstein, 1981; Hudson, 1981; Wikström et al., 1982; Mitsuyama, 1984; Ojeda, Grainger and Day, 1984). In those cases in which autopsy was carried out, the cause of organic dementia was found to be a non-specific atrophy of the cerebrum (Hudson, 1981; Ojeda, Grainger and Day, 1984). The changes of Alzheimer's disease such as neurofibrillary tangles, senile plaques and granulovacuolar degeneration were not present.

The combination of ALS with parkinsonism may occur either familially or sporadically (Schmitt, Emser and Heimes, 1984). In a familial case, post-mortem analysis revealed neurofibrillary tangles in the substantia nigra, locus ceruleus, parahippocampal gyrus and hippocampus. The pedigree suggested a recessive trait (Schmitt, Emser and Heimes, 1984).

Combinations of ALS with other disorders may occur more frequently in familial ALS than in sporadic cases, which may suggest a genetic linkage. About 10–15% of ALS cases are familial, with the most frequent pattern of inheritance being autosomal dominant. Siddique et al. (1991)

have recently shown evidence of a gene causing familial ALS on chromosome 21. Genetic analysis, by examining restriction fragment length polymorphism of familial Alzheimer's disease with onset before age 65 years, demonstrated linkage to DNA markers in the proximal region of the long arm of chromosome 21 (Strittmatter and Appel, 1990). There is also some evidence to link complex I deficiency and associated mitochondrial DNA aberration in Parkinson's disease (Di Monte, 1991; Hattori *et al.*, 1991). However, preliminary studies of a few cases of Guam ALS/PDC have not shown any genetic linkage.

5.6 ETIOLOGICAL PERSPECTIVES OF WESTERN PACIFIC NEUROLOGICAL DISORDERS

5.6.1 Genetic cause

The Spanish occupation of Guam led Chamorros to declare that 'foreigners brought to the island rats, flies, mosquitoes, and strange diseases' (Safford, 1903). Resistance by the Chamorros to attempts to 'civilize' them led eventually to the violent death and 'martyrdom' of Padre Sanvitores. Continuous warring developed between the Chamorros and their Spanish conquerors, and the so-called 'reduction' acted synergistically with devastating epidemics of introduced diseases in 1688 and 1700. It is estimated that by 1710 the Chamorro numbers had been reduced to a mere 3600 of the original population of 50 000 to 100 000 (Mulder, Kurland and Iriarte, 1954). Some of these escaped north to the island of Rota. Subsequently, the Guam population increased as a result of the addition of Spanish, Mexican and Filipino immigrants, and intermarriage with the remaining Chamorros.

The dramatic fall in population, and subsequent isolation, may have caused dissemination and pooling of genetic traits through selection. Descriptions of a genetic basis for such vulnerability in other mammals based on a similar calamitous fall in population have been given (O'Brien, Roelke and Marker, 1985).

There has been an intense search for a genetic cause of ALS/PDC since the early 1950s. Familial aggregation was recognized by the Chamorros for many years, but formal genetic studies were not initiated until 1958 with the establishment of a registry to determine if first-degree relatives and spouses were at greater risk for developing disease (Plato *et al.*, 1967). Analysis of 126 patients and 126 controls, matched for age, sex, marital status and village of residence, with 25 years of follow-up of 2212 living 0.5 relatives and 189 spouses failed to reveal any significant differences that would support a genetic hypothesis for ALS/PDC (Plato *et al.*, 1986). Other studies to identify genetic markers, including blood groups, serum proteins, red cell enzymes, HLA antigens, immuno-globulin allotypes and dermatoglyphics, and calculation of in-breeding coefficients and segregation analysis, have had similar negative findings (Plato, Cruz and Kurland, 1969; Reed, Torres and Brody, 1975; Hoffman *et al.*, 1977; Blake *et al.*, 1983; Garruto *et al.*, 1983).

The following circumstances suggest that genetics alone cannot account for the high prevalence of ALS/PDC among Chamorros on Guam and the other Western Pacific foci:

1. three different populations are involved;
2. there appears to be an excess of ALS and PDC among Filipinos who settled on Guam as young adults (Garruto, Gajdusek and Chen, 1981); and
3. the remarkable shift from a predominance of ALS to that of PDC and the increase in age at onset of both ALS and PDC over the past 30 years (Lavine *et al.*, 1991).

Thus, while strong consideration should be given to a genetic predisposition in the development of Western Pacific ALS/PDC, a genetic mechanism alone cannot account for the changing clinical features and pattern of distribution.

5.6.2 Environmental considerations

The cumulative epidemiologic data tend to support the hypothesis that exposure to some environmental factor(s) leads to development of ALS/PDC in the geographic isolates of the Western Pacific, although establishing causality has remained elusive. Two major hypotheses have been proposed to account for the unusual occurrence of ALS/PDC, both dealing with the neurotoxic consequences of exposure to environmental toxins.

CYCAD HYPOTHESIS

One candidate as the source of an exogenous toxin has been the seed of the false sago palm, *Cycas circinalis*. The cycad seed was identified as a potential cause of ALS on Guam as a result of Whiting's observation during field studies in Umatac and Yigo (Whiting, 1963). *Cycas circinalis* is a member of the order Cycadales, the palm-like evergreens that flourish in subtropical and tropical climates. The seeds of *Cycas circinalis* have been known to be highly toxic for humans since ancient times. Some populations learned how to process the seeds for food so that the effects of acute toxicity could be avoided. Among the Chamorros of

Guam a ritual of prolonged soaking developed; and during times of famine, especially following typhoons and in times of conflict such as World War II, cycad became an important source of carbohydrate in the diet. The freshly ground cycad seed was also used as a medicinal, particularly in the form of a poultice applied to ulcers and other lesions of the skin. Induction of carcinogenesis as a result of topical application of cycad nut extract to skin ulcers in mice, assumed to be due to the effects of cycasin, has been demonstrated (O'Gara, Brown and Whiting, 1964). Spencer, Ohta and Palmer (1987), and Spencer *et al.* (1987a) have reported that unwashed cycad was used as a medicinal in the other high-incidence foci, namely the Irian Jaya focus in western New Guinea, as a poultice, and the Kii Peninsula of Japan, as a 'tonic' made from dried seeds of *Cycas revoluta*.

Two toxins have now been identified in *Cycas circinalis*. One is cycasin (methylazoxymethanol β-D-glucoside), a major toxic component of the cycad seed (2–4%). Cycasin is metabolized by plant and animal β-glucosidases to methylazoxymethanol (MAM), a potent cytotoxin and carcinogen. The neurotoxicity of cycasin may be related to the intracellular production of the potent alkylating agent, MAM, a chemical with the ability to alter cell function irreversibly and progressively long after exposure has ceased (Polsky, Nunn and Bell, 1972). This toxin can be removed by adequate soaking when the seeds are prepared for consumption. However, in periods of stress and hunger, as in the Japanese occupation of Guam during World War II, water for soaking, and time (several days, as recommended), were often not available, so exposure to the toxin may have increased considerably.

A second water-soluble toxin that has been identified is α-amino-β-methyl-aminopropionic acid, or β-*N*-methylamino-L-alanine (BMAA). The neurotoxicity of BMAA has been demonstrated when applied to explants of the central nervous system (Nunn *et al.*, 1987; Weiss, Koi and Choi, 1989). Using large doses of a purified synthetic L-isomer of BMAA, Spencer and colleagues reported that rhesus monkeys developed an illness with skeletal muscle weakness as in human ALS and possibly PDC (Spencer *et al.*, 1986; Spencer, 1987).

It has been suggested that BMAA is an excitotoxic amino acid (Ross, Seelig and Spencer, 1987). Some investigators have proposed that a neurotoxic metabolite of BMAA, perhaps formed peripherally, may be the active neurotoxin. Because millimolar concentrations are required *in vitro* to demonstrate toxicity, and the predicted brain levels at which BMAA is neurotoxic *in vivo* are of the same magnitude, these data are consistent with direct neurotoxic effect of BMAA and argue against it acting via a peripherally formed metabolite (Duncan *et al.*, 1991).

In a recent study from Spencer's laboratory, it was found that the

119

traditionally processed (washed) cycad flours obtained from Chamorro residents of Guam still retain variable quantities of cycasin (Kisby, Ellison and Spencer, in press). The residual cycasin was approximately 10 times that of residual BMAA. On the basis of the cycasin content, the ingestion of such flour would result in an estimated human exposure to milligram amounts of cycasin per day. It has been suggested that MAM, the aglycone of the cycad carcinogen, cycasin, may react with naturally occurring amino acids to produce derivatives that have neurotoxic properties similar to those of the glutamate agonist, N-methyl-D-aspartate (NMDA) (Kisby, Ellison and Spencer, in press).

Another possible mechanism that could account for cycad toxicity is via the pollen of *Cycas circinalis*; specimens from Guam recently have been found to contain both cycasin and BMAA (L.T. Kurland and A.A. Seawright, unpublished data). Cycad pollens from other parts of the world studied to date contain smaller quantities of BMAA but no cycasin. It is postulated that the pollen could be a mechanism for transporting these toxins to the nasal mucosa and thereby to the nerve fibers, which could carry them to the neurons of the olfactory bulb. From there, it is conceivable that the toxin could affect the entorhinal cortex, the amygdala and hippocampus and other areas of the central nervous system. Olfactory neurons are the only central neurons in direct contact with the external environment. This transport mechanism could explain the serious loss of neurons with neurofibrillary tangle degeneration in the olfactory bulb as well as the hippocampus and other parts of the brain. The loss of odor identification in a large proportion of patients with early PDC and some with early ALS on Guam apparently reflects cell loss in the olfactory bulb (Doty, Perl and Steele, 1991).

It should be noted that, in spite of extensive study, evidence of an association between cycads and motor system dysfunction is limited. Experimental data in support of an association between cycads and ALS/PDC come from feeding experiments by Dastur (1964) and from the work of Spencer *et al.* (1986, 1987b), employing high dietary levels of BMAA. At least two groups have undertaken long-term feeding studies employing unprocessed cycad meal and have been unable to identify any behavioral changes or relevant neuropathology (Sieber *et al.*, 1980; Garruto, Yanagihara and Gajdusek, 1988). Furthermore, there are other regions around the world such as Indochina (Poilane, 1924), India (Bryant, 1783), Malaya (Keng, 1972) and Australia (Maiden, 1897; Harvey, 1945) where cycad seed consumption by humans has been common for centuries, without any reports of increased risk for developing ALS/PDC. However, the process of flour production in these areas generally includes crushing the seed into small particles, which may permit more thorough washing than does the process used on

Guam. Also, studies by Whiting (1963) and those reported by Reed and Brody (1975) showed that over 80% of the Chamorro population had exposure to cycad. Case-control comparisons among Chamorros and Filipino migrants on Guam have not shown a significant difference in this exposure (Reed *et al.*, 1966; Reed and Brody, 1975). The process of soaking the cycad seeds varied greatly so that reconstruction of the history which would indicate levels of exposure to residual cycasin and BMAA is not feasible after so many years.

ALUMINUM HYPOTHESIS

As early as 1961, Kimura *et al.* (1963) reported a high prevalence of ALS in two villages in the Kii Peninsula of Japan and observed that ALS occurred in areas where river and drinking water were low in certain minerals. During the next decade, Yase and colleagues, working in both the Kii Peninsula and on Guam, postulated a possible mechanism involving manganese and other metals in these disorders (Yase, 1972; Yoshimasu *et al.*, 1980). In all three foci, reports of low environmental levels of calcium and high levels of aluminum began to appear (Garruto, Gajdusek and Chen, 1980; Gajdusek and Salazar, 1982; Shiraki and Yase, 1975; Garruto *et al.*, 1984a). However, recent studies on Guam have shown an adequate calcium and magnesium content of water and food grown in the soil of areas such as Umatac, where ALS/PDC is particularly prevalent (Zolan and Ellis-Neill, 1986).

With respect to calcium, Yanagihara *et al.* (1984) reported that serum parathyroid hormone (PTH) levels were mildly elevated in 6 of 16 Guam ALS patients and in 5 of 33 PDC patients. Levels of PTH were related to the mobility status of the patients. Intestinal absorption of calcium was decreased in only 2 of 16 ALS and 4 of 33 PDC patients. Although the authors stated that hypocalcemia was commonly observed among the patients, none of the ALS and PDC patients had serum calcium levels lower than the normal range for Chamorros and laboratory controls. It is likely that the slight changes observed in calcium metabolism were related to the decreased mobility associated with the neurological dysfunction.

Nevertheless, the observations by Kimura *et al.* (1963) and Yanagihara *et al.* (1984) initiated a series of studies on calcium and magnesium deficiency in rabbits and primates. According to these models, it is postulated that chronic deficiency of calcium and magnesium causes secondary hyperparathyroidism with mobilization of calcium and other excess metals (e.g. aluminum) from the bone, leading to motor neuron disease (Yase, 1978). In addition, it has been suggested that parathyroid hormone causes enhanced gastrointestinal absorption of aluminum and deposition in several tissues, including cerebral gray matter (Mayor et al., 1977).

Garruto et al. (1989) have reported the results of a study of the effects of a low-calcium, high-aluminum diet on motor neuron pathology in juvenile cynomolgus monkeys. They found that such an unbalanced diet caused degenerative changes, 'compatible with those of early ALS and Parkinson's disease', in motor neurons of the spinal cord, brainstem, substantia nigra and cerebrum. The neurofibrillary pathology was most frequently seen in animals fed the low-calcium diet supplemented with aluminum and manganese in comparison with the animals fed on a low-calcium diet alone. These findings suggest that aluminum excess may be of greater importance than calcium deficiency alone with respect to neurodegenerative disorders (Garruto, 1991). Moreover, aluminum appears to accumulate in affected nerve cells in concentrations that are more than 200 times higher than normal amounts (300–600 parts per million *vs.* 1–2 parts per million) (Perl et al., 1982, 1986). This has also been noted using advanced laboratory techniques (Perl et al., 1986; Garruto et al., 1984b; Linton et al., 1987; Piccardo et al., 1988). Aluminum has been shown to have neurotoxic effects. Injection of aluminum salts into rabbits and cats (but not mice, rats or monkeys) is reported to produce neurofibrillary tangles (McLachlan, 1986). In addition, high concentrations of aluminum in Alzheimer's neurofibrillary tangles and neuritic plaques have been observed (Perl and Brody, 1980; Candy et al., 1986). However, Markesbery, Lovell and Ehmann (1990), using laser microprobe mass analysis (LAMMA) as described by Perl et al. (1986), examined a large number of neurofibrillary tangle-containing neurons and neurofibrillary tangle-free neurons from former Alzheimer's disease patients. They report 'comparison of the nucleus and cytoplasm of neurofibrillary tangle-containing neurons with neurofibrillary tangle-free neurons revealed no significant difference in aluminum content'. Furthermore, a recent study using nuclear microscopy, a new analytic technique involving million-volt nuclear particles, failed to demonstrate the presence of aluminum in plaque cores in untreated brain tissue from Alzheimer's disease (Landsberg, McDonald and Watt, 1992).

5.7 COMMENT

During the past 40 years, the multidisciplinary study of hyperendemic foci of ALS and PDC in the Western Pacific has led to the recognition of the three major forms of ALS, i.e. sporadic (classical), familial and Western Pacific forms, and has enhanced our understanding of other neurodegenerative disorders such as Parkinson's disease and Alzheimer's disease. However, the elucidation of cause, means of prevention and treatment of ALS, PDC and dementia alone (which may all be clinical variants of a single disease entity) remain elusive. Recent observations of olfactory deficits and disturbances of supranuclear ocular movement in patients with PDC and the possible relationship of a pigmentary retinopathy to ALS/PDC suggest that the spectrum of neurodegenerative disease on Guam is broader than previously recognized.

The incidence of ALS appears to be declining in all three Western Pacific foci (Guam and Rota, the Kii Peninsula of Japan and Irian Jaya in New Guinea). The prevalence of PDC remains high on Guam and Rota. Dementia without parkinsonism is being observed more frequently, especially in the older female population of Guam. The age of onset for both ALS and PDC has increased during the past 30 years. The remarkable changes in age of onset and the character of ALS/PDC strengthen the evidence in favor of an environmental factor in the pathogenesis of these diseases to which exposure may have decreased after the 1940s. Furthermore, migration studies indicate that there is a long latent period between exposure to the exogenous agent(s) and onset of the disease. The long latent period and the uncertainty of the types of environmental exposure have made it difficult to identify a specific etiologic agent. The neurological sequelae of cycad toxicity and aluminum excess are being investigated in animal models. It is also conceivable that environmental factors such as cycad or mineral toxicity acting on a genetically susceptible population may be responsible for the Western Pacific neurodegenerative disorders. However, the fact that the three populations affected appear to be quite dissimilar genetically argues against the concept of a single-gene hypothesis.

In the future, the following areas of research should add a great deal to a better understanding of the Western Pacific neurodegenerative diseases. Effort should be made to carry out intensive general medical, neurological and electrophysiological studies to define precisely the spectrum of neurodegenerative diseases before they disappear. Prompt autopsies will provide tissues for ultrastructural and neurochemical studies. Recent advances in molecular neurosciences involving genetic linkage studies, mitochondrial DNA and respiratory enzyme complex need to be applied to the Guam population. As the genes carrying familial ALS and Alzheimer's dementia both appear to be linked to chromosome 21, there is merit in exploring this with the Guam disease. Alternatively, environmental factors that may adversely affect mitochondrial function resulting in chronic neuronal injury also warrant investigation.

ALS–parkinsonism–dementia complex on Guam

ACKNOWLEDGMENTS

The authors wish to thank Jim Naessens for assistance with statistical analysis and Laura Long for editorial assistance in the preparation of this manuscript.

REFERENCES

Arnold, A., Edgren, D.C. and Palladino, V.S. (1953) Amyotrophic lateral sclerosis: fifty cases observed on Guam. *J. Nerv. Ment. Dis.*, **117**, 135–9.

Blake, N.M., Kirk, R.L., Wilson, S.R. *et al.* (1983) Search for a red cell enzyme or serum protein marker in amyotrophic lateral sclerosis and parkinsonism–dementia of Guam. *Am. J. Med. Genet.*, **14**, 299–305.

Brody, J.A. and Kurland, L.T. (1973) Amyotrophic lateral sclerosis and parkinsonism–dementia in Guam, in *Tropical Neurology* (ed. J.D. Spillane), Oxford University Press, Oxford, pp. 355–74.

Brody, J.A., Edgar, A.H. and Gillespie, M.M. (1978) Amyotrophic lateral sclerosis. No increase among U.S. construction workers in Guam. *J. Am. Med. Assoc.*, **240**, 551–2.

Bryant, C. (1783) *Flora Diaetetica or History of Esculent Plants, Both Domestic and Foreign*, London.

Burnstein, M.H. (1981) Familial amyotrophic lateral sclerosis, dementia, and psychosis. *Psychometrics*, **22**, 151–7.

Campbell, R.J., Steele, J.C., Cox, T.A. *et al.* (1993) Pathologic findings in the retinal pigment epitheliopathy associated with the amyotrophic lateral sclerosis/parkinsonism–dementia complex of Guam. *Ophthalmology*, **100**, 37–42.

Candy, J.M., Klinowski, J., Perry, R.H. *et al.* (1986) Aluminosilicates and senile plaque formation in Alzheimer's disease. *Lancet*, **i**, 354–7.

Charcot, J.M. and Joffroy, A. (1869) Deux cas d'atrophie musculaire progressive. *Arch. Physiol. Norm. Pathol.*, **2**, 354–67 and 629–49.

Chen, K.-M. and Chase, T.N. (1986) Parkinsonism–dementia, in *Handbook of Clinical Neurology*, Vol. 49, *Extrapyramidal Disorders* (eds P.J. Vinken, G.W. Bruyn and H.L. Klawans) Elsevier Science Publishers, Amsterdam, pp. 167–83.

Chen, K.-M., Makifuchi, T., Garruto, R.M. *et al.* (1982) Parkinsonism–dementia in a Filipino migrant: a clinicopathologic case report. *Neurology*, **32**, 1221–6.

Chen, L. (1981) Neurofibrillary change on Guam. *Arch. Neurol.*, **38**, 16–18.

Cox, T.A., McDarby, J.V., Lavine, L. *et al.* (1989) A retinopathy on Guam with high prevalence in Lytico-Bodig. *Ophthalmology*, **96**, 1731–5.

Dastur, D.K. (1964) Cycad toxicity in monkeys: clinical, pathological, and biochemical aspects. *Fed. Proc.*, **23**, 1368–9.

Di Monte, D.A. (1991) Mitochondrial DNA and Parkinson's disease. *Neurology*, **41** (Suppl. 2), 38–42.

Doty, R.L., Perl, D.P. and Steele, J.C. (1991) Odor identification deficit of the parkinsonism–dementia complex of Guam: equivalence to that of Alzheimer's and idiopathic Parkinson's disease. *Neurology*, **41** (Suppl. 2), 77–80.

124

References

Duncan, M.W., Villacreses, N.E., Pearson, P.G. *et al.* (1991) 2-amino-3-(methylamino)-propionic acid (BMAA) pharmacokinetics and blood–brain barrier permeability in the rat. *J. Pharmacol. Exp. Therapeut.*, **258**, 27–35.

Eldridge, R., Ryan, E., Rosario, J. *et al.* (1969) Amyotrophic lateral sclerosis and parkinsonism–dementia in a migrant population from Guam. *Neurology*, **19**, 1029–37.

Gajdusek, D.C. (1984) Environmental factors provoking physiological changes which induce motor neuron disease and early neuronal ageing in high incidence foci in the Western Pacific, in *Research Progress in Motor Neuron Disease* (ed. F.C. Rose), Pitman Books, London, pp. 44–69.

Gajdusek, D.C. and Salazar, A.M. (1982) Amyotrophic lateral sclerosis and parkinsonism syndromes in high incidence among the Auyu and Jakai people of West New Guinea. *Neurology*, **32**, 107–26.

Garruto, R.M. (1991) Pacific paradigms of environmentally-induced neurological disorders: clinical, epidemiological and molecular perspectives. *Neurotoxicology*, **12**, 347–78.

Garruto, R.M. and Yase, Y. (1986) Neurodegenerative disorders of the western Pacific: the search for mechanisms of pathogenesis. *Trends Neurosci.*, **9**, 368–74.

Garruto, R.M., Gajdusek, D.C. and Chen, K.-M. (1980) Amyotrophic lateral sclerosis among Chamorro migrants from Guam. *Ann. Neurol.*, **8**, 612–19.

Garruto, R.M., Gajdusek, D.C. and Chen, K.-M. (1981) Amyotrophic lateral sclerosis and parkinsonism–dementia among Filipino migrants to Guam. *Ann. Neurol.*, **10**, 341–50.

Garruto, R.M., Yanagihara, R. and Gajdusek, D.C. (1985) Disappearance of high-incidence amyotrophic lateral sclerosis and parkinsonism-dementia on Guam. *Neurology*, **35**, 193–8.

Garruto, R.M., Yanagihara, R. and Gajdusek, D.C. (1988) Cycads and amyotrophic lateral sclerosis/parkinsonism dementia. *Lancet*, **ii**, 1079.

Garruto, R.M., Plato, C.C., Myrianthopoulos, N.C. *et al.* (1983) Blood groups, immunoglobulin allotypes and dermatoglyphic features of patients with amyotrophic lateral sclerosis and parkinsonism-dementia of Guam. *Am. J. Med. Genet.*, **14**, 289–98.

Garruto, R.M., Yanagihara, R., Gajdusek, D.C. *et al.* (1984a) Concentrations of heavy metals and essential minerals in garden soil and drinking water in the Western Pacific, in *Amyotrophic Lateral Sclerosis in Asia and Oceania* (eds K.-M. Chen and Y. Yase). National Taiwan University, Taipei, pp. 265–329.

Garruto, R.M., Fukatsu, R., Yanagihara, R. *et al.* (1984b) Imaging of calcium and aluminum in neurofibrillary tangle-bearing neurons in parkinsonism-dementia of Guam. *Proc. Natl. Acad. Sci. USA*, **81**, 1875–9.

Garruto, R.M., Shankar, S.K., Yanagihara, R. *et al.* (1989) Low-calcium, high-aluminum diet-induced motor neuron pathology in cynomolgus monkeys. *Acta Neuropathol.*, **78**, 210–9.

Gass, J.D.M. and Lewis, R.A. (1976) Subretinal tracks in ophthalmomyiasis. *Arch. Ophthalmol.*, **94**, 1500–5.

Goto, S., Hirano, A. and Matsumoto, S. (1990) Immunohistochemical study of the striatal efferents and nigral dopaminergic neurons in parkinsonism–dementia complex of Guam in comparison with those in Parkinson's and Alzheimer's diseases. *Ann. Neurol.*, **27**, 520–7.

Guiroy, D.C., Miyazaki, M., Multhaup, G. *et al.* (1987) Amyloid of neurofibrillary tangles of Guamanian parkinsonism-dementia and Alzheimer disease share an identifiable amino acid sequence. *Proc. Natl. Acad. Sci. USA*, **84**, 2073–7.

Guiroy, D.C., Miyazaki, M., Garruto, R.M. *et al.* (1990) Amyloid of neurofibrillary tangles of Guamanian amyotrophic lateral sclerosis contains low molecular weight proteins. *Ann. Neurol.*, **28**, 228.

Haddock, R.L. (1973) *A History of Health on Guam*, 2nd edn, Cruz Publications, Agana, Guam.

Harvey, A. (1945) Food preservation in Australian tribes. *Mankind*, **3**, 191–2.

Hattori, N., Tanaka, M., Ozawa, T. and Mizuno, Y. (1991) Immunohistochemical studies on complex I, II, III, and IV of mitochondria in Parkinson's disease. *Ann. Neurol.*, **30**, 563–71.

Hirano, A., Malamud, N. and Kurland, L.T. (1961) Parkinsonism–dementia complex, an endemic disease on the island of Guam. II. Pathological features. *Brain*, **84**, 662–79.

Hirano, A., Kurland, L.T., Krooth, R.S. *et al.* (1961) Parkinsonism–dementia complex, an endemic disease on the island of Guam. I. Clinical features. *Brain*, **84**, 642–61.

Hirano, A., Malamud, N., Elizan, T.S. *et al.* (1966) Amyotrophic lateral sclerosis and parkinsonism-dementia complex on Guam. *Arch. Neurol.*, **15**, 35–51.

Hoffman, P.M., Robbins, D.S., Gibbs Jr, C.J. *et al.* (1977) Histocompatibility antigens in amyotrophic lateral sclerosis and parkinsonism–dementia on Guam. *Lancet*, **ii**, 717.

Hudson, A.J. (1981) Amyotrophic lateral sclerosis and its association with dementia, parkinsonism, and other neurological disorders: a review. *Brain*, **104**, 217–47.

Ito, H., Hirano, A., Yen, S.-H. *et al.* Demonstration of β amyloid protein-containing neurofibrillary tangles in parkinsonism–dementia complex on Guam. *Neuropathol. Appl. Neurobiol.* (in press).

Keng, H. (1972) Cycad seeds as food in Malaya. *Malay. Nat. J.*, **25**, 101–3.

Kimura, K., Yase, Y., Higashi, Y. *et al.* (1963) Epidemiological and geomedical studies on amyotrophic lateral sclerosis. *Dis. Nerv. Syst.*, **24**, 155–9.

Kisby, G.E., Ellison, M. and Spencer, P.S. Content of the neurotoxins cycasin (methylazoxymethanol β-D-glucoside and BMAA (β-N-methylamino-L-alanine) in cycad flour prepared by Guam Chamorros. *Ann. Neurol.* (in press).

Koerner, D.R. (1952) Amyotrophic lateral sclerosis on Guam: a clinical study and review of the literature. *Ann. Intern. Med.*, **37**, 1204–20.

Kurland, L.T. (1957) Epidemiologic investigations of amyotrophic lateral sclerosis. 3. A genetic interpretation of incidence and geographic distribution. *Proc. Staff Meet. Mayo Clin.*, **32**, 449–62.

Kurland, L.T. and Mulder, D.W. (1954) Epidemiologic investigations of amyotrophic lateral sclerosis. 1. Preliminary report on geographic distribution, with special reference to the Mariana Islands, including clinical and pathologic observations. *Neurology*, **4**, 355–78 and 438–48.

Kurland, L.T., Hirano, A., Malamud, N. and Lessell, S. (1961) Amyotrophic lateral sclerosis in Guam. *Clin. Neurol.*, **1**, 301–6.

Landsberg, J.P., McDonald, B. and Watt, F. (1992) Absence of aluminium in neuritic plaque cores in Alzheimer's disease. *Nature*, **360**, 65–8.

Lavine, L., Steele, J.C., Wolfe, N. *et al.* (1991) Amyotrophic lateral sclerosis/parkinsonism–dementia complex in southern Guam: Is it disappearing? In *Advances in Neurology*, Vol. 54, *Amyotrophic Lateral Sclerosis and Other Motor Neuron Diseases* (ed. L.P. Rowland). Raven Press, New York, pp. 271–85.

Lepore, F.E., Steele, J.C., Cox, T.A. *et al.* (1988) Supranuclear disturbances of ocular motility in Lytico-Bodig. *Neurology*, **38**, 1849–53.

Linton, R.W., Bryan, S.R., Griffis, D.P. *et al.* (1987) Digital imaging studies of aluminum and calcium in neurofibrillary tangle-bearing neurons using secondary ion mass spectrometry. *Trace Elements Med.*, **4**, 99–104.

McLachlan, D.R. (1986) Aluminum and Alzheimer's disease. *Neurobiol. Aging*, **7**, 525–32.

Maiden, J.H. (1897) Plants reported to be poisonous to stock in Australia. *Agr. Gaz. New South Wales*, **8**, 1–24.

Malamud, N., Hirano, A. and Kurland, L.T. (1961) Pathoanatomic changes in amyotrophic lateral sclerosis on Guam: special reference to the occurrence of neurofibrillary changes. *Arch. Neurol.*, **5**, 401–15.

Markesbery, W.R., Lovell, M.A. and Ehmann, W.D. (1990) Aluminum determination in Alzheimer's disease by laser microprobe mass analysis (abstract). *J. Neuropathol. Exp. Neurol.*, **49**, 317.

Matsumoto, N., Yase, Y. and Yasui, M. (1972) Preliminary survey of motor neuron disease in Ilocos Norte, Philippine Islands. *Wakayama Med. Rep.*, **15**, 181–5.

Matsumoto, S., Hirano, A. and Goto, S. (1990) Ubiquitin-immunoreactive filamentous inclusion in anterior horn cells of Guamanian and non-Guamanian amyotrophic lateral sclerosis. *Acta Neuropathol.*, **80**, 233–8.

Mayor, G.H., Keiser, J.A., Makdani, D. *et al.* (1977) Aluminum absorption and distribution: effects of parathyroid hormone. *Science*, **177**, 1187–9.

Mitsuyama, Y. (1984) Presenile dementia with motor neuron disease in Japan: clinico-pathological review of 26 cases. *J. Neurol., Neurosurg. Psychiatr.*, **47**, 953–9.

Mulder, D.W. and Kurland, L.T. (1954) Amyotrophic lateral sclerosis in Micronesia. *Proc. Staff Meet. Mayo Clin.*, **29**, 666–70.

Mulder, D.W., Kurland, L.T. and Iriarte, L.L.G. (1954) Neurologic diseases on the island of Guam. *U.S. Armed Forces Med. J.*, **5**, 1724–39.

Nunn, P.B., Seelig, M., Zagoren, J.C. *et al.* (1987) Stereospecific acute neuronotoxicity of 'uncommon' plant amino acids linked to human motor-system diseases. *Brain Res.*, **410**, 375–9.

O'Brien, S.J., Roelke, M.E. and Marker, L. (1985) Genetic basis for species vulnerability in the cheetah. *Science*, **227**, 1428–34.

O'Gara, R.W., Brown, J.M. and Whiting, M.G. (1964) Induction of hepatic and renal tumors by topical application of aqueous extract of cycad nut to artificial skin ulcers in mice. Proceedings of the Third Conference on the Toxicity of Cycads. *Fed. Proc.*, **23** (6, Part I), 1383.

Ojeda, V.J., Grainger, K.M.R. and Day, T.J. (1984) Familial motor neuron disease associated with non-specific organic dementia. A clinico-pathological study of a family. *Med. J. Aust.*, **141**, 430–3.

Perl, D.P. and Brody, A.R. (1980) Alzheimer's disease: X-ray spectrometric evidence of aluminum accumulation in neurofibrillary tangle-bearing neurons. *Science*, **208**, 297–9.

Perl, D.P., Gajdusek, D.C., Garruto, R.M. *et al.* (1982) Intraneuronal aluminum accumulation in amyotrophic lateral sclerosis and parkinsonism–dementia of Guam. *Science*, **217**, 1053–5.

Perl, D.P., Munoz-Garcia, D., Good, P.F. *et al.* (1986) Calculation of intracellular aluminum concentration in neurofibrillary tangle (NFT) bearing and NFT-free hippocampal neurons of ALS/parkinsonism–dementia (PD) of Guam using laser microprobe mass analysis (LAMMA). *J. Neuropathol. Exp. Neurol.*, **45**, 379.

Piccardo, P., Yanagihara, R., Garruto, R.M. *et al.* (1988) Histochemical and x-ray microanalytical localization of aluminum in amyotrophic lateral sclerosis and parkinsonism–dementia of Guam. *Acta Neuropathol.*, **77**, 1–4.

Plato, C.C., Cruz, M.T. and Kurland, L.T. (1969) Amyotrophic lateral sclerosis/parkinsonism–dementia complex of Guam: further genetic investigations. *Am. J. Hum. Genet.*, **21**, 133–41.

Plato, C.C., Reed, D.M., Elizan, T.S. *et al.* (1967) Amyotrophic lateral sclerosis/parkinsonism–dementia complex of Guam. IV. Familial and genetic investigations. *Am. J. Hum. Genet.*, **19**, 617–32.

Plato, C.C., Garruto, R.M., Fox, K.M. *et al.* (1986) Amyotrophic lateral sclerosis and parkinsonism–dementia of Guam: a 25-year prospective case–control study. *Am. J. Epidemiol.*, **124**, 643–56.

Poilane, M. (1924) Les cycas d'Indochine. *Rev. de Bot. Appliq. (and d'Agr. coloniale)*, **4**, 472–3.

Polsky, F.I., Nunn, P.B. and Bell, E.A. (1972) Distribution and toxicity of α-amino-β-methylaminopropionic acid. *Fed. Proc.*, **31**, 1473–5.

Reed, D.M. and Brody, J.A. (1975) Amyotrophic lateral sclerosis and parkinsonism–dementia on Guam, 1945–1972. I. Descriptive epidemiology. *Am. J. Epidemiol.*, **101**, 287–301.

Reed, D.M., Torres, J.M. and Brody, J.A. (1975) Amyotrophic lateral sclerosis and parkinsonism–dementia on Guam, 1945–1972. II. Familial and genetic studies. *Am. J. Epidemiol.*, **101**, 302–10.

Reed, D.M., Plato, C.C., Elizan, T. and Kurland, L.T. (1966) The amyotrophic lateral sclerosis/parkinsonism–dementia complex: a ten-year follow-up on Guam. I. Epidemiological studies. *Am. J. Epidemiol.*, **83**, 54–73.

Rodgers-Johnson, P., Garruto, R.M., Yanagihara, R. *et al.* (1986) Amyotrophic lateral sclerosis and parkinsonism-dementia on Guam: a 30-year evaluation of clinical and neuropathological trends. *Neurology*, **36**, 7–13.

Ross, S.M., Seelig, M. and Spencer, P.S. (1987) Specific antagonism of excitotoxic action of 'uncommon' amino acids assayed in organotypic mouse cortical cultures. *Brain Res.*, **425**, 120–7.

Safford, W.E. (1903) Guam and its people. *Am. Anthrop.*, **4** (Oct–Dec), 707–29.

Schmitt, H.P., Emser, W. and Heimes, C. (1984) Familial occurrence of amyotrophic lateral sclerosis, parkinsonism, and dementia. *Ann. Neurol.*, **16**, 642–8.

Shankar, S.K., Yanagihara, R., Garruto, R.M. *et al.* (1989) Immunocytochemical characterization of neurofibrillary tangles in amyotrophic lateral sclerosis and parkinsonism–dementia complex of Guam. *Ann. Neurol.*, **25**, 146–51.

Shiraki, H. and Yase, Y. (1975) Amyotrophic lateral sclerosis in Japan, in *Handbook of Clinical Neurology*, Vol. 22 (eds P.J. Vinken and G.W. Bruyn). Elsevier, New York, pp. 353–419.

Siddique, T., Figlewicz, D.A., Paricak-Vance, M.A. *et al.* (1991) Linkage of a gene causing familial amyotrophic lateral sclerosis to chromosome 21 and evidence of genetic locus heterogeneity. *New Engl. J. Med.*, **324**, 1381–4.

Sieber, S.M., Correa, P., Dalgard, D.W. *et al.* (1980) Carcinogenicity and hepatotoxicity of cycasin and its aglycone methylazoxymethanol acetate in nonhuman primates. *J. Natl. Cancer Inst.*, **65**, 177–89.

Snow, B.J., Peppard, R.F., Guttman, M. *et al.* (1990) Positron emission tomographic scanning demonstrates a presynaptic dopaminergic lesion in lytico-bodig. The amyotrophic lateral sclerosis–parkinsonism–dementia complex of Guam. *Arch. Neurol.*, **47**, 870–4.

Spencer, P.S. (1987) Guam ALS/parkinsonism–dementia: a long-latency neurotoxic disorder caused by 'slow toxin(s)' in food? *Can. J. Neurol. Sci.*, **14**, 347–57.

Spencer, P.S., Ohta, M. and Palmer, V.S. (1987) Cycad use and motor neurone disease in the Kii Peninsula of Japan. *Lancet*, **ii**, 1462–3.

Spencer, P.S., Nunn, P.B., Hugon, J. *et al.* (1986) Motor neurone disease on Guam: possible role of a food neurotoxin. *Lancet*, **i**, 965.

Spencer, P.S., Palmer, V.S., Herman, A. *et al.* (1987a) Cycad use and motor neurone disease in Irian Jaya. *Lancet*, **ii**, 1273–4.

Spencer, P.S., Nunn, P.B., Hugon, J. *et al.* (1987b) Guam amyotrophic lateral sclerosis–parkinsonism–dementia linked to a plant excitant neurotoxin. *Science*, **237**, 517–22.

Strittmatter, W.J. and Appel, S.H. (1990) Alzheimer's disease, in *Current Neurology*, Vol. 10 (ed. S.H. Appel), Year Book Medical Publishers, Chicago, pp. 357–94.

Syralden, P., Nitter, T. and Mehl, R. (1982) Ophthalmomyiasis interna posterior: report of a case caused by the reindeer warble fly larva and review of previous reported cases. *Br. J. Ophthalmol.*, **66**, 589–93.

Tillema, S. and Wynberg, C.J. (1953) 'Endemic' amyotrophic lateral sclerosis on Guam: Epidemiological data, preliminary report. *Doc. Med. Georg. Trop.*, **5**, 366–70.

Torres, J., Iriarte, L.L.G. and Kurland, L.T. (1957) Amyotrophic lateral sclerosis among Guamanians in California. *Calif. Med.*, **86**, 385–8.

Uebayashi, Y. (1980) Epidemiological investigation of motor neuron disease in the Kii Peninsula, Japan, and on Guam: the significance of long survival cases. *Wakayama Med. Rep.*, **23**, 18–27.

Weiss, J.H., Koh, J.–Y. and Choi, D.W. (1989) Neurotoxicity of BMAA and BOAA on cultured cortical neurons. *Brain Res.*, **497**, 64–71.

Whiting, M.G. (1963) Toxicity of cycads. *Econ. Bot.*, **17**, 271–302.

Wikström, J., Paetau, A., Palo, J. *et al.* (1982) Classic amyotrophic lateral sclerosis with dementia. *Arch. Neurol.*, **39**, 681–3.

Yanagihara, R., Garruto, R.M., Gajdusek, D.C. *et al.* (1984) Calcium and vitamin D metabolism in Guamanian Chamorros with amyotrophic lateral sclerosis and parkinsonism–dementia. *Ann. Neurol.*, **15**, 42–8.

Yase, Y. (1972) The pathogenesis of amyotrophic lateral sclerosis. *Lancet*, **ii**, 292–6.

Yase, Y. (1978) The basic process of amyotrophic lateral sclerosis as reflected in Kii Peninsula and Guam. *Proceedings of the 11th World Congress on Neurology. International Congress Series 434* (eds W.A. den Hartog Jager, G.W. Bruyn and A.P.J. Heijstee), Excerpta Medica, Amsterdam, pp. 413–27.

Yoshimasu, F., Yasui, M., Yase, Y. *et al.* (1980) Studies on amyotrophic lateral sclerosis by neutron activation analysis. 2. Comparative study of analytical results on Guam PD, Japanese ALS, and Alzheimer's disease cases. *Psychiat. Neurol. Jap.*, **34**, 75–82.

Zhang, Z.–X., Anderson, D.W., Lavine, L. *et al.* (1990) Patterns of acquiring parkinsonism-dementia complex on Guam: 1944 through 1985. *Arch. Neurol.*, **47**, 1019–24.

Zimmerman, H.M. (1945) *Monthly report to Medical Officer in Command*, U.S. Naval Medical Research Unit No. 2.

Zolan, W.J. and Ellis-Neill, L. (1986) *Technical Report No. 64*, University of Guam.

6 The natural history of amyotrophic lateral sclerosis

BENJAMIN RIX BROOKS, DAVID LEWIS,
JON RAWLING, MOHAMMED SANJAK,
DARYN BELDEN, HISHAM HAKIM,
YAN DE TAN, ROBERT SUFIT,
JAMES GAFFNEY and ROXANNE DEPAUL

6.1 INTRODUCTION

A complete understanding of the natural history of the clinical features of amyotrophic lateral sclerosis (ALS), both in the individual and within a group of affected individuals, is necessary for the optimal conduct of therapeutic trials (Brooks, 1985, 1989). The precise clinical endpoints required to permit statistical planning include determination of (1) the precision of a test measurement; (2) its biological variation over a short time span as a measure of reproducibility; and (3) the population standard deviation of the test measurement at the end of the various sampling periods in order to define sample size, trial duration and mode of statistical analysis (Capildeo and Orgogozo, 1988). We will outline the strategies to be applied when trying to determine the best measures of change in individual patients or groups of patients with ALS over different time periods (Brooks *et al.*, 1986, 1991; Festoff *et al.*, 1988). In addition, we will present preliminary experience with a model trying to predict the future course of ALS by analyzing specific measures over a 3-month period early in the course of the disease.

6.2 SYMPTOM DEVELOPMENT IN ALS

The natural history of motor neuron loss may be described for each individual and for groups of affected individuals by qualitative and quantitative techniques linked to a time scale (Caroscio *et al.*, 1987; Kuther, Struppler and Lipinski, 1987; Munsat, Andres and Skerry, 1989). Symptom accrual may be defined for each individual as clinical changes due to muscle weakness and atrophy that occur after loss of 70–80% of motor neurons. We analyzed the development of paralysis in poliomyelitis patients following onset of fever and pain (Brooks, 1991). We pooled the data from 78 patients with leg onset of poliomyelitis and determined by a modification of life table analysis the rapidity with which poliomyelitis spread to the opposite leg, to either arm or to involve the bulbar structures. Hematogenous spread allows for multi-focal onset in the central nervous system. However, poliovirus inoculated naturally by hematogenous spread or experimentally by direct injection into the central nervous system extends through the nervous system by axonal transport (Jubelt, Narayan and Johnson, 1980). Analysis of data from a large group of patients with leg onset indicates that spread of clinical symptoms in a population of patients shows a gradient from the site of initial involvement. We proceeded to employ this method to analyze the natural history of symptom development in large groups of patients with amyotrophic lateral sclerosis of the Charcot variant and found different rates of symptom accrual depending on the site of onset and the age or gender of the patient.

6.2.1 Natural history of symptom development in ALS

The onset of symptoms in ALS patients occurs when approximately 80% loss of motor neurons is achieved, similar to poliomyelitis. Symptoms due to lower motor neuron loss will accrue according to a function dependent upon the time it takes for motor neuron groups to lose neurons down to the 20% threshold at which symptoms are obvious to the patient (Sobue et al., 1983).

Patients who eventually developed probable or definite ALS by the El Escorial World Federation of Neurology Criteria for the Diagnosis of Amyotrophic Lateral Sclerosis have been followed at the University of Wisconsin ALS Clinical Research Center for up to 7 years. Confirmation of the diagnosis was performed by at least two neurologists following neurological and neurophysiological examinations over several months. A questionnaire was completed on entry to the registry and updated at 18-month intervals by all patients. Complete information on the accrual of bulbar and limb symptoms was available on 702 patients who had completed at least two follow-up questionnaires. The time of symptom development was verified by

1. direct patient interview;
2. medical record review;
3. physician interview; and/or
4. spouse or family member interview.

Statistical analysis was performed by a modification of life table analysis (Kalbfleisch and Prentice, 1980; Lee, 1980; Cox and Oakes, 1984; Friedman, Furberg and DeMets, 1985). Symptom development is a function of the site of onset as well as gender and age of the patient.

6.2.2 Topographical effects on symptom development

LIMB ONSET

The cumulative percentages of ALS patients who develop weakness and atrophy in arms, legs or the bulbar musculature are presented as a function of time following the onset of the first symptoms of ALS in Figure 6.1. Contralateral arm symptom accrual in 174 unilateral leg-onset ALS patients was significantly slower than symptom accumulation in both the opposite leg for 3 years of disease ($P < 0.003$) and the ipsilateral arm for 2 years of disease ($P < 0.03$). Ipsilateral arm symptom accrual in unilateral leg-onset ALS patients was significantly ($P < 0.03$) faster than contralateral arm symptom accrual. The symptom accrual in the opposite arm compared with contralateral leg or ipsilateral leg of 213 unilateral arm onset ALS patients was significantly ($P < 0.001$) faster than bulbar symptom accrual during the first 5 years of disease. In comparison with bulbar symptom accrual, the symptom development in other limbs (opposite leg, ipsilateral arm, and contralateral arm) of ALS patients following unilateral leg onset was significantly faster ($P < 0.04$) for the first 5 years of disease (Brooks et al., 1990, 1991).

BULBAR ONSET

Cranial motor neuron symptom accrual in unilateral arm-onset ALS patients was significantly ($P < 0.04$) faster than bulbar symptom accrual in unilateral leg-onset ALS patients at 2, 3 and 4 years of disease (Figure 6.1). In 96 bulbar ALS patients with speech onset, swallowing symptom accrual was significantly ($P < 0.001$) faster than both arm and leg symptom accrual for the first 4 years of disease. By way of contrast, there was no significant difference in arm symptom accrual compared with leg symptom accrual in bulbar-onset ALS patients. However, limb (arm plus leg) symptom accrual in bulbar-onset ALS patients was significantly ($P < 0.01$) faster than bulbar symptom accrual in unilateral limb (arm or leg) onset ALS patients for 6 years of follow-up. Sample-size determinations for clinical trials based on symptom development are not efficient in terms of time or patients (Fleiss, Tytun and Ury, 1980; Gubbay et al., 1985).

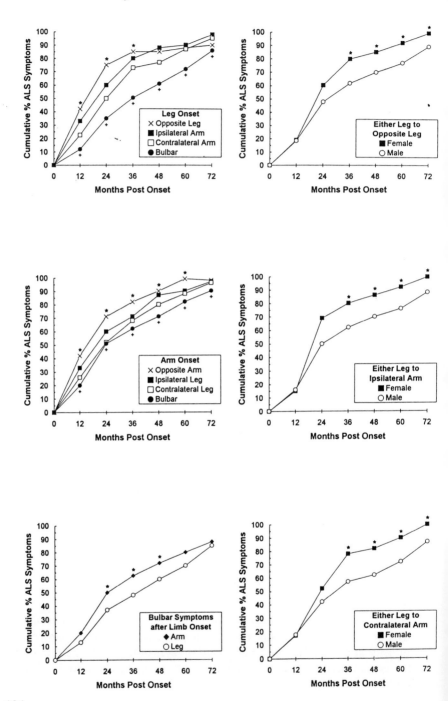

134

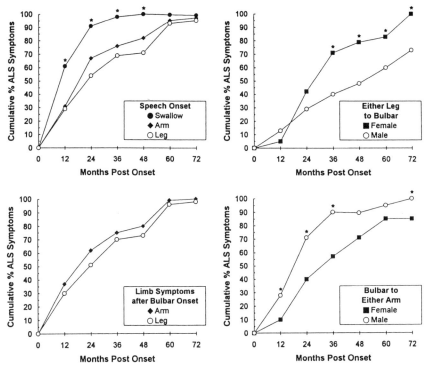

Figure 6.1 Symptom development in sporadic ALS. Symptom development was assessed in 174 unilateral leg-onset, 213 unilateral arm-onset and 96 speech-onset ALS patients in the figures in the left panel. Statistical analysis was performed as described in the text. * Statistically significant change of leg to opposite leg relative to arm, arm to opposite arm relative to leg or speech to swallowing relative to either limb. ⁺ Statistically significant change of bulbar symptom development relative to arm or leg symptom development. Symptom development was assessed in 290 male and 193 female ALS patients in figures in the right panel. Statistical analysis was performed as described in the text. *Statistically significant change of leg to opposite leg, ipsilateral arm, contralateral arm or bulbar musculature in females or bulbar musculature to arm in males.

6.2.3 Gender effects on symptom development

FEMALE EFFECTS

Female ALS patients who had leg onset demonstrated, from the third year onward, a higher proportion of symptom spread to other regions than male ALS patients. Compared with male ALS patients having unilateral leg onset, female patients developed significantly ($P < 0.02$)

increased opposite leg symptoms, increased ipsilateral arm symptoms, increased contralateral arm symptoms and increased bulbar symptoms (Brooks *et al.*, 1991).

MALE EFFECTS

A marked contrast occurs in male ALS patients following bulbar onset. Male ALS patients with bulbar onset manifested significantly ($P < 0.01$) more symptom spread to arms in the first 3 years of disease (Brooks, 1991; Brooks *et al.*, 1991).

6.2.4 Age effects on symptom development

YOUNG ALS

The proportion (25%) of 98 young ALS (yALS) patients with right arm onset is significantly ($P < 0.05$) higher than in older sporadic ALS (oALS) patients (14%), but other sites are not disproportionately represented. The progression of symptoms in the bulbar region following arm or leg onset is identical in young ALS and older sporadic ALS patients. However, symptom progression from the bulbar region or legs to involve the arms or from the arms to involve the legs is significantly faster ($P < 0.005$) in young ALS patients than in older sporadic ALS patients (Figure 6.2) and possibly could correlate with more rapid axonal transport in younger animals (Brooks, 1991).

6.2.5 Symptom development in familial ALS

AUTOSOMAL DOMINANT FAMILIAL ALS

Probands from 57 families with familial ALS (fALS) were studied and compared with sporadic ALS patients. The proportion of patients with bulbar, arm or leg onset was similar in both familial and sporadic ALS (sALS). Symptom development in familial ALS patients who had bulbar or arm onset was identical to that seen in sporadic ALS patients. However, familial ALS patients with leg onset manifested a slower development of symptoms in the opposite leg, the ipsilateral arm or to either arm, than sporadic ALS patients (Figure 6.2).

6.2.6 Mechanisms and neural substrates of symptom spread

These findings suggest that neuronal degeneration occurs within contiguous areas, which are more quickly involved than non-contiguous

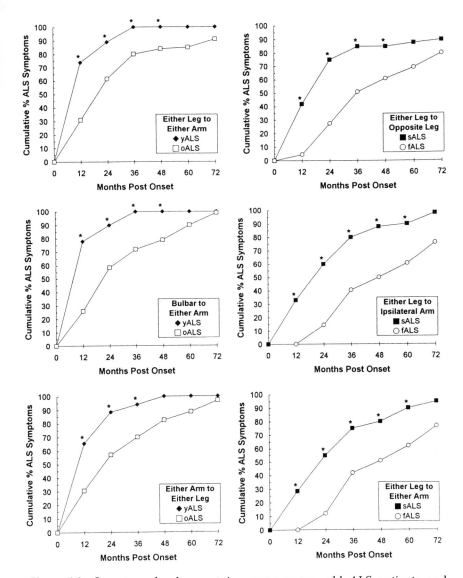

Figure 6.2 Symptom development in young versus old ALS patients and familial ALS. Symptom development was assessed in 98 young ALS patients (< 40 years) compared with 385 old ALS patients (≥ 40 years) in the figures in the left panel. Statistical analysis was performed as described in the text. * Statistically significant change of leg to either arm, bulbar to either arm, or either arm to leg in young ALS patients compared with old ALS patients. Symptom development was assessed in 57 autosomal dominant familial ALS patients compared with 483 sporadic ALS patients in the figures in the right panel. *Statistically significant change of either leg to opposite leg, ipsilateral arm or either leg to either arm in sporadic ALS patients compared with familial ALS patients.

137

The natural history of ALS

areas. The local spread to contiguous areas of motor neuron function is faster in the brainstem and cervical and lumbar regions. The more rapid limb involvement following bulbar onset is more dramatic in males than females. On the other hand, the more rapid onset of opposite leg, either arm or bulbar involvement in females with leg onset raises issues concerning the gender effects on the mode of development of the degeneration. However, these observations do not immediately allow distinction among degenerative, toxic or infectious etiologies as well as possible loss of factors that limit disease expression. The more rapid rostral–caudal versus caudal–rostral involvement might argue for axonal transport rather than diffusion as a possible mechanism, but rapid-onset symmetrical spinal cord anterior horn disease may be mediated by rostral–caudal spread of infectious agents via the central canal (Jackson et al., 1987; Brooks, 1991).

SEGMENTAL AND ROSTRAL–CAUDAL SPREAD

By presenting the course of ALS in this fashion, we can see for the first time that segmental symptom development in an ALS population (arm to contralateral arm, leg to contralateral leg, speech to swallowing) occurs faster and to a greater extent than distal symptom accrual (arm to ipsi- or contralateral leg, leg to ipsi- or contralateral arm, speech to arm or leg) (Tan, Dolan and Brooks, 1988; Brooks, 1991). Moreover, symptom accrual in the spinal cord occurs faster than bulbar symptom accrual in ALS patients with either unilateral arm or leg onset. Furthermore, when bulbar symptom accrual does occur following limb onset, it occurs faster in the second, third and fourth years of disease in patients following unilateral arm onset than in those with unilateral leg onset. In addition, ipsilateral distal spinal cord symptom development (leg to ipsilateral arm; arm to ipsilateral leg) occurs faster in the first 3 years of disease following leg onset but not arm onset. Although caudal–rostral spread within the spinal cord and from the cervical spinal cord to the bulbar region appears faster than rostral–caudal spread within the spinal cord, limb symptom development occurs faster subsequent to bulbar onset than bulbar symptom development following limb onset. At this time, such gradients of symptom development support, more directly, the concept of the spread of a disease process following asymmetric regional onset rather than a simple concept of selective vulnerability (Swash, 1980; Swash et al., 1986). However, in many ALS patients EMG changes may antedate clinical weakness and atrophy, suggesting that symptom accrual is a function of the balance between denervation and reinnervation in a region after the initiation of the disease process (Swash and Ingram, 1988). In this case, spread of

138

disease measured by symptom accrual may reflect loss of one or more factors that limit disease expression in anatomically contiguous regions (contralateral spread before rostral or caudal spread). The loss of disease-limiting factors is equivalent to the spread of inhibitors of these disease-limiting factors as measured by the symptom accrual methodology. Thus, the presence of EMG changes that antedate clinical weakness and atrophy, as well as anatomical evidence of multifocal motor neuron disease loss, suggests that the exact neural substrates for the observed changes need further study correlating the clinical findings antemortem with morphometric studies post mortem (Tsukagoshi *et al.*, 1979; Swash and Ingram, 1988; Swash *et al.*, 1988).

6.3 STRENGTH AND FUNCTION CHANGES IN ALS

The symptom, weakness, and the sign, atrophy, are present in muscles when 80% of the spinal cord motor neurons are lost (Sobue *et al.*, 1983). In order to develop these symptoms and signs, strength will be lost presymptomatically before strength loss is measured by manual muscle testing (John, 1984; Swash and Ingram, 1988; Aitkens *et al.*, 1989). Several clinical centers have systematically measured strength and function changes in ALS patients prior to the development of symptoms documented by classical clinical scales (Sobue *et al.*, 1983; Munsat *et al.*, 1988; Brooks *et al.*, 1992; Munsat, 1992; Ringel *et al.* in press). Muscle strength has been analyzed in comparison with strength in age- and gender-matched control subjects (Brooks *et al.*, 1992) or in comparison with strength in the entire ALS population (Munsat *et al.*, 1988; Brooks *et al.*, 1992; Ringel *et al.*, in press).

6.3.1 Muscle strength in control subjects

Isometric muscle strength was measured in 10 upper extremity and 10 lower extremity muscles in male and female control subjects and compared with literature values (Jones, 1947; Beasley, 1961; Edwards *et al.*, 1977; Montoye and Lamphiear, 1977; Danneskiold-Samsoe *et al.*, 1984; Murray *et al.*, 1985; Bohannon, 1986a; Shaunak *et al.*, 1987; Hall, Froster-Iskenius and Allanson, 1989). Care was taken to minimize fatigue and to maximize effort and reproducibility (Johansson, Kent and Shepard, 1983; Sanjak *et al.*, 1987; Patterson and Baxter, 1988; Fillyaw *et al.*, 1989). Males are stronger than females in absolute strength after the second decade (Figure 6.3). Hamstring strength, in particular, decreases after the fifth decade in both males and females compared with younger subjects. Quadricep strength decreases in females after the second decade.

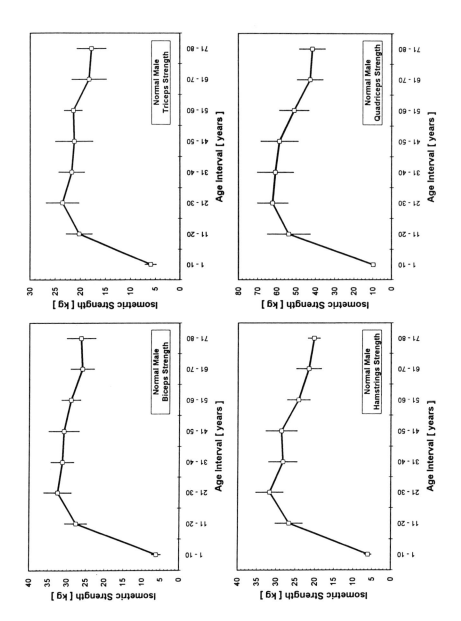

Figure 6.3 Isometric muscle strength in normal males and females as a function of age. Experimentally obtained ($n = 120$) and literature-based measurements ($n = 1586$) were combined when the experimentally measured normative values were shown to overlap literature values. Upper extremity flexors (biceps) and extensors (triceps) muscles are averaged and compared with lower extremity flexors (hamstrings) and extensors (quadriceps). Upper and lower extremity

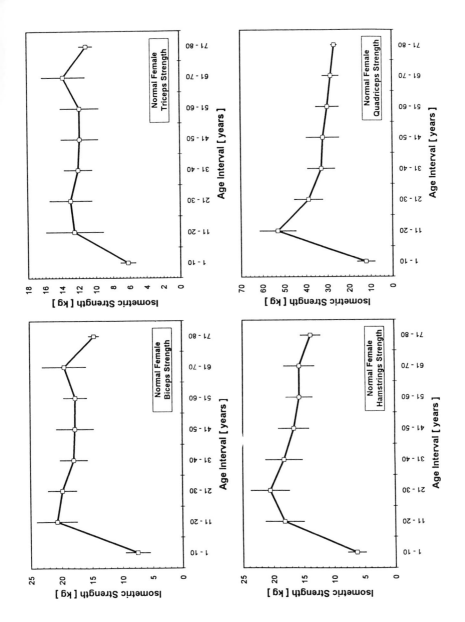

strength is increased in males compared with females after the second decade. Upper extremity strength does not commonly decrease in males and females with aging. Lower extremity strength significantly decreases in males and females after the fifth decade. Lower extremity strength decreases in the female quadriceps significantly after the second decade.

6.3.2 Muscle strength in ALS patients

Isometric muscle strength in ALS patients in the Wisconsin Database ($n = 117$), presented as a percentile of age- and gender-matched control subjects, declines slightly more rapidly in flexors than extensors in both the upper and lower extremities (Figure 6.4). This difference is greatest for the quadriceps and hamstrings but is not statistically significant because of the large population standard deviation (Wiles and Karni, 1983). Hamstring strength correlates best with walking and decreases in parallel with the ability to walk (Sufit et al., 1987; Brooks et al., 1989). The change over time in isometric muscle strength as a percentile of normal shows a dramatic decrease late in the course of the disease when less functioning muscle is available. This accelerated loss late in the disease process correlates best with loss of function because less than 20% of the strength across joints is employed for the functional activity of the joint (Munsat et al., 1988; Munsat, Andres and Skerry, 1989; Kelly et al., 1990).

Isometric muscle strength, presented as individual arm and leg megascore plots as a function of time after onset of disease in the Wisconsin Database ($n = 117$), indicates that the absolute amount of strength does not automatically determine the length of follow-up (Figure 6.5). In addition, the change in arm and leg megascore over time is not perfectly linear in all patients but may have inflection points at the beginning of isometric strength loss after prolonged stable strength. In addition, strength may show transient increases for variable periods. A second inflection point may occur when the muscles are weakest and can demonstrate very little change. The length of follow-up is not a function of the site of onset (bulbar, arm or leg). Overall, however, the slope of the loss of arm or leg strength for the population of ALS patients is best described by a linear regression slope (Figure 6.6). Individual rates of arm and leg strength loss may not be ideally linear but may approximate linear change. When the least-squares regression linear slope of strength loss in the arms or legs is plotted for individuals as a function of time after onset of disease, it is apparent that the rate of loss is quite stable within a broad range after the first year of disease. Within the first year of diagnosis there is a much wider range of rate of loss than after the first year (Figure 6.6). The rate of arm strength loss occurs within a slightly narrower range than the rate of leg strength loss.

6.3.3 Strength–function relationships in ALS patients

Presymptomatic changes in strength and function in ALS patients have been studied over periods as short as 6–12 months and as long as 12–48 months. In the following section information is presented on the

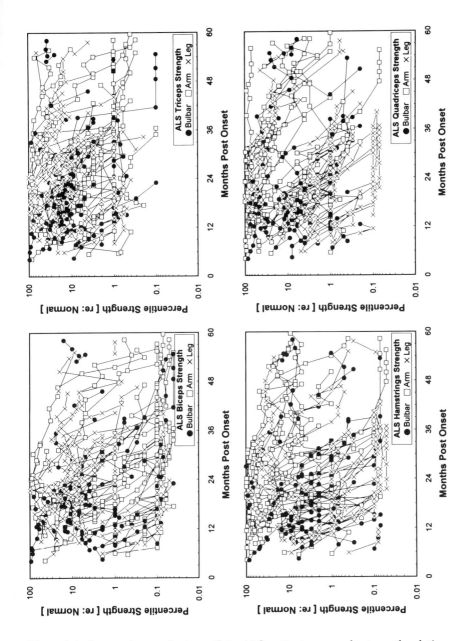

Figure 6.4 Isometric muscle strength in ALS patients – muscle strength relative to normal subjects. Biceps, triceps, hamstrings and quadriceps muscle strength is transformed as a percentile of the age and gender-matched control database (see Figure 6.3). Muscle strength is presented logarithmically to accentuate the rapid decline in muscle strength near the terminal phase of ALS in patients with bulbar, arm or leg onset.

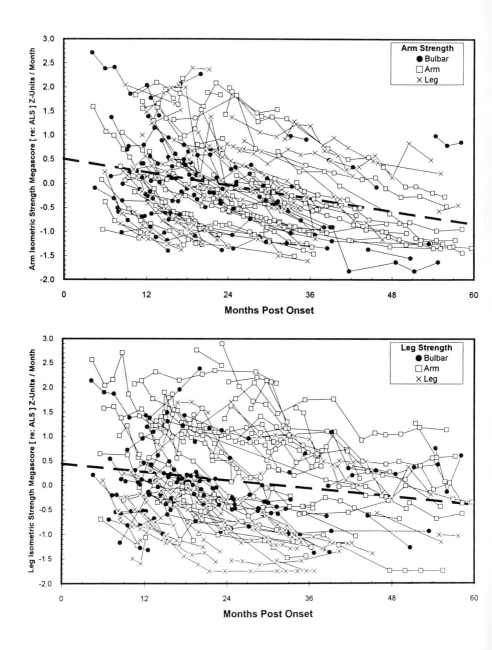

Figure 6.5 Isometric muscle strength in ALS patients – arm and leg megascores relative to ALS population. Arm and leg megascores for Wisconsin ALS patients (*n* = 117) plotted as a function of the site of onset (bulbar, arm or leg) and time after onset of disease that the patient was studied.

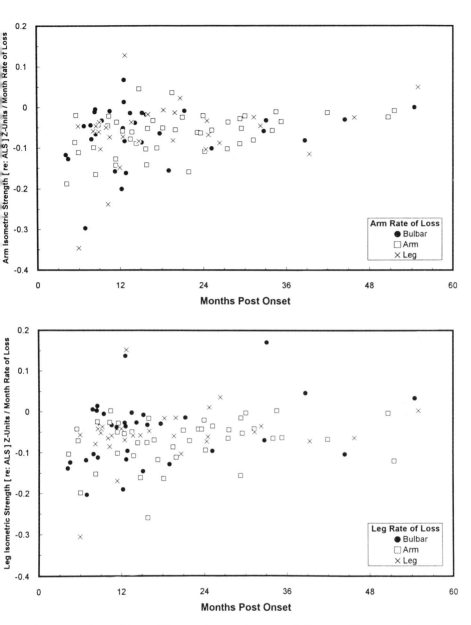

Figure 6.6 Rate of loss of isometric muscle strength (arm and leg megaslopes). Arm and leg megaslopes for Wisconsin ALS patients (*n* = 117) plotted individually at the first time point that the patient was tested following the onset of disease. Note that rate varies most widely in the first year of disease (incident cases) compared with the relatively stable rate after the first year of disease. Bulbar-onset disease patients show a wide range of observed rate of decline throughout the follow-up course compared with arm-onset patients.

significant changes that may occur in ALS patients over the short study period. We have:

1. determined the change in strength and function longitudinally over time in a carefully defined population of ALS patients;
2. correlated strength with function cross-sectionally over the entire studied ALS population;
3. correlated changes in strength with changes in function longitudinally over time in individuals within the studied ALS population;
4. assessed the role of laterality (right vs. left) in strength and function both cross-sectionally and longitudinally over time;
5. assessed the role of rostral–caudal relationships (upper extremity vs. lower extremity) in strength and function cross-sectionally and longitudinally over time;
6. defined the most sensitive independent measures of strength and function that may be used clinically in short therapeutic trials of new drugs.

TEST PROCEDURES

Strength and function were tested as previously described (Elkins, Leden and Wakim, 1951; Andres, Skerry and Munsat, 1989; Amundsen, 1990a,b). Fixed isometric dynamometry was used for all strength testing (Brooks et al., 1991). Hand grip strength was measured with a Jamar dynamometer (Schmidt and Toews, 1970; Mathiowetz, Wiemer and Federman, 1986; Niebuhr and Maraion, 1987; Mathiowetz, 1990). Forced vital capacity (FVC) as a measure of pulmonary function was assessed with a Respiradyne respirometer (Braun, 1987). Timed repetition of 'pa', 'pata', 'pepper' and 'ticker' was used as a measure of bulbar function (Dworkin and Aronson, 1986; DePaul and Abbs, 1987; DePaul et al., 1988). The Purdue pegboard test was used for distal upper extremity function. Timed rapid alternation of the forearm from pronation to supination was used to test proximal upper extremity function. Tests for proximal leg function included a timed sit to stand, 15-foot walk and 360° turn. Distal leg function was tested by measuring the rate of foot tapping by the seated patient.

Z-TRANSFORMATION AND MEGASCORE FORMULATION

Statistical analysis was performed on a DEC Station using SAS version 6.07. All raw values were converted to Z-scores (Andres et al., 1988; Munsat et al., 1988; Finison, 1989):

$$Z = \frac{\text{raw score} - \text{population mean of score}}{\text{population standard deviation of score}}$$

We concluded that our sample population in the short study period was not statistically different from a typical ALS patient population in the Wisconsin Database ($n = 117$) or the combined University of Wisconsin–University of Colorado (WICO) ALS Natural History Database ($n = 253$) by comparing demographic characteristics or the means and standard deviations of isometric muscle testing data of our sample population (Brooks *et al.*, 1992). We therefore used the means of the larger data set when calculating Z-scores for the isometric muscle tests. For tests for which we had no values from the larger data set, we used the means and standard deviations of our data set. Megascores were obtained by averaging composite Z-scores of anatomically related measurements (arm, leg, proximal and/or distal upper and/or lower extremities). The megascores were analyzed cross-sectionally (csa) for the entire studied population independently of time. Megaslopes (slopes) were calculated for each patient by least-squares linear regression of megascore values over time. Megaslopes were analyzed in order to perceive differences in strength–function relationships within individual patients over time and the entire studied population over time. The statistical level of significance chosen was a two-sided *t*-test with $P < 0.05$. Corrected for multiple comparisons by the Bonferroni technique, this level of statistical significance became $P < 0.001$ (Lewis *et al.*, in press).

6.3.4 Strength changes over time

All measures of strength in muscles innervated by motor neurons at the level of the cervical spinal cord decreased significantly ($P < 0.001$) over the 6 ± 3 months period of follow-up (Table 6.1). Of all the measures of strength in muscles innervated by motor neurons at the level of the lumbosacral spinal cord, only ankle dorsiflexion was shown to decrease significantly over the time period studied ($P < 0.001$). Isometric muscle strength in jaw, lip and tongue muscles has demonstrated hierarchical involvement in ALS patients, with tongue strength being much less than lip strength relative to age- and gender-matched control subjects (Dworkin, 1980; Dworkin, Aronson and Mulder, 1980; DePaul *et al.*, 1988). In the short-term study, bulbar musculature isometric strength did not change significantly during the follow-up period.

6.3.5 Function changes over time

No measure of upper extremity function was found to decrease significantly over the time period studied. Of all measures of lower extremity function, only the timed 15-foot walk decreased significantly over the period of study ($r^2=0.059$, $P < 0.0005$). Bulbar function, which

Table 6.1 Correlation of measures with months on study

Variable	P-value	r^2	Variable	P-value	r^2
Ankle dorsiflexion	0.0001	**0.1402**	Elbow flexion	0.0001	**0.0873**
Knee extension	0.0101	0.0383	Ticker	0.6824	0.0020
Hip flexion	0.0062	0.0433	Pa	0.3115	0.0053
FVC	0.0083	0.0562	Pata	0.9342	0.0000
Right pegboard	0.0135	0.0312	Right grip	0.0005	**0.0700**
Left pegboard	0.0078	0.0363	Left grip	0.0001	**0.1150**
Walking	0.0005	**0.0591**	Left shoulder extension	0.0001	**0.1010**
Right Ram	0.1514	0.0225	Right shoulder extension	0.0002	**0.0765**
Left Ram	0.1195	0.0259	Left elbow flexion	0.0001	**0.1217**
Right Tap	0.0715	0.0377	Right elbow flexion	0.0037	0.0487
Left Tap	0.0750	0.0364	Right ankle dorsiflexion	0.0001	**0.1042**
Stand	0.0147	0.0665	Left ankle dorsiflexion	0.0001	**0.1530**
Turn clockwise	0.0317	0.0514	Right knee extension	0.0079	0.0408
Turn anticlockwise	0.0084	0.1069	Left knee extension	0.0208	0.0310
Pegboard	0.0083	0.0356	Right Hip flexion	0.0043	0.0470
RAM	0.0962	0.0295	Left Hip flexion	0.0154	0.0340
Left Prox	0.0072	0.1334	Leg c dorsiflexion	0.0001	**0.0916**
Papata	0.8155	0.0003	Leg s dorsiflexion	0.0063	0.0431
Pepper-ticker	0.4564	0.0062	Hand grip	0.0001	**0.0985**
Bulbar	0.9569	0.0000	Shoulder extension	0.0001	**0.0956**
Pepper	0.3384	0.0103			

Significant findings are in bold ($P < 0.001$).

has been shown to decline at a slower rate than arm and leg function, did not decrease significantly over the time period studied. In the short-term study, FVC did not change significantly during the follow-up period.

6.3.6 Correlations of strength and function

In the cervical region, strength was found to correlate with function, both proximally and distally, for cross-sectional analysis (csa) ($P < 0.0001$, $P < 0.0001$) but not for analysis by slopes ($P < 0.2242$, $P < 0.3424$) (Table 6.2). Proximal upper extremity (pUE) strength correlated with distal upper extremity (dUE) strength both cross-sectionally ($P < 0.0001$) and by slopes ($P < 0.0001$) (Table 6.3). Proximal upper extremity function correlated with distal upper extremity function cross-

Table 6.2 Strength–function correlations (r^2)

	Strength			
	pUE	*dUE*	*pLE*	*dLE*
Function				
pUE				
csa	**0.4751**			
Slopes	0.0022			
dUE				
csa		**0.6619**		
Slopes		0.0301		
pLE				
csa			**0.2619**	
Slopes			0.0258	
dLE				
csa				**0.3118**
Slopes				0.1865

Significant findings are in bold ($P < 0.001$).

Table 6.3 Regional strength and function correlations (r^2)

	Strength			Function	
	dUE	*dLE*		*dUE*	*dLE*
pUE			pUE		
csa	**0.7139**		csa	**0.5954**	
Slopes	**0.5960**		Slopes	0.1403	
pLE			pLE		
csa		**0.4335**	csa		**0.7603**
Slopes		**0.9149**	Slopes		0.0498

Significant findings are in bold ($P < 0.001$).

ectionally ($P < 0.0001$) but not by slopes ($P < 0.0714$) (Table 6.3). All measures of strength in the cervical region correlated significantly with strength of the contralateral limb both cross-sectionally ($P < 0.0001$) and for slopes ($P < 0.0001$) except for grip, which was not significant by slopes ($P < 0.0454$) (Table 6.4). Both proximal and distal arm function correlated cross-sectionally with function of the contralateral limb ($P < 0.0001$). However, only proximal arm function correlated for analysis by slopes ($P < 0.0001$) (Table 6.5).

In the lumbosacral region, strength was found to correlate with function, both proximally and distally, for cross-sectional analysis ($P < 0.0001$) but not for analysis by slopes ($P < 0.26$, $P < 0.19$) (Table 6.2).

Table 6.4 Strength laterality correlations (r^2)

| | Right | | | |
	pUE	*dUE*	*pLE*	*dLE*
Left				
pUE				
csa	**0.7558**			
Slopes	**0.7668**			
dUE				
csa		**0.6232**		
Slopes		0.1269		
pLE				
csa			**0.8242**	
Slopes			0.2311	
dLE				
csa				**0.6171**
Slopes				**0.7140**

Significant findings are in bold ($P < 0.001$).

Table 6.5 Function laterality correlations (r^2)

| | Right | | | |
	pUE	*dUE*	*pLE*	*dLE*
Left				
pUE				
csa	**0.7903**			
Slopes	**0.4166**			
dUE				
csa		**0.7584**		
Slopes		0.0139		
pLE				
csa			**0.9125**	
Slopes			**0.5700**	
dLE				
csa				**0.6893**
Slopes				**0.6102**

Significant findings are in bold ($P < 0.001$).

Proximal lower extremity strength correlated with distal lower extremity strength for both cross-sectional analysis ($P < 0.0001$) and for analysis by slopes ($P < 0.001$). Proximal lower extremity function correlated with distal lower extremity function cross-sectionally ($P < 0.0001$), but not by

Table 6.6 Rostral–caudal strength and function correlations (r^2)

	Strength			Function	
	pLE	*dLE*		*pLE*	*dLE*
pUE			pUE		
csa	**0.2194**	**0.4426**	csa	**0.1716**	**0.1466**
Slopes	**0.8605**	**0.7409**	Slopes	0.0163	0.4172
dUE			dUE		
csa	**0.1025**	**0.4777**	csa	0.0383	0.1047
Slopes	**0.3760**	0.2931	Slopes	0.0748	0.1602

Significant findings are in bold ($P < 0.001$).

slopes ($P < 0.4430$) (Table 6.3). Distal leg function correlated with distal function of the contralateral limb both cross-sectionally ($P < 0.0001$) and for slopes ($P < 0.0001$) (Table 6.4).

Proximal upper extremity strength correlated significantly with proximal and distal lower extremity strength both cross-sectionally ($P < 0.0001$) and by slopes ($P < 0.0001$). Distal upper extremity strength correlated significantly with proximal lower extremity strength both cross-sectionally ($P < 0.0001$) and by slopes ($P < 0.001$). Distal upper extremity strength correlated with distal lower extremity strength cross-sectionally ($P < 0.0001$) but not by slopes ($P < 0.002$). Proximal upper extremity function correlated with proximal lower extremity function cross-sectionally ($P < 0.0001$), but not by analysis of slopes ($P < 0.55$). Distal upper extremity function did not correlate with distal lower extremity function cross-sectionally ($P < 0.063$) or by slopes ($P < 0.065$). Bulbar function correlated cross-sectionally with only proximal arm function ($P < 0.001$) and with no other functional measurement by slopes (Table 6.6).

Previous quantitative studies of ALS have analyzed the relationship between strength and function in different CNS regions strictly on a cross-sectional basis (Andres *et al.*, 1986, 1987, 1988; Munsat *et al.*, 1988; Munsat, Andres and Skerry, 1989; Munsat, 1992; Ringel *et al.*, in press). Some functional tests have been excluded from further analysis on the basis that they added no new information to existing groups of functional and isometric tests. While many test items may correlate cross-sectionally when followed in individuals over time, the change in Z-score may not correlate with strength and function. For example, in our study the pegboard test was strongly correlated with a high significance to grip cross-sectionally ($P < 0.0001$, $r = 0.6619$). However, when slopes were analyzed this correlation disappeared ($P = 0.3424$, $r = 0.0301$).

The natural history of ALS

In the clinical arena, monitoring the disease status of patients is done most thoroughly and efficiently by testing only independent measures. Employing this method of analysis of individual slopes in the short-term Wisconsin ALS population identified the following variables as independent over the time period studied:

- strength and function at all anatomical locations;
- function between different sites on the same limb;
- distal function between right upper extremity and left;
- function between upper and lower limbs;
- distal strength between right upper extremity and left;
- proximal strength between right lower extremity and left;
- distal strength between upper and lower limbs.

6.3.7 Sample size determinations with different megascore formulations

In therapeutic trials of new drugs, it is preferable to analyze measures that decline the most rapidly in order to obtain the highest sensitivity (Lachin, 1981; Shafer and Olarte, 1982; Schoenberg, 1984; Brooks *et al.*, 1987, 1990, 1991; Miller, 1989a,b). However, it is also necessary to ensure specificity by eliminating false improvements of function or strength (De Boer, Boukes and Sterk, 1982; Bohannon, 1986; Agre *et al.*, 1987). In the past, independent measures of strength and function have been combined into megascores in an attempt to eliminate over-recognition of chance improvements in strength or function. This, in effect, is sacrificing sensitivity for specificity. Ideally, a single measurement could be found that decreases both rapidly and consistently. The combination of a sensitive and specific measure of disease status allows for efficiency in design of procedures to test new therapeutic modalities.

In the Wisconsin Database ($n = 117$), arm and leg megascores plotted over time by patient (Figure 6.5) indicate a wide variability in the individual change in strength over time. The mean slope of the group of individual values averaged over specific intervals [-0.02 ± 0.09 (standard deviation) Z units/month] declines much less rapidly than the mean of individual slopes averaged over the same time period (Table 6.7). Individual rates of decline in arm and leg megascores (megaslopes) are relatively stable over a broad range of values 12 months after the onset of disease (Figure 6.6). The early wider variability of rates of decline as a function of time studied after disease onset is a particularly important variable in clinical trials that may enter variable numbers of new or incident cases compared with prevalent cases (Ringel *et al.*, in press). Using analysis by standardized difference, we identified sensitive and specific measures of patient status in different formula-

Table 6.7 Megaslope rate of strength loss (Z units/month ± SD) in ALS patients employing megaslopes derived from different muscle combinations in arm and leg according to site of onset of disease

Muscle combinations	Site of onset			
	Arm (n = 51)	Leg (n = 32)	Bulbar (n = 34)	All (n = 117)
Ten muscles				
Arm$_{WICO}$	−0.059 ± 0.048	−0.068 ± 0.096	−0.068 ± 0.070	−0.064 ± 0.070
Arm$_{Tufts}$	−0.070 ± 0.058	−0.081 ± 0.120	−0.083 ± 0.084	−0.077 ± 0.087
Leg$_{WICO}$	−0.060 ± 0.058	−0.061 ± 0.075	−0.041 ± 0.069	−0.055 ± 0.067
Leg$_{Tufts}$	−0.070 ± 0.058	−0.081 ± 0.120	−0.083 ± 0.084	−0.077 ± 0.087
Six muscles				
Arm$_{WICO}$	−0.059 ± 0.050	−0.074 ± 0.118	−0.066 ± 0.072	−0.066 ± 0.070
Arm$_{Tufts}$	−0.071 ± 0.063	−0.089 ± 0.151	−0.082 ± 0.088	−0.079 ± 0.102
Leg$_{WICO}$	−0.060 ± 0.055	−0.052 ± 0.068	−0.050 ± 0.083	−0.058 ± 0.068
Leg$_{Tufts}$	−0.078 ± 0.065	−0.061 ± 0.081	−0.059 ± 0.096	−0.068 ± 0.079
One muscle				
Handgrip$_{WICO}$	−0.044 ± 0.064	−0.081 ± 0.159	−0.073 ± 0.085	−0.063 ± 0.106
Handgrip$_{Tufts}$	−0.063 ± 0.094	−0.116 ± 0.229	−0.108 ± 0.127	−0.091 ± 0.155
Dorsiflexion$_{WICO}$	−0.074 ± 0.109	−0.015 ± 0.068	−0.053 ± 0.129	−0.052 ± 0.105
Dorsiflexion$_{Tufts}$	−0.079 ± 0.117	−0.016 ± 0.072	−0.057 ± 0.138	−0.056 ± 0.112

tions of arm and leg megascores comprising distal muscles alone, four proximal muscles and distal muscles or nine proximal muscles and distal muscles (Brooks *et al.*, 1992; Lewis *et al.*, in press).

6.3.8 Megaslopes comprising different muscle combinations

The sensitivity of single distal muscles to change over time is not as good as that of combinations of proximal and distal muscles. The standard deviation decreases as increasing numbers of muscles are combined, but the maximal efficiency is achieved after six muscles are combined (Lewis *et al.*, in press; Ringel *et al.*, in press). The efficiency is not apparent in the megaslopes. We compared the arm and leg megaslopes determined with the Tufts ALS standard population (n = 176; 20 ± 13 months of observation) and the combined University of Wisconsin–University of Colorado (WICO) ALS standard population (n = 253; 11 ± 8 months of observation). The most important determinant of the efficiency is the standard deviation of the megaslope of strength loss. Strength loss in the arms and legs is not statistically different regardless of which muscle combinations or databases are employed. However, the sample size required to demonstrate a 30% slowing of the rate of progression of strength loss in ALS patients is markedly decreased by employing

Table 6.8 Sample size required for each treatment group to detect a 30% reduction ($\alpha \leq 0.05$, $1-\beta = 0.80$) in the rate of strength loss by ALS patients employing megaslopes derived from different muscle combinations in arm and leg according to site of onset of disease

	Site of onset			
Muscle combinations	Arm (n = 51)	Leg (n = 32)	Bulbar (n = 34)	All (n = 117)
Ten muscles				
Arm$_{WICO}$	116	352	187	213
Arm$_{Tufts}$	123	386	180	225
Leg$_{WICO}$	165	270	510	258
Leg$_{Tufts}$	169	265	456	251
Six muscles				
Arm$_{WICO}$	129	440	209	266
Arm$_{Tufts}$	138	498	202	287
Leg$_{WICO}$	122	308	493	241
Leg$_{Tufts}$	123	309	468	238
One muscle				
Handgrip$_{WICO}$	381	678	233	498
Handgrip$_{Tufts}$	391	679	243	502
Dorsiflexion$_{WICO}$	383	3411	1028	698
Dorsiflexion$_{Tufts}$	382	3396	1021	696

multiple muscles in the megaslope determinations (Table 6.8). Moreover, the site of onset also affects sample-size requirement. Arm-onset patients as a group have a smaller standard deviation for the determined megaslope and require a smaller sample size to show clinically significant effects. The effect of site of onset was not apparent in the smaller studies previously published (Munsat *et al.*, 1988; Munsat, 1992).

6.3.9 Effect of database size on sample-size calculations

The mean of the individual megaslope of isometric strength loss is particularly robust, particularly in the combination of arm muscles derived from the cervical region of the spinal cord. To test what errors could occur by studying smaller groups of patients for short periods of time compared with the Wisconsin Database ($n = 117$), we calculated the sample size required to demonstrate a 30% decrease in the rate of decline of arm and leg strength in ALS patients over a 6-month period using the original Wisconsin Database ($n = 117$) and the new short-term database studied for 6 ± 3 (standard deviation) months ($n = 37$). The sample-size calculations based on the arm megaslope mean and

Table 6.9 Sample size required for each treatment group to detect a 30% reduction ($\alpha \leq 0.05$, $1-\beta = 0.80$) in the rate of strength loss by ALS patients employing megaslopes derived from six muscles in arm and leg according to length of natural history observation period

	12 ± 10 months[a] (n = 117)	6 ± 3 months (n = 37)
Six muscles		
Arm$_{WICO}$	266	322
Leg$_{WICO}$	241	966

[a] Length of observation period employed to define megaslopes.

Table 6.10 Megaslope rate of strength loss (Z units/month ± SD) of arm and leg in incident and prevalent ALS patients

	< 12 months[a] (n = 37)	≥ 12 months (n = 70)
Six muscles		
Arm$_{WICO}$	-0.099 ± 0.089*	-0.047 ± 0.052
Leg$_{WICO}$	-0.079 ± 0.072*	-0.043 ± 0.61

* $P < 0.0005$.
[a] Time that patient began isometric testing after onset of ALS.

standard deviation are only slightly affected by the change in sample size and period of observation (Table 6.9). The leg megaslope mean and standard deviation result in sample-size estimates that are not in keeping with the larger database. Therefore the arm megaslope is quite robust but the leg megascore is not. Thus, historical databases may be subject to biases owing to differences in the number of patients and the proportion of patients with different sites of disease onset. These different biases may not affect the slope of disease-induced loss of muscle strength but will affect population standard deviations that will be used to calculate sample sizes for clinical trials.

6.3.10 Effect of time after onset that isometric strength is measured on sample-size calculations

The rate of strength loss is significantly greater in the arm ($P < 0.0001$) and the leg ($P < 0.0005$) of ALS patients studied within the first 12 months of onset than in patients studied after the first 12 months of disease (Table 6.10). The marked increase in the rate of strength loss is

The natural history of ALS

Table 6.11 Sample size required for each treatment group to detect a 30% reduction ($\alpha \leq 0.05$, $1-\beta = 0.80$) in the rate of strength loss by ALS patients employing megaslopes derived from six muscle combinations in arm and leg according to time after onset of ALS that patient natural history is measured

	< 12 months (n = 37)	≥ 12 months (n = 70)
Six muscles		
Arm$_{WICO}$	142	215
Leg$_{WICO}$	146	352

associated with a marked increase in the standard deviation of this measurement for the population. Nevertheless, patients studied in the first 12 months of disease will permit a marked efficiency in sample size for both arm and leg strength loss (Table 6.11). After 12 months measuring the rate of strength loss in the arms the required sample size increases by only 50%, while measuring the rate of strength loss in the legs increases the required sample size by 141%.

6.4 PREDICTING THE COURSE OF ALS

The Wisconsin Database was employed to develop a test of the description of the course of ALS by the following parameters:

- slope of simple average of all arm muscles in kg;
- slope of simple average of all leg muscles in kg;
- slope of mega Z-score for arm muscles based on standard (Tufts) ALS population;
- slope of mega Z-score for leg muscles based on standard (Tufts) ALS population;
- slope of mega Z-score for arm muscles based on gender- and age-controlled population;
- slope of mega Z-score for leg muscles based on gender- and age-controlled population;
- slope of simple average of percentile strength based on gender- and age-controlled population of arm muscles;
- slope of simple average of percentile strength based on gender- and age-controlled population of leg muscles.

The hypothesis to be tested was whether the course of ALS in the first 3 months of measurement could predict those patients who would have a fast decline over the entire period studied. One published study eliminated the slopes of patients who did not show decline over the period studied and the slopes of those patients who had already lost significant amounts of strength and would not decline further (Munsat et al., 1988). This study has been used inappropriately to imply that historical controls may be used in phase II and possibly phase III clinical therapeutic trials in ALS patients. We did not exclude any megascores in the model described here.

The data set was derived from the raw strength measurements at each time point for 10 muscles (right and left) in the arms and legs (shoulder extensor, flexor; arm extensor, flexor; hand grip; hip extensor, flexor; leg extensor, flexor; ankle dorsiflexor). The derived data at each time point include the following:

- derived simple averages of the kg strength over the limbs (right and left arm; right and left leg) at each time point;
- Z_{ALS} megascores based on an ALS standard population (right and left arm; right and left leg) at each time point;
- Z_{Con} megascore based on an age- and gender-matched population (right and left arm; right and left leg) at each time point;
- derived simple averages of the strength percentiles of age- and gender-matched normals (right and left arm; right and left leg) at each time point.

6.4.1 Least-squares overall slope determination

These simple averages of kilogram isometric strength, mega Z-scores of isometric strength and simple averages of isometric percentage over time were used to obtain a linear estimate by the least-squares method of the slope of change in each of these measures in the arms or the legs for each patient:

- slope [simple average of kg strength change per month per limb (averaged over right and left limbs)] over the entire period of study;
- slope [mean Z_{ALS} score strength change per month per limb (transformed over right and left limbs based on standard ALS population] over the entire period of study;
- slope [mean Z_{Con} score strength change per limb (transformed over right and left limbs) change per month based on gender- and age-controlled population] over the entire period of study;
- slope [simple average of percentile strength per month per limb (averaged over right and left limbs) per month based on gender- and age-controlled population] over the entire period of study.

6.4.2 Simple average slope in 3-month periods

In addition, the simple averages of the slopes in 3-month periods were calculated for each measure:

- mean kg strength change per limb (averaged over right and left limbs) per month over 3 months;
- mean Z_{ALS} score strength per limb (transformed over right and left limbs) change per month over 3 months;
- mean Z_{Con} score strength per limb (transformed over right and left limbs) change per month over 3 months;
- mean percentile strength per limb (averaged over both limbs) per month over 3 months.

6.4.3 Derived slopes

The overall slopes derived by the least-squares method and the 3-month slopes derived by simple averaging were placed in the final data set for analysis with demographic data including age at testing, gender, months of disease prior to testing, months that the patient had been followed for testing, maximal average percentile strength in first 3 months of testing in arms or legs. Descriptive statistics of the above measures as well as other demographic data were prepared for the entire combined data set, males and females separately, fast decliners described by the Z_{ALS} megascore slope over the entire study and fast decliners defined by the simple average of the Z_{ALS} megascore in the first 3-month study period (Table 6.12). Both unweighted and weighted (by month of follow-up) linear regressions of the data were prepared using SAS ASSIST on a Digital DEC 5 000/200 workstation employing SAS version 6.07.

6.4.4 Descriptive statistics

The following variables were analyzed:

Age   years
MOI   maximum months in study
MOO   months of disease prior to start of study
SZALS_A   overall slope of Z_{ALS} arm score
SZALS_L   overall slope of Z_{ALS} leg score
SZCON_A   overall slope of Z_{Con} arm score
SZCON_L   overall slope of Z_{Con} leg score
SSAKG_A   overall slope of simple average of kg arm strength
SSAKG_L   overall slope of simple average of kg leg strength

Table 6.12 Loss of arm and leg strength: comparison of statistical transformation

Parameter	Total	Males	Females
Number	117	75	42
Age	55.4 ± 12.9	55.1 ± 13.3	55.9 ± 12.2
MOI	10.2 ± 6.6	10.4 ± 6.8	9.7 ± 6.2
MOO	30.2 ± 42.9	31.3 ± 36.5	28.4 ± 52.4
MAXP_A3[a]	14.7 ± 19.4	11.8 ± 17.2	19.8 ± 21.9
MAXP_L3[a]	24.7 ± 24.7	21.4 ± 21.1	30.6 ± 25.9*
ALSM_A3[b]	−0.06 ± 0.13	−0.06 ± 0.17	−0.05 ± 0.10
SZALS_A[b]	−0.06 ± 0.07	−0.06 ± 0.07	−0.05 ± 0.08
SZCON_A[b]	−0.08 ± 0.10	−0.07 ± 0.08	−0.09 ± 0.12
SSAKG_A[c]	−0.28 ± 0.63	−0.31 ± 0.65	−0.24 ± 0.58
SSAPER_A[d]	−0.55 ± 1.58	−0.44 ± 1.32	−0.72 ± 1.94

[a] Mean maximum strength as a percentile of normal age- and gender-matched controls in arm (A) or leg (L) during first 3 months of observation.
[b] Mean megaslope for arm (A) defined as megascore units per month charge ± standard deviation for first 3 months of observation [ALSM_A3 (based on Tufts ALS patient population)] or the entire year of observation [SZALS_A (based on Tufts ALS patient population) or SZCON_A (based on age- and gender-matched control population)].
[c] Mean slope for arm (A) loss of simple average of isometric muscle strength as kg per month change ± standard deviation for the entire year of observation (SSAKG_A).
[d] Mean slope for arm (A) loss of simple average of isometric muscle strength as percentile units per month ± standard deviation for the entire year of observation (SSAPER_A (based on age- and gender-matched control population)].

SSAPER_A	overall slope of simple average of percentile arm strength
SSAPER_L	overall slope of simple average of percentile leg strength
ALSM_A3	simple average of Z_{ALS} arm score in the first 3 months
ALSM_L3	simple average of Z_{ALS} leg score in the first 3 months
MAXP_A3	maximum average arm percentile strength in the first 3 months
MAXP_L3	maximum average leg percentile strength in the first 3 months

6.4.5 Gender differences

The Wisconsin Database contains 75 males (64.3%) and 42 females (35.6%). They differed in none of the measured variables except for the maximum percentage strength relative to normal at the start of the study. Females had a significantly ($P < 0.005$) higher maximum percentage strength controlled for gender and age than males (Table 6.12).

6.4.6 Lowest coefficient of variation

The data transformation with the lowest overall coefficient of variation for the population was Z_{ALS}. The smaller population standard deviation provides the model based on this transformation with an efficient means to estimate sample sizes required for clinical therapeutic trials.

6.4.7 Linear regression model of course of ALS

The course of ALS defined as the mean slope of change for the ALS population was modeled in a stepwise procedure for each of the following variables.

DEPENDENT VARIABLE DEPENDING ON THE MODEL

SSAKG_A	overall slope of simple average of kg arm strength
SSAKG_L	overall slope of simple average of kg leg strength
SZALS_A	overall slope of Z_{ALS} leg score
SZALS_L	overall slope of Z_{ALS} arm score
SZCON_A	overall slope of Z_{Con} arm score
SZCON_L	overall slope of Z_{Con} leg score
SSAPER_A	overall slope of simple average of percentile arm strength
SSAPER_L	overall slope of simple average of percentile leg strength

INDEPENDENT VARIABLE DEPENDING ON THE MODEL

Age	years
KGA_A3	simple average of mean kg arm slope in the first 3 months
KGA_L3	simple average of mean kg leg slope in the first 3 months
ALSM_A3	simple average of Z_{ALS} arm score in the first 3 months
ALSM_L3	simple average of Z_{ALS} leg score in the first 3 months
CONM_A3	simple average of Z_{con} arm score in the first 3 months
CONM_L3	simple average of Z_{con} leg score in the first 3 months
PER_A3	simple average of mean percentile arm slope in the first 3 months
PER_L3	simple average of mean percentile leg slope in the first 3 months

MAXP_A3   maximum average arm percentile strength in the first
              3 months
MAXP_L3   maximum average leg percentile strength in the first
              3 months

WEIGHT DEPENDING ON THE MODEL

MOF   Final month on study

6.4.8 Weighted model

The weight used was the number of months that each patient was studied. The initial 3-month slope has a direct positive effect in the predictive model. The maximum strength in this time period as a percentage of normal has a mild negative effect (Table 6.13). Stepwise correlation analysis demonstrates that the major predictive variable for the rate of strength loss in ALS is the slope in the first 3 months of observation (66–88%), with the exception of the percentile transformation in the arm, where the maximum strength in the first 3 months was a

Table 6.13 Linear regression equation parameter estimates for simple weighted model for strength loss in ALS

Overall slope	Intercept	Three-month slope effect	Three-month percentile strength effect	Age effect
SA$_{kg}$arm	0.0416	**0.0798**	−**0.0040**	−0.0046
SEM	0.1248	0.0161	0.0014	0.0022
SA$_{kg}$leg	0.4434	**0.2440**	−**0.0076**	−0.0087
SEM	0.2955	0.0276	0.0029	0.0051
Z$_{ALS}$arm	0.0050	**0.1766**	−**0.0008**	−0.0008
SEM	0.0238	0.0233	0.0003	0.0004
Z$_{ALS}$leg	0.0013	**0.2390**	−**0.0009**	
SEM	0.0103	0.0292	0.0003	
Z$_{Con}$arm	0.0024	**0.1118**	−**0.0013**	−0.0009
SEM	0.0311	0.0183	0.0003	0.0005
Z$_{Con}$leg	−0.0004	**0.1264**	−**0.0010**	
SEM	0.0123	0.0238	0.0004	
SA$_{\%tile}$arm	0.5231	**0.0862**	−**0.0276**	−0.0100
SEM	0.2611	0.0132	0.0029	0.0046
SA$_{\%tile}$leg	1.5743	**0.1940**	−**0.0256**	−0.0221
SEM	0.5437	0.0256	0.0052	0.0095

Bold designates significance at $P > 0.0001$. SEM, standard error of the mean.

Table 6.14 Linear regression equation parameter partial and model r^2 for simple weighted model for strength loss in ALS

Overall slope	Three-month slope effect	Three-month percentile strength effect	Age effect
SA_{kg}arm			
Partial	**0.0802**	**0.0255**	0.0166
Model	**0.0802**	**0.1057**	0.1223
SA_{kg}leg			
Partial	**0.2275**	**0.0215**	0.0088
Model	**0.2275**	**0.2491**	0.2578
Z_{ALS}arm			
Partial	**0.1703**	**0.0293**	0.0113
Model	**0.1703**	**0.1996**	0.2108
Z_{ALS}leg			
Partial	**0.1986**	**0.0314**	
Model	**0.1986**	**0.2300**	
Z_{Con}arm			
Partial	**0.1208**	**0.0425**	0.0094
Model	**0.1208**	**0.1633**	0.1726
Z_{Con}leg			
Partial	**0.0935**	**0.0286**	
Model	**0.0935**	**0.1222**	0.1222
$SA_{\%tile}$arm			
Partial	**0.1142**	**0.2430**	0.0123
Model	**0.1142**	**0.3570**	0.3695
$SA_{\%tile}$leg			
Partial	**0.1696**	**0.0720**	0.0167
Model	**0.1696**	**0.2416**	0.2583

Bold designates significance at $P < 0.0001$.

major predictor of the overall rate of loss of strength (66%) (Table 6.14). The age of the patient was not a significant variable for the Z_{ALS} or Z_{Con} transformations but did have a small (3–8%) effect on the simple average (SA) hilogram and percentile transformations. The effect of the 3-month slope was significant ($P < 0.0001$) for all transformations. The effect of the maximum strength as a percentage of normal was significant only in the percentile transformation. The age effect was not statistically significant.

6.4.9 *Post hoc* identification of rapid decliners

Using the Z_{ALS} arm score slope we defined 33 patients (28%) with a negative slope. The mean decline for these patients was nearly three times that of the population as a whole. Using the Z_{ALS} leg score we defined 28 patients (24%) with a negative slope. The mean decline for these patients was nearly twice that for the population as a whole.

6.4.10 *Pre hoc* identification of rapid decliners

Because the linear regression model suggested that the 3-month slope may be a good predictor of the overall slope, we identified 26 rapid decliners on the basis of the initial 3-month Z_{ALS} score slope. Using Z_{ALS} arm scores, 5 of these 26 patients did not have a rapid overall strength decline. This constitutes a false-positive rate of 19%. We did identify 21 patients who continued to have a rapid overall strength decline for a true-positive rate of 64%. Using the Z_{ALS} leg scores, 16 patients were found to have rapid strength loss in the first 3 months. Of these patients, four were found not to have overall negative Z_{ALS} score slopes, which constitutes a false-positive rate of 25%. We did identify 12 of 28 patients who continued to have a rapid decline over the entire period of study for a true-positive rate of 43%. The 19–25% false-positive rate of identifying rapid progressors with this strategy does not permit us to gain efficiency in short-term clinical trials trying to increase the change in a short observation period while maintaining the same population standard deviation. Moreover, it is not *a priori* clear whether therapeutic agents would be likely to work in rapidly progressing patients to the same extent as in moderately or slowly progressing patients.

6.5 FUTURE DIRECTIONS IN THE NATURAL HISTORY OF ALS

6.5.1 Can historical controls be used in clinical trials?

While time to failure analysis may be used to describe survival and symptom development in ALS over time periods of several years, time to failure analysis is not as robust as analysis of the slope of decline in muscle strength measured presymptomatically by isometric dynamometry. The latter techniques have been introduced in several international centers and statistical analyses are currently under way (Conradi, DeJong and Steiner, personal communications). The current analyses and modeling have looked at linear models over short time periods (Brooks *et al.*, 1992; Munsat, 1992; Ringel *et al.*, in press). Studies have indicated that slopes of decline are robust over short time periods, but biases may exist in terms of the percentage of patients with different sites of onset, which will affect the standard deviation of the study population over time and the efficiency of sample-size estimates for clinical therapeutic trials. The site of onset issue is the single most important bias that may vary from center to center in terms of the types of patients entered into clinical trials. Until the mathematics of modeling can better predict the effect of site of onset, parallel placebo-controlled trials are absolutely necessary to prevent both type I and type II errors (Friedman, Furberg and DeMets, 1985).

6.5.2 Issues to be addressed in future studies

The current models of ALS progression do not allow for the clinically apparent facts of relatively stable strength and stable function in some CNS regions prior to more rapid decline. This effect may be the normal to symptomatic inflection point. This clinical occurrence results from the redundancy of strength in muscle groups relative to the strength required for the function provided by the muscle group. None of our models yet adequately accounts for this state of change in the progression of ALS. A second inflection point occurs when more than 80–90% of the total possible strength in a muscle group is lost. At this point, using percentile transformations, we see a more rapid loss of strength and function. This is the acceleration inflection point, which is inadequately studied by current models and may reflect the important relationship between residual strength and function that most clinically affects patients. Although isometric models capture the symptomatic inflection point and the acceleration inflection point in the course of ALS may be appropriately studied by this method, many patients demonstrate normal isometric strength early in the course of the disease but have abnormalities that may be identified by isokinetic dynamometry (Sufit *et al.*, 1987; Brooks *et al.*, 1989). It will require appropriate application of new technologies such as isokinetic dynamometry to appropriately capture what may be the presymptomatic inflection point in the course of ALS that is not at all garnered by current clinical assessment strategies.

The natural history of ALS is an appropriate target of clinical scientific investigation. The tools that must be brought to bear include intelligence, clinical insight, new physiological measuring devices of strength and the development of mathematical models that will provide hypotheses that can be tested in the context of therapeutic trials that endeavor to stem the tragically ingravescent course of this disease.

ACKNOWLEDGMENTS

The concepts described in this chapter derive from many conversations over the last several years with Theodore Munsat, Tufts University School of Medicine; Steven Ringel and James Murphy, University of

References

Colorado; Roberto Guiloff, Charing Cross–Westminster Medical School; Micheal Swash, London Hospital; Adrian Williams, University of Birmingham Medical School; Forbes Norris, Pacific Medical Center; and Donald Mulder, Mayo Clinic.

The diligent assistance of Kathy Roelke, RN, Jennifer Parnell and Jennifer Tamulevich in monitoring and analyzing the Wisconsin Natural History Database and the assistance of Trisha Stanton in preparing the manuscript are gratefully appreciated.

This work was supported in part by grants from the Muscular Dystrophy Association, Regeneron Pharmaceuticals, Department of Veterans Affairs and National Institutes of Health Institute of General Medical Sciences General Clinical Research Center (M01RR03186).

REFERENCES

Agre, J.C., Magness, J.S., Hull, S.Z. *et al.* (1987) Strength testing with a portable dynamometer: reliability for upper and lower extremities. *Arch. Phys. Med. Rehabil.*, **68**, 454–8.

Aitkens, S., Lord, J., Bernauer, E. *et al.* (1989) Relationship of manual muscle testing to objective strength measurements. *Muscle Nerve*, **12**, 173–7.

Amundsen, L.R. (1990a) Measurement of skeletal muscle strength: an overview of instrumented and non-instrumented systems, in *Muscle Strength Testing: Instrumented and Non-instrumented Systems* (ed. L.R. Amundsen), Churchill Livingstone, New York, pp. 1–24.

Amundsen, L.R. (1990b) Isometric muscle strength testing with fixed-load cells, in *Muscle Strength Testing: Instrumented and Non-instrumented Systems* (ed. L.R. Amundsen), Churchill Livingstone, New York, pp. 89–122.

Andres, P.L., Skerry, L.M. and Munsat, T.L. (1989) Measurement of strength in neuromuscular diseases, in *Quantitation of Neurologic Deficit* (ed. T.L. Munsat), Butterworths, Boston, pp. 87–100.

Andres, P.L., Hedlund, W., Finison, L. *et al.* (1986) Quantitative motor assessment in amyotrophic lateral sclerosis. *Neurology*, **36**, 937–41.

Andres, P.L., Thibodeau, L.M., Finison, L.J. and Munsat, T.L. (1987) Quantitative assessment of neuromuscular deficit in ALS. *Neurol. Clin.*, **5**, 125–41.

Andres, P.L., Finison, L.J., Conlon, T. *et al.* (1988) Use of composite scores (megascores) to measure deficit in amyotrophic lateral sclerosis. *Neurology*, **38**, 405–8.

Beasley, W.C. (1961) Quantitative muscle testing: principles and applications to research and clinical services. *Arch. Phys. Med. Rehabil.*, **42**, 398–406.

Bohannon, R.W. (1986) Test–retest reliability of hand-held dynamometry during a single session of strength assessment. *Phys. Ther.*, **66**, 206–9.

Bohannon, R.W. (1986) Upper extremity strength and strength relationships among young women. *J. Orthop. Sports Phys. Ther.*, **8**, 128–33.

Braun, S.R. (1987) Respiratory system in amyotrophic lateral sclerosis. *Neurol. Clin.*, **5**, 9–31.

Brooks, B.R. (1985) Test protocol development: further preliminary experience with the effects of TRH in ALS. *Muscle Nerve*, **8**, 460–5.

Brooks, B.R. (1989) A summary of the current position of TRH in ALS therapy. *Ann. NY Acad. Sci.*, **553**, 431–61.

Brooks, B.R. (1991) The role of axonal transport in neurodegenerative disease spread: a meta-analysis of experimental and clinical poliomyelitis compares with amyotrophic lateral sclerosis. *Can. J. Neurol. Sci.*, **18**, 435–8.

Brooks, B.R., Beaulieu, D., Erickson, L. *et al.* 1986 Pilot studies and clinical therapeutic trials in amyotrophic lateral sclerosis. *Muscle Nerve*, **9** (Suppl. S5), 90–4.

Brooks, B.R., Sufit, R.L., Montgomery, G.B. *et al.* (1987) Intravenous thyrotropin releasing hormone in patients with amyotrophic lateral sclerosis: dose–response and randomized concurrent placebo-controlled pilot studies. *Neurol. Clin.*, **5**, 143–58.

Brooks, B.R., Sufit, R.L., Clough, J.A. *et al.* (1989) Isokinetic and functional evaluation of muscle strength over time in amyotrophic lateral sclerosis, in *Quantification of Neurologic Deficit* (ed. T.L. Munsat), Butterworths, Stoneham, pp. 143–54.

Brooks, B.R., DePaul, R., Tan, Y.D. *et al.* (1990) Motor neuron disease, in *Controlled Clinical Trials in Neurology* (eds B.S. Schoenberg and R. Porter), Marcel Dekker, Norwood, pp. 249–81.

Brooks, B.R., Sufit, R.L., DePaul, R. *et al.* (1991) Design of clinical therapeutic trials in amyotrophic lateral sclerosis, in *Advances in Neurology*, Vol. 56 (ed. L.P. Rowland), Raven Press, New York, pp. 521–46.

Brooks, B.R., Roos, R., Samaha, F. *et al.* (1992) Natural history of amyotrophic lateral sclerosis: effect of data transformation (Z score, simple average, percentile) on sample size requirements for placebo-controlled therapeutic trials (abstract P169). *Ann. Neurol.*, **32**, 272.

Capildeo, R. and Orgogozo, J.-M. (eds) *Methods in Clinical Trials in Neurology: Vascular and Degenerative Brain Disease*, Stockton, London.

Caroscio, J.T., Mulvihill, M.N., Sterling, R. and Abrams, B. (1987) Amyotrophic lateral sclerosis: its natural history. *Neurol. Clin.*, **5**, 1–8.

Cox, D.R. and Oakes, D. (1984) *Analysis of Survival Data*, Chapman & Hall, London.

Danneskiold-Samsoe, B., Kofod, V., Munter, J. *et al.* (1984) Muscle strength and functional capacity in 78–81 year old men and women. *Eur. J. Appl. Physiol.*, **52**, 310–18.

De Boer, A., Boukes, R.J. and Sterk, J.C. (1982) Reliability of dynamometry in patients with a neuromuscular disorder. *Eng. Med.*, **11**, 169–74.

DePaul, R. and Abbs, J.H. (1987) Manifestations of ALS in the cranial motor nerves – dynametric, neuropathologic and speech motor data. *Neurol. Clin.*, **5**, 231–50.

DePaul, R., Abbs, J.H., Caligiuri, M. *et al.* (1988) Hypoglossal, trigeminal, and facial motorneuron involvement in amyotrophic lateral sclerosis. *Neurology*, **38**, 281–3.

References

Dworkin, J.P. (1980) Tongue strength measurement in patients with amyotrophic lateral sclerosis: qualitative vs. quantitative procedures. *Arch. Phys. Med. Rehabil.*, **61**, 422–4.

Dworkin, J.P. and Aronson, A.E. (1986) Tongue strength and alternate motion rates in normal and dysarthric subjects. *J. Commun. Disord.*, **19**, 115–32.

Dworkin, J.P., Aronson, A.E. and Mulder, D.W. (1980) Tongue forces in normals and in dysarthric patients with amyotrophic lateral sclerosis. *J. Speech Hearing Res.*, **23**, 828–37.

Edwards, R.H.T., Young, A., Hosking, G.P. and Jones, D.A. (1977) Human skeletal muscle function: description of tests and normal values. *Clin. Sci. Mol. Med.*, **52**, 283–90.

Elkins, E.C., Leden, U.M. and Wakim, K.G. (1951) Objective recording of the strength of normal muscles. *Arch. Phys. Med. Rehabil.*, **32**, 639–44.

Festoff, B., Smith, R.A., Melmud, S. *et al.* (1988) Tufts quantitative neuromuscular examination and amyotrophic lateral sclerosis in the recombinant age. *Ann Neurol.*, **24**, 138A–139A.

Fillyaw, M.J., Badger, G.J., Bradley, W.G. *et al.* (1989) Quantitative measures of neurological function in chronic neuromuscular diseases and ataxia. *J. Neurol. Sci.*, **92**, 17–36.

Finison, L.J. (1989) Modeling of time strength relationships. *Muscle Nerve*, **13** (Suppl.), S49–S52.

Fleiss, J.L., Tytun, A. and Ury, H.K. (1980) A simple approximation for calculating sample sizes for comparing independent proportions. *Biometrics*, **36**, 343–6.

Friedman, L.M., Furberg, C.D., DeMets, D.L. (eds) (1985) *Fundamentals of Clinical Trials*, 2nd edn, PSG, Littleton.

Gubbay, S.S., Kahana, E., Zilber, N. *et al.* (1985) Amyotrophic lateral sclerosis: a study of its presentation and prognosis. *J. Neurol.*, **232**, 295–300.

Hall, J.G., Froster-Iskenius, U.G. and Allanson, J.E. (1989) *Handbook of Normal Physical Measurements*, Oxford University Press, Oxford.

Jackson, A.C., Moench, T.R., Griffin, D.E. and Johnson, R.T. (1987) The pathogenesis of spinal cord involvement in the encephalomyelitis of mice caused by neuroadapted Sindbis virus infection. *Lab. Invest.*, **56**, 418–23.

Johansson, C.A., Kent, B.E. and Shepard, K.F. (1983) Relationship between verbal command volume and magnitude of muscle contraction. *Phys. Ther.*, **63**, 1260–3.

John, J. (1984) Grading of muscle power: comparison of MRC and analogue scales by physiotherapists. *Int. J. Rehab. Res.*, **7**, 173–81.

Jones, H.E. (1947) Sex differences in physical abilities. *Hum. Biol.*, **19**, 12–19.

Jubelt, B., Narayan, O. and Johnson, R.T. (1980) Pathogenesis of human poliovirus infection in mice. II. Age-dependency of paralysis. *J. Neuropathol. Exp. Neurol.*, **39**, 149–59.

Kalbfleisch, J.D. and Prentice, R.I. (1980) *The Statistical Analysis of Failure Time Data*, Wiley, New York.

Kelly, J.J., Thibodeau, L., Andres, P.L. and Finison, L.J. (1990) Use of electrophysiologic tests to measure disease progression in ALS therapeutic trials. *Muscle Nerve*, **13**, 471–9.

The natural history of ALS

Kuther, G., Struppler, A. and Lipinski, H.G. (1987) Therapeutic trials in ALS – the design of a protocol, in *Amyotrophic Lateral Sclerosis: Therapeutic, Psychological and Research Aspects* (eds V. Cosi, A.C. Kato, W. Parlette, P. Pinelli and M. Poloni), *Adv. Exp. Med. Biol.*, **209**, 265–276.

Lachin, J.M. (1981) Introduction to sample size determination and power analysis for clinical trials. *Controlled Clin. Trials*, **2**, 93–113.

Lee, E.T. (1980) *Statistical Methods for Survival Analysis*, Lifetime Learning, Belmont.

Lewis, D.H., Belden, D., Rawling, J. *et al.* Statistical analysis of strength and function in patients with amyotrophic lateral sclerosis. *Neurology* (in press).

Mathiowetz, V. (1990) Grip and pinch strength measurements, in *Muscle Strength Testing: Instrumented and Non-instrumented Systems* (ed. L.R. Amundsen), Churchill Livingstone, New York, pp. 163–77.

Mathiowetz, V., Wiemer, D. and Federman, S.M. (1986) Grip and pinch strength: norms for 6- to 19-year olds. *Am. J. Occup. Ther.*, **40**, 705–9.

Miller, J.P. (1989) Statistical considerations in clinical trials. *Muscle Nerve*, **13** (Suppl.), S43–S44.

Miller, J.P. (1989) Statistical considerations for quantitative techniques in clinical neurology, in *Quantitation of Neurologic Deficit* (ed. T.L. Munsat), Butterworths, Boston, pp. 69–84.

Montoye, H.J. and Lamphiear, D.E. (1977) Grip and arm strength in males and females, age 10 to 69. *Res. Q.*, **48**, 109–19.

Munsat, T.L. (1992) The natural history of amyotrophic lateral sclerosis, in *Handbook of Amyotrophic Lateral Sclerosis* (ed. R.A. Smith), Marcel Dekker, New York, pp. 65–75.

Munsat, T.L., Andres, P.L. and Skerry, L.M. (1989) The use of quantitative techniques to define amyotrophic lateral sclerosis, in *Quantitation of Neurologic Deficit* (ed. T.L. Munsat), Butterworths, Boston, pp. 129–42.

Munsat, T.L., Andres, P.L., Finison, L. *et al.* (1988) The natural history of motoneuron loss in amyotrophic lateral sclerosis. *Neurology*, **38**, 409–13.

Murray, M.P., Gore, D.R., Gardner, G.M. *et al.* (1985) Shoulder motion and muscle strength of normal men and women in two age groups. *Clin. Orthop.*, **192**, 268–72.

Niebuhr, B.R. and Maraion, R. (1987) Detecting sincerity of effort when measuring grip strength. *Am. J. Phys. Med.*, **66**, 16–19.

Patterson, R.P. and Baxter, T. (1988) A multiple muscle strength testing protocol. *Arch. Phys. Med. Rehabil.*, **69**, 366–8.

Ringel, S.P., Murphy J.R., Alderson, K. *et al.* The natural history of amyotrophic lateral sclerosis. *Neurology* (in press).

Sanjak, M., Paulson, D., Sufit, R. *et al.* (1987) Phisiologic and metabolic response to progressive and prolonged exercise in amyotrophic lateral sclerosis. *Neurology*, **37**, 217–20.

Schmidt, R.T. and Toews, J.V. (1970) Grip strength as measured by the Jama dynamometer. *Arch. Phys. Med. Rehabil.*, **51**, 321–54.

Schoenberg, B.S. (1984) Controlled therapeutic trials in motor neuron disease:

methodologic considerations, in *Human Motor Neuron Disease* (ed. L.P. Rowland), Raven Press, New York, pp. 547–53.

Shafer, S.Q. and Olarte, M.R. (1982) Methodological considerations for clinical trials in motor neuron disease, in *Human Motor Neuron Diseases* (ed. L.P. Rowland), Raven, New York, pp. 559–68.

Shaunak, S., Ang, L., Colston, K. *et al.* (1987) Muscle strength in healthy white and asian subjects: the relationship of quadriceps maximum voluntary contraction to age, sex, body build and vitamin D. *Clin. Sci.*, **73**, 541–6.

Sobue, G., Sahashi, K., Takahashi, A. *et al.* (1983) Degenerating compartment and functioning compartment of motor neurons in ALS: possible process of motor neuron loss. *Neurology*, **33**, 654–7.

Sufit, R.L., Clough, J.A., Schramm, M. *et al.* (1987) Isokinetic assessment in ALS. *Neurol. Clin.*, **5**, 197–212.

Swash, M. (1980) Vulnerability of lower brachial myotomes in motor neuron disease: a clinical and single fiber EMG study. *J. Neurol. Sci.*, **47**, 59–68.

Swash, M. and Ingram, D.A. (1988) Preclinical and subclinical events in motor neuron disease. *J. Neurol. Neurosurg. Psychiat.*, **51**, 165–8.

Swash, M., Leadaer, M., Brown, A. and Swetrehan, K. (1986) Focal loss of anterior horn cells in the cervical cord in motor neuron disease. *Brain*, **109**, 939–52.

Swash, M., Scholtz, C.L., Vowles, G. and Ingram, D.A. (1988) Selective and asymmetric vulnerability of corticospinal and spinocerebellar tracts in motor neuron disease. *J. Neurol. Neurosurg. Psychiat.*, **51**, 785–9.

Tan, Y.D., Dolan, P. and Brooks, B.R. (1988) Symptom progression in amyotrophic lateral sclerosis. *Ann. Neurol.*, **24**, 14A.

Tsukagoshi, H., Yanagisawa, K., Oguichi, N. *et al.* (1979) Morphometric quantification of the cervical limb motor cells in controls and in amyotrophic lateral sclerosis. *J. Neurol. Sci.*, **41**, 287–97.

Wiles, C.M. and Karni, Y. (1983) The measurement of strength in patients with peripheral neuromuscular disorders. *J. Neurol. Neurosurg. Psychiat.*, **46**, 1006–10.

7 Neurophysiology

N.M.F. MURRAY

7.1 INTRODUCTION

Clinical neurophysiological studies are of great importance in the investigation and diagnosis of motor neurone disease (MND). The clinical diagnosis of MND is usually all too straightforward (Rowland et al., 1991) but the prognosis is so gloomy that supportive evidence is highly desirable. The role of the electromyographer is to provide positive evidence for anterior horn cell disease by demonstrating changes of partial denervation in conjunction with normal sensory conduction and normal or near-normal conduction in surviving motor fibres (Lambert and Mulder, 1957; Willison, 1962). It is axiomatic that denervation changes should extend beyond the territory of a single peripheral nerve or root, and it is helpful to demonstrate denervation where there is also evidence for upper motor neurone involvement, for example denervation of the quadriceps in association with a pathologically brisk knee jerk. The recently introduced technique of trans-cutaneous magnetic stimulation of the motor cortex enables the electromyographer to demonstrate abnormal conduction in the cortico-spinal tracts (Barker, Jalinous and Freeston, 1985; Schriefer et al., 1989). In contrast, even the most sophisticated imaging techniques cannot provide reliable evidence of anterior horn cell loss, and only in certain cases can magnetic resonance imaging demonstrate corticospinal tract degeneration.

The electrophysiological abnormalities encountered in MND are not specific to this disease; they may indicate other anterior horn cell diseases such as the spinal muscular atrophies and poliomyelitis, and, if focal, they may reflect a localized lesion of the spinal cord such as syringomyelia or spondylotic myelopathy (Kimura, 1989). Conversely, other disorders, in particular certain multifocal neuropathies, may present with a clinical picture indistinguishable from MND, and nerve conduction studies are of great importance in clarifying the diagnosis here (Lewis *et al.*, 1982; Pestronk *et al.*, 1988; Krarup *et al.*, 1990).

7.2 DIAGNOSTIC CRITERIA FOR MND

The most widely used criteria for electrodiagnosis of MND were set out by Lambert (Lambert and Mulder, 1957; Lambert, 1969). He noted that the pattern of EMG abnormalities that supports the diagnosis of MND includes:

1. fibrillation and fasciculation in muscles of the lower and the upper extremities, or in the extremities and the head;
2. reduction in number and increase in amplitude and duration of motor unit action potentials;
3. normal electrical excitability of remaining fibres of motor nerves, and motor fibre conduction velocity within the normal range in nerves of relatively unaffected muscles and not less than 70% of the average normal value according to age in nerves of more severely affected muscles;
4. normal excitability and conduction velocity of sensory nerve fibres even in severely affected extremities.

Lambert noted that this pattern of abnormalities should distinguish MND from myopathies, localized spinal cord lesions and disease affecting only the upper motor neurones, but not from other diffuse disorders of the anterior horn cells or from certain chronic polyneuropathies. Lambert's criteria have generally stood the test of time remarkably well, but a recent review (Behnia and Kelly, 1991) found that 50 of 133 patients with a clinical diagnosis of MND did not fulfil Lambert's criteria at presentation. The most common reason for this was insufficiently distributed fibrillation potentials (40 patients), but nerve conduction studies were abnormal in 11 patients and F waves abnormal in six. They made several points:

1. Conduction studies may be unreliable in motor nerves with markedly low compound muscle action potential (CMAP) amplitudes.
2. Sensory nerve action potential (SNAP) amplitudes may be abnormal in a small percentage of otherwise typical MND patients, though better controls for elderly subjects are required.
3. Electromyography may not show widespread active denervation early in the disease.
4. Some patients may have a mild polyneuropathy.

In practice, there is rarely much to lose by waiting a few weeks and repeating the electrophysiological study, but some modification of

Lambert's criteria, taking the clinical picture into account, may reduce unnecessary extra investigations and opinions. It may also allow earlier diagnosis and thus, if desired by the patient, earlier entry into experimental treatment trials. Behnia and Kelly (1991) noted that, even with redefinition of Lambert's criteria, more than a quarter of their patients still had non-diagnostic studies at first presentation.

7.3 ELECTROPHYSIOLOGICAL TECHNIQUES

7.3.1 Electromyography

The classic features of partial denervation and reinnervation include fibrillation potentials and positive sharp waves, and a reduced number of motor unit potentials, of increased amplitude and duration, on voluntary activation of the muscle and fasciculations. Fibrillations and positive sharp waves imply loss of the nerve supply to individual muscle fibres; they are generally more profuse in acute denervating lesions than in chronic disorders and are thus less commonly encountered in MND than in acute peripheral nerve injuries, but are more frequent than in chronic spinal muscular atrophies (SMA). The term 'active denervation' is often used when fibrillations are present; this is somewhat misleading since they can be found many years after the onset of a relatively non-progressive disorder such as polio, and in this context they are of no value for differentiating subjects with progressive weakness due to post-polio syndrome from those who are clinically stable (Ravits *et al.*, 1990; Dalakas and Illa, 1991). In MND fibrillations are more frequent in clinically affected than unaffected muscles, but they may occur in a quarter of muscles with normal power (Lambert, 1969).

Reduction in the number of motor units recruited voluntarily mirrors the drop in anterior horn cell numbers; estimates of the decrease in motor units required for clinical weakness to become apparent vary from 25 to 50% (Wohlfart, 1958; Hansen and Ballantyne, 1978).

When the interference pattern is so reduced that individual motor units can be identified during voluntary recruitment, firing at high rates (40–60 per second) in isolation, this indicates good voluntary effort by the patient. Irregular and low firing rates may indicate either reduced effort or coexistent upper motor neurone disease. Increase in the amplitude and the duration of individual motor unit potentials indicates collateral reinnervation of denervated muscle fibres by surviving motor units.

Very broadly, where the denervating process is relatively chronic, individual units will tend to be of long duration, both in their main component and in total duration, taking late components (satellite potentials) into account; on maximum volition the amplitude of the interference pattern may be up to 15 mV, though the number of components is grossly reduced, and spontaneous activity is often sparse. In acute denervating processes and where collateral reinnervation is poor or not established, fibrillation potentials and positive sharp waves are more common and increase in mean motor unit potential duration and amplitude less pronounced. In both acute and chronic anterior horn cell disorders the electromyographic abnormalities may be quite variable from muscle to muscle and within an individual muscle: classic neurogenic features may be present at one site, whereas in an adjacent area the findings may be altogether more suggestive of primary muscle disease. Where there is uncertainty about the nature of the disorder, sampling of more sites and more muscles will usually settle the matter; in general it is more common to encounter 'myopathic' abnormalities in a neurogenic disorder than 'chronic neurogenic' abnormalities in primary muscle disease.

The EMG examination should involve proximal and distal muscles in three limbs, emphasizing muscles that are clinically affected and supplied by nerves in which conduction studies can be performed. Facial and trunk muscle electromyography will be necessary in some cases, guided by the clinical picture.

7.3.2 Fasciculations

Fasciculation potentials have long been recognized as a hallmark of anterior horn cell disease (Lambert and Mulder, 1957; Hjorth, Walsh and Willison, 1973). A fasciculation potential is caused by the spontaneous discharge of a group of muscle fibres, either all or a proportion of those innervated by one anterior horn cell or cranial motor neurone. Depending on the number of fibres contracting and the nearness of the contracting fibres to the skin surface, a visible twitch may or may not be produced by a fasciculation; even those which are not seen may still be perceived by the patient.

Although fasciculations are a particular feature of anterior horn cell disease, they also occur, though less commonly, in peripheral nerve and root diseases, in the muscle pain–fasciculation syndrome and in normal subjects (Hudson, Brown and Gilbert, 1978; Layzer, 1982). In cervical spondylotic myelopathy fasciculations may occur in both upper and lower extremities; whereas this activity in the arms may simply reflect segmental anterior horn cell dysfunction or coexistent radiculopathy, the reason for lower limb fasciculations is less obvious. Ischaemia and lack of inhibition are possible explanations. Interestingly, the fasciculations in the legs may resolve after cervical decompressive surgery (King and Stoops, 1963; Kadson, 1977).

Identification of the benign or malignant nature of a fasciculation may not be easy; benign fasciculations typically occur in the hand and calf muscles and around the eyes; they often occur at a much higher frequency than those associated with anterior horn cell disease, where the interdischarge interval may be very long indeed (Trojaborg and Buchthal, 1965), but the morphology of the individual potential may be simple or complex in either case. Apart from the fasciculation potentials, electromyography and clinical examination are normal in subjects with benign fasciculations.

Fasciculation potentials in anterior horn cell disease are usually outwith voluntary control; the spontaneously discharging potential cannot be readily suppressed and most fasciculating units cannot be activated voluntarily. A recent study of patients with MND showed that approximately 10% of fasciculations are under voluntary control, and these tend to be of less complex morphology than those which cannot be voluntarily activated (Guiloff and Modarres-Sadeghi, 1992). Assuming that a fasciculation potential in MND simply reflects a dying motor neurone, then it is possible that early in the course of disease for a particular motor unit it may both fasciculate and be under voluntary control, the ectopic generation site responsible for the fasciculation being near or above the point of axonal branching. As disease progresses voluntary activation may be lost and ectopic generation may shift to the terminal portion of the motor unit.

The observation and recording of fasciculation potentials is important for the diagnosis of MND, but it may be time-consuming to document their distribution by eye, and painful by EMG needle. In this situation multichannel surface recording of fasciculations may be helpful (Hjorth, Walsh and Willison, 1973; Howard and Murray, 1992). A conventional electroencephalograph is used with eight pairs of plate electrodes, recording activity from the upper and lower segments of the arms and legs over a period of about 20 min. Many more fasciculation potentials are recordable by this means than are seen by the clinical observer or are recordable by a needle electrode. Widespread fasciculations occur in all anterior horn cell diseases and the diagnosis of MND should be reconsidered when fewer than five out of eight recording leads show fasciculations. The proportion of patients with peripheral neuropathies and myelopathies who exhibit widespread fasciculations is much less, and they occur only rarely in other neurological disorders. A paucity of fasciculations in MND may indicate a relatively good prognosis (Norris, 1975).

7.3.3 Single-fibre EMG and macro EMG

Single-fibre EMG (SF EMG)provides important information on the status of the motor unit in MND (Stalberg, Schwartz and Trontelj, 1975; Stalberg and Trontelj, 1979; Stalberg, 1982). The jitter is a measure of the variability on consecutive discharges of the time interval between action potentials of muscle fibres supplied by the same motor unit. Jitter may be abnormal due to disease of the terminal nerve fibre, the neuromuscular junction or the muscle fibre. Abnormal jitter is a particular feature of early reinnervation, when the immature collateral sprouts do not permit stable, sustained conduction. Increased jitter may be associated with impulse blocking, complete failure of conduction along the terminal nerve fibre and thus temporary drop-out of one or more muscle fibre potentials, depending on the site of conduction failure along the nerve twig. In general, jitter and blocking are more prominent in acute denervating conditions such as MND than in more chronic processes such as spinal muscular atrophies.

The fibre density is a measure of the number of single fibre potentials from one motor unit present within the uptake area of the SF EMG electrode. Fibre density is measured by triggering the oscilloscope sweep on one muscle fibre potential, having maximized its amplitude, and then counting the number of time-locked muscle fibre potentials. This is performed for 20 different recording sites within the muscle and a mean value obtained. Essentially fibre density measures the local concentration of muscle fibres within a single motor unit, and increase thus suggests rearrangement of muscle fibres due to collateral sprouting. In general the more chronic the neurogenic disorder, the higher the fibre density; in Kugelberg–Welander disease the fibre density is characteristically more elevated than in MND, whereas jitter and blocking may be less prominent.

Macro EMG records from all of the fibres of the motor unit, using a special electrode with a large recording area (Stalberg, 1983; Stalberg and Sanders, 1984). One channel is used to trigger the oscilloscope from a single fibre potential and a second averages the time-locked response from the 200–500 muscle fibres constituting the motor unit. Macro motor unit potentials (MUPs) are characteristically of large amplitude in MND, particularly in those with slow clinical progression. The macro MUP configuration may be abnormal even when amplitude is normal. Broadly, increase in the amplitude of the macro MUP is evidence for effective reinnervation, and to some extent it mirrors increase in fibre density. Decline in clinical strength as MND progresses may be accompanied by a simultaneous decrease in macro EMG amplitude, possibly because the motor neurone has become 'overloaded' and can no longer support the abnormally large number of muscle fibres that it controls. As expected, in primary muscle disease the macro MUP is usually of low amplitude though it may be within the normal range.

7.3.4 Motor nerve conduction

Motor nerve conduction studies are important for distinguishing MND from other disorders, particularly peripheral neuropathies. Early in the course of MND motor conduction studies are typically normal. As the disease progresses CMAP amplitudes decline, and at this point (when CMAP amplitude is less than 30% of the normal mean value for the nerve) a moderate reduction in motor conduction velocity (MCV) with prolongation of distal motor latency (DML) may be seen. This is due to random loss of fast-conducting fibres and slow conduction in degenerating or poorly myelinated regenerating axons (Ertekin, 1967; Lambert, 1969; Daube, 1982; Koutlidis, de Recondo and Bathien, 1984). Slowing of conduction in a wasted limb is often compounded by the effect of cooling, and some studies have reported MCVs as low as 67% of the lower limit of normal with distal latencies up to 160% of the upper limit of normal.

It is of prime importance when investigating a patient with suspected MND to ascertain that slowing of motor conduction can reasonably be attributed to fibre drop-out and degeneration and/or temperature effect, rather than demyelinating peripheral neuropathy. In chronic inflammatory demyelinating neuropathies (CIDP), in which immunosuppressive therapy may be of great benefit, there is usually widespread, albeit somewhat patchy, slowing of motor conduction, often in the presence of relatively normal CMAP amplitudes. The degree of slowing is more pronounced than in MND, and it may vary from segment to segment, as well as from nerve to nerve; thus slowing may be particularly prominent in the proximal segment of the ulnar nerve but more distal in the adjacent median nerve. There may be a discrepancy between the F latency and conduction in the distal nerve, indicating slowing more proximally, perhaps in motor roots, and conduction block may be prominent (Lewis and Sumner, 1982). Sensory conduction is usually but not invariably abnormal.

A recent study specifically examined motor nerve conduction in well-documented cases of MND, paying due regard to limb temperature and examining both upper and lower limb nerves (Cornblath, Kuncl and Mellits, 1992). Motor nerve conduction velocity, distal latency and F-wave latency were related to distal evoked CMAP amplitude in peroneal, median and ulnar nerves. The authors noted that in nerves with reduced CMAP amplitude MCV rarely fell to less than 80% of the lower limit of normal and distal latency and F latency rarely exceeded 1.25 times the upper limit of normal. Confidence limits were set for expected values of these parameters as a function of CMAP amplitude and these data should be of value in differentiating MND from other illnesses, specifically motor neuropathies.

Ingram, Davis and Swash (1987) used a complex multiple stimulus and collision technique to assess conduction velocity across the range of fibres in the motor nerve, rather than only examining the fastest fibres, as in conventional MCV measurement. They found that MND did not preferentially affect particular neuronal subpopulations; follow-up studies demonstrated that reduction in velocity could exceed 30% of the initial value, as the disease progressed.

Conduction block is not a normal feature of MND, and its detection in a suspected case should alert the electromyographer to the possibility of chronic inflammatory demyelinating polyneuropathy or multifocal motor neuropathy with conduction block (MMN) (Lewis et al., 1982; Pestronk et al., 1988; Krarup et al., 1990; Cornblath et al., 1991; Pestronk, 1991; Sumner, 1991). Conduction block is usually caused by demyelination and is characterized electromyographically by an abnormal decrease in the negative peak amplitude and area of the CMAP on proximal versus distal stimulation of a nerve. In CIDP, conduction block occurs along with marked diffuse slowing of conduction and frequent sensory involvement. In contrast, in MMN slowing of motor conduction is rare other than across regions of partial conduction block, which tend to occur at unusual sites. Sensory abnormalities are rare, but sural nerve biopsy may reveal sensory fibre abnormalities, and it is possible that MMN is in fact a variant of CIDP, rather than a separate entity. Prominent fasciculations and asymmetry of weakness increase the potential for misdiagnosis of MMN as MND.

The diagnosis of conduction block is by no means straightforward when there is associated slowing of motor nerve conduction, causing temporal dispersion of the CMAP to proximal stimulation (Cornblath et al., 1991; Sumner, 1991). Temporal dispersion prolongs the duration of the CMAP and can also result in cancellation of the negative phase of one motor unit action potential by the positive phase of another, as a result of desynchronization. This phenomenon is particularly liable to occur when individual motor unit potentials are few in number and of large amplitude, owing to chronic partial denervation. The result is a reduction in both the amplitude and the area of the CMAP to proximal stimulation, which may easily be misinterpreted. This is a possible explanation for some claims for conduction block in MND (Trojaborg *et al.*, 1990). In practice, it seems likely that there is at least an element of conduction block when the decrement on proximal stimulation of a motor nerve exceeds 50% of the distal CMAP amplitude or area. Transcutaneous stimulation over the spinal column may demonstrate very proximal block when conventional studies are normal (Mills and Murray, 1985).

7.3.5 Repetitive stimulation

Abnormal decremental responses on low-frequency repetitive stimulation have been demonstrated in up to two-thirds of patients with MND (Denys and Norris, 1979; Bernstein and Antel, 1981). Decremental responses of this type occur most commonly in patients with a rapidly progressive disease and are particularly prominent in wasted and fasciculating muscles. Decremental responses are associated with abnormal jitter and impulse blocking on SF EMG and may reflect abnormal conduction in poorly myelinated degenerating and reinnervating nerve fibres. Administration of edrophonium reduces the decrement.

7.3.6 Sensory nerve conduction

Conduction in sensory nerve fibres is classically normal in MND (Lambert and Mulder, 1957; Ertekin, 1967; Lambert, 1969). However, abnormalities of threshold for detection of cutaneous sensation including vibration and temperature have been described (Mulder *et al.*, 1983; Jamal, Weir and Hansen, 1985). More recently, careful studies of the sural nerve sensory action potential using near-nerve recording techniques demonstrated that 9 of 18 patients with MND had abnormally reduced minimum conduction velocity even when maximum conduction velocity and amplitude of the SNAP were normal (Shefner, Tyler and Krarup, 1991). The authors suggested that the abnormality was likely to reflect the presence of slow-conducting regenerating fibres, possibly indicating a dying-back sensory axonopathy rather than a neuronopathy. Interestingly, in nine patients who were retested after an interval of 3 months there was no progression of the sensory nerve abnormality. Mondelli *et al.* (1993) used standard sensory nerve conduction tests in 64 patients with MND; they found minor abnormalities involving SNAP amplitude more than velocity, compatible with either a neuronopathy or an axonopathy. Behnia and Kelly (1991) noted minor sensory conduction abnormalities in a small proportion of their series of patients with otherwise classical MND; these abnormalities tended to reflect either asymptomatic median nerve compression at the wrist or the paucity of reliable normative data on sensory conduction in older age groups, though a mild axonal polyneuropathy seemed the likely explanation in a few.

7.3.7 Somatosensory evoked potentials

Evidence for abnormalities of conduction in central sensory pathways is conflicting. Chiappa (1983) reported normal somatosensory evoked potentials (SEPs), whereas Matheson, Harrington and Hallett (1986) reported abnormal upper limb SEPs in 34% and abnormal lower limb SEPs in 41% of patients with MND. Radtke, Erwin and Erwin (1986) found a similar incidence of lower limb SEP abnormality, though only 2 out of 16 patients had abnormal median SEPs. Recently Zanette *et al.* (1990) examined median SEPs in 26 patients using both mid-frontal and ear-lobe references. Central conduction time was prolonged in three patients, but only with a mid-frontal reference. Half of the patients with amyotrophic lateral sclerosis and progressive bulbar palsy exhibited abnormalities of the early prerolandic potentials, and these findings correlated with clinical evidence for upper motor neurone involvement; patients with progressive muscular atrophy had normal SEPs. The authors suggested that the abnormalities were due to neuronal loss in the motor cortex affecting the generator sites of prerolandic potentials.

7.4 CENTRAL MOTOR CONDUCTION

A technique for high-voltage transcutaneous electrical stimulation of the motor cortex was devised by Merton and Morton in 1980. Anodal shocks of up to 700 V are delivered through a low-output impedance electrical device and the latency and amplitude of the evoked muscle response give a measure of conduction in the corticospinal tracts as well as the peripheral motor nerve. The peripheral component of the motor pathway may be measured by stimulation over the spinal column to excite the motor roots or, indirectly, by use of the formula $1/2(F+M-1)$, where F is the latency of the F wave and M is the latency of the direct muscle response to peripheral muscle stimulation. Subtraction of the peripheral from the total latency gives a measure of conduction in the central motor pathways. The technique has been used to demonstrate moderate prolongation of central conduction in motor neurone disease, often with very low-amplitude responses, and abnormally raised threshold intensity for excitation of the motor cortex (Hugon *et al.*, 1987; Ingram and Swash, 1987).

The chief drawback of transcutaneous electrical stimulation of the cortex is the considerable discomfort it can cause; the technique has now largely been replaced by magnetic stimulation of the cortex, which is essentially pain free (Barker, Jalinous and Freeston, 1985; Hess, Mills and Murray, 1987). The magnetic field generated by the stimulator passes unattenuated through high-resistance structures such as the skull and scalp; therefore the current induced at the skin surface is low and no pain is caused. The magnetic field induces a current within the motor cortex that excites the cortical motor neurones, enabling muscle action potentials to be recorded on a conventional electromyograph.

In a series of 22 patients with MND, central motor conduction (CMC) to abductor digiti minimi (ADM) was assessed by magnetic stimulation of the motor cortex and electrical stimulation over the lower cervical region (Schriefer *et al.*, 1989). CMC was abnormal in 14 patients; responses to brain stimuli were unobtainable in seven patients on one or both sides, and CMC time was prolonged in nine patients. Half of the delayed responses were also of pathologically small amplitude. Subclinical involvement of central motor pathways was demonstrated in two cases; conversely, CMC was entirely normal on both sides of two subjects and on one side in three despite small hand muscle weakness, hyper-reflexia, brisk finger jerks and impaired fine finger movements. In general, correlations between clinical findings and responses to brain stimulation are rather poor in MND, presumably on account of the combination of upper and lower motor neurone involvement.

Eisen *et al.* (1990) used magnetic stimulation of the motor cortex to evaluate 40 patients with MND. In 12 of these patients pseudobulbar signs were prominent, and in these motor evoked potentials could not be elicited. In the other patients, in whom lower motor neurone abnormalities were more prominent, the overall prevalence of MEP abnormalities (latency and/or amplitude) approached 100%. They noted that this high rate of abnormality detection was achieved by examining several muscles rather than hand muscles alone. It should be emphasized that unless the amplitude of the response to brain stimulation is expressed as a percentage of that evoked by peripheral nerve stimulation for the same muscle, a low-amplitude response to brain stimulation does not differentiate between corticospinal tract dysfunction and loss of anterior horn cells (Schriefer *et al.*, 1989).

Recent evidence suggests that the threshold intensity for magnetic stimulation of the motor cortex is abnormally low in some cases, particularly early in the course of the disease, and this may be associated with a more favourable prognosis than elevated threshold (Eisen, 1992). Fasciculations have been reported to be especially frequent in muscles with low cortical thresholds, and both phenomena could reflect increased excitability of diseased anterior horn cells (Caramia *et al.*, 1991). Some fasciculation potentials seem to be elicitable by cortical stimulation, but it is not clear whether these are also under voluntary control.

There are several possible reasons for CMC abnormalities in MND. Loss of cortical motor neurone cells should result in low-amplitude responses to brain stimuli and, by drop-out of larger, faster conducting axons and reduction in the number of the descending impulses onto anterior horn cells, could also cause delay of spinal motor neurone depolarization and thus prolongation of CMC time (Murray, 1992). Central motor delay is typically a feature of demyelination of corticospinal tracts, as in multiple sclerosis, but similar delays may occur in MND and changes should not be regarded as specific (Hess *et al.*, 1987; Murray, 1992). However, in general demyelinating diseases of the central nervous system are associated with prolongation of CMC time whereas disorders associated with loss of cortical motor neurones or their axons tend to cause low amplitude responses and abnormally raised stimulus thresholds without marked delay. In MND central motor conduction studies seem to be especially useful when it is particularly important to ascertain the presence of upper motor neurone involvement. Examples include those patients with a lengthy history, apparently confined to the lower motor neurones, in whom the possibility of SMA is considered. Magnetic stimulation of the cortex may also be helpful in patients with profound peripheral abnormality sufficient to mask any dysfunction of central motor pathways and in certain patients with cervical or lumbar radiculopathy.

7.5 PROGNOSIS IN MND

No single electrophysiological parameter is a reliable predictor of a good or bad prognosis, but the nature and distribution of EMG abnormalities are undoubtedly of value. Indices that suggest acute and severe denervation with little reinnervation tend to predict a rapid progression and include: profuse fibrillation and positive sharp waves; highly unstable polyphasic motor unit potentials, particularly of low amplitude; small CMAPs; and decremental responses to low-frequency stimulation. Very generally, the more widespread the abnormalities, the worse the prognosis is likely to be; a particularly gloomy future is suggested when there is early and severe involvement of bulbar muscles such as the tongue and masseters. Denervation of the diaphragm, the thoracic paraspinal muscles and the rectus abdominal muscles portends the onset of clinical signs of respiratory insufficiency (Kuncl, Cornblath and Griffin, 1988; Cornblath *et al.*, 1987; Saadeh *et al.*, 1993). Absence of recordable muscle responses to magnetic brain stimulation may be evidence for a poor prognosis.

7.6 MONITORING DISEASE PROGRESSION

The use of electrophysiological tests to assess disease progress in MND is becoming increasingly important as clinical trials proliferate. The discomfort inherent in many electrophysiological techniques must be taken into account if assessment is to be performed at all frequently. A successful test should not be too time-consuming, should correlate well with progressive weakness and should not be overdependent on the small hand muscles, which may be severely atrophied relatively early in the course of the disease. A recent study (Kelly, Thibodeau and Andres, 1990) examined a battery of electrophysiological parameters including CMAP amplitude and area, fibrillation density, fibre density and motor unit firing rate. During regular follow-up studies over more than 1 year, CMAP amplitude from tibialis anterior correlated best with strength and showed a strong linear correlation with time.

More complex procedures such as assessment of motor unit numbers (Hansen and Ballantyne, 1978), quantitative analysis of the interference pattern (Hayward and Willison, 1977), SF EMG and macro EMG (Stalberg, Schwartz and Trontelj, 1975; Stalberg and Trontelj, 1979; Stalberg, 1983; Stalberg and Sanders, 1984) provide important pathophysiological data on the balance between denervation and reinnervation but may be less acceptable to the patient when repeated studies are required. The fact that a steady clinical course does not imply a constant denervation–reinnervation ratio is a drawback to all neurophysiological assessment techniques in MND.

7.7 ELECTRODIAGNOSTIC ASPECTS OF DIFFERENTIAL DIAGNOSIS

As has already been noted, the EMG changes of partial denervation are not at all specific to MND and one must rely on the distribution of these abnormalities and associated motor and sensory nerve conduction studies, as well as the history and clinical findings, to confirm the diagnosis. Lambert's criteria may be fulfilled in spinal muscular atrophies, although in the X-linked recessive bulbospinal neuronopathy (Kennedy, Alter and Sung, 1968; Harding et al., 1982) sensory nerve action potentials are frequently absent or of low amplitude, indicating a coexistent sensory neuronopathy. The possibility of a chronic MMN should be considered, and great care taken to exclude proximal conduction block before the diagnosis of sporadic focal SMA is made. In other SMAs the distribution and time course of the abnormalities are essential information for diagnostic purposes, electromyography simply confirming partial denervation (Hashimoto et al., 1976; Harding and Thomas, 1980; Harding, Bradbury and Murray, 1983). Similarly, there are no specific diagnostic EMG findings in other disorders, such as Creutzfeldt–Jakob disease, in which anterior horn cell disease may occur (Kimura, 1989).

Neurophysiology

Post-polio syndrome cannot be reliably differentiated electromyographically from either stable old polio or MND (Ravits *et al.*, 1990; Dalakas and Illa, 1991). Spontaneous activity including fibrillations and fasciculations may be widespread in all three disorders, though it has been noted that neurogenic jitter may be absent in post-polio syndrome. This may suggest that the abnormality in post-polio is more distally situated along the terminal axon than is the case in MND (Ravits *et al.*, 1990). In the author's experience central motor conduction studies using magnetic stimulation of the cortex have been consistently normal in old polio and in post-polio syndrome (unpublished observations).

Primary lateral sclerosis is characterized by exclusively upper motor neurone findings and normal electromyography and peripheral nerve conduction (Russo, 1982); magnetic stimulation of the motor cortex has shown absent or very delayed responses to brain stimulation with CMC times up to 24 ms in hand muscles (upper limit of normal 8.3 ms) (Brown *et al.*, 1992).

The important abnormalities of motor conduction velocity and conduction block that are necessary for electrophysiological confirmation of the diagnoses of CIDP and MMN have already been discussed. Two recently described lower motor neurone (LMN) syndromes may be difficult to distinguish from MND (Pestronk *et al.*, 1990). Distal LMN syndromes present with slowly progressive asymmetric weakness, often commencing in a leg but with little evidence of bulbar or upper motor neurone involvement. Electrophysiologically, absence of conduction block distinguishes them from MMN and there are changes of chronic partial denervation. The majority have a high serum IgM anti-GM1 antibody titre, and some improve with immunosuppression. Proximal LMN syndromes present with asymmetric and mainly upper limb involvement: there is no conduction block and IgM anti-GM1 antibody levels are rarely markedly raised, but a third have a high titre of antibody to the glycolipid asialo-GM1. There is no evidence as yet for clinical or electrical response to immunosuppression.

Most hereditary peripheral neuropathies pose little diagnostic difficulty, but on occasion the peripheral neuropathy associated with acute intermittent porphyria may be confused with MND. This disorder is characterized by attacks of muscle weakness with a subacute onset, sometimes over weeks, and with little or no sensory involvement. The distribution of muscle weakness and wasting is variable: it may be generalized or proximal or distal. Although tendon reflexes are usually depressed or lost there may be retention of the ankle jerks. Electromyography reveals partial denervation changes with normal motor conduction velocities and frequently normal sensory potentials, findings consistent with a predominantly motor axonal neuropathy (Thomas,

184

1987). Lead poisoning produces, at least in adults, a predominantly upper limb peripheral neuropathy of axonal type that may be almost purely motor (Nielson, 1987).

The diagnosis of MND in patients with known cervical and/or lumbar radiculopathy may not be straightforward; demonstration of denervation changes in bulbar and thoracic paraspinal muscles will demonstrate the wide extent of the disease. The occasional occurrence of widespread upper and lower limb fasciculations in cervical spondylotic myelopathy has been reported (King and Stoops, 1963).

Some primary muscle diseases may cause diagnostic difficulties, particularly inclusion body myositis, in which electromyography frequently shows a mixed myopathic and neurogenic picture (Lotz *et al.*, 1989). Dermatomyositis, polymyositis and acid maltase deficiency myopathy may all feature abundant spontaneous activity on electromyography, but the findings are otherwise usually typically 'myopathic'.

7.8 CONCLUSION

Lambert's original criteria for the electrophysiological diagnosis of MND still serve the electromyographer well, with only minor caveats. Due regard must be paid to the effects on nerve conduction of age, muscle atrophy and limb temperature, and the physician should recognize that changes in number and configuration of motor unit potentials may provide perfectly acceptable evidence for denervation, despite absence of fibrillation potentials in some muscles. It is a matter of clinical judgement whether, when the distribution of denervation changes is restricted or Lambert's criteria are not fulfilled for some other reasons, one proceeds to further investigations or elects to observe the patient and to repeat the EMG in due course. Modern imaging techniques, far more acceptable to the patient than those previously available, permit the relatively easy recognition or exclusion of 'surgical' disorders of the spinal cord and roots. Nowadays the electromyographer has a particular responsibility to identify those conditions, often potentially treatable, which can mimic MND but in which imaging is unhelpful and other investigations are more invasive. In particular, peripheral disorders, such as CIDP and MMN, must be identified, and this requires the maintenance of a high level of suspicion. Clearly it will not be appropriate to perform prolonged and painful motor conduction studies in all cases, but it is incumbent on the examiner to test two, perhaps three, motor nerves as a matter of routine in suspected MND, and to be ready to extend the study using proximal stimulation techniques if there is any suspicion of conduction block or other hallmarks of demyelination. Measurement of conduction in central motor pathways using transcranial magnetic stimulation may be of considerable value when

Neurophysiology

clinical evidence for upper motor neurone involvement is weak or equivocal, though it must be recognized that the rate of detection of subclinical abnormalities is not high at present. There is, however, real scope for improvement here, as instrumentation improves and experience accumulates on the relative merits of response variables such as amplitude, latency and threshold intensity.

REFERENCES

Barker, A.T., Jalinous, R. and Freeston, I.L. (1985) Non-invasive stimulation of human motor cortex. *Lancet*, ii, 1106–7.

Behnia, M. and Kelly, J.J. (1991) Role of electromyography in amyotrophic lateral sclerosis. *Muscle Nerve*, **14**, 1236–41.

Bernstein, L.P. and Antel, G.P. (1981) Motor neurone disease: decremental responses to repetitive nerve stimulation. *Neurology*, **31**, 204–7.

Brown, W.F., Ebers, G.C., Hudson, A.J. *et al.* (1992) Motor-evoked responses in primary lateral sclerosis. *Muscle Nerve*, **15**, 626–9.

Caramia, M.D., Cicinelli, P., Paradiso, C. *et al.* (1991) Excitability changes of muscular responses to magnetic brain stimulation in patients with central motor disorders. *Electroencephalogr. Clin. Neurophysiol.*, **81**, 243–50.

Chiappa, K. (1983) *Evoked Potentials in Clinical Medicine*. Raven Press, New York.

Cornblath, D.R., Kuncl, R.W. and Mellits, E.D. (1992) Nerve conduction studies in amyotrophic lateral sclerosis. *Muscle Nerve*, **15**, 1111–15.

Cornblath, D.R., Kuncl, R.W., Rechthand, D.E. *et al.* (1987) The value of rectus abdominal muscle electromyography. *Muscle Nerve*, **10**, 376.

Cornblath, D.R., Sumner, A.J., Daube, J. *et al.* (1991) Conduction block in clinical practice. *Muscle Nerve*, **14**, 869–71.

Dalakas, M. and Illa, I. (1991) Post-polio syndrome: concepts in clinical diagnosis, pathogenesis and etiology, in *Advances in Neurology*, Vol. 56, *Amyotrophic Lateral Sclerosis and Other Motor Neurone Diseases* (ed. L.P. Rowland), Raven Press, New York, pp. 495–511.

Daube, J. (1982) *AAEE Minimonograph No. 18: EMG in Motor Neuron Disease*, American Association of Electromyography and Electrodiagnosis, Rochester, MN, USA.

Denys, E.H. and Norris, F.H. (1979) Amyotrophic lateral sclerosis: impairment of neuromuscular transmission. *Arch. Neurol.*, **36**, 202–5.

Eisen, A. (1992) Transcranial magnetic stimulation in amyotrophic lateral sclerosis and some other disorders affecting pyramidal pathways, in *Clinical Applications of Magnetic Transcranial Stimulation* (ed. M.A. Lissens), Peeters Press, Leuven, pp. 91–104.

Eisen, A., Shytbel, W., Murphy, K. *et al.* (1990) Cortical magnetic stimulation in amyotrophic lateral sclerosis. *Muscle Nerve*, **13**, 146–51.

Ertekin, C. (1967) Sensory and motor conduction in motor neurone disease. *Acta Neurol. Scand.*, **43**, 499–512.

Guiloff, R.J. and Modarres-Sadeghi, H. (1992) Voluntary activation and fibre density of fasciculations in motor neuron disease. *Ann. Neurol.*, **31**, 416–24.

References

Hansen, S. and Ballantyne, J.P. (1978) A quantitative electrophysiological study of motor neurone disease. *J. Neurol. Neurosurg. Psychiatr.*, **41**, 773–83.

Harding, A.E. and Thomas, P.K. (1980) Hereditary distal spinal muscular atrophy. *J. Neurol. Sci.*, **45**, 337–48.

Harding, A.E., Bradbury, P.G. and Murray, N.M.F. (1983) Chronic asymmetrical spinal muscular atrophy. *J. Neurol. Sci.*, **59**, 69–83.

Harding, A.E., Thomas, P.K., Baraitser, M. *et al.* (1982) X-linked recessive bulbospinal neuronopathy: a report of ten cases. *J. Neurol. Neurosurg. Psychiatr.*, **45**, 1012–19.

Hashimoto, O., Asada, M., Ohta, M. *et al.* (1976) Clinical observations of juvenile non-progressive muscular atrophy localized in hand and forearm. *J. Neurol.*, **211**, 105–10.

Hayward, M. and Willison, R.G. (1977) Automatic analysis of the electromyogram in patients with chronic partial denervation. *J. Neurol. Sci.*, **33**, 415–23.

Hess, C.W., Mills, K.R. and Murray, N.M.F. (1987) Responses in small hand muscles from magnetic stimulation of the human brain. *J. Physiol.*, **388**, 397–419.

Hess, C.W., Mills, K.R., Murray, N.M.F. *et al.* (1987) Magnetic brain stimulation: central motor conduction studies in multiple sclerosis. *Ann. Neurol.*, **22**, 744–52.

Hjorth, R.J., Walsh, J.C. and Willison, R.G. (1973) The distribution and frequency of spontaneous fasciculations. *J. Neurol. Sci.*, **18**, 469–74.

Howard, R.S. and Murray, N.M.F. (1992) Surface EMG in the recording of fasciculations. *Muscle Nerve*, **15**, 1240–5.

Hudson, A.J., Brown, W.F. and Gilbert, J.J. (1978) The muscle pain–fasciculation syndrome. *Neurology*, **28**, 1105–9.

Hugon, J., Lubeau, M., Tabarard, F. *et al.* (1987) Central motor conduction in motor neurone disease. *Ann. Neurol.*, **22**, 544–6.

Ingram, D.A. and Swash, M. (1987) Central motor conduction is abnormal in motor neurone disease. *J. Neurol. Neurosurg. Psychiatr*, **50**, 159–66.

Ingram, D.A., Davis, G.R. and Swash, M. (1987) Motor nerve conduction velocity distributions in man: results of a new computer-based collision technique. *Electroencephalog. Clin. Neurophysiol.*, **66**, 235–43.

Jamal, G.A., Weir, A.I. and Hansen, S. (1985) Sensory involvement in motor neurone disease: further evidence from automated thermal threshold determination. *J. Neurol. Neurosurg. Psychiatr.*, **48**, 906–10.

Kadson, D.L. (1977) Cervical spondylotic myelopathy with reversible fasciculations in the lower extremities. *Arch. Neurol.*, **34**, 774–6.

Kelly, J.J., Thibodeau, L. and Andres, P.L. (1990) Use of electrophysiologic tests to measure disease progression in ALS therapeutic trials. *Muscle Nerve*, **13**, 471–9.

Kennedy, W.R., Alter, M. and Sung, J.H. (1968) Progressive proximal spinal and bulbar muscular atrophy of late onset: a sex-linked recessive trait. *Neurology*, **18**, 671–80.

Kimura, J. (1989) Diseases of the motor neurone, in *Electrodiagnosis in Diseases of*

Neurophysiology

Nerve and Muscle, 2nd edn, F.A. Davis Company, Philadelphia, USA, pp. 429–46.

King, R.B. and Stoops, W.L. (1963) Cervical myelopathy with fasciculations in lower extremities. *J. Neurosurg.*, **20**, 948–52.

Koutlidis, R.M., de Recondo, J. and Bathien, N. (1984) Conduction of the sciatic nerve in its proximal and distal segment in patients with ALS (amyotrophic lateral sclerosis). *J. Neurol. Sci.*, **64**, 183–91.

Krarup, C., Stewart, J.D., Summer, A.J. *et al.* (1990) A syndrome of asymmetrical limb weakness and motor conduction block. *Neurology*, **40**, 118–27.

Kuncl, R.W., Cornblath, D.R. and Griffin, J.W. (1988) Assessment of thoracic paraspinal muscles in the diagnosis of ALS. *Muscle Nerve*, **11**, 484–92.

Lambert, E.H. (1969) Electromyography in amyotrophic lateral sclerosis, in *Motor Neuron Disease* (eds F.H. Norris, J.R. Junior and L.T. Kurland), Grune & Stratton, New York, pp. 135–53.

Lambert, E.H. and Mulder, D.W. (1957) Electromyographic studies in amyotrophic lateral sclerosis. *Mayo Clin. Proc.*, **32**, 441–6.

Layzer, R.B. (1982) Diagnostic implications of clinical fasciculation and cramps, in *Human Motor Neuron Diseases* (ed. L.P. Rowland), Raven Press, New York, pp. 23–7.

Lewis, R.A. and Sumner, A.J. (1982) The electrodiagnostic distinctions between chronic acquired and familial demyelinative neuropathies. *Neurology*, **32**, 592–6.

Lewis, R.A., Sumner, A.J., Brown, M.J. *et al.* (1982) Multifocal demyelinating neuropathy with persistent conduction block. *Neurology*, **32**, 958–64.

Lotz, B.P., Engel, A.G., Nishino, H. *et al.* (1989) Inclusion body myositis: observations in 40 patients. *Brain*, **112**, 727–47.

Matheson, J.K., Harrington, H.J. and Hallett, M. (1986) Abnormalities of multimodality evoked potentials in amyotrophic lateral sclerosis. *Arch. Neurol.*, **43**, 338–40.

Merton, P.A. and Morton, H.B. (1980) Stimulation of the cerebral cortex in the intact human subject. *Nature*, **285**, 287.

Mills, K.R. and Murray, N.M.F. (1985) Proximal conduction block in early Guillain–Barré syndrome. *Lancet*, ii, 659.

Mondelli, M., Rossi, A., Passero, F. *et al.* (1993) Involvement of peripheral sensory fibres in amyotrophic lateral sclerosis: electrophysiological study of 64 cases. *Muscle Nerve*, **16**, 166–72.

Mulder, D.W., Bushek, W., Spring, E. *et al* (1983) Motor neuron disease (ALS): evaluation of detection thresholds of cutaneous sensation. *Neurology*, **33**, 1625–7.

Murray, N.M.F. (1992) Invited Editorial: The clinical usefulness of magnetic cortical stimulation. *Electroencephalogr. Clin. Neurophysiol.*, **85**, 81–9.

Nielson, V.K. (1987) Toxic polyneuropathies, in *Clinical Electromyography* (eds W.F. Brown and C.F. Bolton), Butterworths, Boston, pp. 283–303.

Norris Jr, F.H. (1975) Adult spinal motor neuron disease, in *Handbook of Clinical*

Neurology, Vol. 22, *System Disorders and Atrophies* (eds P.J. Vinken and G.W. Bruyn), North Holland, Amsterdam, pp. 1–56.

Pestronk, A. (1991) Invited review: motor neuropathies, motor neuron disorders and antiglycolipid antibodies. *Muscle Nerve*, **14**, 927–36.

Pestronk, A., Cornblath, D.R., Ilyas, A.A. *et al.* (1988) A treatable multifocal motor neuropathy with antibodies to GM1 ganglioside. *Ann. Neurol.*, **24**, 73–8.

Pestronk, A., Chaudhry, V., Feldman, E.L. *et al.* (1990) Lower motor neuron syndromes defined by pattern of weakness, nerve conduction abnormalities, and high titers of antiglycolipid antibodies. *Ann. Neurol.*, **27**, 316–26.

Radtke, R.A., Erwin, A. and Erwin, C.W. (1986) Abnormal sensory evoked potentials in amyotrophic lateral sclerosis. *Neurology*, **36**, 796–801.

Ravits, J., Hallett, M., Baker, M. *et al.* (1990) Clinical and electromyographic studies of postpoliomyelitis muscular atrophy. *Muscle Nerve*, **13**, 667–74.

Rowland, L.P., Santoro, M., Lange, D.J. *et al.* (1991) Diagnosis of amyotrophic lateral sclerosis. *Ann. Neurol.*, **30**, 225–7.

Russo Jr, L.S. (1982) Clinical and electrophysiologic studies in primary lateral sclerosis. *Arch. Neurol.*, **39**, 662–4.

Saadeh, P.B., Fitzpatrick Crisafulli, C., Sosner, J. *et al.* (1993) Needle electromyography of the diaphragm: a new technique. *Muscle Nerve*, **16**, 15–20.

Schriefer, T.N., Hess, C.W., Mills, K.R. *et al.* (1989) Central motor conduction studies in motor neurone disease using magnetic brain stimulation. *Electroenceph. Clin. Neurophysiol.*, **74**, 431–7.

Shefner, J.M., Tyler, H.R. and Krarup, C. (1991) Abnormalities in the sensory action potential in patients with amyotrophic lateral sclerosis. *Muscle Nerve*, **14**, 1242–6.

Stalberg, E. (1982) Electrophysiological studies of reinnervation in ALS, in *Human Motor Neuron Diseases* (ed. L.P. Rowland), Raven Press, New York, pp. 47–59.

Stalberg, E. (1983) AAEE Minimonograph No. 20, Macro EMG. *Muscle Nerve*, **6**, 619–30.

Stalberg, E. and Sanders, D.B. (1984) The motor unit in ALS studied with different neurophysiological techniques, in *Research Progress in Motor Neurone Disease* (ed. C. Rose), Pitman, London, pp. 105–22.

Stalberg, E. and Trontelj, J. (1979) *Single Fibre Electromyography*, The Miravelle Press, Old Woking, Surrey, UK.

Stalberg, E., Schwartz, M.S. and Trontelj, J.V. (1975) Single fibre electromyography in various processes affecting the anterior horn cell. *J. Neurol. Sci.*, **24**, 403–15.

Sumner, A.J. (1991) Separating motor neurone diseases from pure motor neuropathies: multifocal motor neuropathy with persistent conduction block, in *Advances in Neurology*, Vol. 56, *Amyotrophic Lateral Sclerosis and Other Motor Neurone Diseases* (ed. L.P. Rowland), Raven Press, New York, pp. 399–403.

Thomas P.K. (1987) Classification and electrodiagnosis of hereditary neuropathies, in *Clinical Electromyography* (eds W.F. Brown and C.F. Bolton), Butterworths, Boston, pp. 177–205.

Trojaborg, W. and Buchthal, F. (1965) Malignant and benign fasciculations. *Acta Neurol. Scand.*, **41**, 251–4.

Trojaborg, W., Lange, D.J., Latov, N. *et al.* (1990) Conduction block and other abnormalities of nerve conduction in motor neuron disease: a review of 110 patients. *Neurology*, **40** (Suppl. 1), 182.

Willison, R.G. (1962) Electrodiagnosis in motor neurone disease. *Proc. Roy. Soc. Med.*, **55**, 1024–8.

Wohlfart, G. (1958) Collateral reinnervation in partially denervated muscle. *Neurology*, **8**, 175–80.

Zanette, G., Polo, A., Gasperini, M. *et al.* (1990) Far-field and cortical somatosensory evoked potentials in motor neurone disease. *Muscle Nerve*, **13**, 47–55.

PART TWO

8 Early management

TOM HEAFIELD and AMANDA POWELL

8.1 CORRECT DIAGNOSIS

Good early management is dependent upon having the correct diagnosis, as discussed in Chapter 1. The problems of diagnosis and management are such that in most circumstances a skilled interested neurologist should be involved, as experience suggests that vascular or even myasthenia bulbar palsies, cervical spondylosis and treatable motor neuropathies are more likely to be recognized by the specialist; the rarer syndrome of spinal muscular atrophy and the Kennedy variant, which have important prognostic implications, are unlikely to be appreciated by generalists.

8.2 TESTS

The use of tests is discussed in Chapters 1 and 7. One issue is the use of investigations in the cases in which a definite diagnosis can be made on clinical grounds alone. Many clinicians take the 'no stone unturned' approach as the implications of the diagnosis are so serious. In any case the patient will find it hard to accept such a serious diagnosis without tests and at least neurophysiological tests can be justified for documentation even when not strictly necessary.

8.3 SUSPECTED MOTOR NEURONE DISEASE

There will be some patients in whom the diagnosis is suspected but is not certain. As in the management of all cases, communication with the patient in this situation has to be individualized and adapted to cultural norms. It would be the normal practice in the UK not to mention the term MND in this situation unless faced with a patient with a great deal of medical knowledge or with a barrage of enquiries as to the possibilities.

Early management

One would instead explain that the patient had a disorder that affected the motor nerves that was non-compressive, that there was no treatment and that the possibility had to be faced that it might be progressive. Volunteering to arrange a second opinion may be helpful, and indeed the use of a second opinion can be a help in definite cases as well, as it gives the patient the extra reassurance that nothing has been overlooked. After all there is no diagnostic test for the condition.

8.4 DEFINITE MOTOR NEURONE DISEASE

When the diagnosis is definite (Henke, 1968; Newick and Langton-Hewer, 1984; Norris, 1992) most physicians and patients feel that the patient should be told the diagnosis and the implications explained. There are still some societies that feel this inappropriate, and it is not so long since this was not accepted practice in the UK. In an interim phase it was common to tell the relatives a lot more than the patient, but those days are also passing. However, problems still remain and since in the past communication skills have not been overvalued as part of a neurological training it is necessary to give a few pointers.

Such discussions should not take place in public or in a rush. Ideally they should take place at a prearranged time in a private room. Normally a relative should be present, as should the patient's nurse, preferably one who has a background in neurology and ideally a nurse practitioner who deals with motor neurone disease. In a perfect world the general practitioner who has known the patient and family for years should be present, but this is usually impossible to attain.

Information will need to be given in a phased manner and in understandable terms, not all necessarily by the physician. The degree of phasing and the speed at which information is given should be extremely individualized and not prescriptive. It should rely heavily on feedback from the patient and relatives (Brewin, 1991).

It is helpful to have some background information from having met the individual on several occasions previously. This is another reason why doing some tests, even if not wholly necessary, can be helpful; additionally, from one's attitude and expressions one may already have communicated enough to let the patient know that there will not be any easy therapeutic answers. It may also be helpful to have an idea as to what the patient expects the diagnosis to be. For instance there may be inappropriate relief that it is not a form of cancer. One should also know if the patient is still working and in what sort of job and have a feel for the home situation. There will be differences in the family's response, depending on whether the patient is in work or if there are still children at home.

One should give the name of the disease. Although in a sense it is just a label it will give the patient some confidence that the physician knows what is wrong, that it is not a diagnostic mystery, and that he has dealt with such cases previously. It is worth mentioning that the illness is not understood, but in most cases one can be reassuring that there is no significant genetic risk to other members of the family. Occasionally it may also be worth stating that it is not an infectious illness and that there is no risk to others who live with or touch the patient. One should explain that it is a disorder of the motor nerve and that other systems are not affected such that dementia is rare, incontinence is not a feature and hearing and eyesight are not affected. Certainly one should admit that there is no effective medical cure. However, one should cushion that with an emphasis on how the physician, and hopefully the clinical team, will be able to help arrange care. Additionally, research can be mentioned though one should try to avoid planting false hopes. Nevertheless, involvement in drug trials can be looked on in a positive way, as can involvement in other research that involves donating blood samples or, ultimately, tissue.

How much discussion there is about coping with the disability will depend to a large extent on the stage of the illness and anatomically which area is taking the brunt of the illness at the time. One therefore rarely goes into details of gastrostomy or respiratory care in a patient who has presented with a foot drop. On the other hand, even in the early case, if the patient has presented with bulbar problems or respiratory symptoms, then it will be appropriate to discuss these straight away. Indeed the case for interventions such as gastrostomy or respiratory support is very much stronger in patients who are still ambulant. In this centre we would only volunteer discussions on respiratory assistance in a patient in whom respiratory symptoms were a presenting problem. Additionally, we would only press for an early gastrostomy in a patient presenting with bulbar problems with reasonably good limb function.

8.5 GIVING A PROGNOSIS

First of all one has to give an idea as to the likely development of the disease and disability. At least compared with some illnesses it is a relatively predictable disease and one should attempt a reasonable degree of honesty, tempered by the patient's emotional response and questions. One helpful side of the inevitability of progression is that the disability and coping with the handicap can be planned for, for instance

Early management

using home adaptations and aids to daily living (see Chapter 9). On the other hand, one must avoid offering such services too early, and the timing should be dictated by the patient and relatives. However, at present some services are only provided as crisis situations emerge or unfortunately when it is too late to benefit the patient. Deciding whether it is right to discuss the progress of disability over the next year or so, or whether or not one takes the longer view and discusses the eventual level of disability and chances of getting bulbar problems, say, when one presents with weakness in an arm or a leg is highly dependent on the patient's attitude.

As far as giving a prognosis as to life expectancy, it should be accepted that not all patients will ask or wish to know. It is important that patients in the early stages of the illness are not treated as if they are terminally ill. Nevertheless, one should not deny that it is in the end a fatal illness. Despite the fact that the illness progresses inexorably, there is of course a wide variation in survival. Usually average figures, even if it is emphasized that they are average and on a bell-shaped curve, are misinterpreted by the patients such that an average life expectancy of 2–3 years is understood as 2 or 3 years to live. Thus, if forced to use such a definite time period one should always emphasize that it is the average and that the prognosis could be either longer or shorter. If discussions regarding terminal care do arise one should emphasize that the vast majority of patients manage at home until the end with support from community staff, though a few will be admitted to hospice or hospital care but often only for the last week or two.

8.6 SYMPTOMS RESPONDING TO DRUGS IN THE EARLIER STAGES OF MND

8.6.1 Cramp

Cramp is a problem in many patients with motor neurone disease, but it can respond to quinine and to more homeopathic measures used for the treatment of cramp. As with ordinary cramps, stretching of the muscle by either patient or carer can help.

PAINLESS CRAMP

It is not that unusual for painless cramps to occur in motor neurone disease. It can give an almost myotonic appearance, though in our experience EMGs have shown continual motor activity and not

196

myotonic or pseudomyotonic discharges. Occasionally phenytoin appears to help this symptom, though its prognosis seems to be good as it disappears with time.

8.6.2 Fasciculation

This is often not complained of but can be aggravating. In a few patients a beta blocker may have some effect.

8.6.3 Spasticity

Good physiotherapy can be most useful in helping the patient attain the best from weakening muscles. It can also help relieve some spasticity in the few patients where it is a major problem. Lioresol and Dantrolene can be used, though with most patients with MND the spasticity is not great and the increase in weakness from the use of this medication often means that it is unhelpful. It is useful to tell the patient that the exercise will not hasten deterioration, but neither will it restore already lost muscle power.

8.7 PAIN RELIEF

Although motor neurone disease is not seen as an overtly painful disorder, 40% of patients experience pain at some stage. Cramps have been mentioned. Postural problems later in the course of the illness can be in part circumvented by efficient wheelchairs and neck supports, together with information to carers regarding careful positioning and passive exercises. However, in some patients analgesics will also be required.

8.8 DEPRESSION

Signs of endogenous depression are not common with motor neurone disease, though such individuals are often so brave that it may be difficult to tell. However, it does not appear to be so interlinked with the illness as it does with Parkinson's disease. Nevertheless, there will be some patients in whom an antidepressant or an anxiolytic will be appropriate, though such medication is rarely useful in the early stages of getting over the shock of the diagnosis. Depression and anxiety in the carer should also not be overlooked.

197

8.9 CONTINUING SUPPORT

We have found it important to give continuing support, both from the physician and from a multidisciplinary care team, as will be outlined below. We have also found it of use to tell most patients about the lay organization, the Motor Neurone Disease Association, and that they may obtain some personal support as well as sometimes equipment and certainly information from the publications of such societies, though in a very early mild case one has to be careful that the shock will be too much. We have also found it important to inform and educate the family doctor, who is an important figure in the future care of patients and in organizing services (Way and Steiner, 1986). As motor neurone disease is a rare disease it is helpful to give additional information to the general practitioner in many cases and to write sensible pragmatic letters, not assuming experience of this condition. We also find it of help if there is personal contact between not necessarily the physician but a member of the care team and the family doctor.

8.10 COUNSELLING

It has been our experience, and others', that the support of someone experienced with counselling and with motor neurone disease can be of enormous benefit. Some centres have used individuals with a background in psychology and counselling. We have recruited a nurse practitioner who has been trained in counselling skills to deal with patients' problems right from the time of diagnosis, offering subsequent visits following discharge. Obviously in familiar home surroundings without the pressure of the busy ward environment, the 'threat' of white coats and numerous other patients listening into the conversation, many more areas of concern can be covered that the patient usually feels are 'too trivial to bother the doctor' but which cause unnecessary worry, anxiety and misunderstanding. Some units use prediagnostic counselling apparently with benefit. We have tended to use the period before diagnosis as a time to get to know the patient rather than specifically for counselling.

This need for more support for patients became obvious after we had piloted a critical care plan for the care of patients with motor neurone disease. We would like to briefly allude to this plan, which was done on an inpatient basis, though it could be easily modified for outpatient use or a shorter inpatient assessment and the rest done in outpatients. A brief description of the system will also emphasize the multidisciplinary nature of caring for patients with motor neurone disease even at the early stages of the illness and certainly later in the course.

8.11 CRITICAL CARE PLAN

In this department during 1990, as a result of Department of Health interest in combined intervention in patient management by medical and paramedical groups, a proposal to document intervention was established in the form of a collaborative care plan (CCP) for MND.

CCP was first devised in the USA and applied to many general medical acute admissions for conditions such as acute myocardial infarction or fractured neck of femur.

In order to establish a framework for a CCP, members of a multi-disciplinary team, such as physiotherapists and occupational therapists, devised a written protocol for their input once a patient had been diagnosed (Figure 8.1).

Individual assessments are documented and, when acted upon, detailed on a CCP chart, the paperwork incorporating confirmation of assessment and any need for intervention (Figure 8.2). This single document is shared by all members of the team thus avoiding duplication of overlapping features requiring intervention. The additional benefit of this approach is that each member of the team is aware of the intervention of their colleagues and a constant swapping of information occurs. The decision as to which assessments are appropriate is made by clinicians early in the admission so that, for example, patients without speech or swallowing or breathing difficulties are not always assessed by the relevant therapists.

The structure of the team, which combines community and hospital care, demonstrates the link between diagnostic services, and paramedical and specialist referrals. A 'key worker' for each patient to provide liaison between these components is essential (Jowett and Armitage, 1988). In our department, the role is served by the nurse practitioner.

CCP is popular with staff, patients and carers, fosters team spirit and allows good feedback when mistakes are made, e.g. too much video fluoroscopy, poor communication or conflicts between different medical and paramedical groups. In our particular unit it highlighted problems with lack of counselling skills and time offered for this, the need for further explanations regarding disease following discharge, and how important it is to give patients contact names and numbers from various disciplines to reduce some of the isolation that many patients and families feel and the divide between hospital- and community-based services such as social services, housing and even dual systems, such as physiotherapy/occupational therapy, which are represented in both camps.

Many of the problems with delivery of care are difficult to resolve, but financial issues are only a limiting factor in part as in many instances a

CRITICAL MEDIAL PATHWAY DRAFT COPY JULY 1990

Surname ....
Forename ....
Sex ....
Address ....

G. No. ....
DoB ....
Age ....
Consultant ....
Ward ....

OR HOSPITAL LABEL

ADMISSION DATE ....
PROPOSED DISCHARGE DATE ....
ACTUAL DISCHARGE DATE ....

PLEASE CIRCLE/TICK AND DATE WHERE REQUIRED

PRE-ADMISSION ARRANGEMENTS	DAY 1 DATE	DAY 2 DATE	DAY 3 DATE	DAY 4 DATE	DAY 5 DATE	DISCHARGE COMMUNICATIONS
DAY ARRANGED	**AM** HOUSEMAN CLERK	**AM** BLOOD TESTS FBC/ESR LITH HEP PROFILE/CA2+ CPK SUGAR TBH PROTEIN ELECTROPHORESIS B12 VDRL	**AM** LP	**AM** SECOND CONSULTANT REVIEW YES / NO DIAGNOSIS EXPLAINED YES / NO TTO'S YES / NO	? HOME	DATE PATIENT CARERS GP FOLLOW UP
EMG ORDERED YES / NO MYELOGRAM ORDERED YES / NO	NORRIS SCORE					
	PM EMG/NCS (OR BISSESSAR)	**PM** XRAYS PLAIN C/SPINE: L/SPINE: CXR: ANTIGANGLIASE ANTIBODIES	**PM** MYELOGRAM + CF8 OR LP (OR ROLFE) REGISTRAR REVIEW	**PM** ASSOCIATE REFERRALS DATE ENT YES / NO PSYCHIATRY YES / NO REHAB YES / NO HOSPICE YES / NO ANAETHETIC YES / NO OTHER YES / NO ? HOME		
SPEECH THERAPY (IF BULBA INVOLVEMENT) YES / NO	NEURO REG ASSES					
ADMISSION NOTIFICATION DATE						
NURSING INPUT	PHYSICAL SOCIAL EMOTIONAL ASSESSMENT NURSING INTERVENTION YES / NO	NURSING INTERVENTION YES SEE PLAN NO	NURSING INTERVENTION YES SEE PLAN NO	TRANSPORT YES / NO D/N LETTER YES/ NO		

Figure 8.1 Critical medial pathway draft copy, July 1990.

MULTI-DISCIPLINARY MANAGEMENT PLAN

PLEASE TICK/CIRCLE AND DATE WHERE REQUIRED / NR = NOT REQUIRED

OCCUPATIONAL THERAPY DATE REFERRAL YES / NO ASSESSMENT YES / NO CARERS HOME VISIT YES / NO PROPOSED DISCHARGE	INPUT YES / NO DATE	HOME VISIT YES / NO DATE DETAILS	EQUIPMENT REQUIRED YES / NO ITEMS: DATE ORDERED	DISCHARGE PLAN/ ADVICE YES / NO CONTINUED THERAPY REQUIRED	FOLLOW UP YES / NO DATE WHERE	DISCHARGE INFORMATION GIVEN TO PATIENT ☐ CARER ☐ GP ☐
PHYSIOTHERAPY DATE REFERRAL YES / NO ASSESSMENT YES / NO INTERVENTION YES / NO	TREATED YES / NO EQUIPMENT YES / NO ITEMS: DATE:	TREATED YES / NO	TREATED YES / NO	DISCHARGE PLAN/ ADVICE YES / NO	FOLLOW UP YES / NO DATE WHERE	DISCHARGE INFORMATION GIVEN TO PATIENT ☐ CARER ☐ GP ☐
SPEECH THERAPY DATE REFERRAL YES / NO ASSESSMENT YES / NO INTERVENTION YES / NO	DATE SEEN YES / NO COMMUNICATION AID YES / NO REFERRAL ENT YES / NO ASSESSMENT YES / NO	INTERVENTION REQUIRED SPEECH YES / NO DATE SWALLOWING YES / NO DATE	DATE SEEN YES / NO EQUIPMENT REQUIRED YES / NO ITEMS SPECIFIED:	DISCHARGE PLAN/ ADVICE YES / NO	FOLLOW UP YES / NO DATE WHERE	DISCHARGE INFORMATION GIVEN TO PATIENT ☐ CARER ☐ GP ☐
DIETICIAN DATE REFERRAL YES / NO ASSESSMENT YES / NO INTERVENTION YES / NO NUTRITION SISTER REFERRAL YES / NO	ASSESSMENT DATE NORMAL YES / NO MODIFIED YES / NO SUPPLEMENTS YES / NO TUBE FEED YES / NO	EQUIPMENT/FEED YES / NO ORDERED DATE		DISCHARGE PLAN/ ADVICE YES / NO	FOLLOW UP YES / NO DATE WHERE	DISCHARGE INFORMATION GIVEN TO PATIENT ☐ CARER ☐ GP ☐

Figure 8.2 Multidisciplinary management plan.

Early management

change in attitude amongst individuals and agencies involved can lead to significant improvements in the care offered to the patient with MND.

REFERENCES

Brewin, T.B. (1991) Three ways of giving bad news. *Lancet*, **337**, 1207–9.
Henke, E. (1968) Motor neurone disease: a patient's view. *Br. Med. J.*, **4**, 765–6.
Jowett, S. and Armitage, S. (1988) Hospital and community liaison links in nursing: the role of the liaison nurse. *J. Adv. Nursing*, **13**, 579–87.
Newrick, P.G. and Langton-Hewer, R. (1984) Motor neurone disease: can we do better? A study of 42 patients. *Br. Med. J.*, **289**, 539–42.
Norris, E.H. (1992) Motor neurone disease (editorial; comment). *Br. Med. J.*, **304**, 459–60.
Way, J. and Steiner, T.J. (1986) Motor neurone disease: what can the GP do? *Practitioner*, **230**, 149–53.

9　A carer's perspective

ROSALIND PEGG

Motor neurone disease is a particularly cruel disease, robbing sufferers of movement and speech and leading inexorably to death. It makes escalating demands on carers and I, for one, found caring physically exhausting and emotionally draining.

My husband, Steve, was 39 when MND was diagnosed. Our only daughter, Eleanor, was 3. She was just 7 when her father died. Those 4 years, which should have been among the happiest of our lives, were instead blighted by the appalling disability that MND brings and Steve's inevitable death. During those 4 years Eleanor was exposed to traumas that many adults never face in a lifetime, but she also witnessed love, courage, kindness, humour and honesty that I hope she will never forget.

Before he became ill Steve had enjoyed an active outdoor life. We used to walk miles together. He played squash twice a week and refereed football matches each weekend. By Christmas 1986, however, he had begun to sense a weakness in his right hand while playing squash and could not grip his racquet tightly. We assumed it was a sports injury so he rested, but his hand did not improve. He felt well enough to continue with football, though, until he went into hospital for tests in May 1987.

After a couple of days of investigations Steve returned home none the wiser. We waited nearly 2 weeks before he was called back to see the consultant neurologist. We had been given a 5 p.m. appointment, but it was immediately obvious from the crowded waiting room that the clinic was running late. The receptionist asked if we could come back another day. However, a preliminary discussion with our GP had increased our concern for Steve's health and we did not want to postpone the diagnosis. We said we wanted to see the consultant as arranged so we were told to go for a drink and phone back in an hour and a half.

We eventually saw the consultant at 7 p.m. He left us alone in his room while he went off to search, in vain, for some test results. After a brief physical examination he told Steve he had motor neurone disease. I had never heard of it. Steve referred to David Niven and requested more information. We learned that MND is a serious muscle-wasting disease, that the cause is unknown and that there is no treatment and no cure. A few statistics were mentioned and we left.

It was not until I went to the library the next day and read a description of the disease for myself that I realized the true awfulness of the prognosis. It was absolutely shocking. It was as if Steve died then, and I experienced much of the numbness and grief that normally accompany bereavement.

Because Steve looked so fit apart from his hand, we could not believe the diagnosis. In fact, we refused to accept it.

Instead we embarked on a range of 'alternative therapies' and asked for a second opinion. When it came some 5 months later it was the same, but this time we were not surprised. Steve's right hand had become practically useless and he was feeling so tired that he had given up work as a teacher. His left hand was also struggling with fine motor control.

In October 1987 Eleanor saw him fall down the stairs at home. In November, 6 months after the original diagnosis, Steve took Eleanor swimming for the last time. He felt people were giving him strange looks as he struggled with socks and shoes. He typed in his diary:

> In December 1987 I went to lift my sleeping daughter to carry her upstairs to bed. She was too heavy for me. On Christmas Day I drove my car for the last time; my left hand, like my right, now too weak to turn the ignition. In January 1988, after walking 400 metres, I keeled over backwards on the doorstep. Unable to stop myself, I crashed to the ground like a felled elm. In February we went to Cornwall. On the way home I read Eleanor a story for the last time, my croaky voice running out of expression on a dual carriageway near Exeter. In April we visited the Cotswold Wildlife Park. This was the occasion of my public wheelchair debut.

In May 1988, 1 year after Steve's original diagnosis, I gave up my job as a teacher. I did not want to. I had always worked. I could not imagine how we would manage financially. But, perhaps worst of all, I would no longer be able to escape from what was happening at home. I had been finding it increasingly difficult to teach full-time, and to look after Steve, Eleanor and the house. I was going into work late, rushing home at lunchtime to feed and toilet Steve, and leaving early whenever possible. The strain was intolerable because he could not manage for more than a couple of hours without me. The deterioration in his health was relentless. I thought he would be dead by Christmas. I realized I was dispensable at work but indispensable at home. I had to do everything I could to make those last months somehow bearable for us all.

Although I never regretted my decision to care full-time for Steve, I cannot adequately convey the awfulness of watching, in his words, 'Robert Redford fade away, a gulag stranger in his place staring back at me'. By November 1988 (18 months post diagnosis) his speech was practically incomprehensible, even to me, and he could do nothing for himself except move his head. It seemed that no sooner had we mourned the loss of one set of muscles and begun to manage the situation than another group would go and we would inherit a different range of problems. There was nothing to build on. The sands were constantly shifting and it was this unrelenting progressive disability that made adjustment so difficult. We could not plan for the future because of the overwhelming pace of change.

I always felt, no matter how much I did for Steve, that it was never enough because I could not stop him dying and as that was what I wanted above all, I constantly felt my efforts were in vain, that I was failing him. An emotional, irrational reaction? Maybe. But I did not just feel impotent. I used to feel guilty too. Guilty that I could go for a walk, chat with a friend, prepare and eat a meal. I could still do those things but they gave me no pleasure knowing that Steve would never again be able to enjoy them.

There were times when Steve was angry, of course, and there were certainly moments of great frustration, but it is a measure of his character that 2 years after the diagnosis he could type, using a pointer strapped to his head:

> I am quite sane at present but feel physically weaker almost daily. I don't feel bitter about my predicament, however, and I never ask why me? I am sad that I cannot watch Eleanor grow up and that she will not have me around for a friend and guide. I am also very sad to see Ros having to care for me in my helpless state. But, despite these sadnesses, I cannot feel sorry for myself having seen so many children and adults lead briefer and less happy lives than mine.

Steve's courage was inspirational. If he was not bitter then nor could I be. It would be so negative, so demeaning. Moreover, bitterness and anger are very draining and I needed all the energy and inner strength I could muster to make the best of whatever time Steve had left – and not just for his sake, but for mine and Eleanor's too. Besides, other people could barely cope with Steve. His emotional lability, in the early stages, was especially hard to accept. Certain friends drifted away. Those who stayed the course would have found it much harder if I had appeared embittered or depressed. I needed their support so I could not risk alienating them. After all, it was nobody's fault.

The realization that I would need support dawned slowly. My first instinct as a carer was to be completely independent. I felt Steve's increasing disability was so distressing for him, so undignified, that he had enough to bear. I wanted to spare him the further humiliation that I imagined would arise out of being cared for by others. I also felt that by doing things myself, in relative secrecy, I could somehow pretend to the outside world in general, and the family in particular, that life was not so bad.

However, as Steve began to require more attention I had correspondingly less time for other things and I was soon glad of the help the family offered. I began to see that they needed to give help as much as I needed to receive it. By excluding them and insisting on doing everything myself I would actually have made it harder for them to cope, not easier as I had first thought. This was an important lesson – recognizing that I could not manage alone.

As the family began to take responsibility for routine chores I was able to spend more time with Steve. We developed our own coping strategies – our own untutored ways of moving, feeding, communicating – and I began to get an intuitive feel for what Steve wanted, which saved time and effort on both sides.

I acknowledge with the benefit of hindsight, however, that the desire to do everything for Steve myself was misguided. It made him completely dependent on me and, although I sometimes got it wrong, he never really trusted anyone else to get it right. Leaving him for any time was fraught with difficulty, so I rarely left the house for more than half an hour. If I was planning to go for longer he would panic, have problems breathing or fail to be positioned comfortably. This made others nervous of taking responsibility for him. To make matters worse, everyone was so sensitive to Steve's suffering and so anxious not to hurt him that their common sense often deserted them.

For example, to assist communication, we had invented our own alphabet board – a simple grid with the letters arranged in order along five lines. When I pointed to the right line Steve would blink; when I read out the correct letter from that line, he would blink again. Thus letter by letter we spelled out the key words. I became very adept at this and could often predict a word or phrase from the initial letter. Others never quite mastered it. Feeling hot, Steve tried to ask my mother to leave the door open. I quote from his diary:

Peggy got the alphabet board and we tried to converse. We started badly when Peggy pointed to the top line. As I wanted 'd' for door I blinked once – the sign for yes. Peggy said 'Is it your eyes?' I shook my head. After we had repeated this procedure several times Peggy understood why I was blinking and managed to deduce that what I wanted to say began with 'd'. I thought this was a major break-through. It was, however, an isolated success since she then proceeded to guess aloud words beginning with 'd'. How many such words, I asked myself, would you find even in a children's dictionary?'

Communication was not the only problem area. Positioning was another minefield for family volunteers. Once I went out leaving my sister in charge. Steve wrote:

Luckily for me Eleanor stayed at home. Before long I was in a lot of pain so I used the alphabet board to ask Denise to move me. Den said she would try but as she had no idea where to begin I ended up in an even more painful position. Part of the trouble was Den attempting to lift my head before moving my hips and part of the trouble was Den wearing more bangles than a Bantu bride on her wedding night. I tried to show her that my right arm had disappeared underneath me but by this time Den was beginning to panic. Fortunately Eleanor stayed calm. 'Phone Margaret the nurse,' she suggested.

This example demonstrates how Eleanor at 6 was less afraid of Steve's 'ranting' and better able to deal with him than many adults because she was constantly in his company. She was never excluded from helping with his daily care if she wanted to help. Steve appreciated this and it ensured that they retained their close relationship. It also enabled Eleanor to come to terms with her father's illness in a practical way and prepared her for his ultimate death. This example also highlights the need for other helpers to remain in touch with the situation. My sister lived the other side of the country. She visited whenever she could, but each time she arrived things had moved on and she had to steel herself to further deterioration and learn the latest ways of coping. For her and Steve to feel confident about each other they needed to spend much more time together.

Once we really understood the prognosis, we planned to live as normally as possible for as long as possible. For us that meant minimal professional help and no unnecessary aids. We did not want to feel invaded or to turn our house into a nursing home. We wanted our friends and Eleanor's to feel relaxed about visiting. We wanted to establish our own routine and not be bound by someone else's work schedule. We wanted to retain control and flexibility. This may have made us difficult to accommodate at first but ultimately rendered a better service. Our reasons (related to washing, feeding, rest and privacy) for negotiating visits by the primary health care team were readily appreciated when, eventually, we allowed them in.

One of the problems of looking after a loved one at home is the emotional involvement in every aspect of the caring process. Take, for example, the aids that are simply tools of the trade to many in the medical profession. I remember the first time Steve had a plastic splint moulded to support his curling lifeless fingers. I felt physically sick having to fit it. I wanted to cry because he had to submit himself to this. I wanted to spare him the way you want to shield your child from hurt. I felt exactly the same when he had to use a headpointer for typing, a wheelchair, a bottle for passing urine, a gastrostomy tube for feeding, a suction pump, a convene. . . . Each new aid, supplied with the best intention, distressed me. I was confronted with the inescapable truth that things had deteriorated further and I wondered what else he would have to endure.

Of course, I never showed these feelings, or rarely. I did not want Steve to think I was upset, could not cope, would not manage or might finally turn my back on him and his attendant paraphernalia. Instead, I usually gritted my teeth and got on with it, often defusing an awkward or embarrassing moment with humour. It was vital for Eleanor's sake to continue calmly and show how useful the new equipment would be. At her age, she could use the wheelchair for slalom races in the garden and could look upon feeding Steve by gastrostomy tube in much the same way as putting petrol in the car. But, joking apart, however wonderful new aids may be and whatever problems they may solve, professionals must be sensitive about introducing them because for the sufferer and his carer they are yet another reminder of the progressive toll of the disease.

Although we chose initially to manage Steve's condition by ourselves, he did agree to physiotherapy once a week. After a while we contacted the occupational therapist, who supplied implements for eating and drinking, though these were soon redundant. Other pieces of equipment were gradually introduced and we accepted them, reluctantly, if we thought they would actually make life easier. The Motor Neurone Disease Association supplied a useful information pack and their regional care adviser organized a reclining chair from the society's resource bank, which was a godsend. It was one of the few pieces of equipment that remained useful throughout Steve's illness.

Occasionally pieces of equipment were discussed but never materialized, or arrived too late to be of any use. At times the health service seems unable to keep pace with the rate of deterioration in MND patients. I would urge those with influence, therefore, to discriminate positively in favour of MND patients. A piece of equipment can improve their quality of life enormously but they cannot wait months for it. Our speech therapist understood this. She supplied a headpointer for typing and, when it was obvious that Steve's speech was becoming increasingly slurred, she organized the marvellous word processor/voice synthesizer that became his lifeline.

Eighteen months after diagnosis our social worker persuaded me to have a home help because Steve's father, and then my mother, became seriously ill. Proof, if it were needed, of the devastating effect MND has not only on the sufferer but also on those closest to him.

Almost 2 years after diagnosis I was forced to enlist nursing help. I had been washing, dressing, toileting, feeding and moving Steve single-handedly day and night, but one awkward movement sent a shooting pain up his back and he could no longer weight bear. I had to call the district nurse, and when she saw how disabled and dependent Steve had become she insisted on daily visits to help shower and dress him.

Thus a proper pattern of support was established: home care 2 hours a day; district nurse for up to an hour most mornings; GP visiting every 2 weeks or so for symptom control; and physio increasing from one to three sessions a week. The physio was especially beneficial, minimizing stiffness and allowing me to move and dress Steve without causing him pain. Although I learned to do all the exercises I did not do them effectively because I was trying to do everything else as well. When the nurses came I still did all the lifting and moving, making it ever more difficult to be relieved of this responsibility.

During this time we had over a dozen different nurses. I hated each new visitor to the shower room because I had to explain everything all over again and they were of little use until they had been several times. Gradually the number of different nurses reduced to the same four or so and in the final months it was usually the same two with whom we had struck up a special relationship. I became pleased, relieved even, to see them, and they have remained very supportive. I did not like working with so many different nurses in the beginning and I never thought it was fair on Steve. I think it is essential for a small support team to be established consisting of people with whom there is genuine empathy. With MND, in spite of the physical disability, the intellect and personality remain unchanged, but communication can be so severely limited that all other helpers must cooperate very closely with the principal carer over a longish period to build confidence and trust all round.

This was why I never contemplated respite care for Steve. I could not abandon him to people who did not know him. Unless I was with him,

209

which would not have benefited me, he would not have been able to communicate his needs adequately. So it is unlikely Steve would have gained anything from respite care, though this is a personal perspective and does not necessarily apply to other sufferers. He would not have enjoyed the unlimited individual attention he received at home and he would not have had immediate access to the things that mattered most – Eleanor, his writing, his music, books. . . .

However tired I was, I always knew that caring would come to an end one day and I would be able to resume something like a normal life. While Steve was ill all that mattered was looking after him and Eleanor to the best of my ability. I had little time or energy for anything else. I did not mind, but what I needed, in order to keep going, was a good night's sleep. Steve would become uncomfortable in one position and, unable to move himself, would groan or alert me with his alarm. I used to move him all day and between two and eight times a night throughout his illness. I did not have an unbroken night for more than 3 years.

I would have liked someone to spend time getting to know us and our routines with a view to eventually relieving me overnight. I think I could have put up with anything if I had known that once in a while I could have been assured of a complete night's rest. As it was, some nights were intolerable. No sooner had my head hit the pillow than Steve would be asking for another move. There were times when I was rougher than I should have been, when I wept with exasperation, or cried myself to sleep from sheer exhaustion. I came close to breaking point a couple of times but somehow I always pulled back. Unfortunately, though, it did not seem possible to provide the kind of home relief that I felt would be appropriate.

For the last 4 months of his life Steve remained in bed, getting up only to use the commode or for an occasional shower. He still needed to be moved frequently but he had little energy left for the writing that had previously absorbed him. He was fed and had his drugs administered by gastrostomy tube. I had to use a suction pump regularly to remove the excess saliva that pooled in his mouth and the thick mucus that clogged his throat. He required constant attention. In addition to the spasms and other problems associated with moving, and the loss of speech which we regretted most but had grown accustomed to, Steve could not swallow at all and was very frightened of choking. His breathing was very shallow, which made him feel faint at times. He was often painfully constipated and required degrading manual evacuation. Later, possibly as a result of infection, he became doubly incontinent. I knew I could not manage much longer like this with just an hour of nursing help a day, but I did not want to admit it. Steve was also very concerned. When the nurse arrived one morning he was ready with the following message on his voice synthesizer.

> I hope that someone hears this before the situation goes too far. Everyone admires the way Ros has been coping since I've been ill. No one else could have done better. However, she's now reached a point where she is neglecting me. More importantly, she's neglecting herself. This neglect is not deliberate, of course, but results from Ros attempting to do everything without very much help. We are grateful for any help we've received but I feel it's time to review our situation otherwise someone will have to find me a residential hospital bed, Eleanor a foster home, and Ros a place for psychiatric treatment.
>
> I am resigned to die soon, to go somewhere for everlasting respite care, but I hope my wife and daughter will live long and healthy lives. I'm afraid that if there is no one to help Ros she will work herself into illness. In recent months I've observed signs that she is not the organised, easy-going, vivacious carer she used to be. I know that Ros still loves me. Why else would she put up with me? But love is no longer enough.

The outcome of this cry from the heart was three or four visits from Crossroads, an organization that cares for carers. The first time their sitter came I succeeded in having a bath without being disturbed. Another time I was able to browse in the supermarket and once I managed to meet my parents for a quick lunch. It could have worked but, as it transpired, it was too little, too late.

One afternoon in April 1991 a sudden alteration in Steve's breathing pattern and a tell-tale change of colour alerted me to the fact that he was nearing his death. The doctor confirmed this. For the first time in 4 years I was told it would be no trouble to arrange for a night nurse immediately. I refused. I had never sat with anyone who was dying; I had never even seen a dead person before, but I was not afraid. After everything we had been through together I had no doubt that I would cope. I did not want to share Steve and his final hours with a stranger. Although I had been close to confessing I could not go on, I was certain, now the end was in sight, that I could do anything for Steve in those last precious moments of intimacy.

I filled the room with flowers from the garden. Eleanor and I read to him from an advance copy of the book he had written during his illness. Later I played Steve some of his favourite music, including pieces he had chosen for his funeral. At that point he seemed to drift. I climbed into bed with him and held him gently. He died in my arms and I cuddled him for a long time. When I felt ready, I called the doctor.

Steve died exactly as he had wanted – at home, with just Eleanor and me. It was peaceful and painless. I was very sad and elated simultaneously. I felt as if I has done everything I could. In the end, there was no guilt. I had an almost intoxicating sense of relief.

Steve once wrote, 'Motor neurone disease has made me entirely dependent on the help of others. As each muscle in my body mutinies against the orders sent out by my brain I'm locked in solitary confinement on death row'.

But he was not alone. There were many times when I, as his carer, felt imprisoned with him. The difference was that I had a stay of execution and I'm on remission now, but I frequently remind myself that however hard it is to care for someone with MND it is a million times worse to have the disease. And, for the victims, there is sadly no reprieve.

10 *Coping with the disability of established disease*

JIM UNSWORTH

10.1 INTRODUCTION

The heterogeneous nature of motor neurone disease, symptom classification and life expectancy are covered elsewhere in this book. The physical impairments seen commensurate with the neurological progression of the disease are broadly predictable but the services offered to an individual can have a marked impact on both the level of disability and handicap conferred. To the non-specialist, motor neurone disease is an uncommon diagnosis and poor or inadequate provision of information, support and counselling in the early stages is sadly the rule rather than the exception. An average family practitioner would see only one new case of motor neurone disease every 25 years or so and given the short, sometimes aggressive course that is often seen there is little chance to gain confidence and expertise. I would strongly advocate the use of specialist centres for early confirmation of diagnosis, backed up with a consistency of approach that can provide accurate information, counselling and support which is focused towards inter-agency and interdisciplinary collaboration, and the setting of attainable therapeutic or rehabilitation goals and their delivery. Honesty is vitally important and patients will quickly expose inconsistencies in the approach of the clinical team which can damage the relationship that must provide a central basis for the treatments offered. People should be offered the information available about voluntary support agencies such as the Motor Neurone Disease Association, although it is an individual decision whether or not they use them.

From both sides of the consultation, it is easy to focus on the loss of function and disabilities which occurs during the progression of the disease; it is more difficult to be open, frank and realistic whilst at the same time concentrating on the abilities and potential which remain. Try to remember that people are living with motor neurone disease, not dying from it.

10.2 SYMPTOMS AND TREATMENT

Historically, symptoms and physical signs have been empirically grouped and although obviously the reader must be aware of the better prognosis in 'progressive muscular atrophy', there is overlap especially during the later course of the disease with 'amyotrophic lateral sclerosis' giving a mixed picture reflecting upper and lower motor neurone degeneration. Bulbar dysfunction occurs in over 80% of affected individuals. For the purposes of this text, the distinctions are not important and I will concentrate on the functional consequences of the neurological deterioration.

10.2.1 The upper limb

Asymmetrical weakness of one arm is a common presenting feature of motor neurone disease. Normally this starts in the hand and progresses centrally although occasionally the shoulder may have been involved at first. The weakness normally becomes symmetrical and is most commonly lower motor neurone in type. Diagnostic anecdotes include presentation because of an inability to dress or undress because of a loss of dexterity, a sudden inability to wind clockwork devices because of the weakness in pro and supination and shoulder girdle pain. Although cramps are relatively rare at presentation, 40% of patients will experience significant abnormal cramp-like sensation in their muscles at some stage in the disease and the biceps, quadriceps and peroneal muscles are the commonest sites.

Unless a person's job or hobby demands great dexterity, functional impairment is not normally significant until the long flexors of the fingers are involved. This is compromised by weakness in the fingers and wrist extensors and although grip can be improved by orthotic intervention this is seldom helpful in the medium term. A working wrist splint which holds the wrist in about 20° of extension will maximize the remaining function in the long flexors. Although it may be tempting to add active extension of the digits to produce a 'lively' splint, these devices are difficult to manufacture to an individual's requirements, and cumbersome and need constant modification to keep pace with the changing pattern of weakness. Encouraging the passive extension of the metacarpo–phalangeal and interphalangeal joints hourly will prevent contractures, and avoid maceration of the palm which can be accompanied by excoriation as the fingernails dig into the palm. If the individual is unable to perform passive exercises independently these should be performed by a friend or carer after initial supervision by a trained therapist, ideally at least twice daily. A Bespoke plastic or plaster night resting splint can be a useful adjunct to therapy which will help preserve function if combined with adaptations and advice as detailed later.

10.2.2 The elbow

Weakness of pro and supination is common, making feeding and other complex tasks difficult. This is often accompanied by weakness of the elbow flexors and shoulder girdle. No formal orthotic intervention is helpful but support against gravity for the arm can maximize function. At its most simple this could be a wheeled coaster to help with writing or desk work, or one of the more complex mobile arm supports such as those supplied by district wheelchair services or the commercially available devices. In my experience, swivelling wheelchair or armchair arms are unlikely to add to an individual's abilities because of the restricted range of movement that results from these arrangements.

10.2.3 The shoulder

It is usual for the weakness in motor neurone disease to spread to the shoulder but, as mentioned above, it can occasionally start there. Simple tasks such as grooming, washing, shaving, feeding and dressing become difficult. A painful shoulder disrupts sleep and greatly interferes with both independent and assisted transfers. The most easily prevented disability is that of a secondary frozen shoulder or adhesive capsulitis (Kumar *et al.*, 1990). Greater awareness has made this much less common and a full range of passive movements, taking less than five minutes, performed twice daily is effective prophylaxis. If the condition is untreated it tends to be more persistent than 'idiopathic' frozen shoulder but will still respond to therapy and manipulation. If augmented by an intra-articular injection of corticosteroid with local anaesthetic (25 mg of Triamcinolone hexacetonide plus 5 ml lignocaine 1%) relief is hastened.

If there is weakness of the shoulder girdle, gleno-humeral subluxation can be significant. This is often accompanied by disruption of the rotator cuff, subacromial bursitis, sometimes with acromioclavicular joint pain. It is very important that the diagnosis is appropriately made and swiftly treated. Local therapeutic techniques (megapulse, ultrasound, interferential etc.) have a place in the management of this more complex disorder but the anatomical disturbance will normally lead to persistent discomfort. Support for the shoulder can be useful. I have found no benefit in the long term in using a 'figure of eight' bandage. It is however possible to unload the gleno-humeral or subacromial joints to a degree

215

either by using a 'muffler' slung around the neck (although it is impossible to disguise this device and most people are reluctant to use it) or a tailored, elasticated fabric or neoprene, shoulder support. Supporting straps across the body must be positioned to give optimal mechanical advantage. Unfortunately this seldom provides lasting relief. Simple pain killers and non-steroidal anti-inflammatory drugs may be prescribed and can work well. A suprascapular nerve block is effective in relieving intractable shoulder pain (Black *et al.*, 1990).

Gleno-humeral subluxation may be measured by palpating the subacromial space with and without traction on the lower arm. Subjectively this can then be assessed in 'finger breadths' or objectively by measuring the distance from the tip of the acromium to the lateral epicondyl with and without traction. Although superspinatous or subacromial pain is rare in isolation, injection with steroid and local anaesthetic is helpful. More commonly the problem is less well defined anatomically, and in my experience injection to the structures around the shoulder, with or without a suprascapular nerve block, offers the best hope of relief. Ideally, the patient sits on the edge of an examining couch with the affected arm extended and internally rotated behind their back. The subacromial space and anterior aspect of the shoulder joint are infiltrated with local anaesthetic and steroids. With practice this is both untraumatic and effective. The procedure may be repeated as appropriate depending on the relief conferred, taking into account the individual's prognosis and the likelihood of developing side effects. It is important to exclude as far as possible cervical root pain as a contributory factor for any discomfort in the upper limb (Hawkins *et al.*, 1990).

10.2.4 The spine

Cervical and lumbar pain are common in motor neurone disease. Poor posture when seated and a loss of tone in the cervical region with a decrease in head control are important contributory factors. Lumbar pain is classically postural and occasionally presents because of an exaggerated lumbar lordosis. Much more commonly there is a loss of the lumbar lordosis aggravated if not caused by a poor seating position. This is important especially for people who are obligate wheelchair users, who may be unable to change their position throughout the course of a whole day. Most people find a lumbar corset restrictive and as diaphragmatic breathing is important in motor neurone disease, these should be avoided if possible. Sculpted back supports for wheel and easy chairs are easy to fabricate or can be purchased. Pre-existing back problems can be exacerbated by the loss of paraspinal musculature and it is not uncommon for surgery to have been performed for a mistaken diagnosis of prolapsed intervertebral disc at the onset of the disease.

The invaluable experience gained in a unit that has dealt with motor neurone disease for some time cannot be understated and the expertise of physiotherapists in providing local pain management techniques and occupational therapists in correctly seating people is of paramount importance here.

Although variable, both in extent and progression, lack of head control is common. This is normally manifest by a flopping forwards of the head and is frequently associated with bulbar symptoms and signs. This results in dribbling of saliva. A cervical collar is often recommended to relieve the symptoms of neck pain and correct the adopted position. These tend to be difficult if not impossible to don and doff independently and the fear of choking or asphyxiating is very common. It is necessary to exert force on the mandible to keep the head erect with such a device and this will compromise already weakened muscles of mastication. There are several types of collar available and individual clinical circumstances will dictate which is appropriate. While travelling in a car there can be a significant risk of neurological damage from even minor collisions. A reasonably firm or well fitting collar should be strongly recommended for use at all such times. Although it is difficult to predict which individuals would benefit from its use, the MNDA head support developed with the help of the Motor Neurone Disease Association at Mary Marlborough Lodge in Oxford has proved invaluable in the management of poor head control in a large number of patients with motor neurone disease. The spring tension and dimensions of the chin support can be adjusted and it is much less restrictive than a standard collar although of course conferring no protection during travel (see Figure 10.1). As with all specialized orthoses the device is ineffective unless fitted by experts. The use of circumferential head bands (e.g. the Lee's head support) either mounted on an aluminium support frame strapped to the back, or more commonly attached to a wheelchair, has been advocated. As with all such devices some people find benefit, while others are intolerant of them.

10.2.5 The ankle

Motor neurone disease occasionally presents with asymmetrical progressive (lower motor neurone type) footdrop and tripping or stumbling will be the main complaint. It is often difficult to ascend or descend stairs safely. Most commonly this progresses to become bilateral and predominantly upper motor neurone in type. This predisposes to falling and without the protection afforded by being able to cushion the fall

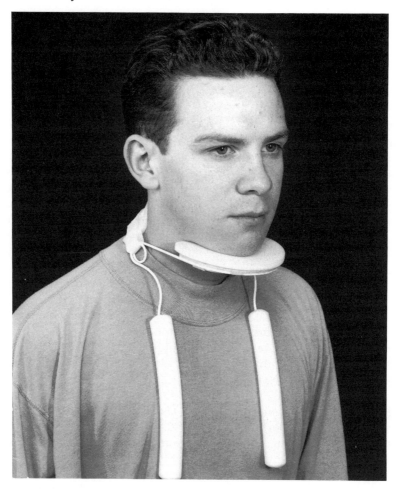

Figure 10.1 MNDA head support.

with outstretched arms it is dangerous and demoralizing. The hypertonia is often more marked than the weakness, and responds variably to antispasmodics (Baclofen, Dantrolene, Diazepam) which can compromise the function in the upper limbs.

There are a battery of ankle foot orthoses available from a light spring loaded device, plastic or polythene ankle foot orthoses through to bespoke items which can be cast and made of more durable materials (e.g. a high density polythene or ortholene), fabricated to give enough medial or lateral support to stabilize an ankle drifting into varus or valgus. If the active equinus deformity is significant, then it may be

218

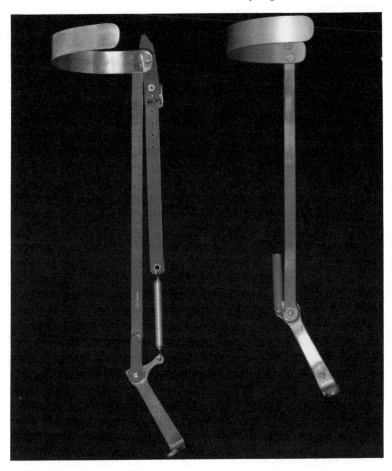

Figure 10.2 Below knee irons with external and concealed springs.

necessary to have a strap across the ankle to hold the foot into the splint. Below knee irons with either a backstop or concealed spring device fitted to the calliper have been used effectively especially in male patients. The scope of these devices is however limited because of weight. A selection of these ankle foot supports is shown in Figures 10.2 and 10.3.

10.2.6 The knee

It is more common to have increased than decreased tone at the knee and therefore dynamic orthotic devices are less useful. If the muscular imbalance around the knee has aggravated a pre-existing arthritic

219

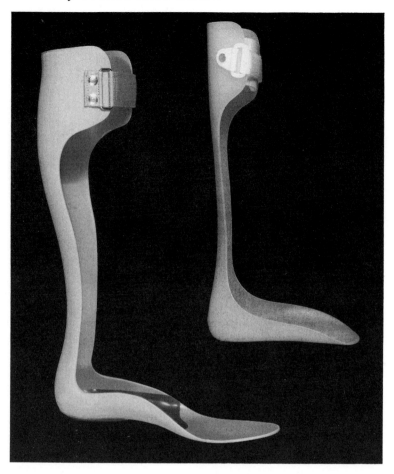

Figure 10.3 Bespoke ortholene and stock polythene ankle foot orthoses.

condition, then local treatment as appropriate may be helpful. If the problem is one of weak quadriceps and an inability to lock the knee, then occasionally a hinged (Stanmore type) knee ankle foot orthosis (KAFO) with a set back knee mechanism will stabilize the stance phase of gait. Any advantage given is normally short-lived and provision should only be made with care as the device can contribute to falls if inappropriately prescribed. Mobility and transferring ability can be improved using a KAFO with a locking knee mechanism. Some support can be given if the knee is painful from either a 'Tubigrip' or neoprene knee support. Occasionally a valgus support brace is provided but again, I seldom find these helpful. When orthotic support is required

220

above the ankle, given the tendency to fall, the danger in doing so and the progressive nature of motor neurone disease, it is only rarely that corrective orthotic management is warranted.

10.3 ACTIVITIES OF DAILY LIVING

People's requirements will constantly change throughout the course of the disease and it is important that any assessment of aids or adaptations which are designed to confer independence in the activities of daily living is appropriately and realistically targeted to produce a rapid and effective result. Delay is unacceptable and can easily represent a missed opportunity.

10.3.1 Sleeping

Sleep disturbance is common in motor neurone disease, especially later in the course of the condition. Muscle cramps and pains in the neck, shoulders and legs are a common feature of the disease. A combination of (normally) unimpaired sensation and significantly reduced mobility lead to difficulties in turning or changing position voluntarily in bed. Sometimes a comfortable night's sleep can be gained just by trying different types of mattress, with and without pressure redistributing overlays. Particular care must be taken because although pressure sore formation is rare, a poor night's sleep is common. Examples of overlays include the Spenco, Propad, Ripple and Roho devices. Different sleeping positions need to be experimented with and a fixed backrest is simple to construct and less liable to slip than pillows. Alternatively, a pneumatic or electrically operated adjustable backrest, which can be controlled by the 'patient', allows more independence. Beds are available which will both turn the individual or give them complete control of their position (Disabled Living Foundation, 1992). Antispasmodics or sedative drugs can be used (vide supra), and occasionally quinine-related drugs will ease cramps. Analgesics are seldom effective in relieving night pains.

As dependence increases, help may be needed to use a urinal, bed pan or commode or gain access to the toilet during the night. The appropriate positioning or provision of equipment can greatly help. Shoulder pain can disturb sleep and once this is recognized it can be treated.

Nocturnal hypoventilation with drowsiness and fatigue on waking must be identified and its medical and mechanical management is discussed elsewhere.

It is helpful to discuss early on with couples whether or not they wish to sleep in the same room or bed. Due consideration must be given to the supporting partner's health and welfare. It is however surprising how infrequently people complain about disturbance because of their spouse's requirements.

10.3.2 Transfers

Safe transferring is essential and an individual assessment by a trained and experienced physiotherapist is invaluable. The pattern of weakness or spasticity will greatly determine recommended transfer techniques. It cannot be stressed too much that the transfers need to be safe, both for the transferred and transferrer. Due consideration must be given to the help available and the abilities of the people providing help. The accessibility, heights and relationships of easy chair, wheelchair, toilet, bath, bed, motor car etc. all need to be borne in mind. It is often sufficient to have been instructed in the correct mechanical principles and ergonomics underlying safe transfer. For people who can still take weight through their legs a turning disc can be a very effective aid. Even late on in the course of the disease the spasticity in the legs can still be used to effect standing transfer. There are a wide range of hoists and slings available and a thorough knowledge is required before undertaking any assessment (Cochrane, 1990). Hydraulic, portable hoists are difficult to push over carpet when loaded. Electric hoists can be portable or mounted on overhead tracking. A well thought out hoisting system can greatly enable both user and carer. The benefits that this confers are enormous, but unfortunately time and financial constraints sometimes lead to the recommendation of a less comprehensive system.

Probably the most difficult transfer to achieve safely is into and out of a motor car. Given a choice of car, it would be possible to pick one of ideal height (indeed some have variable height suspensions), with large doors (two or three door cars tend to have larger doors than four or five door models) (Darnborough and Kincade). Only a minority of people with motor neurone disease can use a sliding board safely for transfer and it is sometimes necessary to use either a rotating car seat or even a roof mounted car hoist.

10.3.3 Dressing and clothing

Where possible the maximum independence should be preserved for dressing and an awareness of the problem and an open mind will often provide a solution early on in the disease. When people are still mobile it is common to have difficulty in fastening or undoing buttons. If the button is replaced by Velcro but resewn on as a cosmetic rather than functional item, the normal appearance of a shirt or blouse can be retained but with the convenience of easy fastening. Ambulant men might have difficulty undoing their trouser zips which can even lead to incontinence. The addition of a 'ring pull' on the zipper allows an individual to hook their thumb for closure and opening and can avoid great personal embarrassment.

The use of bibs to collect rather than control salivation is common; these can be replaced by a more cosmetically acceptable 'polo neck' with a false bib front. Wide or larger shoes may be needed to accommodate orthoses and depending on the individual's disability, other dressing aids can be useful. Further reading is advised (Cochrane, 1989).

10.3.4 Bathing

It is important to make sure that existing bathing or washing facilities are both accessible and safe. This may require the simple addition of a non-slip surface to a bath or shower base, or the provision of appropriate grab rails. After determining whether independent, supervised or assisted techniques are appropriate (now and in the future) equipment and structural adaptations can be recommended. Major adaptations can be a worthwhile investment and these should be anticipated rather than being a response to a crisis. Where it is appropriate modifications to the existing equipment are obviously preferable, and simple devices are available to make any transfer in and out of a bath safe. Sliding boards and bath seats can help, but as the weakness progresses more complex equipment may be needed. The majority of showers over bathtubs are difficult to use for people with motor neurone disease and an ordinary shower tray is both too small to accommodate safe seating and relatively inaccessible because of the lip. A custom built level access shower that is non-slip and (shower chair) accessible allows both independent and assisted bathing in safety and comfort. However, it is often impossible to fit these because of the flooring and drainage, so a modular shower unit is preferable. Specially adapted baths can help with transfer problems but in general it is more appropriate to provide an effective hoisting system.

10.3.5 Shaving

Having established that a clean shaven man does not wish to grow a beard nor a bearded one wish to keep it, then weakness in the arms and shoulder girdles obviously presents problems with shaving. If it is acceptable then the lightest possible electric shaver is the most appropriate implement. The hazards of wet shaving are willingly accepted by some people out of personal preference. Mobile arm supports can help, and if neck movement remains good, then a shaver fixed in front of the individual gives the opportunity for a close shave. If these manoeuvres are difficult or dangerous and help is available, either a wet or dry shave can be easily accomplished with assistance.

10.3.6 Dental hygiene

There have been many attempts to provide an automated mechanism for tooth brushing. None are wholly successful but for people with good head control and limited use of their arms, an (electric) toothbrush can be fixed and the head moved around it. This is not normally satisfactory as the limited cleaning effected is not adequate. If the individual can use mobile arm supports with an electric toothbrush this may help. The advice and treatment of an experienced dental hygienist is strongly recommended, especially for people with bulbar dysfunction, because food residue in the cheeks and on the palate combined with a tendency to mouth breath leaves a dry and unpleasant taste. Mouthwashes, lozenges and good advice on head and neck positioning are all important. As with most other problems awareness and experience count for much.

10.4 ELIMINATION

Establishing a regular bowel habit and pattern of micturition will be not only possible but useful later on in the disease. Perineal access can be a problem even quite early on in the disease and this needs to be approached sensibly. Continence and the independent management of bladder and bowel function are important in the maintenance of dignity and self-esteem. Conversely, problems with incontinence or the inability to adequately toilet oneself can be demoralizing. As sphincter sensation and function are not normally affected it is normally lack of mobility or access that causes problems.

10.4.1 Bladder

Often the first problem manifest in attempting urination is the inability to remove clothes or gain perineal access. Simple adaptations to trouser zips have been discussed earlier and consideration needs to be given as to whether or not a dress or skirt would be easier for a woman to use with appropriate underclothes. For men, both ambulant and non-ambulant, a sheath drainage system can provide reassurance and will allow them to void urine without assistance or away from home provided the bag is emptied frequently and the seal at the base of the penis is adequate. With the use of devices to provide supra-pubic pressure, fixation, or adhesion, in-dwelling catheters should be avoidable. Catheters are needed more frequently in women, as no equivalent satisfactory external device is available. Until too weak it is possible to use a female urinal or a slipper bedpan either from a bed or easy chair (it is more difficult in a wheelchair when a special cut out cushion may be required). Frequently people will decrease their fluid intake in order to reduce the amount of urine that they need to void and thereby lessen the problem. This in itself is not without hazard and can certainly exacerbate constipation and general ill health through dehydration. Where regular support is available and acceptable, a toileting schedule can maintain continence.

10.4.2   Bowels

Immobility combined with a decreased fluid input and difficulty in eating foods that have a high fibre content, sometimes aggravated by medication, can predispose to, or worsen, constipation. Not only is this uncomfortable and distressing for the individual but it also makes bowel movements unpredictable, irregular and tedious. Good dietetic advice early in the course of the disease with the maintenance of a regular bowel habit will greatly help.

It is important to maintain a good fluid balance and avoid opiate or related analgesics. If it is not possible to take an adequate amount of fibre by normal dietary means then it may be helpful to add bran to food. Commercially available stool bulking agents such as Isphagula husk (Fybogel, Isogel, Regulan) may be used in conjunction with substances which increase the water content of the stool by osmosis (Lactitol, Lactulose) or a faecal softener and mild stimulant such as Co-danthramer. If good advice is given early enough then constipation can normally be avoided without the use of stimulant laxatives although occasionally these may be unavoidable. For established constipation or the regularization of bowel habit, glycerine suppositories can be used to initiate defecation. Enemata should not be necessary.

10.4.3   Toilets

Simple seat raisers on the toilet combined with sturdy rails or side supports can maintain independence in toileting and personal hygiene for some time although cleaning can be difficult because of weakness or impaired perineal access. It is unusual to benefit from the use of toilet paper holders or similar devices and unless it is possible to have a partner or carer who is prepared to perform these intimate functions without causing undue embarrassment, the most acceptable alternative is to try one of the semi-automated combined 'wash and blow dry' toilet adaptations.

10.5 MOBILITY

Progression of the disease inevitably leads to a decrease in mobility, which can be helped by the addition of a walking aid to a simple walking stick, which may have a moulded (Fischer type) handle. Tri- and quadropods are more stable but with the typical clinical picture of motor neurone disease, gripping these devices is difficult. Many people feel safe with a walking frame and the more easily propelled Rollator is normally preferred to a standard Zimmer. A 'walkabout', such as the Metco trolley, can be extremely useful and a mobility assessment should include the opportunity to try both gutter and pulpit type frames.

The majority of people with motor neurone disease will require a wheelchair at some stage in their condition. Only a minority can self-propel and those who do normally 'scoot' along with their feet. If a self-propeller is required, and if one is recommended, it should be as ergonomically efficient as possible. The majorlty of chairs required are for transit or are electrically powered. A transit chair is normally propelled by an attendant and the individual may spend many hours sitting in it. It is important to recognize that a change of position is very difficult for people with advanced motor neurone disease and so short-term assessments have their limitations. The seating should be as anatomically correct, accommodating and comfortable as possible. The provision of a lumbar support, sacral pad, ramped base and lateral support is required, and expert advice and follow up is needed from the local wheelchair services. Occasionally people will feel more comfortable when an insert is provided such as the Spenco or Burnet body support. If there is a danger of pressure sores or in case of discomfort, a pressure relieving cushion can be supplied. This can be made from simple, or scored, foam of differing densities, a gel or pneumatic (Roho type) device. As mentioned above, for female users, cushions may need to be sculpted to enable urination.

The environment within which an electrically powered chair is to be used needs to be carefully appraised and the recommendations about appropriate seating mentioned above are relevant here. If an outdoor powered chair is to be recommended then in the clinician's eyes there must be a full explanation of any risk with contraindications clearly stated. It is possible to control the powered wheelchair if there is **any** voluntary movement **reliably** present. There is a vast array of equipment available which requires a specialist bioengineering department to be adequately explored and appraised. Surface electrodes or infra-red beams can detect eye movement. Single switch input can be linked with an appropriate and, if necessary, gated direction finding device. 'Manual' access of head or chin switches, or with a swashplate operated by foot movement if possible, can be most effective.

10.6 EATING

The problems with swallowing will be discussed later. The preparation of food is vitally important. Feeding difficulties tend to be related to either physical inability to get the fork or spoon to the mouth or a disturbance in chewing or swallowing mechanisms. If eating is difficult, then towards the end of the meal, fatigue can further compromise the existing impairment and it is important not to base too much on a single examination. If independent feeding is impossible then a sensible approach is needed by the carer as this increasing dependence can be demoralizing for the individual. A close relationship and a calm atmosphere do much to aid mastication and deglutition. Eating assessments are appropriately carried out by an experienced team involving nursing, speech therapy, dietetic and specialized medical elements. To start, consider:

- Table height. This is important and, if the forearm is rested on a tray or table near mouth height, it is easier to get the food to the mouth. Occasionally people eat directly from the plate which can then be mounted on a turning disc.
- Taste of the meal. This can be used as an incentive; a well prepared and enjoyable meal is more likely to be persevered with.
- Temperature. This must be right for the individual. Food that is excessively hot can increase incoordination and spasm. The sucking of ice cubes before a meal, the application of an ice pack around the neck and sub-mandibular area as well as eating ice cream before a meal, seem to help some people.
- Texture of the food. This must be to the individual's requirement and may need experimentation with a blender, food processor or sieve. Problems are normally experienced either with liquids or food that requires excessive chewing. High fibre foods unfortunately can often be difficult to swallow. I am told that a well cooked and blended meal can be as enjoyable to eat as the individual components which are subsequently blended in the mouth but I have no recent experience to confirm or refute this.

The disability of established disease

- Temperance. This may, in this instance, be a virtue as alcohol can exacerbate existing dysfunction, and spirits can precipitate acute muscle spasms.
- Timing. The timing of the feeding routine is important. With the correct positioning of the head a conscious effort is made to take small mouthfuls, chew them thoroughly, pass them to the back of the throat, pause and then try to initiate a swallow. It may be better to take small, nutritious meals frequently and if necessary remain upright for a period after finishing eating to avoid regurgitation.
- Technological solutions are available. The mechanical foot-operated feeding aid developed at Mary Marlborough Lodge in Oxfordshire, the Magpie manipulator, is an example. This device utilizes accurate foot movement to control a spoon which, with little practice, allows an individual to put the food, if appropriately prepared, between the plate and mouth. It has also been used to manipulate other devices. Robotic feeding aids are being developed. The simple concept behind the Handy-1 robot has enabled people with advanced and severely disabling conditions to control what they eat (Topping, 1989), as seen in Figure 10.4.

10.7 SWALLOWING

At any one time, approximately half of the people diagnosed as suffering from motor neurone disease will be experiencing communication and/or swallowing difficulties (Nerwick and Langton Hewer, 1984). When swallowing becomes a problem, normally there are both upper and lower motor neurone components to the clinical picture. The tongue is usually affected first, with the disease progressing to the palate, pharynx and larynx. Poor tongue movement impairs bolus formation and decreases the channelling of fluids and propulsion of solids into the pharynx. Poor palatal lift with a failure of velopharyngeal closure reduces the ability to develop a negative intra-oral pressure which would physiologically lift the hyoid and initiate deglutition. This is worsened by poor lip closure. An orthodontically fitted palatal lift or loop can stimulate this reflex. Although nasal regurgitation is uncommon, it does occur. Cricopharyngeal spasm or incoordination is commonly found in motor neurone disease. It is important to establish the exact nature of the swallowing problem, appreciate the changing picture seen with the disease and advise accordingly.

The parameters that need to be examined for safe and acceptable swallowing have been mentioned above. The importance of a good functional position will bear repeating as will the importance of a calm and controlled atmosphere at all times. Dysphagia or choking at meal

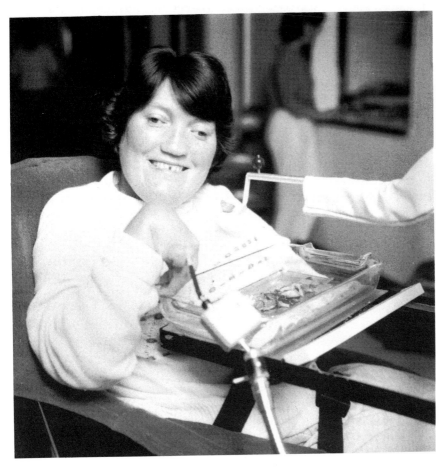

Figure 10.4 The Handy 1 feeding robot (Rehab Robotics, University of Keele).

times is frightening and it is important to train attendants in basic resuscitation techniques so that they are able to manually clear the airway and give assisted coughing, and are proficient in the use of a suction device. The clinician should be aware that fatigue during the course of a meal is an important contributory factor to choking.

It can be particularly distressing not to be able to swallow saliva and a combination of an immobile tongue, loss of automatic swallowing reflex, and poor head position make this only too obvious. The normal salivary volume is in excess of two litres per day and the fluid and electrolyte loss that can occur in marked cases of dribbling is significant. Exercise and techniques to improve lip closure will help. The application of ice as

The disability of established disease

described above is also beneficial, simple clothing adaptations have been suggested earlier and of course a clear explanation of the problems is mandatory. Atropine drops 0.6 mg tds will increase the viscosity and decrease the volume of secretions as will the prescription of a tricyclic anti-depressant. Topical antimuscarinic preparations have been applied using skin patches over the jaw with some effect. The side effects seen with these medications can be significant as the viscous saliva is difficult to clear, foul tasting, and may have an increased tendency to harbour *Candida*. Radiotherapy to the salivary glands is advocated and has been used successfully. It can, unfortunately, aggravate problems with swallowing and must only be recommended by an experienced team. Surgical diversion of the salivary flow, dependent on the intra-oral musculature, can be very valuable and a simple reversal of Wharton's ducts will benefit selected patients. I have had no experience with transtympanic chorda tympani neurectomy, in which partial denervation of the salivary glands is said to be effective in decreasing secretion (Zalin and Cooney, 1974).

If an inability to eat leads to significant or protracted weight loss, dehydration, unmanageable constipation, regurgitation and/or aspiration then a full clinical and radiological assessment of the relevant pathologies may be needed. In experienced hands, the most useful confirmatory investigation is video fluoroscopy. Investigation, however, should not be performed when it will not influence treatment or advice.

If conservative measures have failed, swallowing can be preserved surgically. I believe that for the vast majority of people with motor neurone disease these procedures are not indicated. If the epiglottis fails to protect the airway during swallowing and adduction of the vocal chords is seen to be incomplete at nasendoscopy then Teflon injection into the vocal chords has been recommended. If phonation is absent, a glottic closure or laryngectomy with the fabrication of a permanent tracheostomy will allow safe swallowing. I have no experience of either of these measures. Cricopharyngeal dysfunction can be identified either by manometry or videofluoroscopy (Wilston *et al.*, 1990). Cricopharyngeal myotomy can be very effective for some people and ineffective in others and carries a high morbidity and mortality (Loizou, Small and Dalton, 1980).

If the difficulties in achieving adequate hydration and nourishment by mouth are insurmountable, even after consideration of operative intervention, it is helpful to openly discuss alternatives: the insertion of a fine bore nasogastric tube, which can be made either of soft plastic or woven silk, may be difficult because of the incoordination of bulbar musculature. It is important that the clinician inserting such a device is experienced and it may be necessary to check radiologically that the tube is in place before commencing feeding or hydration. Dietary supplements such as Fortison (standard) or fluids can be fed by gravity or infusion pump. These devices are comfortable (unlike the Ryle's tubes) for long term use but prone to blocking in domiciliary maintenance and need a confident clinician to re-insert them. An oesophagostomy or pharyngostomy will permit the permanent or intermittent introduction of a wider bore tube. The stoma is normally on the left side of the neck and it can be covered effectively with a scarf or cravat. In my experience this is less acceptable than a percutaneous endoscopic gastrostomy (PEG) which is easy to insert and manage. If the patient is able to undergo the endoscopic procedure then the silicone tube left *in situ* will permit the dietary supplement or fluids to be administered directly to the stomach either by gravity or an infusion pump. It is possible in most people to give the bulk of the food and fluids overnight as long as this does not cause problems with nocturnal production of urine. Most medications can be given either in crushed or in syrup form into the tube and it is still possible to take water or ice in the mouth, and indeed if supervised and safe, to eat small amounts of food which can be enjoyed at leisure.

10.8 COMMUNICATION

Throughout the course of motor neurone disease, more than three-quarters of patients will have severe problems with communication or speech (Saunders, *et al.*). The first sign is most often a decrease in articulation skills which will progress to a frank dysarthria, sometimes with nasal speech dysphonia or aphonia. It is important to recognize that the action of bulbar muscles is not the same in swallowing and speech (Bosma and Brodie, 1969). A full and expert speech therapy assessment is required, identifying dysfunction and highlighting compensatory techniques such as the speed of delivery, avoidance of difficult sounds, stress and pausing techniques. The diminished respiratory reserve means that shorter sentences are easier to deliver intelligibly. Again, sucking ice cubes or applying an ice pack (or frozen vegetables!) to the face and throat for three to five minutes, three or four times a day, can helpfully change tone and increase articulation skills. Badly fitting dentures should be replaced and the provision of a palatal lift can improve the quality of speech (Enderby, Hathorne and Servant, 1984).

Where phonation is quiet then a speech amplifier may be used and if absent then an external or intra-oral artificial larynx can compensate assuming the muscles of articulation are sufficiently preferred. It is important to recognize that communication skills need to be taught, not just to the patient, but also to those people at home or work who 'co-own' the communication problem. Lip-reading and signing skills can provide useful prompts and other methods of non-verbal communication have been clearly described.

Even with the best management, communication problems will normally develop as the disease progresses. The signing, lip reading and other 'clues' learned by immediate family and friends will be helpful as speech becomes more difficult. For the age group normally affected by motor neurone disease, symbolic or pictorial communication systems are less useful than text and the spoken word. The spoken word is needed to address a group of people, those who are illiterate, people with impaired vision or small children. If the ability to write is retained then this is a rapid and effective means of communication. Different adaptations are available to make the writing implement easier to grip (Cochrane).

Quite rightly, light writers are universally popular. An alphabetically arranged alternative to the 'QWERTY' keyboard layout is available for some models to aid those without typing skills (Figure 10.5). There are two single line LCD displays, one facing the user and the other facing the person being addressed. There can be memory, printout or speech synthesizer attachments. Keyguards are available which reduce the probability of an incorrect keystroke. The great advantage of these devices is that with practice people can become very proficient in their use and they do allow communication with others who lack special skills.

The addition of speech to a communication system greatly extends its potential and the enormous developments in this field make a comprehensive review beyond the scope of this chapter. The reader is strongly advised to seek expert advice. In the UK there are a number of interdisciplinary teams who provide specialist advice for the recommendation, training in and modification of aids to communication. In general, there is a distinction between recorded, digitized and synthetic speech. Recorded messages can be stored and replayed at will, giving excellent quality but a very limited repertoire. Digitized speech is an abstraction from recorded human voice which the computer then reiterates to form new sentences and messages. This provides a rapid and intelligible device albeit of limited vocabulary. Speech synthesis is the *de novo* generation of electronic speech converting text into phonemes and thence speech, the quality of which depends entirely upon the complexity of the program and the skill of the operator in manipulating the system. The first generation speech synthesizing units delivered a staccato male heavily accented North American voice and

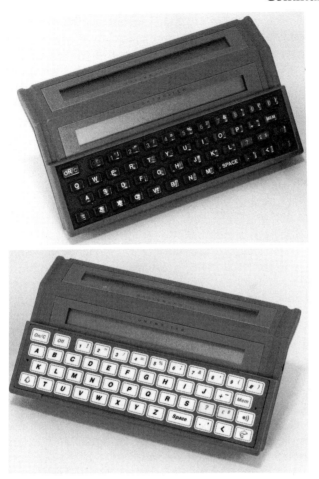

Figure 10.5 'QWERTY' and alphabetical lightwriter keyboard displays.

were difficult to understand in conversation. Later generations are much better and more flexible. The vocabulary is unlimited in these devices but the pronunciation can be a poor 'guess'.

Electronic speech is an important help in communicating. Although sample messages can be stored and replayed at will, spontaneously generated communication is difficult, and it is necessary to educate both the user and listener in the correct interaction to maximize the benefit. Normal eye contact is maintained when communicating, but this is unlikely to be effective as a single approach.

The development of affordable lap-top computers has opened up new possibilities. It allows the use of any of the wide variety of switch inputs

233

with an infinitely variable keyboard layout on the screen that can be accessed using a predictive program (Cochrane). When coupled to a voice synthesizer, the computer can be a very powerful therapeutic instrument. It is simple to modify and mount such a device on a wheelchair and, in addition to a communication aid, text can be stored to be printed off when convenient. The confidence and independence gained is well worth the time spent to achieve it.

10.9   ENVIRONMENTAL CONTROL

The technology to control electrical devices around the home is advancing rapidly and it would not be of help to detail specific devices here. In the UK, the legislation currently in force requires 'hard wired' systems and there is a national budget for the provision of environmental control units managed normally at a regional or sub-regional level. Suitability is agreed following a referral from local community-based clinicians by a regional environmental control assessor and the equipment available via this route is restricted (NHS Supplies Authority). There are available, however, microwave and infra-red activated systems that are being considered for supply, and although the assessment is available, the supply of this equipment falls outside the mandate of the UK environmental control assessors. Use of the equipment varies and standards of clinical practice need to be agreed (Mandelstam, 1992).

It is possible to link together, from a central switching point (which may be mobile and on an electrically powered wheelchair), the control of lights, remote door opener, intercom, internal and external alarm, hands free telephone, remote controlled television, video cassette recorder, Hi-Fi system, cassette, talking book, fan heater, sockets, curtain closing and opening and a page turner. Virtually any electrical appliance is controllable given the resources and technical expertise.

10.10   HOME AND WORK

The deteriorating course of motor neurone disease with the feeling frequently expressed of 'losing ground' forces a change in the individual's relationships with friends, family and workmates (Robertson and Brown, 1992). Within the expert centre providing advice for the affected individual, there must be a nominated key person who can be a point of contact and constancy, will act as an agent or advocate, and will have formal counselling skills and a sufficiently wide knowledge base to access other facilities that may be required to maintain health, wealth and welfare. It matters little if this function is fulfilled by the general practitioner, hospital consultant, therapist, nurse, voluntary support worker or social worker as long as they work as a trusted member of the team. They must have access to detailed knowledge of the locally applicable benefit arrangements and be aware of the pitfalls that will impede any request for equipment or adaptations to the home. Good general advice must be supported by local specialist services. Any major modifications of equipment that are likely to be contentious must be anticipated and the aim is to provide an integrated (interdisciplinary and interagency) pro-active service.

Disputes over the ability to drive have caused more problems in my personal clinical work than any other field with this disease. The dependence on the motor car is so strong that it is seen as a very undesirable step to admit that driving is no longer safe. With appropriate adaptations and advice most people can drive through the majority of their illness using power steering, circumferential mirrors, automatic transmission, foot control, adapted transfer techniques etc. There does come a time, however, when the weakness in the arms, spasticity in the legs and poor head control make driving unsafe and this has got to be freely and frankly discussed.

Employers vary in the amount of support they are willing to provide for an individual; in part this reflects their generosity and in part the value they place on the individual concerned. I have seen examples of whole accounting procedures being computerized to enable a senior partner to continue work, the installation of a new telephone system to facilitate a local businessmen's input into the company and major changes to the fabric of the building in order to render it accessible to a wheelchair user. Sometimes supporting staff are enormously generous and helpful. Unfortunately equally frequently I have seen summary dismissal, arguing about pensionable rights and financial hardship imposed upon families already at breaking point.

10.11 PROGRESSION

Motor neurone disease, with its predictable but generally aggressive course, requires due consideration and sensitivity when providing a service aimed at supporting people and allowing them to maintain their independence and dignity throughout. The relationship between the rehabilitation team and the individual must be based on mutual respect and an understanding of wants, needs and abilities. Although the diagnosis is often made at a time when the people are independent and able, a time when it is too easy to deny problems that may arise in the future, this is a vital time for good advice and forward planning.

The disability of established disease

Normally, by the time a patient with motor neurone disease has been referred to the rehabilitation services, an idea of the rate of progression is apparent. The management of bulbar dysfunction and intercurrent infections, whilst maintaining adequate nutrition, have been important in maintaining quality of life. As early as is possible, I favour an honest and open approach, discussing with the individual the likelihood of intercurrent lower respiratory tract or urinary infection, the danger of aspiration or malnutrition, and the treatments available.

The local facilities available, with reference to both financial resource and expertise, will determine what can be offered or maintained within the home for any individual. Artificial ventilation is a salient example. Life is significantly prolonged by such means but the ethics and health economics of these issues are outside the scope of this chapter.

The use of respite or hospice facilities is welcomed by some individuals or families. I think that a simple 'holiday' admission is a negative and potentially unfruitful stay. If a respite rota is to be arranged then it is more appropriately orientated if an individual is encouraged to bring problems to the unit, and each stay is seen as an interval re-assessment of their overall rehabilitation needs. Thus a seating, sleeping or feeding problem can be approached within their one- to two-week stay. In addition, contact between the key worker, the individual and their family can be reinforced. There should also be an emergency admission facility and I think it is best sited within the unit, providing respite to allow for continuity and to avoid the inappropriate placement of such people in non-specialist units.

Motor neurone disease remains a condition which is (almost) universally fatal. At some stage the majority of people with motor neurone disease want to talk about death. Most are afraid of asphyxiation, inhalation and choking and very few are reassured by the bland statements given to the effect of 'most people die in their sleep'. If the disease progresses, however, and a consistent and compassionate approach which is sensitive to an individual's wishes can be provided, it is my experience that open and frank discussion will eventually take place and that this should naturally involve the patient themselves and only at their behest take account of their spouse's or family's requirements, wishes or views.

I should stress that many of the services, investigations and treatments recommended in this chapter are not solely the provision of rehabilitation service; and that neurology, neurorehabilitation and community units can provide all or part of the required structure. I emphasize again, however, the need for confident, consistent and truly expert clinical appraisal and advice. I feel that partly this must come from centralization of scarce resources in a specialist centre.

236

10.12 USEFUL POINTS OF CONTACT IN THE UK

Disabled Living Foundation
380–384 Harrow Road
London
W9 2HU
Tel: 071 289 6111
Fax: 071 266 2922

Equipment for Disabled
Mary Marlborough Lodge
Nuffield Orthopaedic Centre
Headington
Oxford
Tel: 0865 227600
Fax: 0865 742348

University of Keele
Keele
Staffordshire
ST5 5BG
Tel: 0782 619373

Keep Able Foundation
2 Capital Interchange Way
Brentford
Middlesex
TW8 0EX
Tel: 081 994 6614
Fax: 081 742 2006

Mobility Advice and Vehicle Information Service (MAVIS)
TRRL
Crowthorne
Berkshire
RG11 6AU
Tel: 0344 770456

How to get Equipment for Disability (1990) Michael Mandelstam
Jessica Kingsley Publishers and Kogan Page
for Disabled Living Foundation

REFERENCES

Black, K.P. *et al.* (1990) Suprascapular nerve block – a safer technique (letter). *Anaesthesiology*, **72** (3), 580–1.

The disability of established disease

Bosma, J.F. and Brodie, D.R. (1969) Disability of the pharynx in amyotrophic lateral sclerosis as demonstrated by cineradiography. *Radiology*, **92**, 97–103.

Cochrane, G.M. (ed.) (1989) *Clothing and dressing: Equipment for disabled people.* Oxford RHA.

Cochrane, G.M. (ed.) (1990) *Hoists and lifts: Equipment for disabled people.* Oxford RHA.

Cochrane, G.M. (ed.) *Equipment for disabled people: Communication.* Oxford RHA, pp. 83–5 and 90–9.

Darnborough, and Kincade (eds) *Motoring and Mobility for Disabled People.* Royal Association for Disability and Rehabilitation, pp. 120–5.

Disabled Living Foundation (1992) Beds and bed accessories, in *Disabled-Living Foundation Information Service Handbook.* Section 1A.

Enderby, P.M., Hathorne, I. and Servant, S. (1984) The use of intraoral appliances in the management of velopharyngeal disorders. *BDJ*, Sept, 157–60.

Hawkins, R.J. *et al.* (1990) Cervical spina and shoulder pain. *Clin. Orthop.*, **258** (9), 142–6.

Kumar, R. *et al.* (1990) Shoulder pain in hemiplegia. The role of exercise. *Am. J. Phys. Rehabil.*, **69** (4), 205–8.

Loizou, L.A., Small, M. and Dalton, G.M. (1980) Cricopharyngeal myotomy in motor neurone disease. *J. Neurol. Neurosurg. Psych.*, **43**, 42–5.

Mandelstam, M. (1992) *Environmental control systems: investigating provision.* Report for the Eleanor Hamilton Educational Trust, Disabled Living Foundation.

Nerwick, P.G. and Langton Hewer, R. (1984) Motor Neurone Disease – Can we do better? A study of 42 patients. *BMJ*, **289**, 539–42.

NHS Supplies Authority *Arrangements for the provision of environmental control equipment through the Department of Health.*

Robertson, S.E. and Brown, R.I. (eds) (1992) *Rehabilitation Counselling – Approaches in the Field of Disability.* Chapman & Hall, London.

Saunders, C., Walsh, T.D. and Smith, M. Hospice care in motor neurone disease, in *Hospice – the living idea* (eds Sanders, Summers and Teller) Edward Arnold, pp. 126–55.

Topping, M.J. (1989) *Low cost robot arms as aids to independence for severely disabled people.* Proceedings of DTI International Workshop on Domestic Robots, pp. 303–7.

Wilston, P.J. *et al.* (1990) Videofluoroscopy in motor neurone disease prior to cricopharyngeal myosomy. *Ann R. Coll. Surg. Eng.*, **72** (6), 375–7

Zalin, H. and Cooney, T.C. (1974) Chorda Tympani Neurectomy – a new approach to submandibular salivary obstruction. *Br. J. Surg.*, **61**, 391–4.

11 Respiratory function

FORBES H. NORRIS and ROBERT J. FALLAT

Respiratory muscle paralysis occurs in all cases of the malignant motor neuron disease (MND) amyotrophic lateral sclerosis (ALS). Respiratory involvement can be very acute and severe (Fromm, Wisdom and Block, 1977; Sivak and Streib, 1980; Nightingale et al., 1982; Hill, Martin and Hakim, 1983), though more commonly it takes the slowly progressive course seen in the other skeletal muscles. Acute respiratory failure has been reported in the more benign MND, progressive muscular atrophy (Parhad et al., 1978), though we suspect ALS with death occurring before upper motor pathology in such cases (Mackay, 1963). In our population-based study from 1970 to 1986 in northern California, 4% of the ALS patients had dyspnea on exertion or even shortness of breath at rest as an early manifestation (Norris et al., 1993). Whether such respiratory weakness develops earlier or later in the course of MND, it is usually progressive, and as it progresses the shadow of death descends.

Related complications such as frequent aspiration and then aspiration pneumonitis bring death closer. Aspiration is closely associated with the progressive respiratory weakness because the pharyngeal muscles are usually similarly affected at the same time; moreover the cough is weakened and so reduces the body's natural defense against aspiration. For the clinician with a patient having ALS or another MND and respiratory compromise, the three key functions are breathing, coughing strength and the frequency of aspiration. Aspirate not cleared by coughing will soon lead to pneumonitis. We lose half our ALS patients from the first episode of aspiration pneumonitis and half of the survivors in each subsequent episode because of the difficulty in treating this lung involvement in the presence of weakened breathing and coughing.

Fortunately, this fatal sequence is much less common in the other, more benign MND such as primary lateral sclerosis, progressive muscular atrophy and neuronal Charcot–Marie–Tooth disease. Even in what begins as classic ALS the progression ceases in 10–15% of patients

Respiratory function

(Swank and Putnam, 1943; Norris *et al.*, 1993), as witness Professor Stephen Hawking. Even should adequate strength be lost or critically reduced for breathing and coughing, modern respiratory care can allow many months or even years of satisfactory life for the paralyzed patient if aspiration pneumonitis is absent or overcome (Dicus, 1976).

11.1 MEASUREMENT OF PULMONARY FUNCTION

Objective evaluation of ventilatory function may well be one of the best means of monitoring the progression of MND. Methods range from the simple measurement of respiratory rate to the complex array of equipment to assess sleep (polysomnography) or exercise.

The simplest, most reproducible and clinically useful test is spirometry (Fallat *et al.*, 1979). The inexpensive water-filled or bellows spirometer measures the vital capacity (VC). If done with forced exhalation (FVC) and timed, a measurement of volume exhaled in the first second (FEV_1) gives the best assessment of either airway obstruction or reduced force generation from MND.

Many office spirometers, available for less than $3000, automatically calculate an array of flows along with a flow–volume loop (Figure 11.1). The characteristics of this loop can be of great value in differentiating neuromuscular weakness from airway obstruction and sometimes in identifying the source of the obstruction as pharyngeal or glottal occlusion (flutter waves or sudden descents in flow, Figure 11.1), large-airway (reduction of peak flow and FEV_1) or small-airway disease (curved loop), or combinations of disease.

The maximum voluntary ventilation (MVV) may be one of the earliest manifestations of MND (Fallat *et al.*, 1979), particularly rapid fatigue (myasthenic) states (Mulder, Lambert and Eaton, 1959; Denys and Norris, 1979). However, the MVV is an effort-dependent test and requires maximum technician and patient cooperation.

The maximum expiratory pressure (MEP) developed at the mouth may be reduced before the VC or MVV, but an experienced technician with a properly designed pressure gauge and controlled pinhole leak are required to obtain reliable results. This measurement is also very sensitive to the lung volume at which it is measured (Fiz *et al.*, 1990).

Lung volumes are more complex measurements requiring gas dilution or body plethysmography techniques only available in a pulmonary function laboratory. The inability to exhale below the resting point at the end of a tidal breath (functional residual capacity, FRC) results in a small loss of VC and rise in residual volume, which may frequently be an early sign of MND (Fallat *et al.*, 1979).

240

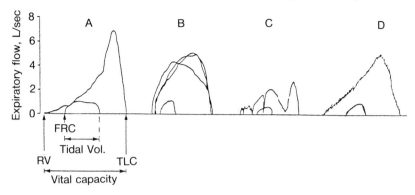

Figure 11.1 Forced vital capacity flow–volume curves from four patients with ALS. The parameters marked in A are FRC, functional residual capacity; RV, residual volume; TLC, total lung capacity. The curvature in expiratory flow in patient A is characteristic of airway obstructive disease and shows no characteristics of MND. (B) A characteristic flow–volume curve with ALS, showing inability to fully exhale, manifest by the initiation of inspiration while the expiratory flows are still quite high. (C) A patient with bulbar ALS, showing erratic effort complicated by sudden loss of flow due to glottic occlusion from muscle incoordination. (D) Another ALS patient, whose relatively normal curve has frequent small oscillations reflecting mild pharyngeal airway interference usually associated with obstructive sleep apnea (adapted from Figure 3, Fallat *et al.*, 1979).

Gas exchange is surprisingly well sustained in MND patients, probably because the neuromuscular metabolic demands fall concomitantly. Diffusing capacity and resting arterial blood gases (ABG) are normal until late in the course of the disease (Fallat *et al.*, 1979). In some patients in whom ventilatory muscles decline before extremity muscles, exercise hypoxemia may be detected. This is measured easily and non-invasively with a pulse oximeter, now routinely available in hospitals and many offices. Carbon dioxide elevation also occurs late in the disease, sometimes while the arterial oxygen is still normal. Hypercarbia can develop even earlier when there is an associated obstructive lung disease or other CNS problem causing respiratory depression.

Sleep is a complex ventilatory adjustment. Mild hypoxemia and slight elevations of carbon dioxide are a normal occurrence during sleep. When the ventilatory system is compromised, and especially when the oropharyngeal muscles are involved, obstructive sleep apnea may occur. There are well-recognized sleep disorders in myotonic dystrophy and advanced cases of Duchenne muscular dystrophy (Smith *et al.*, 1987). Sleep disorder in ALS is not well recognized, perhaps because it has not

241

been well studied. Sleep apnea was the presenting complaint in one ALS case study (Carré *et al.*, 1988). In small series, sleep-related hypoxemia and hypoventilation have been observed (Gay *et al.*, 1991), particularly in bulbar patients (Mazzini *et al.*, 1990). Such events may explain the unexpected nocturnal deaths that sometimes occur in MND patients.

Returning to the simplest of measurements, the FVC, it should be emphasized that this objective measurement of ventilatory function may be monitored indirectly by the patient in the home using either an incentive spirometer or a peak flow meter. Teaching the patient and family to use these devices can be very useful in allaying their fears (especially if the measurement is stable and similar to those obtained at clinic or office visits), and can enable them to be aware of a sudden decline.

11.2 STAGING RESPIRATORY FAILURE

A staging method of evaluating the practical consequences of respiratory and pharyngeal weakness has been reported (Norris and Fallat, 1988), using the FVC and MVV plus rough scores for aspiration and coughing (Table 11.1).

Aspiration occurs occasionally to mild degree in most people, particularly under stress. We score aspiration + as the occurrence of aspiration one or more times per week, usually in drinking clear liquids.

Table 11.1 Guidelines for staging respiratory involvement in MND

Stage	Dyspnea	FVC (%)	MVV (%)	Aspiration[a]	Cough[a]
I	0	90–110	90–110	0	+ + + +
II	Minor	80–95	65–90	±	+ + + +
III	Exertional	60–85	<50	+	+ + +
IV	Speaking	30–70	<25	+	+ +
V	Constant	<30	<15	+ +	+
VI	When Off Ventilator	<20	NM	+ + +	±
VII	No Useful Breathing	<10	NM	+ + + +	0
VIII	Apnea	0	NM	+ + + +	0

Modified from Norris and Fallat (1988).
NM, not measurable.
[a] Scores defined in the text.

242

Aspiration ++ is such an occurrence daily. Aspiration +++ occurs each morning, noon and evening, and sometimes between meals from aspiration of saliva. Aspiration ++++ is constant aspiration of saliva (the patient has a chronic, frequent, soft cough) plus aspiration of swallowed liquids. This category includes aspiration of food.

Cough ++++ is normally strong coughing; the examiner cannot restrain the lower chest while gripping from behind. Cough +++ is a reduction, and the examiner can restrain the chest movement. Cough ++ is readily restrained by the examiner though it is still effective at clearing secretions. Cough + is occasionally ineffective, and repetitive soft coughing follows a single, small aspiration.

Stage I is normal. Stage II is dyspnea with unusual exertion and slight depression in spirometry: the FVC is reduced to 80–95% predicted and the MVV to 65–90%. Coughing strength may seem normal. Stage III is dyspnea with ordinary activities (walking a block) and reduced coughing strength. The FVC will be reduced to 60–85% predicted and the MVV to less than 50%. Stage IV is dyspnea during ordinary speech so that complete sentences cannot be uttered. Dyspnea limits many other functions. The cough is severely weakened and may seem minimal on command though effective reflexly. The FVC will be 30–70% and the MVV less than 25% predicted. Counseling on life support options should begin.

Stage V requires the consideration of tracheostomy: dyspnea is constant when the patient is awake and there is feeble coughing. The FVC will be reduced by more than 70% and the MVV by more than 85% or unobtainable. Unexplained fever heralds aspiration pneumonitis. Stage VI is intermittent inadequate respiration so that artificial respiration may be necessary. The cough is usually inadequate and suctioning removes airway secretions. The FVC measurement is variable, usually less than 1000 cc, with the MVV unobtainable. If an endotracheal tube has been placed, consideration of tracheostomy is essential. Stage VII is absence of effective voluntary respiration. Full-time artificial respiration sustains life. The FVC is less than 500 cc, the MVV unobtainable. The strength for coughing is effectively zero and deep suctioning is required. Stage VIII is absence of any respiratory function, usually evolving as the final stage if the patient does not opt for intubation or continuation of artificial respiration; also in earlier stages should there be massive aspiration or fulminant pneumonitis. Other reversible causes include drug (especially benzodiazepines and neuromuscular blockade) sensitivity and oxygen administration in patients dependent on the oxygen respiratory drive because of hypercarbia.

Respiratory function

11.3.1 Case A: ALS

This man of 48 years noted the gradual onset of unusual fatigue after ordinary exercise in 1982. One year from the onset, there was generalized fasciculation and mild atrophy in several arm muscles but no breathing problem. Stage I was maintained until April 1985, when strength for coughing was reduced (Table 11.2). In other skeletal muscles there was profound weakness with atrophy and hyperreflexia. Babinski's sign was present. By September 1985, stage III appeared, with further weakness in the cough and significant reductions in FVC and MVV. Stage IV developed in September 1986 with aspiration and feeble coughing. Speech was impaired by dyspnea. All arm and leg use was lost and he lived a bed-chair existence. A trial of anticholinesterase (Mulder, Lambert and Eaton, 1959; Denys and Norris, 1979) and aminophylline medication (Aubier *et al.*, 1981; Belsh and Shiffman, 1988) with intermittent positive-pressure breathing (IPPB) was proposed but declined.

By January 1987 further deterioration was consistent with stage V (Table 11.2). He opted for no invasive treatment in the event of further paralysis but did consent to the treatment program proposed earlier. Oxtriphylline administration, frequent IPPB treatments and use of a cuirass respirator during sleep were associated with an increase in FVC from 1100 to 1700 cc. There seemed to be further benefit from

Table 11.2 Respiratory staging in MND: ALS, case A

Date	ALS score[a]	FVC (%)	MVV (%)	Aspiration	Cough	Stage
May 1983	96	100	100	0	++++	I
August 1983	95	100	101	0	++++	I
November 1983	95	102	105	0	++++	I
September 1984	82	(ND)	(ND)	0	++++	I
April 1985	59	87	94	0	+++	II
September 1985	46	80	78	0	++	III
March 1986	41	61	60	0	++	III
September 1986	38	36	36	+	+	IV
January 1987[b]	31	26	32	+++	±	V

From Norris and Fallat (1988); case summary in the text.
ND, not done.
[a] ALS score from Norris (1990).
[b] Ten days before death.

isoetharine (Bronkosol) inhalations. Respiratory improvement was maintained in the next week, but the discomfort of the treatments and further loss of other functions caused him to request termination of this therapy. Transition to stage VI seemed imminent, so a morphine sulfate infusion was begun (Norris, 1992). Little change occurred for 36 h, then carbon dioxide narcosis led rapidly to stages VII and VIII, and death within 4 h. The necropsy confirmed ALS.

11.3.2 Case B: ALS

This 43-year-old pilot noted arm muscle twitching and weakness in July 1982. In October, the spirometry was normal (Table 11.3). A program of active daily exercises plus anticholinesterase medication with pyridostigmine (Mulder, Lambert and Eaton, 1959; Denys and Norris, 1979) was associated with relatively little deterioration in the next year and stage I pulmonary function was maintained until the spring of 1985. In May significant declines were found in spirometry and his speech was dysarthric, his arms useless and the legs very weak.

By October there was further decline to respiratory stage III, and this progression continued to stage IV in January 1986. We began discussion of life support measures, and by April it was apparent that a decision

Table 11.3 Respiratory staging in MND: ALS, case B

Date	ALS score[a]	FVC (%)	MVV (%)	Aspiration	Cough	Stage
October 1982	96	101	94	0	++++	I
February 1983	93	106	123	0	++++	I
June 1983	93	101	121	0	++++	I
November 1983	89	101	125	0	++++	I
February 1984	86	101	118	0	++++	I
May 1984	79	97	105	0	++++	I
September 1984	82	90	109	0	++++	I
November 1984	76	88	101	0	++++	I
February 1985	71	88	105	0	++++	I
May 1985	68	81	90	0	++++	II
July 1985	63	76	85	0	++++	II
October 1985	43	56	50	+	+++	III
January 1986	38	44	44	++	++	IV
April 1986[b]	25	(ND)	(ND)	++	+	V

From Norris and Fallat (1988); case summary in the text.
[a] ALS score from Norris (1990).
[b] Died 8 days later.

against ventilation would make death imminent if such progression continued through stage V. He made that decision and was supplied with morphine injections to use at home to maintain his comfort (Norris, 1992). Death occurred during a nap 8 days later.

11.4 MONITORING AND TREATMENT OF RESPIRATORY CHANGES

The staging of respiratory failure in MND has value, but individual patients often require more careful observation and treatment. Monitoring respiratory function can be useful in making treatment decisions from the time of diagnosis. ALS patients frequently do not complain of respiratory symptoms since significant impairment of gas exchange does not occur until the function is reduced to 50% or less. Obtaining spirometry including FEV_1, FVC and MVV, as well as MIP and MEP, will provide a baseline and in some cases indicate much more severe reduction in lung function than was suspected from the patient's symptoms or physical findings.

Table 11.1 points to some of the decisions one can make from the simple VC measurement. As the FVC falls below 80% predicted, it is worthwhile considering using an incentive spirometer, which provides the patient not only with a means of exercising the respiratory muscles and keeping the lungs inflated but also a home monitoring device. If the spirometer reading declines, that may indicate problems such as atelectasis, airway obstruction or a decline in muscle function.

If there is any element of airway obstruction, or even if there is no objective evidence for obstruction but the MND patient is a cigarette smoker, it is probably worthwhile starting aerosolized bronchodilators (most MND patients who are smokers, and certainly all ALS patients, should be counseled on giving up that evil habit). When underlying obstructive airways disease is present, the above decisions are better made using the FEV_1 rather than the FVC for guidance.

As the vital capacity falls below 50%, indicating considerable loss of muscular function, intermittent positive-pressure breathing (IPPB) treatments may be beneficial. Our routine is to have the patient hyperinflate with room air to 35 or 40 cmH_2O several times a day. This procedure can be included during a 10- to 15-min treatment with a bronchodilator aerosol. The other advantage of instituting IPPB treatments in the home at this time is that it gives patients an opportunity to work with ventilators, better preparing them to think and make decisions about more invasive treatments in the future.

As the FVC falls below 30%, approaching 1 liter, significant interference with gas exchange can be expected. We routinely would obtain ABG, but more efficient and less invasive would be measurement of the oxygen saturation using pulse oximetry, particularly when the patient is lying down or even asleep, which is when more significant hypoxemia may occur (Fallat, Norris and Holden, 1987). If at this stage the patient is hypoxemic, i.e. Po_2 less than 50 torr, or oxygen saturation is less than 85–88%, then supplemental oxygen should be started using a nasal cannula or mask. If the Pco_2 is elevated above 50 torr, it is a time to discuss with the patient the future possibility of the need for more continuous ventilatory support and tracheostomy.

Our past experience has been predominantly with invasive naso-tracheal intubation or tracheostomy. Patients with sleep apnea have taught us that partial ventilatory support via a nasal mask with either continuous positive airway pressure (CPAP) or alternating or bimodal pressure application (BIPAP) can effectively maintain ventilation (Berthon-Jones and Sullivan, 1987). Similar success has been achieved using these techniques in young muscular dystrophy patients (Corbas-cio et al., 1990; Renardel et al., 1990; Baydur et al., 1990). These tech-niques may have value in ALS patients who do not have predominant bulbar involvement with secretory and aspiration problems that would prevent the consideration of this less invasive, nasal mask approach. This technique may prove to be beneficial, particularly in those MND patients who demonstrate ventilatory problems during sleep – an area still to be fully evaluated. Intermittent abdominal pressure during exhalation may be used with or without nasal ventilation as yet another non-invasive method to provide ventilatory support to a variety of MND patients (Bach and Alba, 1991).

More often in ALS patients, the abnormalities of gas exchange become apparent only with the onset of an acute event such as atelectasis, bronchial pneumonia or aspiration. The acute event frequently makes it necessary to make a decision for or against intervention with intubation that may not be as rational as a decision made earlier in anticipation of this event, when abnormal ABG or ear oximetry were first found. Nevertheless, it is unusual for patients to make decisions about tracheostomy without first having endured one of these more serious clinical events, which introduce the patient to great respiratory discomfort. Since each of these is potentially reversible and would certainly be treated in a patient without ALS, our view is that the ALS patient with a desire to live should be offered the same vigorous therapy.

Frequently, even after intubation and mechanical ventilation have been instituted, when the underlying complication is resolved, the patients may be able to be extubated and to return home free of any mechanical assistance. It is important, however, to maintain such a patient on IPPB treatments with bronchodilators. Theophylline and related medications not only help with any element of airway obstruction, but also improve respiratory muscle strength and endurance (Aubier *et al.*, 1981; Belsh and Schiffman, 1988).

When the predominant involvement from ALS is in the muscles of swallowing, it may be necessary to institute invasive treatments even when the vital capacity is adequate. In the past, some patients have had such a severe problem handling secretions, with recurrent aspiration pneumonia, that surgical procedures to close the glottis were done (Montgomery, 1975). Currently, such problems are more commonly managed by tracheostomy and use of a cuffed tube to prevent aspiration but allow the patient to maintain speech. If swallowing is virtually impossible, nasogastric tubes or esophageal catheterization in the neck may be used. More recently, we have turned to the use of direct gastrostomy tubes, which are placed percutaneously without the use of anesthesia or surgery (Russell, Brotman and Norris, 1984).

Once a patient has a tracheostomy, several decisions must be made. Will the patient require continuous mechanical ventilation? Can partial or complete weaning be accomplished? How much oxygen is needed? How often can the balloon be deflated to allow the patient to talk? Many times it is sufficient only for the patients to be on a mechanical ventilator during the night, maintaining adequate ventilation, preventing atelectasis during sleep and allowing rest for the weak, fatigued respiratory muscles. The patients are then able to maintain themselves with their own muscle power during the day. Sometimes, as in the case study below, the patients may wean themselves from the ventilator entirely, but prefer to maintain the tracheostomy because of the security and convenience for handling secretions. In addition, the ventilatory load is decreased as a result of the decreased deadspace.

Fenestrated tracheostomy tubes with an inner cannula allow the patient to be on a ventilator during the night with the inner cannula in place and the cuff inflated. During the day the inner cannula is removed, the cuff deflated, and the tube plugged so that the patient is able to breathe through the mouth and have effective speech (Figure 11.2). If the patient cannot tolerate the added deadspace of the upper airway, then a one-way valve rather than a plug can be placed on the tracheostomy tube.

A number of mechanical ventilators are available, driven by battery as well as by line voltage, for use in the home. As the need for and use of such portable units increases, newer models are being developed with satisfactory monitoring and alarm capabilities.

Humidification of the airway has been considered a very important aspect of maintenance of the airway with a tracheostomy. In our experience, there has been an overemphasis on the use of humidifica-

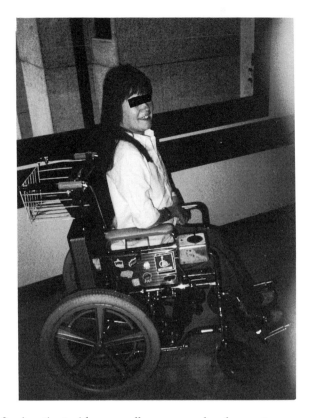

Figure 11.2   A patient with unusually severe and early-onset neuronal Charcot–Marie–Tooth disease. Rapid loss of respiratory strength led to ventilatory failure requiring tracheostomy and artificial ventilation in 1978. Subsequently she was able to reduce the time on the respirator and use it mainly during sleep. The open collar nicely conceals the tracheostomy.

tion, which sometimes leads to excess moisture in the airway and a build-up of secretions; we have found that many patients have tolerated breathing room air via an open tracheostomy during the day without thickening of the mucosa or drying of the mucous membranes. When a ventilator is in use and humidification is desirable, a small humidifier can be added to the system. When oxygen is required, one may use an oxygen 'enricher' to continually generate humidified 40% oxygen.

11.5   HOME CARE OF MECHANICALLY VENTILATED PATIENTS

In the past 15 years, improvements in respiratory care and monitoring have changed our approach to the ALS patient. Preventing respiratory

Respiratory function

Table 11.4 Summary of 30 home ventilator ALS patients[a]

Number (males/females)	21/9	Total: 30
Ages	37–74 years	Mean: 57
Reasons for tracheostomy		
Respiratory failure	26	
Recurrent aspiration	16	
Sleep apnea	1	
Duration of ALS before tracheostomy	6–91 months	Mean: 35
Duration at home	2 weeks to 84 months	Mean: 19

From Fallat *et al.* (1988)

Table 11.5 Pulmonary function at time of tracheostomy in 30 ALS patients

FVC	12–50% of predicted	Mean = 33
P_{O_2}	43–89 mmHg	Mean = 69
P_{CO_2}	30–90 mmHg	Mean = 47
	(seven patients > 50 mmHg)	

From Fallat *et al.* (1988)

failure in the past depended on intermittent manual tests such as spirometry and chest X-ray, or invasive arterial blood gas studies. Patients can now be non-invasively and continuously monitored for hypoxia or hypercapnia, even while asleep. Intubation, tracheostomy and mechanical ventilation can now be routine care for patients who elect to take that option. Mechanical ventilation can be done at home without continuous nursing care, and small, battery-operated ventilators allow mobility (Holden and Stanley, 1987).

In 1978, we discharged to home and the care of the family our first ALS patient with a permanent tracheostomy. Since that time, we have sent home over 40 ALS patients, the first 22 summarized in Table 11.4. The majority of the patients had their tracheostomies because of respiratory failure, while 12 patients had recurrent aspirations, and one had sleep apnea as the primary reason for tracheostomy. A most interesting tracheostomy patient was one with obstructive airways disease who also had intermittent collapse of the oropharyngeal airway, causing acute respiratory embarrassment (see below, case C).

At the time of tracheostomy, as seen in Table 11.5, the FVC was always below 50%, ranging from 12 to 50% of predicted with a mean value of 33%. Oxygenation was usually impaired but seldom was the primary reason for mechanical ventilation; in most cases, it was respiratory distress or a rising P_{CO_2}. The onset of respiratory failure with a need for tracheostomy occurred between 6 and 9 months after the diagnosis of ALS. By the time the patients were discharged to home,

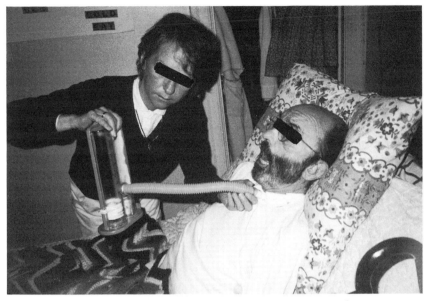

Figure 11.3 Gini encouraging Bill (case C in text) to exercise his respiratory muscles by use of an incentive spirometer attached to the tracheostomy tube.

many of them used the ventilator only nocturnally (seven patients) or intermittently (two patients) and, in one case, not at all.

There are many psychological, financial and physical burdens placed on ALS patients, their families and friends (Bradley, 1982; Fallat *et al.*, 1988). For many, hospitalization is necessary for the final days or weeks of their illness, particularly when it involves complex respiratory and ventilatory problems. Caring for a patient on a ventilator requires planning and preparation by a skilled team working with the families. The adjustments to home care are not easy but, once made, have proven to be worthwhile and preferable to the isolation and loneliness of a hospital room (Norris *et al.*, 1987a; Fallat *et al.*, 1988), as demonstrated by the case of Bill and his friend Gini (Figure 11.3).

11.5.1 Case C: ALS

Bill was a 62-year-old man who first developed hand weakness in January 1981 and was diagnosed as having ALS in July. His pulmonary function tests showed primarily obstructive airways disease, with an FEV_1/FVC of 1.2/3.6 l owing to his 22 years of cigarette smoking. He had no respiratory symptoms and no medications were used, though

251

bronchodilator aerosol improved his FEV_1/FVC to 2.4/4.1 l By June, 1984, his FEV_1/FVC had fallen to 1.7/2.9. The FEV_1 was only 46% predicted; an ABG showed the pH was 7.41, the PCO_2 45 and the PO_2 65 torr, indicating only mild hypoxemia, and dyspnea was not a complaint.

In August 1984, Bill was admitted to the hospital because of a hip fracture and at that time was dyspneic, particularly when supine. Chest X-ray showed basilar atelectasis and his FEV_1/FVC was only 0.6/1.2 l. Following IPPB treatments with metaproterenol aerosol, his FEV_1/FVC improved to 1.2/2.2. Surgical replacement of his right hip was done without complications and only overnight endotracheal intubation with mechanical ventilation. On discharge, he went home with the use of an IPPB device to continue aerosol treatments along with theophylline (300 mg b.i.d.) and an albuterol inhaler as needed.

In November 1984, he was readmitted because of an acute episode of respiratory distress, apparently due to upper airway obstruction from flaccidity of the pharyngeal muscles. After several tracheal intubations, a tracheostomy was performed and the FVC improved to 2.2 l; he was able to breathe easily on his own via the tracheostomy. By January 1985, even with an FVC of 2.0 l, there was intermittent respiratory exhaustion and ventilator assistance was necessary. Bill's close friend, Gini, had extensive training in ventilator and tracheostomy care and at the end of February he was discharged in her care with only daily 1-h visits from a visiting nurse. He was maintained on the ventilator at night and as needed in the day when respiratory distress occurred.

Through May 1987, Bill did very well with only Gini in attendance (Figure 11.3). Two rehospitalizations were then necessary for symptoms of bronchitis, and in June there was need for increased ventilator pressure. He was readmitted with fever and signs of congestive heart failure, which caused him to request termination of artificial respiration. This was done after multiple discussions with Gini, the family and religious advisors. A necropsy revealed severe coronary arteriosclerosis; there was pulmonary edema and a lower lobe pneumonia; the neuropathology showed ALS.

11.6 FAMILY CARE OF THE VENTILATOR-DEPENDENT PATIENT

Such cases as that above illustrate what has become almost a routine in our MND clinic since 1980, mainly of course for ALS patients: instruction of the family in the relevant nursing skills, then discharge home.

One of the most difficult medical and nursing problems is the care of paralyzed, respirator-dependent patients. Some patients with advanced paralysis caused by ALS choose maintenance on a life-support system

Table 11.6 Respirator care at home for the first 20 ALS patients

Case no.	Patient age/sex	Months ALS before	Months home	Chief nurse
1	74/M	52	28	RN
2	64/M	18	21[a]	Son
3	48/M	46	39	RN
4[b]	65/M	17	3	Spouse
5	59/M	36	54	RN
6	54/M	22	60	RN
7	66/M	65	20[a]	RN[c]
8	37/M	26	18[a]	Friend
9	63/F	28	$\frac{1}{4}$[a]	RN
10	64/F	48	14[a]	Spouse
11	47/M	91	48	Spouse[d]
12	59/M	48	3	RN
13	62/F	45	14[a]	Spouse
14	73/M	12	10	Spouse
15	73/F	24	14	Friend
16	64/F	24	12	RN
17	59/M	22	$\frac{1}{2}$	Spouse
18	54/M	48	17	Daughter
19	48/M	21	6	Spouse
20	71/M	10	1	Spouse

Modified from Norris *et al.* (1987a)
[a] Returned to hospital, died later of pneumonia.
[b] Case 4 described in text.
[c] Spouse able to replace herself by professional nurses.
[d] Practical nurses in addition for 17 months.

when respiratory failure develops. In ALS, the usual problems are compounded by the high frequency of emotional lability, drooling and aspiration as a result of oropharyngeal and other upper airway secretions, painful muscle cramps and spasms and other physical causes of pain, even though these patients generally have intact sensibility and mentation, including full consciousness. Since the disease predominantly strikes in the range of 50–70 years (Norris *et al.*, 1992), the sufferer may be the former breadwinner and head of the household. The disease reduces patients to almost total dependence on others for virtually all activities, from scratching the nose, to wiping away a tear, to toileting.

In past years, we have participated in the care of many patients in this predicament, almost all of them in the intensive care unit (ICU) of an acute general hospital. Only rarely were patients treated in their homes, where adequate nursing services were provided through exceptional private insurance plans (cases 1 and 3, Table 11.6), great wealth, or other pre-existing advantages. In 1980, an incident cast new light on this problem.

11.6.1 Case 4: ALS (Table 11.6)

A 60-year-old man had been stricken with steadily progressive paralysis from ALS which, within 15 months, led to progressive respiratory weakness. As sometimes occurs in ALS, the respiratory weakness then worsened rapidly, and it was necessary for him to be admitted on an emergency basis to his community hospital, where he received orotracheal intubation and was placed on artificial respiration. Our telephone consultations with those physicians disclosed no additional therapeutic opportunity, and it appeared likely that the patient would be respirator dependent and confined to the hospital's ICU for the remainder of his life. A tracheostomy was performed.

Approximately 8 weeks after his admission to the hospital, we received an anguished telephone call from the patient's wife, an unprepossessing housewife (age 65). She reported that the community hospital's administrator had told her to prepare to take her husband home within 2 weeks, when his hospital insurance coverage would terminate. We advised that this was inhumane, if not cruel and illegal. We recommended that she lodge a strong protest with the hospital and consider recruiting an attorney for assistance. Not believing that the patient would be discharged under the circumstances, and having other difficult cases to manage at the time, we gave little further thought to this patient until his wife telephoned about 3 weeks later to report that he had been discharged on the date given and was doing quite well at home.

A home visit shortly thereafter revealed that the patient and his wife lived in a small walk-up apartment in a rather seedy neighborhood of expiring small businesses and abandoned shops. At the top of the stairs, a small hall led to a bathroom on the right and a bed-sitting area to the left. Beyond the bed-sitting area there was a kitchen. One corner of the bed-sitting room contained an inexpensive electrically powered bed for the patient. He was totally paralyzed except for the ability to wrinkle his forehead, blink and roll his eyes, and wiggle the fingers of one hand, under which his wife inserted a band of cowbells. If he had an urgent need when she was in the kitchen or bathroom, he could jiggle the cowbells to summon her. On the floor was a Bennett respirator; about six feet of flexible tubing connected it to the tracheostomy tube. A light plastic bucket slung over the tubing was a reservoir for excessive secretions. An electrically powered suction pump was also on the floor, its tubing looped over the head of the bed.

Family care of the ventilator-dependent patient

Seated in the opposite corner of this little room was a much older woman, the wife's mother, apparently in her 90s, who was at least able to go to the toilet by herself, because she did so at one point during the visit. This is part of the conversation with the wife:

'Do you have nurses to help take care of him?'

'The visiting nurses came for about an hour for the first few days, then they said he was stabilized and they haven't come again.'

'Don't you have someone coming in to help you?'

'I don't have anyone to help me. I do it all myself.'

'How about shopping or just getting a little rest by yourself?'

'Well, my daughter stops by for an hour every day on her way home from work, and that gives me a break so I can go out and shop.'

'Other than that, are you the nurse all day long?'

'Yes, I guess I'm it!'

'When do you sleep?'

'I've learned to catnap.'

She and her husband demonstrated the code they had worked out whereby he used his ability to blink to convey certain basic messages such as 'need suction', 'had enough food' (via feeding tube), and so forth, in addition to simple yes and no signals. During the visit, the wife demonstrated competent tracheal suctioning, inflation of the cuff and adjustments in the respirator volume and frequency.

During the next 3 months, the patient probably suffered two episodes of pneumonitis, manifest by fever and purulent bronchial secretions, but he refused offers of re-hospitalization. He signaled that he was receiving better care at home than he had in hospital. Broad-spectrum antibiotics were administered during the first such episode, but he refused antibiotic treatment the second time. A third episode followed within a month, and again he refused antibiotic treatment. His wife found him pulseless when she tried to awaken him from a nap.

Many details have been omitted from this vignette because our purpose now is to demonstrate the feasibility of home care by laymen who have had no previous medical experience and whose training in the necessary techniques has been rudimentary and practical. Moreover, this experience taught that home care of patients who are dependent on respirators may have many advantages, including reduction in the cost of care. For example, in this case the total cost of the electrically powered bed, the Bennett respirator, the suction pump and the associated tubing was less than the cost of 2 days in the ICU. Even more important was the significance of the patient's refusal to return to the hospital. It seemed likely that the home environment and the patient's recovery of some direction of his care, which is sadly uncommon among institutionalized patients, positively affected his morale and outweighed any immediate benefits of hospitalization. We also learned that a spouse who has never manifested any unusual talents or energies can successfully provide a high level of nursing care at home (Holden and Stanley, 1987).

From this single experience, we hypothesized that:

1. institutionalized patients experience immediate and significant morale benefits from returning home;
2. motivated and responsible family members can learn the necessary nursing skills to care for severely paralyzed patients within a relatively short time; and
3. adequate home care can be provided for these patients.

We tested these hypotheses by deliberately undertaking early transfer home of all similarly affected patients if adequate help for home care could be mustered. In the course of this experience, we learned that dedicated friends and neighbors can be included in patient care.

11.7 METHODS

One concern was the motivation and the morale of the patients. As reported elsewhere (Houpt, Gould and Norris, 1977; Armon et al., 1989), we have found ALS patients in general to be psychologically normal and to possess good coping mechanisms. None of these respirator patients or their families required the extensive psychiatric evaluations recommended by Sivak et al. (1982, 1983).

The next concern was the motivation and performance of family members, and later friends, in providing practical bedside care. It helped in our evaluation to encourage them to perform simple tasks at bedside in the hospital. As the home providers' experience increased in this way, it became possible to make realistic assumptions about the level of care they would provide when they were alone with the patient at home. With the exceptions noted below, this is an aspect of treatment that families can usually manage competently. The distance of the patients' homes from our medical centers has not been a consideration: recent patients have lived 42, 89 and 115 miles from our hospitals. In these cases, it has of course been essential to alert local physicians to the pending home care program as soon as possible. Although the alert was met with varying degrees of interest, no resistance was encountered and, in some instances, community physicians have taken over completely.

Consultation was obtained early and routinely in each case with our collaborating services in physical therapy and occupational therapy (with particular attention to devices and aids to assist patients in daily living), as well as nursing home care (discharge planning). Any appropriate medical or surgical consultations were undertaken in addition to the routine investigation and case management by neurology and respiratory specialists and minute-to-minute care by ICU nurses. Psychological problems were frequent in this group of patients, and we were fortunate to have experienced psychiatrists who were available for consultation, as well as an active pastoral service for religious counseling. The trainees in both of these services often saw the patients even if formal consultations had not been requested.

The general aim was to have the patients in the best possible physical and psychological condition prior to transfer home. Sometimes major problems (for example, unresolved aspiration pneumonitis with secondary infection by multiple antibiotic-resistant micro-organisms) necessitated a substantial delay before the home care program could be instituted. In some cases, such complications interrupted the home care preparation, exerting a see-saw effect on patient morale.

We have indicated elsewhere (Norris, Smith and Denys, 1985; Norris et al., 1987b) a wide range of treatments available to palliate if not completely relieve some of the many troublesome symptoms experienced by ALS patients, and of course these were all brought to bear as indicated. Excessive drooling was usually controlled; painful cramps and other muscle spasms were suppressed; emotional problems were alleviated; nutritional problems were corrected by a variety of different approaches, ranging from simple advice about food preparation to percutaneous catheter gastrostomy; abnormal fatigue was sometimes eased by the use of anticholinesterases (Mulder, Lambert and Eaton, 1959) or aminophyllines (Aubier et al., 1981; Belsh and Schiffman, 1988).

Physical therapy instruction in the range of motion (ROM) exercises for the major joints is essential for MND patients. A major cause of pain in these patients, especially in ALS and progressive muscular atrophy, is diffuse upper arm pain, which is increased by certain motions of the shoulder joint. This problem, caused by subluxation, can be almost entirely prevented and is usually corrected by ROM programs. During the in-hospital training of prospective family home care attendants, instruction in the supervision of any possible active exercises by the patient and hands-on practice of relevant ROM therapy was an important topic.

Nothing alarms a family about caring for a patient more than the fear of not knowing what to do 'if something happens'. This fear is particularly great for families of respirator patients, and must be allayed by offering a sufficiently complete and clear explanation, followed by demonstrations, practical 'Do's and Don'ts', and then adequate practice in the hospital. Sometimes, the individual comprehension is increased by a checklist of necessary steps and practices (Holden and Stanley, 1987).

Through trial and error, we found that it was advantageous for the family to spend the better part of each day in the ward or ICU for a minimum of 2 weeks prior to the patient's discharge. During this time, the principal family members, as well as other relatives or friends who were planning to participate at home, took an active part in nursing care, with emphasis on mastering basic adjustment of the ventilator, deep tracheal suctioning and the other essentials of respiratory care. The nurse in attendance was the main instructor for the family. At the same time, the usual level of care provided in the ICU was gradually reduced to what would be provided at home. For example, the usual frequency of ABG determinations was drastically curtailed. Finally, such invasive tests were stopped entirely in favor of simple bedside observation of the patient and attention to the patient's expression of satisfaction with the level of pulmonary support. The entire emphasis shifted from the usual ICU approach, including the use of multiple high technologies, to the simplest and most basic support functions that would be available at home. In the family or other home care group, there were usually one or two members who were the most concerned members and who would be present most of the time. During the 2–4 weeks of training, these individuals progressed from observation to active administration of care at the bedside, while the nurse officially on duty pretended to be doing something else.

One benefit of having consultants and technicians from other services involved in this program was that during their training the home care providers could be observed and criticized by staff members from different disciplines and backgrounds. In this manner, the most complete picture possible of the adequacy of the home care program was obtained and major deficiencies were remedied as they were detected. This was obviously advantageous before the move home, although corrective measures were often necessary later.

Most of these families were able to afford private nurses for one or two 8 h shifts per day during at least the first few days at home. We encouraged them to take advantage of such assistance in order to provide a reassuring framework of professionalism at home. We did not encourage long-term use of professional nursing services for most patients because of the rapidity with which professional home nursing can devour any remaining insurance coverage or financial savings. However, as shown in Table 11.6, some families opted for this support at home. For example, when the patient's spouse was working and that income was essential for continuation of the home care program, it was necessary for a professional nurse to be in attendance during the spouse's working hours, not only to provide care but to support the patient's morale during the spouse's absence. Rather than attempt to promulgate any preconceived notion, we attempted to be flexible and to learn from each patient about useful adaptations that might be applied in subsequent cases. It is particularly important to emphasize the necessity of individualizing all recommendations for equipment and treatment, and remaining open to alterations in any part of the treatment program as circumstances change.

It is also important to consider the preparation of the home. This was undertaken, usually by the respiratory therapy service in the patient's community, in the week before the patient's transfer home. Equipment such as an electrically powered adjustable bed, a commode and a back-up electrical supply in case of power failure all had to be provided and suitably arranged before the transfer. We usually sent home with the patient the same ventilator, tubing, manual ventilation bag and other respiratory equipment that was used in our hospital, plus a month's supply of any medications, tubing feeding mixtures and other necessities. The chief home care provider (designated the 'chief nurse' in Table 11.6) was asked to make telephone reports at least on alternate days throughout the first 2 weeks of home care.

11.8 RESULTS

Table 11.6 shows that 12 of the first 20 patients were successfully cared for at home by family and friends. Eight other patients were also well cared for at home, but with extensive professional nursing. Similar experience has been obtained in over 46 cases. Without exception, the patients who did transfer to the home care program expressed great appreciation of the return home. They all stated, in varying ways, that the occasional lapses in professionalism at home were more than compensated by the recovery of a sense of direction of their own care and by the pleasure of being surrounded by family and friends rather than hospital professionals. 'Home' for the patients in cases 12 and 13 were caravans or mobile homes. In some cases the home nursing care was not actually provided by family but by concerned friends (Table 11.6). This bespeaks a degree of interest and dedication not readily found in most circumstances, but it also indicates that there are more options for home care than we would have considered in the past.

Table 11.6 shows that 75% of the ALS patients in our first 20 home care cases were male, a male predominance that seems to have leveled off at 70% in subsequent experience. The general ALS population is only about 57% male (Norris *et al.*, 1993), so it appears that more men than women opt for continuation of life with such chronic care.

Respiratory function

Numerous fatalities have occurred in this group of patients. The outcome in case 4 is cited above. In case 2, we considered that a reduction in the patient's respirator use was possible and admitted him for supervised 'weaning', but in 2 weeks he developed antibiotic-resistant pneumonia, from which he died. In case 8, the patient returned to his community hospital for a projected period of several weeks while his friends were reorganizing their support program; he contracted and died from antibiotic-resistant pneumonia. In case 10, the patient was admitted to the community hospital for investigation of gastrointestinal symptoms and died within a week from a similar pneumonia.

Three of the patients (cases 3, 14 and 15), after different periods of respirator-dependent living, expressed strong desires, confirmed in each case by family and friends, and by psychiatry consultation in case 3, to try living without the use of artificial ventilators; all of these patients died. In cases 12, 16 and 17, the patients died from pneumonia; two of them refused antibiotic treatment. The respirator support was stopped in case 1 after the patient experienced a week of unexplained coma.

11.9 DISCUSSION

Sivak, Gipson and Hanson (1982) and Sivak, Cordasco and Gipson (1983) reported successful home care of six respirator-dependent ALS patients. There are major similarities in our experiences, but two important differences. First, they selected cases after 'careful, long-term psychological evaluation' of both patients and families, whereas our experience suggests that most patients and their families can cope with home care. Second, Sivak did not consider home nursing by friends. In our experience, de-institutionalization should be feasible in most ALS cases. Comparable success in home care of respirator-dependent patients, usually having less malignant and less trying conditions than terminal ALS, was reported by Burr et al. (1983) and by Splaingard et al. (1982). These authors also found that concerned laymen could be readily trained in respirator care. Further useful details in methodology have been described by Peters and Viggiano (1988).

It may be premature to suggest that happier outcomes might have been obtained for the patients in cases 2, 7, 8, 10 and 13 if they had remained home rather than returning to hospital. Nevertheless, the close association in time between the patients' re-institutionalization and the development of fatal antibiotic-resistant pneumonias seems significant.

The dollar costs of continued in-hospital care are currently being evaluated against the home care costs. A striking example was case 4, in which the spouse provided all of the nursing care. The total cost of all the essential equipment was less than that of a day or two in the hospital. In cases 8 and 15, devoted friends became the principal nurses at home and there were similar striking reductions in costs, over 95% as compared with the in-hospital period. Burr *et al.* (1983) have documented the enormous savings in home care of other patients.

11.10 SUMMARY

Monitoring respiratory functions in MND is important and usually becomes critical in ALS. Spirometry is the best practical technique although other, more detailed tests are becoming widely used. Several treatments are available as breathing and coughing strength fail. When a critical point is reached, nasotracheal intubation/tracheostomy must be considered. Artificial ventilation is usually the next stage unless catastrophic decline has not already occurred from complicating aspiration, pneumonia or other problems. If tracheostomy and continued artificial respiration are chosen, permanent institutionalization is no longer necessary; severely paralyzed, artificially ventilated patients can be managed satisfactorily at home. Motivated relatives or even friends can be trained within weeks in the necessary care techniques. Such patients are better off at home as a result of improved morale and possibly by removal from the hospital germ environment. Symptomatic therapy in the home environment is a major medical resource even when curative therapy is lacking in fatal diseases.

ACKNOWLEDGMENTS

Drs Eric Denys, Philip Calanchini, Ronald Elkin and Harvey Tucker were major clinical collaborators. Katherine Kandal, Everett Stanley and Michael Snow assisted with the pulmonary functions and also worked in the home care program, directed by Dolores Holden, RN, and Linda Elias, RN. Dr Barbara Frances was of great help in preparing the manuscript.

Forbes Norris, MD (May 1928–June 1993), a physician–athlete–researcher, who dedicated his life to the search for the cause and cure for ALS, sadly passed away after he finished writing the manuscript for this chapter. His immense contribution to the understanding and treatment of ALS will always be remembered.

(S.M. Chou, MF, PhD)

Respiratory function

REFERENCES

Armon, C., Kurland, L.T., Beard, C.M. and O'Brien, P.C. (1989) Antecedent psychological and adaptational difficulties in patients with amyotrophic lateral sclerosis in Rochester, Minnesota, 1925 to 1987 (abstract). *Ann Neurol.*, **26**, 138.

Aubier, M., De Troyer, A., Sampson, M. *et al.* (1981) Aminophylline improves diaphragmatic contractility. *New Engl. J. Med.*, **305**, 249–52.

Bach, J.R. and Alba, A.S. (1991) Intermittent abdominal pressure ventilator in a regimen of noninvasive ventilatory support. *Chest*, **99**, 630–6.

Baydur, A., Gilgoff, I., Prentice, W. *et al.* (1990) Decline in respiratory function and experience with long-term assisted ventilation in advanced Duchenne's muscular dystrophy. *Chest*, **97**, 884–9.

Belsh, J.M. and Schiffman, P.L. (1988) Theophylline reduces respiratory muscle fatigue in patients with amyotrophic lateral sclerosis (abstract). *Neurology*, **38** (Suppl. 1), 270–1.

Berthon-Jones, M. and Sullivan, C.E. (1987) Time course of ventilatory response to CO_2 with long term CPAP. *Am. Rev. Resp. Dis.*, **135**, 144–7.

Bradley, W.G. (1982) Respiratory support in amyotrophic lateral sclerosis (letter). *Ann. Neurol.*, **12**, 466.

Burr, B.H., Guyer, B., Todner, I.D. *et al.* (1983) Home care for children on respirators. *New Engl. J. Med.*, **309**, 1319–23.

Carre, P.C., Didier, A.P., Tiberge, Y.M. *et al.* (1988) Amyotrophic lateral sclerosis presenting with sleep hypopnea syndrome. *Chest*, **93**, 1309–12.

Corbascio, M., Granata, C., Capelli, T. *et al.* (1990) Mechanical ventilation in Duchenne muscular dystrophy to counter vital capacity loss (abstract). *J. Neurol. Sci.*, **98** (Suppl.), 341.

Denys, E.H. and Norris, F.H. (1979) Amyotrophic lateral sclerosis: impairment of neuromuscular transmission. *Arch. Neurol.*, **36**, 74–80.

Dicus, R.G. (1976) *How I live with ALS.* Amyotrophic Lateral Sclerosis Society of America, Woodland Hills, California.

Fallat, R.J., Norris, F.H. and Holden, D. (1987) Respiratory monitoring and treatment: objective treatments using non-invasive measurements. *Adv. Exp. Med. Biol.*, **209**, 191–200.

Fallat, R.J., Jewett, B., Bass, M. *et al.* (1979) Spirometry in amyotrophc lateral sclerosis. *Arch. Neurol.*, **36**, 747–80.

Fallat, R.J., Norris, F.H., Holden, D. and Kandal, K. (1988) Ethical and practical issues of home management of respiratory failure with mechanical ventilation, in *Amyotrophic Lateral Sclerosis* (eds T. Tsubaki and Y. Yase), Elsevier, Amsterdam, pp. 271–7.

Fiz, J.A., Texido, A., Izquierdo, J. *et al.* (1990) Postural variation of the maximum inspiratory and expiratory pressures in normal subjects. *Chest*, **97**, 313–14.

Fromm, G.B., Wisdom, P.J. and Block, A.J. (1977) Amyotrophic lateral sclerosis presenting with respiratory failure. *Chest*, **71**, 612–14.

Gay, P.C., Westbrook, P.R., Daube J. *et al.* (1991) Effects of alterations in pulmonary function and sleep variables on survival in patients with amyotrophic lateral sclerosis. *Mayo Clin. Proc.*, **66**, 686–94.

References

Hill, R., Martin, J. and Hakim, A. (1983) Acute respiratory failure in motor neuron disease. *Arch. Neurol.*, **40**, 30–2.

Holden, D. and Stanley, E. (1987) Practicalities of home care for respiratory patients with amyotrophic lateral sclerosis, in *Realities in Coping with Progressive Neuromuscular Diseases* (eds L. I. Charash, R.E. Lovelace, S.G. Wolf *et al.*), Charles Press, Philadelphia, pp. 84–90.

Houpt, J.L., Gould, B.S. and Norris, F.H. (1977) Psychological characteristics of patients with amyotrophic lateral sclerosis. *Psychosom. Med.*, **39**, 299–303.

Mackay, R.P. (1963) Course and prognosis in amyotrophic lateral sclerosis. *Arch. Neurol.*, **8**, 117–27.

Mazzini, L., Mora, G., Pasetti, C. *et al.* (1990) Respiratory sleep disorders in amyotrophic lateral sclerosis (ALS) (abstract). *J. Neurol. Sci.*, **98** (Suppl.), **340**.

Montgomery, W.A. (1975) Surgical laryngeal closure to eliminate chronic aspiration. *New Engl. J. Med.*, **292**, 1390–1.

Mulder, D.H., Lambert, E.H. and Eaton (1959) Myasthenic syndrome in patients with amyotrophic lateral sclerosis. *Neurology*, **9**, 627–31.

Nightingale, S., Bates, D., Bateman, D.E. *et al.* (1982) Enigmatic dyspnoea: an unusual presentation of motor neurone disease. *Lancet* **ii**, 933–5.

Norris, F.H. (1990) Charting the course in amyotrophic lateral sclerosis, in *Progress in Clinical Neurologic Trials, I: Amyotrophic Lateral Sclerosis* (ed. F.C. Rose), Demos, New York, pp. 83–92.

Norris, F.H. (1992) Motor neuron disease: treating the untreated. *Br. Med. J.*, **304**, 459–60.

Norris, F.H. and Fallat, R.J. (1988) Staging respiratory failure in ALS, in *Amyotrophic Lateral Sclerosis: Recent Advances in Research and Treatment* (eds T. Tsubaki and Y. Yase), Exerpta Medica (Internat. Congr. Series No. 769), Amsterdam, pp. 217–22.

Norris, F.H., Smith, R.A. and Denys, E.H. (1985) Motor neuron disease: towards better care. *Br. Med. J.*, **291**, 259–62.

Norris, F.H., Smith, R.A., Denys, E.H. *et al.* (1987a) Home care of the paralyzed respirator patient with amyotrophic lateral sclerosis, in *Realities in Coping with Progressive Neuromuscular Diseases* (eds L.I. Charash, R.E. Lovelace, S.G. Wolf *et al.*), Charles Press, Philadelphia, pp. 72–83.

Norris, F.H., Smith, R.A., Denys, E.H. *et al.* (1987b) The treatment of amyotrophic lateral sclerosis. *Adv. Exp. Med. Biol.*, **209**, 175–82.

Norris, F.H., Shepherd, R.M., Denys, E.H. *et al.* (1993) Onset, natural history and outcome in subtypes of idiopathic adult motor neuron disease. *J. Neurol. Sci.* (in press).

Parhad, I.M., Clark, A.W., Barron, K.D. and Staunton, S.B. (1978) Diaphragmatic paralysis in motor neuron disease. *Neurology*, **28**, 18–22.

Peters, S.G. and Viggiano, R.W. (1988) Home mechanical ventilation. *Mayo Clin. Proc.*, **63**, 1208–13.

Renardel, A., Guillou, C., Foucoult, P. *et al.* (1990) Early use of nocturnal ventilation in DMD (abstract). *J. Neurol. Sci.*, **98** (Suppl.) 139.

Russell, T.R., Brotman, M.J. and Norris, F.H. (1984) Percutaneous gastrostomy. *Am. J. Surg.*, **148**, 132–7.

Respiratory function

Sivak, E.D. and Streib, E.W. (1980) Management of hypoventilation in motor neuron disease presenting with respiratory insufficiency. *Ann. Neurol.*, **7**, 188–91.

Sivak, E.D., Cordasco, E.M. and Gipson, W.T. (1983) Pulmonary mechanical ventilation at home: a reasonable and less expensive alternative. *Resp. Care*, **28**, 42–9.

Sivak, E.D., Gipson, W.T. and Hanson, M.R. (1982) Long-term management of respiratory failure in amyotrophic lateral sclerosis. *Ann. Neurol.*, **12**, 18–23.

Smith, P.E.M., Calverly, P.M.A., Edwards, R.H.T. *et al.* (1987) Practical problems in the respiratory care of patients with muscular dystrophy. *New Engl. J. Med.*, **316**, 1197–206.

Splaingard, M.L., Frates, R.C., Harrison, G.M. *et al.* (1982) Home positive pressure ventilation: twenty years' experience. *Chest*, **84**, 376–82.

12 *Nutritional support*

J.K. RAWLINGS and S.P. ALLISON

ABOUT PATIENTS WHO ARE UNABLE TO EAT

. . . It becomes our duty to adopt some artificial mode of conveying food into the stomach, by which the patient may be kept alive while the disease continues . . .

Hunter (1793)

12.1 INTRODUCTION

Although methods of giving nutritional support have been available for many years, there appears to be no consensus concerning the place of this form of palliative treatment in patients with motor neurone disease. Some neurological departments still pay scant attention to this aspect of the condition, and it is therefore difficult for patients and their families to obtain consistent advice. Eating difficulties not only interfere with the intake of fuel to maintain normal body function, but also distressingly with an important means of social and family contact. It should be possible to maintain the social aspects of eating longer, if the metabolic necessities are maintained by artificial means. It is the purpose of this chapter to describe not only the methods available for giving nutritional support, remembering that such techniques also allow easy administration of fluid and medicines, but to argue a rational approach to the problem addressing the question: 'Which patients should be treated and how?'

12.2 CONSEQUENCES OF WEIGHT LOSS

Assuming that a patient starts with a normal weight for age and height, measurable physiological defects start to occur after loss of 10% of the body weight, and after 15% weight loss may become very marked indeed (Wilmore, 1977). There is increased muscle fatiguability, impairment of muscle strength and wasting of the fast-twitch muscle fibres (Russell *et al.*, 1984). Respiratory function is impaired, with decreased V_{O_2} max and decreased exercise tolerance. Extreme weight loss causes mood changes, with apathy and depression. It could therefore be argued that such changes impose an unnecessary additional burden on MND patients experiencing an increasing struggle to move, swallow and breathe.

12.3 EATING AND SWALLOWING DIFFICULTIES

The incidence of bulbar palsy with dysphagia in this condition is discussed elsewhere in this book. Its management varies from unit to unit, from those who take an almost entirely nihilistic view to those who have a well-organized programme of supportive care. A recent report of 10 years' experience at St Christopher's Hospice (O'Brien, Kelly and Saunders, 1992) describes the management of 124 patients over this time. Severe swallowing difficulties were present in only a proportion of patients at the time of admission. Nineteen per cent were able to feed unaided. A further 24% were able to do so if food was specially prepared, and the remainder needed help. Twenty-one per cent were able to swallow all foods, 42% semisolids only and 27% liquidized or puréed foods. Two per cent were able to manage liquids only and 8% required feeding via a tube. The report also emphasizes that attention to feeding is only a part, if an important one, of the comprehensive management of this condition, and that full involvement of the family is vital. Their patients died of respiratory failure and none perished from 'choking'.

Such retrospective studies of selected groups of patients are of value, but no substitute for a prospective study of an unselected group over the whole natural history of the condition. In collaboration with Dr David Jefferson, we started such a study in June 1991. At initial diagnosis or presentation to the clinic, the patient is seen by a sympathetic dietitian. A history is taken of previous weight and current eating, drinking, swallowing and chewing capacity. A retrospective dietary history is also taken recording, particularly, any changes in the type of food eaten. The current weight is then measured and recorded. A 3-day food intake diary is also kept by the patient or the family at home. The idea that the disease may ultimately involve some difficulty with eating is introduced gently and the family are invited to contact the dietitian by phone should eating difficulties be encountered. Measurements of weight and food intake are repeated every 3 months. Of 22 successive patients referred to the clinic, seven have died in the first year, only one of whom required nutritional support with a gastrostomy. Of the remaining 15, seven have developed swallowing problems and have been referred to the speech therapist in an attempt to overcome these difficulties and to learn techniques allowing them to manage semisolid food (see below). Two patients are managing with proprietary oral nutritional supplements; one has a gastrostomy, three are about to have one placed, and one has refused the procedure. Only when swallowing difficulties begin to be encountered is the idea of a gastrostomy introduced to the patient and family. We convey the idea that this is not just a last ditch resort, but a means of giving supplementary nutrition and medicines, even though small amounts can still be swallowed. Adopting this approach, we find that patients ask for help sooner. Instead, therefore, of struggling desperately to swallow sufficient food and drink to maintain themselves, they can eat small amounts for enjoyment and for social and family reasons, while maintaining a normal nutritional state by means of gastrostomy tube feeding. It is an error to suppose that dysphagic patients can simply maintain their weight by taking longer over meals. Our data show that even minor swallowing difficulties result in a lower intake. The patient just gets tired of trying, or perhaps eats so slowly that the sense of satiety is reached inappropriately early. Of the three possible causes of weight loss – muscle wasting from the disease, an increase in metabolic rate due to the disease, and decreased food intake – the last is clearly the most important. All of our patients who have not yet experienced swallowing symptoms are maintaining their weight, or even increasing it as a result of inactivity. Those with any degree of dysphagia show a clear fall in total energy intake and have all lost weight until appropriate measures are taken to provide supplementation by oral or artificial means. Although the study is incomplete, the value of having a dietitian as a member of the caring team is already very clear.

12.4 PROTOCOLS FOR THE MANAGEMENT OF DYSPHAGIA

12.4.1 Identify the problem

The patient must be weighed on each visit and the remembered weight recorded. The family should be invited to make contact directly should they be concerned about any feeding difficulties. Food intake diaries over 3 days may provide helpful additional information, particularly for research purposes, but are not absolutely necessary. Measured weight can be related to the remembered weight of the patient or converted to body mass index, i.e. weight (kg) divided by height squared (m) (normal range 18–25).

The anthropometric measurements of mid-arm circumference and triceps skinfold thickness can not only be related to normal tables for the patient's weight and sex, but also give an idea of the relative change in muscle and fat (Elia, 1992). Such body compositional measurements can also be supported by the bioimpedance technique (Elia, 1992). When the measurement of height is difficult, the demispan, i.e. the distance between the suprasternal notch and the web of the middle two fingers with the hand outstretched, correlates very well with height (Lehmann *et al.*, 1991). Reference tables for this measurement and its relation to weight have been established.

12.4.2 Early dysphagia

Speech therapists should be involved in the assessment and the management of this. The protocols used by the Nottingham Speech Therapy Department are shown in Tables 12.1 and 12.2.

12.4.3 Moderate dysphagia

The deficit of energy and protein intake from meals can be made up by proprietary food supplements, which can be sipped between meals. The subject of tube feeding should be introduced at this point.

12.4.4 Severe dysphagia

NASOGASTRIC TUBE FEEDING

The development of fine-bore tubes made of improved plastics and introduced by means of a guide-wire has revolutionized nasogastric and nasoenteral feeding (Silk, 1987). Such devices are easier to use, more comfortable in position and less prone to cause oesophagitis than the old wider bore tubes. The complications of nausea, abdominal distension, discomfort and diarrhoea, so often a feature of the old bolus methods of feeding, can be overcome by continuous, controlled and slow infusion using a pump, either overnight or during periods of the day when the patient is at rest. This technique may be valuable for short periods of feeding, but has a number of disadvantages. Although fine-bore tubes can be removed by day and replaced in the evening in hospital, and sometimes at home if the patient or family is particularly competent, in

Table 12.1 Treatment techniques – immediate

Poor lip closure
  Close their lips normally
  Use spouted beaker
  Alter posture to upright position
Poor tongue elevation
  Avoid stodgy, sticky or crumbly foods
  Place food towards back of mouth
  Use syringe or long-handled spoon
  Check oral hygiene following meal
Poor tongue lateralization
  Check oral hygiene
  Position food centrally
  Use a straw for liquids
Delayed/absent swallow reflex
  Use thickened chilled liquids if delayed
  Use alternative means of feeding
  Teach supraglottic swallow
Reduced pharyngeal peristalsis
  Avoid dry and lumpy foods
  Alternate food with sip of water
Reduced laryngeal closure
  Tip head forward during swallow
  Teach supraglottic swallow

---

most cases the tube is kept in place and appears as a blemish on the face that is unacceptable to many patients. In contrast, a gastrostomy is hidden under the clothes and is not apparent to others. Whether weighted or not, the tubes are also frequently displaced, being either regurgitated into the pharynx or pulled out accidentally. If the patient is being treated at home, then replacement may be problematical. Studies have shown (Silk, 1987) that, in hospital, the average life of a tube *in situ* without being displaced is less than a week. Two recent studies have highlighted the advantages of percutaneous endoscopic gastrostomy over nasogastric tubes in the management of neurological patients. In a series of 30 patients with persistent vegetative state from neurological injury, Wicks *et al.* (1992) showed that, at the time these patients were converted from nasogastric to gastrostomy feeding, 67% were malnourished due to a high rate of tube displacement and feed regurgitation. After gastrostomy insertion, all patients achieved a normal body mass index with a low complication rate for the procedure. Park *et al.* (1992) carried out a prospective, randomized, controlled 28-day study of 40 inpatients with a minimum 4-week history of dysphagia secondary to

Table 12.2   Developing a swallowing routine

1. Place a certain amount of food or drink in the mouth. This should not be so small that the patient cannot feel it in his mouth or so large that it is difficult to swallow all at once.
2. Ask the patient to close his lips. If there is difficulty, support the jaw with the back of your hand to assist this.
3. Encourage the patient to move his tongue and teeth in a chewing motion. Chewing may be weak and ineffective and therefore overchewing each mouthful is advisable.
4. Once chewing has been completed, ask the patient to pause, leaving the food in the mouth for a second.
5. The food should be swallowed with a strong swallow, as this will be more effective than a gentle swallow. The patient should be asked to swallow a second time to clear any debris from the mouth.
6. Pause before putting more food in the patient's mouth and repeating this procedure.
7. At the end of the meal, ask the patient to cough forcefully to clear anything that is still in his mouth or throat.
8. Check the patient's mouth after a meal to remove any food that may have accumulated in his cheeks or on the roof of the mouth. This prevents food sliding down later and causing coughing and irritation.
9. Leave the patient sitting in an upright position for half an hour following a meal as regurgitation of food can be uncomfortable as well as dangerous.

neurological disorders, including motor neurone disease. Treatment failure occurred in 18 of the 19 nasogastrically fed patients and in none of the gastrostomy group. The mean duration of feeding before displacement of the tube in the nasogastric group was only 5.2 days. Although no complications occurred in the nasogastric group and three minor problems in the gastrostomy group, the latter received a significantly greater proportion of their prescribed feed, i.e. 93% *vs.* 55% in the nasogastric group. They also gained significantly more weight.

12.4.5   Gastrostomy and jejunostomy

The needle catheter jejunostomy technique (Page *et al.*, 1979; Rombeau *et al.*, 1989) is of particular value in situations where gastrostomy is impossible or contraindicated. It does, however, necessitate a general anaesthetic with a mini-laparotomy for its insertion via a cannula, which is first tunnelled between the layers of the jejunal wall before entering the bowel lumen. The bowel is then stitched to the anterior abdominal wall and the wound closed. We have employed this technique successfully in several patients, using the same tube for many months at a time. Its advantage is that it cannot be associated with reflux. Its disadvantage is that it requires a laparotomy both for initial placement and for replacement. The problems of local infection and the principles of management are the same as for gastrostomy.

The technique of percutaneous endoscopic gastrostomy (Ponsky, Gaudere and Stellato, 1983; Ponsky et al., 1985; Rombeau et al., 1989) has revolutionized the management of neurological swallowing problems and is now the technique of choice in the management of patients with this condition. Its success depends not only on the skilled insertion of the tube using strict protocols, but also on the careful education of the patient and the family in its management at home, the involvement of the district nurse and the general practitioner, the appropriate organization and funding to deliver equipment and supplies of feed to the patient's home, and careful follow-up with instructions for action in case of dysfunction of the tube or complications, as well as a hot-line contact phone number in case of difficulty. We have recently audited our 4-year experience of percutaneous endoscopic gastrostomy and compared the results with those published from the Mayo Clinic in 1988 (Nelson et al., 1986). In the Mayo Clinic series, although tubes were inserted with technical skill and minimal complications, all patients had at least one complication after discharge, possibly reflecting a lack of a coordinated follow-up policy by a single team. Our own experience is that there is a learning curve, so that we are now able to avoid some of the problems encountered initially. More than 50% of the complications encountered were managed at home, without a visit to the hospital, and most of the remainder could be managed during an outpatient visit, although in a few cases, particularly where the tube needed replacement, a short period of hospital admission was necessary.

There are broadly two types of gastrostomy. The first method requires the establishment of a fibrous track with either the insertion of a wide-bore gastrostomy tube surgically or the use of a wide-bore percutaneous endoscopic gastrostomy. After 2–3 weeks this can be removed and a button- or a balloon-type gastrostomy inserted from the outside. This technique has two main advantages: firstly, it can easily be replaced at home; and secondly, in the case of the button type, the external opening is flush with the skin. This is particularly useful in children and mentally handicapped patients who might otherwise pull at or remove a longer tube.

The alternative type is the fine-bore gastrostomy, which requires endoscopy for its insertion or replacement. Our experience of the fine-bore type is so good that we have continued to use it. One of our patients, for example, has had the same tube in place for 2½ years. Since success is heavily dependent upon careful technique and management, we have set out the protocols that we employ below.

12.5 PROTOCOL FOR INSERTION AND MANAGEMENT OF PERCUTANEOUS ENDOSCOPIC GASTROSTOMY (PEG)

All patients are referred to the dietitian in charge of long-term management, who with the endoscopist discusses with the patient and family the advantages and risks of having a PEG; the procedure is described and consent obtained. Preoperative investigations include coagulation screen, full blood count and chest X-ray. The patient receives nil by mouth from midnight, an intravenous cannula is inserted and a 48-h course of a third-generation cephalosporin (e.g. cefuroxime 750 mg tds) is started 1 h before the procedure.

In the endoscopy theatre, the patient receives Diazemuls 5–10 mg intravenously. If respiratory difficulties are anticipated, an anaesthetist should be at hand. The room is darkened and a gastroscope passed. The second operator perceives the endoscope light through the abdominal wall and infiltrates the skin, subcutaneous tissues and stomach wall with local anaesthetic, aiming for the light with the needle. A cannula is then passed, through which a nylon line is threaded. This is grasped with the endoscope biopsy forceps and drawn back through the mouth. The gastrostomy tube is attached and pulled down by the operator until the line and gastrostomy tube is drawn out through the abdominal wall. A flange on the tube fits snugly against the mucosa of the stomach and a second flange is attached to the external portion of the tube and slid down to touch the abdominal skin. The tube, thus anchored, has the hub attached to it, the whole is covered by a light dressing and the patient returned to the ward, where the usual post-operative observations are made. After 6–24 h the gastrostomy is infused firstly with water and then with feed, using gradually increasing rates from 30 to 150 ml per hour by continuous pumping. In most cases, a defined formula whole-protein proprietary feed containing 1 kcal/ml is effective. Elemental or peptide preparations offer no advantage. In some cases a fibre-containing feed is helpful to maintain normal bowel function. Few adults benefit from a lactose-free preparation. Osmolar concentration is less important than osmoles administered per unit time in the causation of diarrhoea. Dietetic guidance should be sought concerning the appropriate dose of feed for a particular patient. This will usually be about 30 kcal/kg per day and 0.15–0.2 g of nitrogen per kg per day.

The patient and family are then given a formal programme of training, by the dietitian in charge of the service, until full competence and confidence are established. This usually takes 5–7 days. The district nurse is also invited to join this process. The general practitioner is also contacted and asked to prescribe the feed on an EC10 form, which can then be dispensed by any pharmacy, including those commercial companies which provide a home enteral delivery service. There is no standard system to pay for the hardware, but most health authorities agree to pay for the plastic sets required, while the company providing the feeds will usually lend or lease the pumps. Each hospital or district should establish its own clear policy in these matters. Further advice and help may also be obtained from the Motor Neurone Disease Association.

Discharge from hospital is associated with a period of anxiety for the patient and family. Support must therefore be available. A domiciliary visit by the dietitian is helpful, a 'hot-line' phone number should be available at all times, and a programme of regular outpatient follow-up by the dietitian or nutrition nurse carried out. The patient should carry a card advising that any problem should be referred to the responsible team. Many of the difficulties we have encountered have been the result of inexpert if well-meaning intervention by others.

A number of problems may occur:

1. Some patients find the constant attachment to the pump and drip psychologically intolerable. Periods of freedom are therefore required. Some patients give themselves continuous feeding overnight with small bolus feeds via a syringe by day. Gravity feeding, with its unreliable rate of administration, and large bolus feeds, is less satisfactory, as both increase the risk of reflux and diarrhoea.
2. The rate of administration of feed is limited by two factors. Firstly, above a certain rate, say 125 ml of feed per hour, the patient may complain of reflux. Secondly, in patients with respiratory muscle weakness, the increased metabolic rate (+15%) associated with too rapid infusion causes breathlessness.
3. Other complications may be divided into early and late. In our audit of 24 patient-years of gastrostomy feeding in 49 consecutive patients (27% MND), 67% were able to return home. Four patients died within 30 days, one from PEG-related aspiration pneumonia. Twenty-two of the 45 patients surviving more than 30 days experienced 41 complications. Fifty-three per cent of these were resolved by a telephone discussion or by a dietitian home visit. The remainder required a hospital visit. There were 21 cases of mechanical problems, e.g. tube blockage, 12 cases of gastrointestinal symptoms such as nausea, reflux, vomiting, constipation or diarrhoea. There were only six cases of early- and two of late-onset local sepsis, all responding to

antibiotics. There were 15 late deaths, 14 due to progress of the underlying disease and one due to gastric perforation by the PEG. Six patients subsequently returned to oral feeding. We concluded that follow-up by a single, small nutrition team and careful observation of standard protocols were as important as skilled insertion of the PEG, in order to maximize benefit and minimize both anxiety and complications. This system also facilitates the solution of any difficulties that arise and the appropriate treatment of any complications if and when they occur.

After discharge, the following protocols are observed and copies of these are given to the patients.

12.5.1   Protocol I: General aftercare

FLUSHING THE TUBE

To prevent blocking, the tube must be flushed at regular intervals, i.e.

- after the administration of medication;
- after each feed or, when continuous feeding, every 6–8 h.

To maintain patency when the tube is not being used, the tube should be flushed *at least* once a day.

It is recommended that a 50-ml syringe of a suitable liquid, e.g. lukewarm tap water, is used to flush the tube.

Medication should be administered in a liquid form and *not* at the same time as the feed.

BODY CARE

The presence of a gastrostomy tube should not alter normal body care. When bathing, showering or swimming, the Luer lock connector on the top of the tube should be closed. For cosmetic reasons, it may be advisable to cover the tube with a waterproof dressing when swimming.

SKIN CARE

The skin around the gastrostomy set should be cleansed daily with a mild soap and water. It is normal to see some encrustation around the tube. A build-up of debris can be cleansed using a swab soaked with hydrogen peroxide. The doctor should be informed if the exit site of the wound becomes reddened and inflamed, if there is leakage of fluid, or if there is abdominal pain.

CHANGE OF DRESSING

If a dressing is used, it should be changed daily during the first week and once or twice per week subsequently.

12.5.2 Protocol II: Instructions for setting up feed for gastrostomy and jejunostomy patients, for pump-assisted feeding using feeding reservoir

Careful hygiene, i.e. hand washing, should be observed.

REQUIREMENTS

- feed in bottles or cans;
- feeding reservoir with attached giving set;
- pump;
- cleaning solution;
- adapter if required;
- syringe for flushing with warm water.

PROCEDURE

1. Before opening bottle, shake well.
2. Close clamp on giving set and open the cap of the feeding reservoir.
3. Fill the feeding reservoir from the bottles or cans.
4. Close the cap.
5. Hang the feeding reservoir above the pump so that there is a loop of giving set above the pump.
6. Put the chamber into the pump drip chamber guide.
7. Release the roller clamp on the giving set and allow the feed to run slowly to about 1″ from the end of the tube.
8. Stretch the silicone tube segment and wrap around the pump rotor.
9. Thread tubing through the tubing guide.
10. Close the clamp.
11. Check that the chamber is not filled to more than one-third or one-half of maximum.
12. Clean the hub with cleaning solution.
13. Attach the giving set to the gastrostomy tube.
14. Set the pump to the required rate and start.

Nutritional support

Opened bottles or containers with any remaining feed may be carefully covered and refrigerated for up to 24 h only. Never use feed that has been opened for longer than 24 h.

12.5.3 Protocol III: Discontinuing the feed

REQUIREMENTS

- 20-ml syringe;
- cleaning solution;
- gauze;
- clean receptacle (i.e. cup, glass or jug).

PROCEDURE

1. Assemble equipment.
2. Wash hands.
3. Draw up 20 ml of lukewarm water from clean utensil.
4. Close gastrostomy tube clamp and remove giving set.
5. Clean connection site with gauze and cleaning solution.
6. Open gastrostomy tube clamp, attach adapter and then syringe and instil water in order to flush the tube free of any material that might coagulate and block it.
7. Close the clamp, remove the syringe and adapter and apply bung.
8. Giving sets and reservoirs are designed for single use and should be changed every 24 h. If for water only, sterilize in a suitable detergent.

12.5.4 Protocol IV: Managing problems

FLUID STOPS FLOWING

1. Check giving set line is not kinked.
2. Check clamps (both giving set and gastrostomy tube) are fully open.
3. Flush gastrostomy tube with warm water. If there is resistance, do not continue. Clamp off the gastrostomy tube, remove the feed, come to the hospital or, if unable, leave till working hours and ring hospital.

DAMAGE OR CRACK IN EQUIPMENT

1. Giving set. Do not use. Discard and run through a new one.
2. Gastrostomy tube. Do not use. Apply clamp, wrap in impregnated

swab with disposable cloth. Come to hospital during working hours for repair or ring hospital, particularly if on medication.

THE FLUID HAS RUN THROUGH QUICKLY

The pump rate is set too fast. Do not worry; apart from feeling full you will come to no harm. Disconnect giving set, flush gastrostomy tube, do not put up another feed. Stay sitting up for at least 4 h. If feeling sick or actually being sick, you may phone the hospital.

THE FLUID HAS RUN TOO SLOWLY

If still within the time limit, i.e. 6 h into feed and three-quarters remains, speed up slowly. Increase rate by 50 ml per hour.

MAINS POWER FAILURE

Batteries will take over automatically and will last for several hours. If this time elapses, remove giving set from the pump and control fluid flow using giving set clamp, or give feed by bolus injection.

YOU FEEL UNWELL

Take your temperature. If above 37°C, phone hospital and arrange visit. Stop feed if still in progress. Do not discard; take feed fluid with you to hospital so that it may be cultured.

DIARRHOEA DEVELOPS

Slow feed infusion rate. Diarrhoea should subside over the next 6–12 h. If diarrhoea persists, phone hospital or arrange visit. Stop the feed and take it with you.

STARTING ON MEDICATION

If you are started on drugs by your GP, let him know about your gastrostomy tube (if he does not already know). Most drugs can be made into liquid form and so can be passed down your tube via a syringe. If you wish to self-medicate (i.e. you have a headache), do not worry; the chemist will help you choose a suitable soluble form of pain relief which can also be passed down your tube via a syringe. It is important to remember to flush drugs with your 20-ml syringe and warm water after each medication.

Nutritional support

BATHING AND SWIMMING

You will come to no harm if you have a bath or go swimming. Just remember to dry your skin around and under the flat disc and also the tube itself.

GOING OUT FOR THE NIGHT

If you wish to go out and have your feed during the day or early evening, you can afford to miss the odd night altogether, but not two consecutively.

12.6 SUMMARY AND CONCLUSIONS

The main cause of weight loss in motor neurone disease is diminished food intake through dysphagia and not primary muscle wasting from the disease itself. Undernutrition and weight loss are associated with depression and diminished muscle and cardiorespiratory function adding to the problems of the underlying disease. All motor neurone disease patients should be carefully monitored in terms of weight and food intake so that appropriate intervention can take place before serious weight loss has occurred. Initial management is via the speech therapist and oral supplements. When dysphagia becomes more severe, the patient should be offered percutaneous endoscopic gastrostomy, which is now the treatment of choice in this condition. Successful gastrostomy feeding depends on skilled insertion of the PEG, the careful observance of standard protocols, adequate training of the patient and family in the use of the equipment, and careful follow-up involving a skilled dietitian or nurse to whom the patient and family have ready access by telephone. The district nurse and the general practitioner should be involved and a proper plan made for prescribing and funding feeds and equipment, which may be delivered to the patient's home by a commercial feed delivery service. Feeding is only part of a well-coordinated overall management, which should be sensitive to the patient and family's wishes and anxieties.

REFERENCES

Elia, M. (1992) Body composition analysis: an evaluation of 2 component models, multicomponent models and bedside techniques. *Clin. Nutr.*, **11**, 114–27.

Hunter, J. (1793) A case of paralysis of the muscles of deglutition, cured by an artificial mode of conveying food into the stomach. *Trans. Soc. Improv. Med. Chir. Know.*, **1**, 182.

278

References

Lehmann, A.B., Bassey, E.J., Morgan, K. *et al.* (1991) Normal values for weight, skeletal size and body mass indices in 890 men and women aged over 65 years. *Clin. Nutr.*, **10**, 18–22.

Nelson, J.K., Palumbo, P.J. and O'Brian, P.C. (1986) Home enteral nutrition: observations of a newly-established program. *Nutr. Clin. Pract.*, **1**, 193–9.

O'Brien, T., Kelly, M. and Saunders, C. (1992) Motor neurone disease – a hospice perspective. *Br. Med. J.*, **304**, 471–3.

Page, C.P., Carlton, P.K., Andrassy, R.J. *et al.* (1979) Safe cost-effective post-operative nutrition: defined formula diet via needle catheter jejunostomy. *Am. J. Surg.*, **138**, 939.

Park, R.H.R., Allison, M.C., Lang, J. *et al.* (1992) Randomised comparison of percutaneous endoscopic gastrostomy and nasogastric tube feeding in patients with persisting neurological dysphagia. *Br. Med. J.*, **304**, 1406–9.

Ponsky, J.L., Gaudere, M.W.L. and Stellato, I.A. (1983) Percutaneous endoscopic gastrostomy. Review of 150 cases. *Arch. Surg.*, **118**, 913–4.

Ponsky, J.L., Gaudere, M.W.L., Stellato, I.A. *et al.* (1985) Percutaneous approaches to enteral alimentation. *Am. J. Surg.*, **149**, 102–5.

Rombeau, J.L., Cauldwell, M.D., Forlaw, L. *et al.* (1989) *Atlas of Nutritional Support Techniques*. Little, Brown, Boston.

Russell, D.M., Walker, P.M., Leiter, L.A. *et al.* (1984) Metabolic and structural changes in muscle during hypocaloric dieting. *Am. J. Clin. Nutr.*, **39**, 503–513.

Silk, D.B.A. (1987) Towards the optimisation of enteral nutrition. *Clin. Nutr.*, **6**, 61–74.

Wicks, C., Gimson, A., Vlavianos, P. *et al.* (1992) Assessment of the percutaneous endoscopic gastrostomy feeding tube as part of an integrated approach to enteral feeding. *Gut*, **33**, 613–16.

Wilmore, D.W. (1977) *The Metabolic Management of the Critically Ill*. Plenum Publishing, New York.

13 *Terminal care*

DAVID OLIVER

13.1 INTRODUCTION

As there is at present no cure for motor neurone disease the care of a patient is palliative, reducing the effects of the disease, controlling and easing the symptoms, allowing the patients to maintain whatever powers they still have and enabling patients and their families to live as full a life as possible. It is not always clear when palliative care merges into terminal care, when death is expected and not far off, and thus in discussing the terminal care of a patient with motor neurone disease it is important to outline the many and varied ways in which palliation can be achieved.

The care that can be offered to a patient with motor neurone disease will involve the 'whole patient', considering physical, emotional/psychological, social and spiritual aspects. Often these aspects are inter-related, and careful interdisciplinary assessment is needed to enable the patient's, and the family's, care to be maximized.

13.2 PHYSICAL PROBLEMS

There are a great many physical problems facing a patient with motor neurone disease, and often there are multiple inter-related symptoms. All these need to be carefully assessed, as it is only after diagnosis of the symptom that the appropriate treatment can be started. The assessment of each symptom will include a careful history and examination, and often several disciplines need to be involved.

After assessment there is a need to explain the symptom and the problem to the patient. This can relieve anxiety and allow patients to express their fears more easily. Some symptoms, in particular emotional lability, may not only cause distress in their own right but lead to anxiety about possible mental deterioration. A patient may need to be prompted to talk about these anxieties and careful explanation of the physical cause of the symptom is a major part of effective treatment.

281

Terminal care

Only after assessment and explanation can treatment be started. The various symptoms will be considered separately.

13.2.1 Dyspnoea

Sixty per cent of patients experience dyspnoea (Saunders, Walsh and Smith, 1981). As this symptom may be exacerbated by anxiety, a calm and confident approach by the carers is essential, and careful positioning, especially of the neck, is important.

Opioids are very helpful in reducing the distress of dyspnoea. A carefully titrated dose of an opioid can be titrated against the effectiveness of the control of the symptom, starting at a low dose such as 5 mg of oral morphine elixir every 4 h or morphine sulphate slow-release tablets 10 mg 12-hourly. An oral antiemetic, such as prochlorperazine or metoclopramide, may be needed during the first few days, but can then be stopped. An aperient, such as lactulose and sennoside or codanthramer, is necessary to prevent constipation.

Used in this way opioids are effective in controlling this distressing symptom, and they can be used safely. O'Brien, Kelly and Saunders (1992) found that 88% of their patients receiving hospice care received opioids on at least one occasion. The mean dose was only 30 mg of oral morphine equivalent per 24 h and the mean duration of use was 58 days. The response was assessed as good in 81% of the patients when the indication was dyspnoea.

Opioids can also be used in the control of an acute episode of breathlessness. An intramuscular injection of diamorphine, chlorpromazine and hyoscine will relieve the distress of acute breathlessness effectively.

Diazepam, as an oral dose of 5–10 mg at night, may be helpful in easing dyspnoea. A suppository or enema of diazepam can be effective in the relief of acute breathlessness when an injection is not possible and can be given by a family member or untrained carer.

Antibiotics may be considered in the treatment of a chest infection in the early stages of the disease. However, as the disease progresses careful consideration of the appropriateness of antibiotic treatment will be needed and the control of the symptoms by an opioid with an anticholinergic, such as hyoscine, may be more appropriate.

13.2.2 Pain

Pain is a distressing symptom experienced by many patients, estimates varying from 40% (Saunders, Walsh and Smith, 1981) to 64% (Newrick and Langton-Hewer, 1985). Although sensory disturbance has been reported the sensory nerves are not usually affected (Newrick and Langton-Hewer, 1985).

There are three different types of pain that can be found in a patient with motor neurone disease:

1. Musculoskeletal: from stiffened joints with restricted movement and altered muscle tone. The shoulders may be particularly affected. Careful positioning and physiotherapy, including regular passive movements to reduce stiffness, are helpful. Non-steroidal anti-inflammatory drugs are helpful and intra-articular injections of steroids and local anaesthetic are useful, particularly in the shoulder.
2. Skin pressure: a patient who is less mobile and unable to change position may experience pain. Regular turning and movement are essential to relieve this discomfort. Opioid analgesics, such as morphine elixir or morphine sulphate slow-release tablets, are very effective. Seventy-four per cent were found to have a good response to opioids and no patient was not helped by opioids (O'Brien, Kelly and Saunders, 1992). Regular administration may be necessary, although some patients may only require a dose at night.
3. Muscle cramps: occurring in spastic muscles. Diazepam or quinine bisulphate can be helpful and other muscle relaxant drugs may be helpful (see Muscle stiffness below).

13.2.3 Dysphagia and drooling

Swallowing problems were found to occur in 58% of patients (Saunders, Walsh and Smith, 1981), and were caused not only by the involvement of motor nuclei in the medulla causing muscle weakness but also by muscle spasticity and incoordination in the hypopharynx and pharynx.

Careful slow feeding is necessary and semisolid foods are often easier to swallow than liquids. On admission to a hospice 37% of the patients with motor neurone disease needed to be fed and a further 19% needed help or supervision (O'Brien, Kelly and Saunders, 1992). Sixty-nine per cent of the patients needed semisolids or liquidized or puréed foods. Many beverages, from tea to whisky, can be frozen into ice cubes and taken more easily in this form.

The dribbling of saliva is a very distressing symptom to both patient and family. Thirty-eight per cent of patients admitted to a hospice (O'Brien, Kelly and Saunders, 1992) and 20% of a survey of outpatients (Newrick and Langton Hewer, 1984) complained of drooling. Sublingual hyoscine tablets can be very helpful. For severe symptoms intramuscular hyoscine or hyoscine in a continuous subcutaneous infusion using a syringe driver can be very helpful. Antidepressants, with anticholinergic action, such as amitriptyline can also be helpful. Suction pumps may be of help to some patients.

Many patients fear choking, and 17% of patients in one survey complained of regular choking (Newrick and Langton Hewer, 1984). Although a sudden respiratory collapse can occur, choking, with obstruction of the airways, is very rare. Post-mortem examination of 19 patients showed the airways to be entirely free of foreign matter (O'Brien, Kelly and Saunders, 1992).

The feelings of choking and respiratory distress can be reduced by careful positioning and the control of salivation. If the feelings become very distressing an injection of diamorphine to reduce the cough reflex and lessen anxiety, and hyoscine to reduce the secretions, relax smooth muscle and act as an amnesic, should be given. If a patient has developed problems with swallowing these injections should be easily available. Diazepam, as an enema, may be used to relieve the distress if an injection cannot be given, and a family member may be able to give an enema at home when professional carers are not immediately available in the emergency situation.

A gastrostomy may be considered for some patients with feeding difficulties and the percutaneous endoscopic technique can allow a feeding gastrostomy to be formed with less discomfort or distress than a laparotomy (Ponsky and Gauderer, 1989).

13.2.4 Dysarthria

Seventy-five per cent of patients develop speech problems (Saunders, Walsh and Smith, 1981), and in a large survey of patients on admission to a hospice 36% had unintelligible or no speech (O'Brien, Kelly and Saunders, 1992). Simple measures, such as ensuring the listener is in front of the patient to ease communication and using short and concise speech, can be helpful. Assessment by a speech therapist can allow the most of the remaining speech and allow the correct use of speech aids.

13.2.5 Constipation

A patient who is inactive and taking a diet low in roughage is prone to constipation and 65% of hospice patients complained of this (O'Brien, Kelly and Saunders, 1992). Aperients, such as a faecal softener, for example lactulose, and a peristaltic stimulant such as sennoside B can be helpful. Rectal measures, such as suppositories, enemata or manual evacuation, may be necessary.

Diarrhoea is often due to constipation with overflow, and this must be excluded by a rectal examination. Anti-diarrhoeal agents may be necessary if there is intercurrent disease.

13.2.6 Muscle stiffness

Spastic muscles can become uncomfortable. This can often be eased by careful positioning and regular passive movements (Oliver, O'Gorman and Saunders, 1986). Muscle relaxant drugs, such as diazepam, baclofen and dantrolene sodium, can be helpful. However, the dose may need very careful adjustment to allow a balance between spasticity and flaccidity, as relief of spasticity may be seen as increased weakness by the patient and reduce mobility.

13.2.7 Sore eyes

The weakness of eye muscles may lead to a reduction of eye blinking, and the eyes may feel sore and become secondarily infected. Lubrication of the eyes with hypromellose eyedrops can be useful, and any infection should be treated with appropriate antibiotic eyedrops.

13.2.8 Hunger and thirst

Hunger can often be alleviated by careful and appropriate feeding so that a reasonable diet can be taken. In the terminal stages of the disease an opioid, such as oral morphine, may be helpful in reducing hunger pangs.

13.2.9 Tiredness

Many patients complain of a feeling of tiredness and lethargy. Activity should be encouraged, but not to overextend the reduced strength of a patient. Listening and sharing the patient's, and his family's, concerns may be all that can be done, so that the feelings can at least be accepted. Corticosteroids have been suggested to increase the feelings of well-being, but in the long term weakness may be increased, together with other side-effects.

13.2.10 Insomnia

Insomnia affected 48% of the patients on admission to a hospice (O'Brien, Kelly and Saunders, 1992) and careful assessment of the cause of insomnia is essential as sleep may be disturbed by pain, fear, discomfort or insecurity. Regular positioning is helpful, and it is important to ensure that the patient can attract the attention of carers easily, such as by the use of an easily operated buzzer, thus decreasing the feelings of insecurity. Benzodiazepines and opioid analgesics may be considered to reduce stiffness and pain.

13.2.11   Bed sores

Bed sores are not common as the regular changes in position necessitated by the preservation of normal sensation reduce the risks. In the large survey only 16% of patients developed bed sores (Saunders, Walsh and Smith, 1981). Prevention, by regular repositioning and good skin care, is important. The treatment of an established bed sore is by the locally favoured method.

13.2.12   Urinary problems

Difficulties in passing urine may occur if the musculature of the abdominal wall becomes weakened. Incontinence is rarely due to motor neurone disease but may occur because of immobility. Investigation may be necessary, in particular to exclude urinary tract infection. Urinary catheterization may be necessary on occasions for convenience in an immobile patient.

13.2.13   Oedema

Ankle oedema may occur in an immobile patient and the raising of the legs, a shaped control stocking or a diuretic may be helpful. However, the ensuing diuresis may cause urinary problems. Persistent or severe oedema may be due to intermittent disease and further investigation is then necessary.

13.3   EMOTIONAL/PSYCHOLOGICAL PROBLEMS

Any person facing a life-threatening illness and progressive disability will have fears and anxieties. If these are not shared and occur with increasing isolation, fear and depression may ensue.

The fears that come to the fore may be of a very individual nature for each person, relating to their past experience of life and personality. However, certain fears may be more common.

13.3.1   Fears of the diagnosis

Many people on learning of the diagnosis of motor neurone disease may be unsure and ignorant, but on reading or listening to more details of the condition fears may increase. A particular fear is of choking. Many of the articles and books on motor neurone disease, particularly in the popular press, talk of choking and 'choking to death'. As shown previously, there is no evidence for respiratory obstruction (O'Brien, Kelly and Saunders, 1992) and good symptom control and care reduce the risk of distress in the terminal stages.

One survey showed that 68% of patients were aware of the nature of motor neurone disease and its likely progression and a further 25% knew the diagnosis but were unaware of the progression to death (O'Brien, Kelly and Saunders, 1992).

Time may be necessary to allow patients and their families to talk of these fears and then attempt to reassure if they are unwarranted.

13.3.2 Fear of disability and dependence

Anyone facing increasing disability will be unsure and fearful of the future. The fear of possible increasing disability and dependence can be profound and cannot be ignored. All the professional carers can do is listen and try to help the patient make the most of his abilities, physical and mental, even as the losses of abilities increase. Specific fears, such as of incontinence, may need to be addressed.

13.3.3 Fears of dying

Many adults have never been with anyone when they are dying and this can cause fear as death approaches. There are many myths, such as of 'death throes', which may occupy someone's mind and it is important to stress what can be done to control distressing symptoms, such as respiratory difficulties or pain.

13.3.4 Fears of physical changes

Many patients fear mental incapacitation or incontinence, although these are rare as part of motor neurone disease. It may take time and confidence for a patient to talk of these concerns, and they must be accepted and talked about rather than dismissed.

13.3.5 Fears of death

All of us have very differing views of death, varying from oblivion to a certainty of 'heaven'. Each patient will have their own belief system and resulting anxieties, and these concerns need to be shared. This may be with members of the family, the medical or nursing team or a specific clergyman. There are no easy answers but listening and accepting is essential.

These fears need to be expressed and the mood of a patient will vary. In motor neurone disease when communication and the expression of emotion is reduced by dysarthria, mood changes and swings are very common. These may be exacerbated if others consider a person who is disabled by this loss of expression or control of emotion to be of reduced intelligence.

Anxiety can often be helped by careful control of other symptoms, a calm confident approach and listening with explanation. Anxiolytics can be helpful, such as benzodiazepines. In an emergency situation of severe panic an injection of diamorphine, chlorpromazine and hyoscine can be given.

It is often very difficult to differentiate the natural sadness of a person with a progressive disabling illness from a true depressive illness. Antidepressants can be helpful if there is evidence of true depression, but the starting dose should be lower than normal and increased slowly, to reduce the risk of side-effects.

Although medication can be helpful it is more important to listen to the patient's concerns and encourage them to be shared within the family.

13.4 SOCIAL PROBLEMS

Most patients are part of a larger family and everyone needs to be involved and included in the patterns and plans of care. There may be particular areas of concern within a family.

13.4.1 Diagnosis

Family members may also be unsure and frightened about the diagnosis of motor neurone disease, and share the same fears as the patient. Moreover, if the family has been told separately from, and perhaps more fully than, the patient, communication within the family may be lost (Carey, 1986). O'Brien, Kelly and Saunders showed that, although 68% of patients were fully aware of the diagnosis, 82% of the main carers were fully aware. These differences in knowledge can cause great friction and separate couples and families at a time when they need to be close and sharing their concerns together (Oliver, 1986, 1989).

Many families fear that motor neurone disease is a hereditary disease. As the genetic component of the disease is small most families can be reassured on this point.

13.4.2 Communication

Communication may be an area of distress within a family as dysarthria and emotional lability reduce patients' ability to communicate their needs and fears. Coupled with increasing physical dependency and anxiety this can lead to increasing isolation within a family. It is essential to ensure that communication is continued so that feelings and fears can be shared.

13.4.3 Isolation

Isolation can occur in a relationship where one member knows more than the other and deceit starts. This can be prevented by openly sharing the details of the diagnosis with the patient and his family together, rather than separately. Isolation can occur within the larger family and the community at large as increasing disability restricts activities away from the home and also leads to friends and family avoiding contact as they are frightened or embarrassed by the illness.

13.4.4 Finances

Families may also have financial problems as the patient's disability increases and enforces early retirement or long-term sickness. A spouse may also be forced to give up employment to care for the patient. These financial worries need to be addressed.

13.4.5 Fear of death

There will also be a variation in a family's attitudes to death and family members may have their own particular fears, of pain, choking or death itself. These need to be shared and everyone needs to be involved in these discussions. Children in particular may feel very excluded but need to be involved and their particular needs addressed.

13.4.6 Sexuality

As the disease progresses the patient and his/her partner may fear a loss of sexual performance. Although there is rarely a loss of erectile ability there may be a need to reassess the capability for intercourse as disability increases. These changes may cause increasing stresses within the relationship and sensitive discussion of the area of sexuality and sexual needs is needed. Alterations in previous sexual behaviour, such as changing sexual positions for intercourse or the consideration of mutual masturbation as an alternative way of expressing closeness, may need to be considered.

It is important to allow and facilitate communication within the family, allowing the sharing of feelings and involvement in the care and plans. Preparations may be necessary, including the making of a will, consideration of funeral arrangements or particular visits to renew friendships, to relive past experiences or for reminiscence. Long-standing aims may be fulfilled, and in this way a family can continue to function together and grow together, even as the illness progresses.

Time becomes precious and needs to be used to the full. Many of the discussions and preparations may need to be considered earlier in the disease when perhaps speech and communication are easier. The carers themselves also need time for themselves. There is great stress on carers when coping with a severely disabled person (Livingstone, 1985; Anderson, 1987), and carers need time to rest and meet others. A time of relief, even for a few hours, will allow carers to continue in their care of the patient (Kinsella and Duffy, 1979).

13.5 SPIRITUAL CONCERNS

When considering the total care of a patient with motor neurone disease it is important to consider the spiritual issues – those concerning the spirit or higher moral qualities (Saunders, 1988). This may, or may not, be linked to a specific religious attitude, and many people without a religious faith will have concerns and worries arising from the area of life concerned with moral values and deeper beliefs.

The issues that may need to be considered include the 'search for meaning' (Saunders, 1988), which can be expressed as 'why me?' There are no easy answers but we may need to sit and share with patients as they make their own journeys of growth through loss (Roche, 1989). Often all we can do is listen and share. Sometimes a team member may enable a patient to communicate the fears and make their own connections within their experiences (Roche, 1989).

Fears of dying and death may also be expressed. These may be of a very practical nature, such as the fear of pain, but may be deeper fears of the 'afterlife' and of oblivion. Again often all that can be done is to listen and enable a patient to make some sense of their condition for themselves.

13.6 INTERDISCIPLINARY TEAM APPROACH

To optimize the care of a patient with motor neurone disease it is essential that an interdisciplinary team approach is undertaken. Close collaboration between team members is important to coordinate care, and it has been suggested that one person should should be designated as the 'key worker', who could act as an intermediary and personal agent for the patient, facilitating the package of care provided by the various professionals involved (Newrick and Langton Hewer, 1984).

13.6.1 Physiotherapy

Physiotherapy has an important role in the continuing care of the patient with motor neurone disease, and regular exercising can help to maintain independence and reduce the problems caused by weakened muscles. Active and passive movements can help to maximize power, decrease stiffness, prevent contractions, maintain joint mobility and minimize the effects of disuse atrophy (Oliver, O'Gorman and Saunders, 1986).

The physiotherapist can also help in enabling the patient to be as comfortable as possible, by finding the best position, especially of the neck and head (Henke, 1968). Breathing exercises to maintain chest expansion and encourage the increased use of diaphragmatic breathing can be helpful (Oliver, O'Gorman and Saunders, 1986).

In all these treatment programmes patients and their families can be actively involved (Oliver, O'Gorman and Saunders, 1986), and regular physiotherapy several times a day is preferable to brief sessions with a professional on an irregular basis (Norris, Smith and Denys, 1985).

13.6.2 Occupational therapy

The many aids to daily living that are available to allow a disabled patient to remain functioning at home can be provided after an assessment by an occupational therapist. The need for aids is continually changing and reassessment is needed as the patient's disability worsens. There may be an increasing need for systems to retain some control over the environment and in this way maintain independence; for instance, environmental control systems such as Possum should be considered.

13.6.3 Speech therapy

Speech therapy can be helpful in allowing the most to be made of remaining speech, and regular reassessment throughout the illness is essential as the speech deteriorates. Aids to communication range from a portable communicator, such as a Lightwriter, to a microprocessor connected to a television monitor or a speech simulation system.

13.6.4 Dietitian

Dietary advice on the choice and preparation of food and drink allows a balanced diet acceptable to both patients and their families. Dietary supplements may be helpful, and further advice on enteral feeding will be necessary if a gastrostomy has been fashioned.

13.6.5 Social worker

Disability and progressive illness causes many differing stresses to both patients and families. Relationships within the family are put under stress and the established roles within the family are altered. The involvement of a social worker may be helpful in providing counselling and support for everyone involved in these changing situations. Financial advice and help in claiming the social benefits may be provided by the social worker.

Other agencies may be involved in the care of a patient and family: clergy or appropriate religious minister to help with spiritual issues; wheelchair and aid specialists for help with equipment; the voluntary agencies, such as the Motor Neurone Disease Association, to provide equipment and financial help. However, it is essential not to ignore the resources of patients and their families. Any help that is offered should be to complement and help patients and their families and not remove their role.

13.7 TERMINAL STAGES

As a patient becomes less well there is a need to review all the needs of both patient and family. This is an extension of the regular review outlined above and all the aspects of care must be considered – physical, emotional, social and spiritual. The aim as the terminal stages are reached must be to anticipate crises and hopefully to prevent crises by careful symptom control.

Communication becomes even more important: communication by the patient of his/her needs and fears; communication within the family to share their own fears and concerns; communication between patient and family and the professional carers; communication amongst the professional carers. Information and plans must be shared among all those involved – family and professionals – and information should be available for other professionals who may become involved if the usual professional carers are unavailable.

The major cause of death in motor neurone disease is respiratory failure. Often the deterioration is over a short period and the clinical picture is of acute or acute-on-chronic respiratory failure. In a series of 113 deaths in the hospice setting 40% deteriorated suddenly and died within 12 h, 18% died within 24 h, 24% within 3 days, 17% within 7 days and only 2% lived for more than a month after the sudden deterioration (O'Brien, Kelly and Saunders, 1992).

Although this respiratory distress may be described as 'choking', post-mortem examination showed that the airways were free of foreign matter and that the 'choking attack' is one of respiratory distress and not respiratory obstruction (O'Brien, Kelly and Saunders, 1992).

The control of these symptoms has been outlined above. There may be an increasing need for opioid medication, to control pain, dyspnoea or discomfort, and in the large series 89% of the patients received opioids with a mean parenteral diamorphine equivalent of 4 mg as a 4-hourly dose during the terminal stages (O'Brien, Kelly and Saunders, 1992).

Injections of an opioid may be necessary if because of dysphagia or weakness oral medication is not possible. Moreover, in an acute episode of breathlessness, pain or panic, an injection of an opioid, such as diamorphine, to provide analgesia and reduce the cough reflex, chlorpromazine as a sedative and an anticholinergic such as hyoscine (scopolamine) to provide smooth muscle relaxation, reduce secretions and act as sedative and amnesic, can allow control of the situation and relief to the patient within minutes. An enema of diazepam can also be helpful, and could be given by a non-professional carer.

In this way the distress of an acute episode can be reduced quickly and, as hyoscine often leads to amnesia of the period of distress, on recovery the patient may not recollect the distress. It is important to control the symptoms and relieve the distress quickly, for both patient and family.

The medication, and information about the use of the drugs, should be easily available. At home it is often helpful to have a small supply of the relevant medication available so it can be given without delays. Thus, if a professional carer is called to help in a crisis situation everything that is needed is quickly available, even if the professional has not normally been involved in the patient's care and is not prepared for this eventuality. In the UK the Motor Neurone Disease Association has produced a box to keep the necessary medication in and leaflets on its use so that medication can be ready for use in a crisis. This 'Breathing Space Kit' was introduced in 1992 and is part of a wider project to support and help patients and families as death approaches.

On occasions there is a need to continue with parenteral injections as the patient's deteriorating condition does not allow the use of oral medication. In some patients it is possible to reduce the need for regular 4-hourly injections by using a continuous subcutaneous infusion using a syringe driver (Oliver, 1985, 1988). This method of drug administration causes little distress to the patient, and the syringe containing the medication is changed only every 24 h so that the strain on nursing services is reduced (Oliver, 1988). Diamorphine or morphine can be given as analgesic, haloperidol or methotrimeprazine as antiemetic and sedatives and hyoscine to reduce salivation and lung secretions.

As well as the practical measures needed to control the symptoms of the patient as the illness deteriorates it is important to continue to reassess all the other aspects of care. Many of the fears of both patient and family may become more pronounced and need to be heard and shared. Some fears can be allayed and others may only be shared.

It is often necessary for there to be discussion about the place of death. This will often not be easy to discuss but it may be easier to openly talk about the options when communication is easier than waiting for a crisis. The main possibilities can be:

- Hospital: an acute medical or neurological ward may not be entirely suitable for the terminal care of a very disabled patient. There may be less experience of palliative care and the ward will often be aiming to cope with diagnosis and treat acute problems. However, if a patient is well known on a ward, and patient, family and staff are agreeable, this may be a suitable option.
- Home: with the support of the primary health care team and extra help at home. There is a need to provide adequate care and support for both patient and family. A 'key worker' will be helpful, to coordinate the care.
- Hospice: many hospices are able to take patients with motor neurone disease for terminal care. However, a hospice is not just a building but a concept of care – controlling symptoms, helping patients to live as full a life as possible and supporting the patient and family. Thus hospice care can be offered at home, with the extra support to the primary health care team that a specialist nurse providing extra advice on symptom control and support can provide; in a day hospice, allowing carers a break for a day and encouraging the patient to be as active as possible as well as providing assessment and treatment of symptoms; hospice inpatient care for terminal care, rehabilitation, respite care or symptom control. All the possibilities need to be discussed fully within the family and the main professional carers so that the most suitable and acceptable package of care can be arranged.

13.8 CONCLUSIONS

The aim in caring for a patient who is deteriorating with motor neurone disease is to care for the 'whole' patient in the context of the family. It is necessary to respond to their needs and ensure coordination of care so that as the illness progresses distress is kept to a minimum. With good palliative care and the involvement and preparation of the patient and family, death may be easier to face. However death can hardly ever be seen to be 'good', and whatever preparations have been made there is a time of loss, of sadness and grieving.

In the care of the patient the aim is to allow as good a living as possible, encouraging and allowing a patient to live until he dies.

REFERENCES

Anderson, R. (1987) The unremitting burden on carers. *Br. Med. J.*, **294**, 73.

Carey, J.S. (1986) Motor neuron disease – a challenge to medical ethics: discussion paper. *J. Roy. Soc. Med.*, **79**, 216–20.

Henke, E. (1968) Motor neurone disease – a patient's view. *Br. Med. J.*, 4, 765–6.

Kinsella, G.J. and Duffy, F. (1979) Psychosocial readjustment in the spouses of aphasic patients. *J. Rehab. Med.*, **11**, 129–32.

Livingston, M.G. (1985) Families who care. *Br. Med. J.*, **291**, 919–20.

Newrick, P.G. and Langton-Hewer, R. (1984) Motor neurone disease: can we do better? A study of 42 patients. *Br. Med. J.*, **289**, 539–42.

Newrick, P.G. and Langton-Hewer, R. (1985) Pain in motor neuron disease. *J. Neurol. Neurosurg. Psychiatry*, **48**, 838–40.

Norris, F.H., Smith, R.A. and Denys, E.H. (1985) Motor neurone disease: towards better care. *Br. Med. J.*, **291**, 259–62.

O'Brien, T., Kelly, M. and Saunders, C. (1992) Motor neurone disease: a hospice perspective. *Br. Med. J.*, **304**, 471–3.

Oliver, D.J. (1985) The use of the syringe driver in terminal care. *Br. J. Clin. Pharmacol.*, **20**, 515–16.

Oliver, D.J. (1986) Motor neurone disease – a challenge to medical ethics (letter). *J. Roy. Soc. Med.*, **79**, 685.

Oliver, D.J. (1988) Syringe drivers in palliative care: a review. *Palliative Medicine*, 2, 21–6.

Oliver, D.J. (1989) *Motor Neurone Disease*. Royal College of General Practitioners, Exeter.

Oliver, D.J., O'Gorman, B. and Saunders, C. (1986) Motor neurone disease, in *Cash's Textbook of Neurology for Physiotherapists* (ed. P.A. Downie), Faber & Faber, London.

Ponsky, J.L. and Gauderer, M.W.L. (1989) Percutaneous endoscopic gastrostomy: indications, limitations, techniques and results. *World J. Surg.*, **13**, 165–70.

Terminal care

Roche, J. (1989) Spirituality and the ALS patient. *Rehabilitation Nursing*, **14**, 139–41.

Saunders, C. (1988) Spiritual Pain. *J. Palliative Care*, **4**, 29–32.

Saunders, C., Walsh, T.D. and Smith, M. (1981) A review of 100 cases of motor neurone disease in a hospice, in *Hospice: the Living Idea* (eds C. Saunders, D.H. Summers and N. Teller), Edward Arnold, London, pp. 126–47.

14 *The role of patient and carer associations*

PETER CARDY

14.1 THE HALL OF MIRRORS

The experience of MND/ALS for the majority of people may be likened to entering a hall of mirrors. The diagnosis itself distorts familiar reality, pushing out of shape ideas about time and life organization. However carefully and sensitively the diagnosis is given, it amounts to a sentence of death, and this is how it is often perceived irrespective of the words that are actually said. The diagnosing physician feels that he has little to offer the patient and carers, beyond the diagnosis itself. The typically rapid progression of the disease means that the patient has to adapt to a rapidly changing series of multiple disabilities, any of them severe enough to be a major life change, while simultaneously trying to learn the complexities of health and social care systems that are not designed to cope with multiple, rapidly advancing disabilities.

This widespread experience had led, by 1992, to the formation of about 40 MND/ALS associations around the world, of which those in the UK and the USA were the biggest by several orders of magnitude. A number of regional international networks exist, and a worldwide alliance has been established. This chapter focuses on the role of the associations in two main areas: patient care and research.

14.2 VARIETY AND COMMON PURPOSES

These associations take a variety of forms: most are independent, though some work under the umbrella of a national neuromuscular association; some are concerned mainly with care, others with supporting research; most are national, though some countries have several independent associations specialized by function or regions. Most include the following functions:

- self-help and mutual support;

The role of patient and carer associations

- publicity/public education;
- professional education;
- practical care for patients;
- support of research.

The character of the associations is surprisingly similar, in spite of the differences in size and resources, not only because the problems presented by the disease are similar throughout the world, but also because many associations have been established by learning from each other. Even though this was to begin with haphazard, some common features have resulted.

Differences are to be expected as a result of the structure of relevant institutions in each country, or in the framework of law within which the associations operate. The major American association is not, because of the insurance structure of the health service, a direct provider of equipment and aids to daily living, even if the logistical problems of such a large continent could be overcome. By contrast, even though the UK health services are almost wholly paid for out of taxation, there is both a need for and the means of lending substantial amounts of equipment in the UK. Again, most countries have some form of legal recognition for non-profit, disinterested associations that work for the public good or are defined as 'charitable' as in the UK. Compliance with these laws can require a division between relief or educational activities and the funding of research, leading to a degree of specialization between organizations, as in the Netherlands.

14.3 THE ASSOCIATIONS AND THE PROFESSIONAL COMMUNITY

The major activity common to all the associations is providing information. Although mortality from the disease is higher than from better known conditions such as multiple sclerosis or muscular dystrophy, the rapid trajectory and small living populations of patients mean that there has been little public understanding or knowledge concerning the disease. This is in itself a source of distress, and a catalyst for activity. The health and related professional groups which can offer most to people with MND also lack a widespread body of knowledge and practice, and this often provides an early meeting ground for voluntary workers and professionals.

Without appropriate care and disease management, the short lives of people with MND and the lives of their immediate carers are marked by insecurity, dread and bereavement. The search for appropriate physical aids and financial support is frustrating and full of disappointments. These are most obvious when equipment arrives after the need for it has been superseded by advancing disability, or indeed after the death of the patient. The associations place great emphasis on speeding the provision of help to match the pace of the disease. Not unnaturally this can lead to friction with the providing services before an accommodation is found that enables specific and general priorities to be harmonized. Neurologists and other health professionals can play an important part in helping to defuse understandable anger, and convert it to constructive activity, by recognizing lay people as allies in a common cause.

A few of the associations employ their own professionally qualified staff, while others have them involved as voluntary workers; this is an important means of bridge-building. For the vast majority of health and social care professionals, even of diagnosing clinicians, their encounters with MND will be few and brief. The many individual experiences of MND/ALS found in each of the lay associations form a unique pool of accumulated experience of the entire course of the disease which can be tapped to advantage. In this condition more than most others, the patient and close carers are themselves the leading experts in the disease management. Only they can say, in the absence of any fundamental treatment, how much inconvenience is worth tolerating in order to maintain personal dignity; or how much dignity can be sacrificed to gain comfort or ease from distress. With their extensive patient contact, the associations are an indispensable source of help in establishing care programmes.

14.4 THE RESEARCH

The role of the lay associations in research, an invariable concern, is rather different. Research on MND/ALS is so complex, particularly in basic science, that investigators in one discipline cannot always follow the argument in other fields. The span of necessary research is so broad, from fundamental questions about the nervous system as a whole, to the development of specific technical aids, that no single scientist can possibly grasp it. Similarly, the initiative for research springs from many sources: the inspiration of scientists working in apparently unrelated fields; the response of social investigators to problems raised for policy or practice by the catastrophic personal and social problems caused by the disease; technological research commissioned to find solutions to particular deficiencies; even research driven and funded by patients with theories or observations.

Given this broad array of research possibilities, what constructive part can be played by associations composed mainly of lay people, most of whom will have no scientific background? The most important contribution that every association is able to make is to provide stimulus and encouragement to researchers in what has so far been a quest without decisive results. Like everyone else, scientists work best when they are acknowledged and rewarded. The simple fact that research is carried out on MND is, regardless of outcome, a source of hope to many people with the disease even though they know it is unlikely to benefit them personally. By reporting research questions and findings to lay people, scientists receive recognition, even celebrity status. Through meetings with people in appalling adversity, the humanitarian purpose of an apparently abstract quest is reinforced. Raising awareness of the disease and the search for its roots among the general public has a similar effect among the scientific and clinical communities and, as demonstrated by HIV and AIDS, raises both the public and professional prestige of an unpromising area.

14.5 A DROP IN THE OCEAN?

Funding, doubtless the most obvious form of lay support for research, is not necessarily the most practical. The UK association's policy is to share its resources equally between practical care and research; some associations do not fund research, and in some countries there are dual associations (in the Netherlands and Australia for example) that support patient care or research separately. Taking the research funds of all the associations together, these amounted in 1992 to no more than US$3 million annually, enough to support perhaps 50 substantial projects, or provide 15–20 programme grants. To put this in perspective, after the expenditure of many millions of research dollars over a couple of decades, by the end of 1991 less than two dozen individuals worldwide were actually receiving gene therapy for various diseases. Gene therapy may ultimately be a single component of the MND picture. Barring the discovery of a single key to the disease, the lay associations will be minor funders by comparison with the National Institutes of Health in the USA or the Medical Research Council in the UK.

In practice this makes their funds more, not less important: to fund pilot studies; to support sound but speculative research; to keep research teams together between major grants; to fund one or other side of clinical/basic science collaborations; to provide continuity of focus in institutions with broader interests; to fund travel or equipment costs ancillary to mainstream research. Careful use of limited money can produce disproportionately large effects.

Another special contribution that can be made by all the associations is illustrated by the work in several countries on familial MND, in finding families and encouraging them to participate. Many families look to the associations for support and reassurance – some indeed have been created by affected families – and many individuals see that the only contribution that they can make to the fight against MND/ALS is to participate personally in research.

14.6 PATIENTS' PARTICIPATION

The associations can also support this and other areas of research by the encouragement of tissue donation, pre and post mortem. Cultural attitudes vary from country to country, of course, and some very strong taboos operate. The UK Association in 1991 gave a very public launch to a programme on avoiding distressful death and as a result has gained confidence that it can address issues regarded as taboo or simply distasteful. There are ethical considerations of course, but most of the practical issues are less to do with this than with the marketing of a very important idea. However, it would not be right for any of the associations to promote tissue donation energetically unless it is clear that there are good arrangements for accepting tissue, and confidence that it can be well used.

As research advances, the importance of building large series of well-documented patients grows. The number of clinical trials at present taking place is small worldwide, but seems likely to expand rapidly in the near future, when numbers of well worked-up cases and controls will also be vital. Here again the associations have a major part to play in encouraging participation and educating their members.

The UK association changed its membership rules so that, in joining, members give permission for basic details to be passed on to 'approved researchers'. Similar practices are no doubt possible elsewhere, within the limitations of data protection legislation. In most associations, not only in MND/ALS but in other dread diseases, the proportion of actual patients in membership is relatively small. In the UK, on the other hand, contact with patients through direct services is relatively high, upwards of 50% of the total patient population, with 1200 new contacts in the course of 1992, close to the theoretical UK rate of new diagnoses. Services are provided unilaterally and universally by the Motor Neurone Disease Association to patients; there is no requirement for them to reciprocate in any way whatsoever. It would be a major policy departure to do so without clear potential benefits.

14.7 AN EDUCATED COMMUNITY

In order to recruit members and others to support or take part in research, it is necessary to work for an educated community of patients and carers, and here also the associations and investigators need each other's help. In many diseases with no cure and no treatment, patients will be prepared to give their time and support to research, offering everything from finance to *in vivo* brain biopsies. Morally and practically it is essential that they and their care-givers are under no illusion about the likelihood of rapid results, and that they understand the processes and basic questions of research.

If patients are to take the risk of receiving a placebo instead of the active compound, they must know why therapeutic trials must often be randomized, blind and controlled. If populist theories are not to distract attention and resources from real science, they must know why commonsense observations do not often withstand scrutiny. If they are to donate tissue before or after death, they must know that it is a gift worth giving and that it will be properly used.

The Motor Neurone Disease Association in the UK requires its grant-holders to report on their work for the lay audience, but it also invites them to write for its magazine, to speak to members' meetings and to brief the media and influential supporters. Only one distinguished investigator has declined in recent years, giving as his reason that, once you start explaining research, the patients simply want more and more information. This antediluvian failure to recognize MND as the property of those who endure it is at the root of the artificial divide between research and care that has split so many disease-specific associations in the UK and elsewhere.

14.8   RESEARCH – PART OF THE CARE

In conditions such as MND, research is as much part of care as the limited therapeutic services now available. To acknowledge this also implies recognition that the interests of present and future patients need to be taken into account in research priorities. Among the considerations of the Motor Neurone Disease Association's peer review panel for research are relevance to MND; and to what extent patients will benefit directly from the research, now or later. Given two proposals of equal scientific merit, that which offers benefit to patients will be favoured. In recognition of the commitment made by families to a study of inherited MND in Britain, the Association decided to step in when external funding unexpectedly ended, rather than allow it to take its chance in the grants lottery.

This is in no sense to challenge intellectual and methodological rigour; it is indeed a stricter discipline to ground research in the human condition rather than in synthetic detachment. In this as in other fields of scientific endeavour at the close of the twentieth century, it is an urgent necessity to reconcile the differences that have been allowed to grow up between science and society. It should be emphasized that non-scientists can not only participate in the scientific process, but also influence it in a perfectly legitimate way.

14.9 JOINERS AND NON-JOINERS

It will not do to be smug about this, however. There are limitations to involvement in research via the membership of lay associations. Participants tend to be the most vocal, those most desperately seeking a solution, those who are angry or optimistic. Voluntary recruitment to research through public appeal appears to produce the same or strongly overlapping membership – that is, people who join associations!

Nevertheless, this is a potentially valuable means of additional recruitment and of cross-checking data; even the best health service records are no more, and sometimes much less, reliable than those of voluntary organizations. The other principal key to better recruitment lies with neurologists. Recent experiences with voluntary recruitment to a large epidemiological study in the UK and a major clinical trial in Europe show that where neurologists are ambivalent or do not offer clear opportunity or invitation to participate, recruitment is slow and patchy. Both clinicians and lay associations therefore have a part to play in recruitment to neuroscience.

There is an obvious and important extra logistical dimension to recruitment of MND/ALS patients, which has strangely been over-looked; that is the generally rapid trajectory of the disease. Not only is progression from diagnosis to death rapid, with the obvious loss of potential recruits, but passage through the phases of reaction to the disease – anger, action, acceptance, perhaps – is correspondingly speedy. There is thus only a very small window of opportunity through which to reach patients when they are not only **able** to offer participation, but **willing** to do so. This must reinforce the view that both associations and clinicians have a part to play in reaching through this window.

14.10 THE SUPPORTING FRAMEWORK

There are other ways in which the lay associations can contribute to research. In technology and bioengineering, for example, lay members are in a unique position to offer practical feedback on most valued developments. The UK Motor Neurone Disease Association has conducted a poll of members, both patients and carers, to establish an order of priority for a series of technical developments shortlisted by market research groups also drawn from among its members. Similarly, at the annual international symposium sponsored by the International Alliance of MND/ALS Associations, the resonance between medical science and patient care/disease management has been underlined by holding parallel conferences, with migration between sessions. The value of this forum is implicit in the worldwide attendance, and in the information exchanges and practical collaborations that ensue. Domestically there is a similar response to meetings of grant-holders and others involved in, or contributing to, research, including health professionals. Although special sessions on MND are routinely included in neuroscience meetings, these do not provide the multidisciplinary opportunities offered by specialist meetings. An intensive workshop supported by lay bodies led to the formulation of the diagnostic criteria now adopted by the World Federation of Neurology.

This by no means exhausts the possibilities for involvement of lay associations in the business of science and research in MND. The way is indeed open for more extensive and imaginative collaborations, which recognize the distinct but complementary interest of scientists and people with MND. If it is true that research is too important to leave to researchers, it is also the case that it is too urgent and complex to leave to the capricious pursuit of knowledge or half-informed speculation. There is a powerful role available to the lay associations in helping to map out the ground for research; but this can only be done with the active consent and enthusiasm of the research community. If the path to the roots of MND were obvious, it should have been taken by now: but researchers and lay associations together can make the search more thorough and systematic. MND is an unspeakable disease that draws pity from the most hardened observer. To eliminate it is a great scientific and humanitarian endeavour which will – which must – one day yield to our combined struggle.

PART THREE

15   *Classical pathology*

MARCO ROSSI

15.1   INTRODUCTION

Motor neurone disease (MND) encompasses the **sporadic** (**'classical'**), the familial, the Mariana Islands and other 'types' (Kuncl *et al.*, 1992).

The multifarious clinical and pathological presentations of sporadic or **'classical'** MND were described over 100 years ago as separate entities:

1. progressive muscular atrophy (PMA) (Aran, 1850; Duchenne, 1853; Charcot and Joffroy, 1869);
2. progressive bulbar palsy (Duchenne, 1860; Charcot, 1870);
3. amyotrophic lateral sclerosis (ALS) (Charcot, 1874).

Soon afterwards, however, they were linked as possible manifestations of the same disease spectrum (Dejerine, 1883). 'Primary lateral sclerosis' involving solely the upper motor neurone was also described in that period (Charcot, 1865; Erb, 1875).

Pathological findings of subsequent large series of cases have highlighted the wide spectrum of pathological findings (Hughes, 1982), thus supporting the notion that the disease may in fact be a syndrome.

This chapter will strictly deal with the pathological features common to 'classical' MND and to its three main clinical 'subtypes', namely ALS (upper and lower motor neurone involvement), bulbar palsy (lower brainstem motor neurone involvement) and PMA (spinal cord lower motor neurone involvement).

Most frequently, the disease affects both upper and lower motor neurones; however, for convenience, pathological changes in the spinal cord, brainstem, forebrain, nerve roots and peripheral nerves and muscles will be described separately. Pathological evidence of involvement of sensory pathways will also be addressed. Clinical and other non-pathological findings are described elsewhere in this book.

Classical pathology

15.2 SPINAL CORD

Degeneration of both crossed and/or uncrossed **pyramidal** tracts is a pathological feature of MND, although morphological changes are more easily appreciable in the former in more subtle cases.

Macroscopically, the cord may appear normal on external examination; however, even in the fresh state, horizontal sections may show evidence of greyish white discoloration in the region occupied by the crossed corticospinal tracts in the posterior part of the lateral funiculi (Brownell, Oppenheimer and Hughes, 1970; Hughes, 1982).

The Marchi impregnation technique (Smith, 1956) is the most suited to demonstrate recent tract degeneration (up to 15 or more months [Smith, Strich and Sharp, 1956; Smith, 1960]). Degenerating fibres have been traced with this technique from motor cortex to the internal capsule, cerebral peduncles and spinal cord (Figure 15.1) (see also illustrations in Oppenheimer, 1984).

In cases of long or relatively long survival or where the Marchi technique is not routinely used, loss of fibre tracts is demonstrated by myelin stains such as Loyez (degenerated tracts are pale and normal myelin blue), luxol (degenerated myelin stains very pale and normal

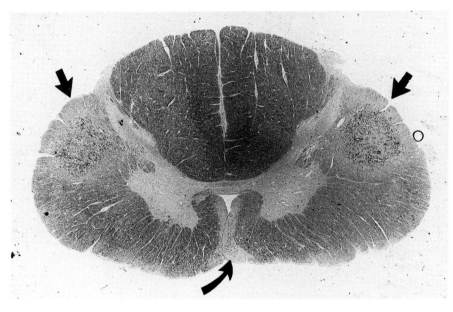

Figure 15.1   **MND**: Marchi-impregnated spinal cord showing degenerated cross (straight arrows) and uncrossed (curved arrow) pyramidal tracts (black) (cervical cord, Marchi ×10).

myelin azure/light blue) or Weigert–Pal (areas of long-standing degeneration are pale and normal myelin black).

Microscopically, there is loss of motor neurones (Tsukagoshi *et al.*, 1979) which is most apparent at cervical (Plate 1) and lumbar level. The whole gamut of changes from chromatolysis, spheroid formation, shrinkage (Kusaka and Hirano, 1985), atrophy and neuronophagia of motor neurones may be seen in rapidly progressive cases. On occasion, an empty space is left after the disappearance of the neurone. Excessive lipofuscin in remaining neurones may be present. *Pari passu* with the loss of neurones, astrocytes increase in number and become hypertrophic, and in some cases the site of neuronal loss may be marked by a gliotic 'scar'.

Chromatolysis and axonal spheroids (both easily discerned by light microscopy) are thought to be among the earliest degenerative changes of lower motor neurones (Hirano and Inoue, 1980; Higgins *et al.*, 1983); however, these changes have also been described in 3/9 normal cords (Kusaka and Hirano, 1985). The unwary may mistake one for the other. Chromatolytic neurones are best demonstrated with a Nissl stain (Plate 2a and b); the cytoplasm is large and 'swollen' with a pale central area merging with azure/bluish-staining Nissl substance at the periphery; vacuolation of the cytoplasm may be present.

Chromatolysis similar to that seen after axotomy occurs in more rapidly progressive cases but not in 'chronic' MND (Hirano, 1982). Chromatolytic neurones and spheroids contain accumulation of phosphorylated neurofilaments (Manetto *et al.*, 1988; Munoz *et al.*, 1988; Leigh *et al.*, 1989; Matsumoto *et al.*, 1989).

Spheroids were first described as argyrophilic globules (measuring > 63 μm in diameter) in neuronal processes including the proximal axon of anterior horn cells (usually lumbar) and brainstem motor neurones (Carpenter, 1968). They were noted to be more numerous in the more acute MND cases (Inoue and Hirano, 1980). With Bodian or Holmes silver stains they are reddish brown in colour (Carpenter, 1968) (Plate 2) and may be surrounded by myelin (Hirano, 1982) but should not be confused with recently described pericapillary rosettes found in ageing spinal cords (Plate 2d) (Sasaki and Maruyama, 1992).

Hirano *et al.* (1984) found spheroids in myelinated axons and lower motor neurone cell bodies. They were composed of bundles and randomly oriented 10-nm filaments and included mitochondria, vesicles and fragments of smooth endoplasmic reticulum. Spheroids were present not only in 'acute' cases but also in more chronic ones, although their numbers were smaller.

The significance of the formation of axonal spheroids may lie in an abnormality of slow axonal transport and, in a unique study of the

309

motor branch of the median nerve involving volunteer MND patients, Breuer *et al.* (1987) demonstrated diminished retrograde transport speed, which could impair communication between axon terminals and perikarya.

Spheroids may be an early marker of pathological changes and may also give an insight into the pathogenesis of MND. In this respect, spheroids have been obtained in different ways in various MND experimental and other models (Mitsumoto and Bradley, 1982; Miyata, 1983; Mitsumoto and Boggs, 1987; Cummings *et al.*, 1990). Study of conditions such as the hereditary accelerated canine spinal muscular atrophy (Cork *et al.*, 1982, 1990) or even a spontaneous MND of pigs (Higgins *et al.*, 1983) may also be useful to unravel the pathogenesis of MND.

It has also been shown that nuclei and cytoplasm of lower motor neurones **shrink** during the early stages of MND (e.g. atrophy), but sometimes post-mortem artefact can also lead to shrinkage of neurones, thus creating diagnostic difficulties.

Neuronophagia consists of phagocytic microglial cells clustered around neurones. According to Oppenheimer (1984), it is more easily detectable in the brainstem motor nuclei.

Fine cytomorphological details of neurones can be obtained with the Golgi techniques, including a variant developed for routine use (Pugh and Rossi, 1991, 1992). However, the spinal cord has been particularly difficult to study, largely for unknown reasons, the difficulty consisting in the paucity of impregnated neurones and processes. In a limited Golgi–Cox mercury impregnation of spinal cord neurones, Kato, Hirano and Donnenfeld (1987) for the first time reported a reduced number of cell processes, poorly developed dendrites, abnormal axons sometimes with lack of normal increase in thickness in the first myelinated segment and also fusiform swellings in cell processes in lumbar motor neurones. The conclusion was that loss of dendrites may be a significant pathological feature of MND. Atrophy of cell processes of large motor neurones in the anterior horns has also been reported following more conventional silver staining (Nakano and Hirano, 1987).

15.2.1 Changes other than 'motor'

Although neurones in the posterior horns and Clarke's nucleus (Mannen, Iwata and Toyokura, 1982; Schroder and Reske-Nielsen, 1984), loss of neurones in the Clarke's column and even 'regular' involvement of Clarke's nucleus have also been described (Averback and Crocker, 1982). Degeneration of the anterolateral (spinocerebellar) and posterior (sensory) funiculi of the spinal cord has been confirmed (Brownell, Oppenheimer and Hughes, 1970; Swash et al., 1986, 1988).

The intermediolateral column of the thoracic spinal cord is generally thought to be unaffected (Brownell, Oppenheimer and Hughes, 1970; Hughes, 1982). However, clinical (Steiner, Sethi and Rose, 1984) and pathological evidence (Kennedy and Duchen, 1985; Oyanagi et al., 1991) suggests that impairment of autonomic function with underlying slight loss of cholinergic neurones may occur. A significant accumulation of phosphorylated neurofilaments (thought to be indicative of degeneration) has also been shown in these neurones (Itoh et al., 1992).

The Onuf's nucleus (innervating bladder and bowel sphincters) is said to be spared in MND (Mannen, Inata and Tick, 1977), but recently Bunina bodies and conglomerate inclusions have been described in three patients (Kihira et al., 1991).

15.2.2 Changes of unknown significance

Heterotopic neurones in the ventral outflow and lateral corticospinal tract regions have been found to be more numerous in MND (Kozlowski et al., 1989), although the significance of their presence is unclear.

A lymphocytic infiltration in the spinal cord of almost 80% of MND cases, particularly in relation to pyramidal tracts, was found in one series (Troost et al., 1989); in a subsequent study most of the cells were found to be CD8 lymphocytes (Troost, Van Den Ord and De Jong, 1990). Increased expression of HLA-DR antigens, particularly in the corticospinal tracts, was found, the suggestion being made that an antigen-specific cytotoxic T-cell reaction may cause or contribute to neuronal degeneration. Other authors have instead sustained that increased expression of class I and II major histocompatibility antigens is associated with the presence of phagocytes in degenerating white matter and not with degenerating motor neurones or muscle fibres. T-cell-mediated immune response may be stimulated by neuronal degeneration and thus contribute to ongoing damage (Lampson, Kushner and Sobel, 1990).

Altered cerebral glucose utilization has been reported in MND (Dalakas et al., 1987), and increased erythrocyte glucose transporter activity as well as altered muscle fructose metabolism has been found (Poulton and Rossi, 1991; Virk et al., 1991; Karim et al., in preparation).

15.2.3 Inclusions in lower motor neurones

Hirano bodies have been found in lower motor neurones (Schochet et al., 1969; Chou, 1979). These structures are eosinophilic, ovoid with

311

Classical pathology

faint striations and measure 10–30 μm in length and 8 μm across. They are composed of parallel filaments 60–100 nm long. Their pathogenesis and significance are unknown.

Hirano *et al.* (1984) also found **corpora amylacea** (polyglucosan bodies) within axons closely related to spheroids.

Bunina bodies (Hirano, 1982) have been considered quite specific for the various types of MND. They are small (1–2 μm) granular inclusions found in the cytoplasm of large lower motor neurones in classical (50% of cases), familial and the Marianas MND (Tomonaga, Saito and Yoshimura, 1978; Hirano and Iwata, 1979). They are acidophilic (Plate 2e) and stain light blue with luxol (Plate 2f) and blue after cresyl fast violet is added (Kluver–Barrera stain) (Plate 2g and h). They are composed of dense amorphous granular material often surrounding a lighter area containing 10-nm filaments. Normal cytoplasmic components are present at their periphery.

They have also been found in the reticular formation in a patient with MND and dementia (Nakano, Hashizume and Tomonaga, 1990). Ubiquitin has been localized at the level of 15-nm filaments in Bunina body-related structures and focal aggregates of fine filamentous structures (skeins). These structures are negative with neurofilament, Tau and high molecular weight microtubule-associated proteins (Matsumoto, Hirano and Goto, 1990; Murayama *et al.*, 1990). A close relationship between filamentous inclusions and Bunina bodies has been hypothesized (Lowe *et al.*, 1988; Murayama *et al.*, 1990). Migheli *et al.* (1990) in an immunogold study found that ubiquitinated cytoplasmic inclusions are located at the level of neurofilament-negative 10–15 nm filament bundles and in round small bodies without membranes.

Conglomerate inclusions consist of intracytoplasmic accumulations of neurofilaments with distinct rims (Kihira *et al.*, 1991).

Basophilic inclusions in sporadic and other MNDs have been described (Kusaka, Matsumato and Imai, 1990; Matsumoto *et al.*, 1992). These were shown to be ubiquitin-negative anilinophilic bodies with distinct rims. Under electron microscopy, filamentous structures (12–25 nm in diameter) with electron-dense ribosome-like granules were observed. These inclusions were found to be similar to those observed in 'Juvenile' (Mortara *et al.*, 1984) MND. Chou (1979) reported that they were frequently associated with Bunina bodies.

Lewy body-like hyaline eosinophilic inclusions (Chou, 1979) are usually found in anterior horn neurones in familial MND with posterior column and spinocerebellar tract involvement (where they contain a network of 10-nm haphazardly oriented neurofilaments), but they have also been found in sporadic MND, where they may also be observed in the brainstem motor nuclei and Clarke's column (Sasaki *et al.*, 1989).

312

They are situated in the perikarya and dendrites; usually single, intracytoplasmic (Okazaki, 1983), round or oval and hyaline but without concentric rings as in true Lewy bodies. They are silver positive and Kluver–Barrera negative; the central core stains with toluidine blue and for ubiquitin but not for cytoskeletal proteins. Under the electron microscope they are composed of randomly arranged linear structures with a variable number of vesicles and no limiting membrane and rare filaments.

Other inclusions have been described. Averback (1986) reported **paracrystalline arrays** with 5-nm electron-dense subunits discernible with the light microscope that had the staining properties of proteins and surrounded by capillary basement membrane, probably situated within pericapillary astrocytes. He also described astrocytic fibrillary bodies without paracrystalline arrangement.

Various other morphological features such as honeycomb structures, dense filamentous aggregates, dense granular deposits and stubby mitochondria have been found in anterior motor neurones (Kusaka and Hirano, 1985).

15.3 BRAINSTEM

Clinical brainstem involvement varies between 19% (Rosen, 1978) and 28% (Carpenter, McDonald and Howard, 1978) of cases of MND. Clinical involvement of the XII (most frequent), V and VII motor nuclei in MND has been described (DePaul, 1988).

In cases with brainstem involvement, the XII nerve may be clearly atrophic. Reduction in the total number of myelinated fibres (with increase in small myelinated fibres with evidence of sprouting) in the XII nerve has been reported in a morphometric study (Atsumi and Miyatake, 1987).

Lawyer and Netsky (1953) found pathological changes in the nucleus ambiguus (motor to the larynx through fibres in the IX, X and XI nerves) in 83%, and Malamud (1968) in 68%, whilst in the XII they were 94% and 90% respectively.

Microscopically, neurone loss and astrocytosis may be present at the level of the motor nuclei, especially the XII but also the V and VII (Lawyer and Netsky, 1953; Bonduelle, 1975). Decrease in neuronal mRNA in the nucleus ambiguus and hypoglossus has also been described (Hartmann et al., 1989). The nuclei of the III, IV and VI nerves are said not to be involved (Kushner et al., 1984), but this is not invariably the case (Jacobs, Bozian and Heffner, 1981).

Classical pathology

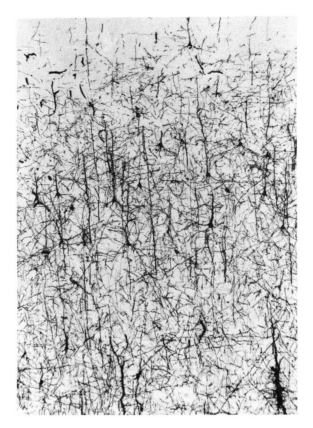

Figure 15.2 **Normal** motor cortex. Note even distribution of impregnated neurones and dendritic network. (Golgi–Cox, paraffin section, 30 μm, ×1000). Compare with Figure 15.3.

15.4 FOREBRAIN

Involvement of the forebrain in MND was first noticed over 100 years ago by Pierre Marie and subsequently confirmed by other authors (Bertrand and Van Bogaert, 1925; Davison, 1941; Friedman and Freedman, 1950). Motor, premotor, sensory and opercular regions were said to be affected mostly by a reduction in the numbers of pyramidal cells (Lawyer and Netsky, 1953; Brownell, Oppenheimer and Hughes, 1970). Degeneration of basal ganglia and substantia nigra has also been reported (Smith, 1960; Brownell *et al.*, 1970; Schoene, 1985).

Macroscopically, the brain is usually normal; however, in patients with upper motor neurone involvement who survive for a long time a

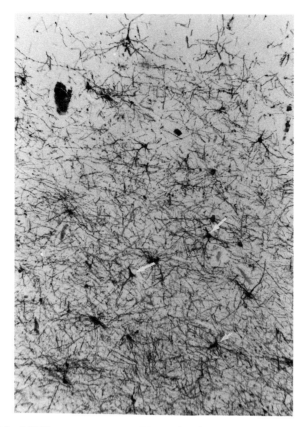

Figure 15.3 **MND** motor cortex. Note the few remaining pyramidal cells (arrows) and reduction of the dentritic arbour of these cells and of the dendritic network in the background. (Golgi–Cox, paraffin section, 30 μm, ×100). Compare with Figure 15.2.

distinct atrophy of the motor cortex is sometimes visible to the naked eye (Plate 3) (Colmant, 1958), although this is rare (Yuasa, Mizushima and Oyanagi, 1980): the present author has only seen one definite case in around 25 autopsies. Various patterns of cerebral atrophy have, however, been described on CT scan (Poloni *et al.*, 1982).

Golgi studies of MND have been few. Various abnormalities of dendrites, including reduced overall network (Rossi *et al.*, 1991; Lafuente *et al.*, 1992), degeneration of Betz cells (Udaka, Kameyama and Tomonaga, 1986) and reduction of impregnated neurones and astrocytosis in the depleted areas (Rossi *et al.*, 1990, 1991, 1992; Rossi, Pugh and Buller, 1991), have been observed (Figures 15.2–15.11). With a simpli-

Classical pathology

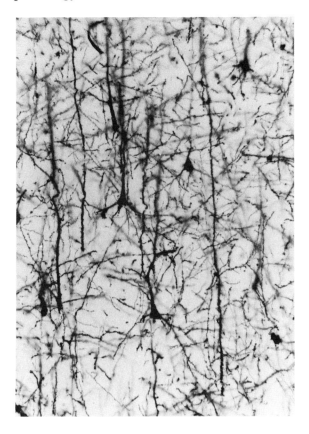

Figure 15.4 **Normal** motor cortex. High-power field demonstrating pyramidal cell bodies, apical and secondary dendrites and a profusion of dendritic spines. (Golgi–Cox, paraffin section, 30 μm, ×280). Compare with Figure 15.5.

fied, consistent and reliable Golgi–Cox paraffin or gelatin technique (Pugh and Rossi, 1991,1992) it is now possible to study neocortical areas of interest from the size of a gyrus to that of an entire hemisphere for the presence of impregnated structures. At the same time, conventional neurohistological stains and immunohistology (Plate 4), polarization (Plate 5), and phase contrast on the same sections or adjacent sections, and electron microscopy (Figure 15.12) can be performed.

Immunocytochemical studies have failed to demonstrate cytoskeletal pathology in Betz cells, with one exception in a patient who demonstrated atrophy of the precentral gyrus and argentophilic cytoplasmic inclusions in Betz cells and other pyramidal neurones in the primary motor area and in lower motor neurones (Murayama, Bouldin and

316

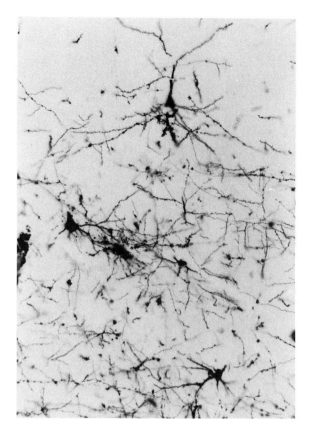

Figure 15.5 **MND**: motor cortex. Obvious paucity of impregnated pyramidal cells and marked reduction of their dendritic branching. (Golgi–Cox, paraffin section, 30 μm, ×280). Compare with Figure 15.4.

Suzuki, 1992). Betz cells contained abnormally phosphorylated neurofilaments and ubiquitination related to granule-associated filaments and neurofilaments.

Astrocytosis has been demonstrated mostly in layers II and III and occasionally in layers IV and V of the motor cortex (Kamo *et al.*, 1987; Pugh and Rossi, 1991,1992; Rossi *et al.*, 1990,1991,1992; Rossi, Pugh and Buller, 1991) (Plate 4); additionally, astrocytic clusters (> 20 cells) were also found. Astrocytosis has also been found to affect premotor (Figures 15.10 and 15.11) and sensory cortex (Figures 15.6–15.9) (Rossi, Pugh and Buller, 1991; Rossi *et al.*, 1991, 1992), and widespread subcortical astrogliosis has been demonstrated (Kushner, Stephenson and Wright, 1991; Rossi, Pugh and Buller, 1991; Rossi *et al.*, 1991, 1992).

Classical pathology

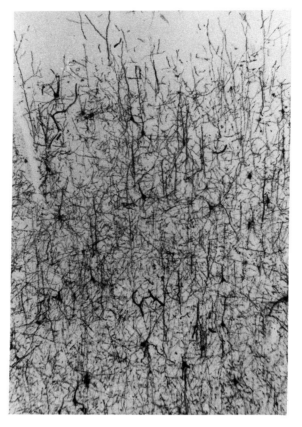

Figure 15.6 **Normal** sensory cortex. Note even distribution of impregnated neurones and dendritic network. (Golgi–Cox, paraffin section, 30 μm, ×110). Compare with Figure 15.7.

In a Marchi study of seven MND patients, Smith (1960) found degenerating fibres not only in the precentral gyrus and paracentral lobule but also in the post-central gyrus, parietal and frontal gyri and to a lesser extent in other parts of the brain.

Some patients with MND (familial and sporadic) may also suffer from **dementia** (mostly 'frontal'). These patients show loss of neurones in more superficial cortical layers (II and III) at the level of the frontal and temporal lobes, but in some the brainstem and basal ganglia may also be affected (Neary *et al.*, 1990). A patient with MND with frontal lobe dementia (Ferrer *et al.*, 1991) also showed reduced dendritic arborization, varicosities and amputations of pyramidal and non-pyramidal neurones in layers II and III on rapid Golgi preparations. Pyramidal cells

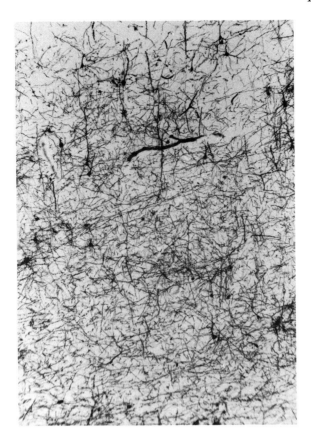

Figure 15.7 **MND**: sensory cortex. Note fewer pyramidal cells and reduction of the dendritic arbour of these cells and of the dendritic network. (Golgi–Cox, paraffin section, 30 μm, ×110). Compare with Figure 15.6.

also showed a decrease in the number of dendritic spines. It was hypothesized that these abnormalities were 'hidden' contributors to the development of dementia. Findings in this case were akin to those found by the same group (Ferrer and Gullotta, 1990) in cortical biopsies of cases of Alzheimer, Pick and Creutzfeldt–Jakob diseases, thus eliminating the possibility of autopsy artefacts. Furthermore, a very recent Golgi and calcium-binding protein immunocytochemistry study of four patients with dementia and amyotrophy confirmed the damage to layers II and III and to dendrites and pyramidal and non-pyramidal neurones (Ferrer, 1992).

Dementia of Alzheimer's type is also said to occur in the families of about 15% of patients with classical MND (Hudson, 1981). Cortical and

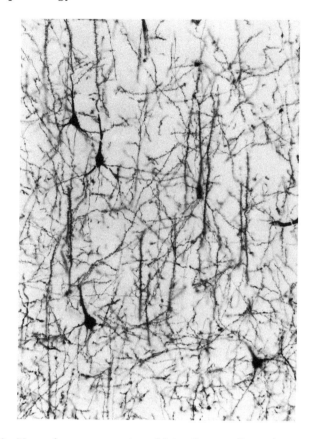

Figure 15.8 **Normal** sensory cortex. Note the excellent demonstration of dendritic spines and dendrites. (Golgi–Cox, paraffin section, 30 μm, ×280). Compare with Figure 15.9.

anterior horn spongiform changes in MND are a not uncommon feature in cases of juvenile MND (Cruz-Sanchez and Tolosa, 1991) and in patients with dementia. Spongiform change may possibly be a common feature shared by these MND patients and those with 'amyotrophic' Creutzfeldt–Jakob disease (Cruz-Sanchez and Tolosa, 1991). The latter usually have a relatively long survival but their disease cannot be transmitted to experimental animals, thus raising doubts as to their correct diagnostic label (Cruz-Sanchez, Lafuente and Cervos-Navarro, 1987; Cruz-Sanchez *et al.*, 1988).

In summary, from evidence reported thus far, it appears that motor cortex but also other neocortical areas and basal ganglia structures are affected in MND. It is possible that neurones functionally related to Betz

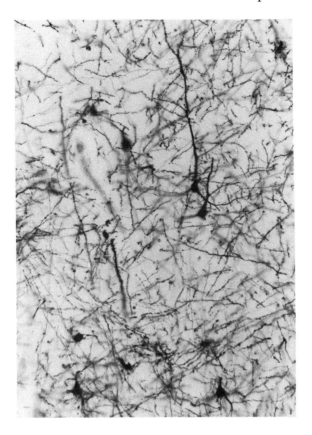

Figure 15.9 **MND**: sensory cortex. Note fewer pyramidal cells and reduction of the dendritic arborization. (Golgi–Cox, paraffin section, 30 μm, ×280). Compare with Figure 15.8.

cells may degenerate through a mechanism of transynaptic degeneration (Smith and Arnason, 1977).

15.5 SPINAL NERVE ROOTS

Macroscopically, the most common finding is thinning and grey discoloration of the anterior nerve roots, which is obvious at autopsy, especially when these are compared with the dorsal roots (Plate 6). Changes are usually more evident at cervical and lumbar level.

Microscopically, it may be possible to ascertain, often even without morphometric analysis, that the number of myelin tubes is reduced (Plates 7 and 8). However, in two patients Inoue and Hirano (1980)

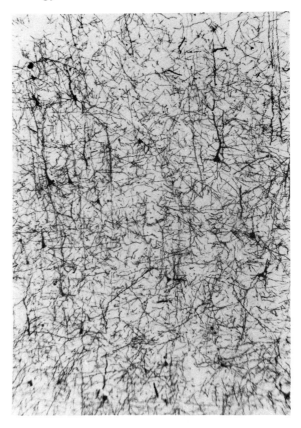

Figure 15.10 **Normal** premotor cortex. Note even distribution of impregnated neurones and dendritic network. (Golgi-Cox, paraffin section, 30 μm, ×110). Compare with Figure 15.11.

found that the total number of myelinated fibres was within normal limits but that there was a decrease in the number of the large myelinated fibres and an increase in small and medium-size myelinated fibres. This could be suggestive of 'atrophy' of large myelinated fibres.

Evidence of degeneration and regeneration of motor fibres at cervical level has been described (Hanyu *et al.*, 1982), as was degeneration of the sensory pathways, dorsal root ganglia and mixed nerves (Dyck *et al.*, 1975; Kawamura *et al.*, 1981; Bradley *et al.*, 1983).

Glial outgrowth along spinal nerve roots ('glial bundles') consists of closely packed astrocytic processes joined by punctated and gap junctions (Hirano, 1982). These bundles are surrounded by basal lamina and by collagen with Schwann cells and myelinated axons situated

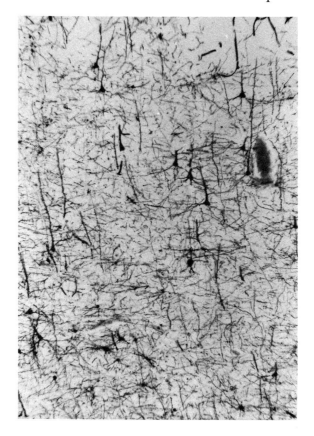

Figure 15.11 **MND**: premotor cortex., Note the reduction in the dendritic network (not as marked as that in the motor and sensory cortex) (Golgi–Cox, paraffin section, 30 μm, ×110). Compare with Figure 15.10.

between the fibres. Glial bundles have been considered to be one of the characteristics of Werdnig–Hoffmann disease, but they have recently also been described in MND (Ghatak and Nochlin, 1981). It is not known whether glial bundles are rare in MND or if they have been overlooked.

15.6 PERIPHERAL NERVES

Changes in peripheral nerves in MND have been documented in a relatively small number of studies (reviewed by Perrie *et al.*, in press). For example, Bradley *et al.* (1983), in a study of various peripheral nerves, showed loss of large myelinated fibres. Dyck *et al.* (1975) in a study of the deep peroneal nerve demonstrated statistically significant

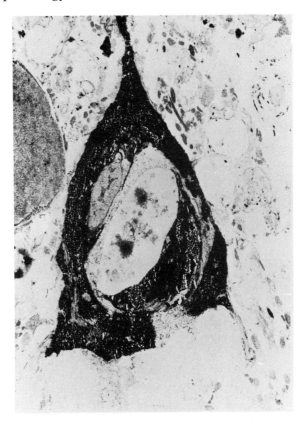

Figure 15.12 **Normal** motor cortex pyramidal cell showing intracytoplasmic impregnation extending into the apical dendrite (top) (Golgi–Cox, electron microscopy, ×1100).

abnormalities in teased nerve preparations in MND *vs.* controls. Ovoids and balls, representing myelin (and indirectly 'axon') degeneration, were a frequent finding in MND. However, both Dyck *et al.* (1975) and Bradley *et al.* (1983) were unable to demonstrate a statistically significant difference in the total number of myelinated fibres in the nerves studied. Focal myelin thickening in a peripheral nerve in a MND patient was shown by Drac (1989). Kawamura *et al.* (1981) found a decrease in the number of large myelinated fibres in the anterior and posterior roots (less severe). Pathological evidence in favour of the involvement of axons in peripheral nerves of MND has also been adduced (Woolf, Serrano and Johnson, 1969; Atsumi, 1981; Perrie *et al.*, in press).

The author's group (Perrie *et al.*, 1991, and in press) has carried out a

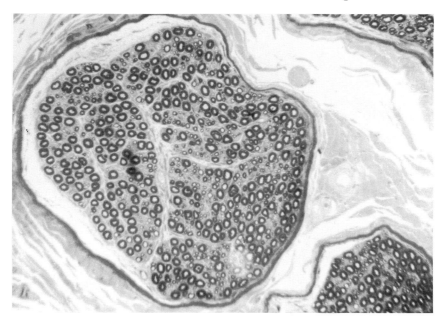

Figure 15.13 **Normal** femoral nerve (osmium impregnation, paraffin section, ×400).

morphometric study of large motor nerves and in particular femoral nerves impregnated with osmium with a new technique in which the whole cross-section of nerve is embedded in paraffin wax. Femoral nerves from eight fresh MND autopsies were matched with eight control cases without known neurological disorder. Loss of both large and small myelinated fibres was noted in some areas of the MND cases (Figures 15.13 and 15.14). Electron microscopy showed myelin irregularities including focal areas of separation (Figure 15.15) (an element of which could be due to post-mortem artefact) and thinly myelinated axons, indirect evidence of remyelination (Figure 15.16). Teased femoral and other nerves showed an increase of myelin abnormalities, including wrinkling or crenation of myelin in several of the fibres (Figure 15.17), further myelin degeneration (Figure 15.18) and indirect evidence of axonal degeneration (Figure 15.19).

Staining with a neurofilament antibody revealed, apart from myelin abnormalities, apparent reduction in the immunocytochemical staining of the axoplasm of MND femoral nerve (Plates 9 and 10).

Despite apparent differences between the matched controls and the MND group, the difference was not statistically significant (Figure 15.20) because the variation in the number of myelinated fibres in the normal

325

Classical pathology

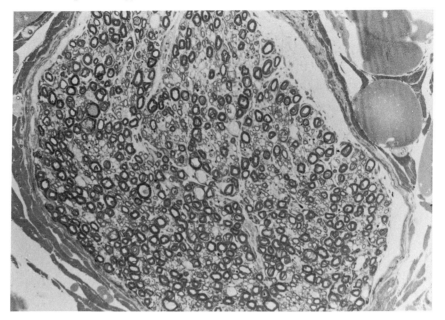

Figure 15.14 **MND**: femoral nerve showing reduction in large and small myelinated fibres in patchy distribution. Note the thinly myelinated axons and the myelin abnormalities (osmium impregnation, paraffin section, ×400).

group was so wide. This is largely because of the variable degrees of degenerative changes that occur in nerves from the age when death from MND occurs. However, an increase in the severity of effect with age could not be demonstrated.

It was concluded that changes in peripheral nerves (including the femoral) are mainly of a qualitative nature and that quantitation would need to be carried out on a much larger sample to avoid the confounding factor related to ageing.

Recently, another spectrum of lower motor neurone syndromes characterized by the presence of circulating autoantibodies (most frequently IgMs) against gangliosides, including GM1, has been described (Shy *et al.*, 1986; Pestronk *et al.*, 1988, 1989, 1990; Santero *et al.*, 1990). Treatment of these cases may lead to some improvement.

It has not yet been decided whether MND is more frequent in patients with cancer, e.g. whether it occurs as a paraneoplastic syndrome (Norris, 1991; Rosenfeld and Posner, 1991). However, cases of lymphoma and MND possibly related to paraproteinaemia have been reported (Younger *et al.*, 1991).

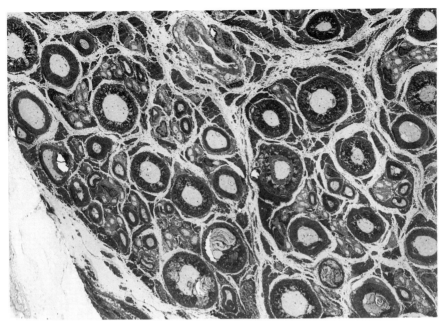

Figure 15.15 **MND**: femoral nerve, see text (electron microscopy, ×1800).

15.7 MUSCLES

Denervation of muscle as a result of loss of anterior motor neurones is a classical finding in MND. Macroscopically, affected muscles show varying degrees of pallor and atrophy.

Microscopic appearances of muscle biopsies in MND have been well described (Dubowitz, 1985; Iwasaki and Kinoshita, 1987; Kimura *et al.*, 1988); however, post-mortem studies on the distribution and severity of muscle changes in muscles throughout the body are wanting (Kristmundsdottir *et al.*, 1990).

In the early stages of the disease there are scattered small groups of atrophic angular fibres which are dark on NADH-TR reaction and show strong acid phosphatase reaction. Once the disease is 'established', there is small-group atrophy and compensatory hypertrophy of surviving fibres (Plate 11), the atrophic fibres being frequently 'wrapped' around hypertrophic ones (Plate 11, top left). Both fibre types become atrophic and partial reinnervation of muscle fibres by surviving motor neurones, initially, partly compensates for the loss, leading to fibre type grouping, but ultimately resulting in large groups of atrophic fibres (Figure 15.21a and b). Increased connective tissue and increased variation in fibre size have also been found (Froes *et al.*, 1987).

327

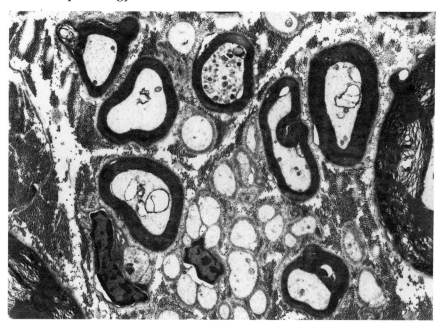

Figure 15.16 **MND**: femoral nerve, see text (electron microscopy, ×7500).

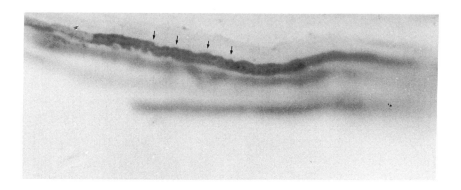

Figure 15.17 **MND**: teased nerve preparation after osmication (×530): 'crenation' of myelin (arrows).

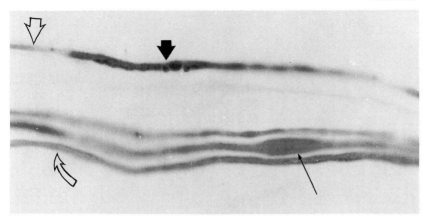

Figure 15.18 **MND**: note fusiform swelling (long straight arrow), early myelin ovoid formation (short broad black arrow), segmental demyelination (open short broad narrow) and thinly myelinated fibre (curved arrow).

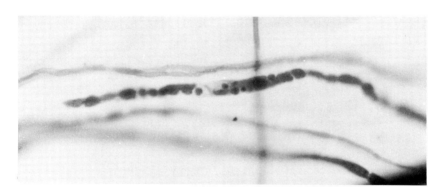

Figure 15.19 **MND**: myelin ovoid formation implying axonal degeneration.

In some cases a mononuclear cell inflammatory infiltrate is seen (Plate 12). A profusion of target fibres, found in denervating conditions (where they affect predominantly type I fibres), may be present in some cases (Plates 11 and 13a and b.) These consist of a normal periphery with a central zone without enzymatic activity that is bordered by a rim of increased activity (Plate 13a). Electron microscopy shows Z-band material and disoriented myofibrils and a paucity of mitochondria in the centre of the 'target' (DeCoster, De Reuck and Vander Eecken, 1976), the ATPase pattern reflecting the presence or absence/disarray of these myofibrils (Plate 13b). Other changes occurring in denervation have been well reviewed (Katsuyoshi, Junzo and Masazumi, 1990).

Classical pathology

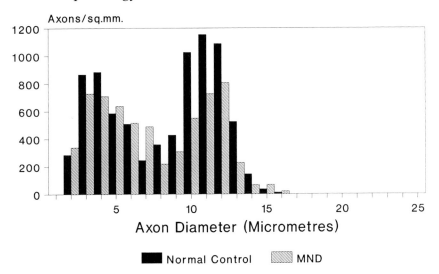

Figure 15.20 Femoral nerve. Myelinated fibres count in eight MND patients and eight matched controls with a Seescan image analyser. The density of myelinated fibres (number/mm²) is as follows (mean ± SD): Controls, 8151 ± 1871 (range 6096–10 662); MND, 6395 ± 1401 (range 4301–7933).

In rapidly progressive cases there may be evidence of muscle fibre necrosis, regeneration, splitting and internal nuclei, thus mimicking a myopathic process. However, in one study, the majority of patients with a disease duration of over 2 years also showed myopathic changes (Achari and Anderson, 1974). In broad terms, fibre atrophy will be prominent in rapidly progressive cases, whereas the concomitant presence of fibre type grouping will be present in the more typical form. Type I grouping has also been linked with longer survival (Patten, Zito and Harati, 1979).

Although showing a basic similarity to ALS, post-polio muscular atrophy (PPMA) is now known to be a distinct disease. Patients who have contracted poliomyelitis many years previously may present with symptoms markedly similar to those of ALS. Biochemical investigations, however, may show differences between the two conditions (Griffiths, Poulton and Perrie, 1991).

15.8 SKIN

Only a few studies have reported on altered skin morphology in ALS (Ono *et al.*, 1986; Ono and Yamauchi, 1992). Abnormalities of the skin include collagen fibres with smaller diameter and reduced collagen

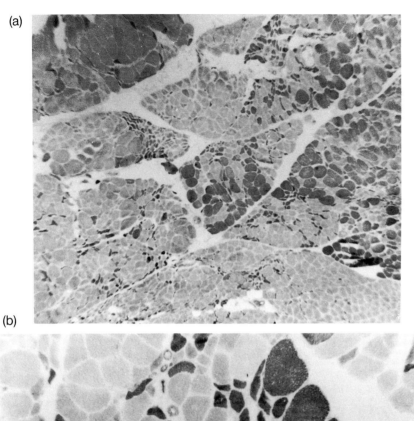

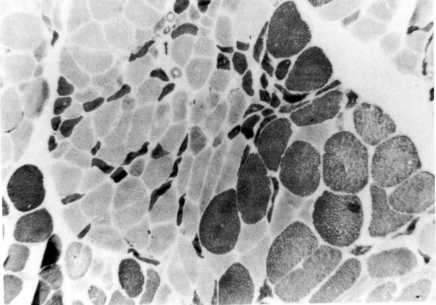

Figure 15.21 (a) **MND** (post-mortem, muscle): fibre type grouping. Pale, type I; dark, type II. Note small groups of atrophic fibres and fibre type grouping (frozen section, ATPase pH 9.4, ×80). (b) **MND**: (high-power of a): note small group of atrophic type II fibres and scattered angulated fibres. Fibre type grouping and hypertrophic type II fibres are also present (×280).

Classical pathology

content that is directly proportional to the duration of the illness. Furthermore, a significant reduction in the content of age-related, stable cross-linked, histidino (hydroxy) droxylysinonorleucine has been found, and this was negatively correlated with the duration of the illness.

15.9 LIVER

On the basis of two cases of hepatic myelopathy with pyramidal tract involvement (Fukuda and Hirayama, 1974) and on a postulate of a possible metabolic cause for the pathological changes in MND, Y. Nakano, Hirayama and Terao (1987), went on to investigate liver biopsies of MND patients and found bizarre giant mitochondria, intramitochondrial paracrystalline inclusions, disorganization of rough endoplasmic reticulum, increase in the endoplasmic reticulum and parasinusoidal fibrosis. Liver function tests showed mild dysfunction.

ACKNOWLEDGEMENTS

I wish to thank Dr F.F. Cruz-Sanchez for helpful discussion. I am indebted to Dr J. deBelleroche for her helpful encouragement on the Golgi work and advice and to Dr T. Steiner for coordinating the activity of our MND group (MCNN/Charing Cross Hospital). Mr B.C. Pugh, Dr W.T. Perrie, Mr G.T. Lee, Dr E.M. Curtis and Ms J.R. Buller, Ms S. Griffiths and Ms J. Sparke of the MCNN are thanked for their cooperation and/or microscopy preparations/photography; their work on MND in this department is contained in the references. Dr M.M. Esiri is thanked for Figure 15.1 and Plate 6.

I wish to thank the Trustees of the Midland Centre for Neurology and Neurosurgery for their support.

REFERENCES

Achari, A.N. and Anderson, M.S. (1974) Myopathic changes in amyotrophic lateral sclerosis. *Neurology*, 47–81.

Aran, F.A. (1850) Reserches sur une maladie non encore decrite du systeme musculaire (atrophie musculaire progressive). *Archives Generales de Medicine*, **24**, 5–35, 172–214.

Atsumi, T. (1981) The ultrastructure of Intramuscular Nerves in amyotrophic lateral sclerosis. *Acta Neuropathol.*, **55**, 193–8.

Atsumi, T. and Miyatake, T. (1987) Morphometry of the degenerative process in the hypoglossal nerves in amyotrophic lateral sclerosis. *Acta Neuropathol.*, **73**, 25–31.

References

Averback, P. (1986) A new type of inclusion body in human spinal cord. *Acta Neuropathol.*, **71**, 106–10.

Averback, P. and Crocker, P. (1982) Regular involvement of Clarke's nucleus in sporadic amyotrophic lateral sclerosis. *Arch. Neurol.*, **39**, 155–6.

Bertrand, I. and Van Bogaert, L. (1925) Rapport sur la SLA-anatomie patologique. *Rev. Neurol.*, **6**, 806–11.

Bonduelle, M. (1975) Amyotrophic lateral sclerosis, in *Handbook of Clinical Neurology* (eds P.J. Vincken, G.W. Bruyn and J.M. DeJong), Elsevier, New York, **22**, 281–338.

Bradley, G.W., Good, P., Rasool, C.G. *et al.* (1983) Morphometric and biochemical studies of peripheral nerves in amyotrophic lateral sclerosis. *Ann. Neurol.*, **14**, 267–77.

Breuer, A.C., Lynn, M.P., Atkinson, M.B. *et al.* (1987) Fast axonal transport in amyotropic lateral sclerosis. An intra-axonal organelle traffic analysis. *Neurology*, **37**, 738–48.

Brownell, B., Oppenheimer, D.R. and Hughes, J.T. (1970) The central nervous system in motor neuron disease. *J. Neurol. Neurosurg. Psychiat.*, **33**, 338–57.

Carpenter, R.J., McDonald, T.J. and Howard Jr, F.M. (1978) The otolaryngologic presentation of amyotrophic lateral sclerosis. *Otolaryngology*, **86**, 479–84.

Carpenter, S. (1968) Proximal axonal enlargement in motor neuron disease. *Neurology*, **18**, 841–51.

Charcot, J.M. (1865) Sclerose des cordons Lateraux de la moelle epiniere chez un femme hysterique atteinte de contracture permanente des quatre membres. *Bull. Med. Hop.*, **2** (Suppl.), 24–42.

Charcot, J.-M. (1870) Note sur un cas de paralysie glossolaryngee suivi d'autopsie. *Arch. Physiol.*, **3**, 247–60.

Charcot, J.-M. (1874) De la sclerose laterale amyotrophique. *Prog. Med.*, **2**, 325–7, 341–2, 453–5.

Charcot, J.-M. and Joffroy, A. (1869) Deux cas d'atrophie musculaire progressive avec lesions de la substance grise et des faisceaux anterolateraux de la moelle epiniere. *Arch. Physiol.*, **2**, 354–67, 629–49, 744–60.

Chou, S.M. (1979) Pathognomy of intraneuronal inclusions in amyotrophic lateral sclerosis, in *Amyotrophic lateral sclerosis: Proceedings of the International Symposium on Amyotrophic Lateral Sclerosis, 2–3 Feb 1978* (eds T. Tsubaki and Y. Toyokura), University of Tokyo Press, Tokyo, pp. 135–76.

Colmant, H.J. (1958) Die myatrophische lateral-sklerose, in *Handbuch der speziellen pathologischen Anatomie und Histologie*, Vol. 13/2b (eds O. Lubarsch, F. Henke and R. Rossle), Springer, Berlin, pp. 2624–92

Cork, L.C., Griffin, J.W., Choy, C. *et al.* (1982) Pathology of motor neurons in accelerated hereditary canine spinal muscular atrophy. *Lab. Invest.*, **46**, 89–99.

Cork, L.C., Price, D.L., Griffin, J.W. *et al.* (1990) Hereditary canine spinal muscular atrophy: canine motor neuron disease. *Can. J. Vet. Res.*, **54**, 77–82.

Cruz-Sanchez, F.F. and Tolosa, E. (1991) Demencias degenerativas tipo no Alzheimer, in *Demencia Senil: Nuevas Perspectivas y Tendencias Terapeuticas* (eds E. Tolosa, F. Bermejo and F. Boller). Springer, Barcelona.

Classical pathology

Cruz-Sanchez, F.F., Lafuente J.V. and Cervos-Navarro J. (1987) Nuevos conceptos sobre la enfermedad de Creutzfeldt-Jakob. *Rev. Esp. Neurol.*, **1**, 269–75.

Cruz-Sanchez, F.F., Lafuente, J.V., Figols, J. *et al.* (1988) Topographical analysis of the neuropathological findings in 16 cases of Creutzfeldt–Jakob disease. *Arch. Neurobiol.*, **51**, 191–6.

Cummings, J.F., de-Lahunta, A., George, C. *et al.* (1990) Equine motor neuron disease: a preliminary report. *Cornell Vet.*, **80**, 357–79.

Dalakas, M.C., Hatazawa, J., Brooks, R.A. *et al.* (1987) Lowered cerebral glucose utilization in amyotrophic lateral sclerosis. *Ann. Neurol.*, **22**, 580–6.

Davison, C. (1941) Amyotrophic lateral sclerosis: origin and extent of the upper motor neuron lesion. *Arch. Neurol. Psych.*, **46**, 1039–56.

DeCoster, W., De Reuck, J. and Vander Eecken, H. (1976) The target phenomenon in human muscle. A comparative light microscopy, histochemical and electron microscopic study. *Acta Neuropathol.*, **34**, 329–38.

Dejerine, J. (1883) Etude anatomique et clinique sur laparalysie labio-glosso-laryngee. *Archives de Physiologie Normale et Pathologique Serie*, **46**, 2180–227.

DePaul, R., Abbs, J.H., Caligiuri, M. *et al.* (1988) Hypoglossal, trigeminal, and facial motoneuron involvement in amyotrophic lateral sclerosis. *Neurology*, **38**, 281–3.

Drac, H. (1989) On the specificity of focal thickenings of myelin in peripheral nerves. *Neuropathol. Pol.*, **27**, 151–68.

Dubowitz, V. (1985) *Muscle Biopsy. A Practical Approach*. Balliere Tindall, London, pp. 221–88.

Duchenne, G.B.A. (1853) Etudes comparee des lesions anatomiques dans l'atrophie musculaire progressive et dans la paralysie generale. *Union Medicale*, **7**, 246–7.

Duchenne, G.B.A. (1860) Paralysie musculaire progressive de la langue, du voile de palais et des levres. *Arch. Gen. Med.*, **16**, 283–96, 431–5.

Dyck, P.J., Stevens, J.C., Mulder, D.W. *et al.* (1975) Frequency of nerve fiber degeneration of peripheral motor and sensory neurons in amyotrophic lateral sclerosis. *Neurology*, **25**, 781–5.

Erb, W.A. (1875) Uber einen weing bekannten spinalen: symptomen complex. *Clin. Wochenschr.*, **12**, 357–9.

Ferrer, I. Dementia of frontal lobe type and amyotrophy. *J. Behav. Neurol.* (in press).

Ferrer, I. and Gullotta, F. (1990) Down's syndrome and Alzheimer's disease: dendritic spine counts in the hippocampus. *Acta Neuropathol.*, **79**, 680–5.

Ferrer, I., Roid, C., Espino, A. *et al.* (1991) Dementia of frontal lobe type and motor neuron disease. A Golgi study of the frontal cortex. *J. Neurol. Neurosurg. Psychiat.*, **54**, 932–4.

Friedman, A.P. and Freedman, D. (1950) Amyotrophic lateral sclerosis. *J. Nerv. Ment. Dis.*, **3**, 1–18.

Froes, M.M.Q., Kristmundsdottir, F., Mahon, M. *et al.* (1987) Muscle morphometry in motor neuron disease. *J. Neuropathol. Exp. Neurol.*, **13**, 405–19.

References

Fukuda, S. and Hirayama, K. (1974) Hepatic myelopathy. *Shinkei Kenkyu Shinpo*, **18**, 563–85.

Ghatak, N.R. and Nochlin, D. (1981) Glial outgrowth along spinal nerve roots in amyotrophic lateral sclerosis. *Ann. Neurol.*, **11**, 203–6.

Griffiths, S.J., Poulton, K.R. and Perrie, W.T. (1991) Histochemical and biochemical aspects of neurogenic muscle changes following poliomyelitis: PPMA or ALS, in *New Evidence in MND/ALS Research* (ed. F. Clifford Rose), Smith-Gordon, London, pp. 29–35.

Hanyu, N., Oguchi, K., Yanagisawa, M. *et al.* (1982) Degeneration and regeneration of ventral root motor fibres in amyotrophic lateral sclerosis: morphometric studies of cervical ventral roots. *J. Neurol. Sci.*, **55**, 99–115.

Hartmann, H.A., McMahon, S., Sun, D. *et al.* (1989) Neuronal RNA in nucleus ambiguus and nucleus hypoglossus of patients with amyotropic lateral sclerosis. *J. Neuropathol. Exp. Neurol.*, **48**, 669–73.

Higgins, R.J., Rings, D.M., Fenner, W.R. *et al.* (1983) Spontaneous lower motor neuron disease with neurofibrillary accumulations in young pigs. *Acta Neuropathol.*, **59**, 288–94.

Hirano, A.H. (1982) Aspects of the ultrastructure of amyotrophic lateral sclerosis, in *Human Motor Neuron Disease, Advances in Neurology*, Vol. 36 (ed. L.P. Rowland), Raven Press, New York.

Hirano, A.H. and Inoue, K. (1980) Early pathological changes of amyotrophic lateral sclerosis: a reappraisal of the spheroid, bunina body and morphometry of the ventral spinal root. *Neurol. Med. Chir.*, **13**, 148–60.

Hirano, A. and Iwata, M. (1979) Pathology of motor neurons with special reference to amyotrophic lateral sclerosis and related diseases, in *Amyotrophic Lateral Sclerosis* (eds T. Tsubaki and Y. Toyokura), Baltimore University Park Press, Baltimore, pp. 107–33.

Hirano, A.H., Donnenfeld, H., Sasaki, S. *et al.* (1984) Fine structural observations of neurofilamentous changes in amyotrophic lateral sclerosis. *J. Neuropathol. Exp. Neurol.*, **43**, 461–7.

Hudson, A.J. (1981) Amyotrophic lateral sclerosis and its association with dementia, parkinsonism and other neurological disorders: a review. *Brain*, **104**, 217–47.

Hughes, J.T. (1982) Pathology of amyotrophic lateral sclerosis, in *Human Motor Neuron Diseases* (ed. L.P. Rowland), Raven Press, New York, pp. 61–73.

Inoue, K. and Hirano, A.H. (1980) Early pathological changes of amyotrophic lateral sclerosis: a reappraisal of the spheroid, Bunina body and morphometry of the ventral spinal root (abstract). *J. Neuropathol. Exp. Neurol.*, **39**, 363.

Itoh, T., Soube, G., Ken, E. *et al.* (1992) Phosphorylated high molecular weight neurofilament protein in the peripheral motor, sensory and sympathetic neuronal perikarya: system dependent normal variations and changes in amyotrophic lateral sclerosis. *Acta Neuropathol.*, **83**, 240–5.

Iwasaki, Y. and Kinoshita, M. (1987) Study on the relationship between the muscular pathology and prognosis in motor neuron disease. *Jpn. J. Med.*, **26**, 335–8.

335

Classical pathology

Jacobs, L., Bozian, D. and Heffner Jr, R.R. (1981) An eye movement disorder in amyotrophic lateral sclerosis. *Neurol.*, **31**, 1282–7.

Kamo, H., Haebara, H., Akiguchi, I. *et al.* (1987) A distinctive distribution of reactive astroglia in the precentral cortex in amyotrophic lateral sclerosis. *Acta Neuropathol.*, **74**, 33–8.

Karim, A.R., Kaur, P., Rossi, M.L. *et al.* Interaction of motor neuron disease plasma with glucose transport (in preparation).

Kato, T., Hirano, A. and Donnenfeld, H. (1987) A Golgi study of the large anterior horn cells of the lumbar cords in normal spinal cords and in amyotrophic lateral sclerosis. *Acta Neuropathol.*, **75**, 34–40.

Katsuyoshi, I., Junzo, T. and Masazumi, A. (1990) Denervation atrophy of skeletal muscle, in *Neuromuscular Disease* (eds M. Adachi and J.H. Sher), Igaku-Shoin, New York, pp. 54–103.

Kawamura, Y., Dyck, P.J., Shimono, M. *et al.* (1981) Morphometric comparison of the vulnerability of peripheral motor and sensory neurons in amyotrophic lateral sclerosis. *J. Neuropathol. Exp. Neurol.*, **40**, 667–75.

Kennedy, P.G.E. and Duchen, L.W. (1985) A quantitative study of intermediolateral column cells in motor neuron disease and the Shy–Drager syndrome. *J. Neurol. Neurosurg. Psychiat.*, **48**, 1103–6

Kihira, T., Yoshida, S., Uebayashi, Y. *et al.* (1991) Involvement of Onuf's nucleus in amyotrophic lateral sclerosis. Demonstration of intraneuronal conglomerate inclusions and Bunina bodies. *J. Neurol. Sci.*, **104**, 119–28.

Kimura, F., Hosokawa, S., Takenaka, M. *et al.* (1988) Morphometrical study on muscle specimens in motor neuron disease. *Rinsho-Shinkeigaku*, **28**, 653–61.

Kozlowski, M.A., Williams, C., Hinton, D.R. *et al.* (1989) Heterotopic neurons in spinal cord of patients with amyotrophic lateral sclerosis. *Neurology*, **39**, 644–8.

Kristmundsdottir, F., Mahon, M., Froes, M.M.Q. *et al.* (1990) Histomorphometric and histopathological study of the human cricopharyngeus muscle: in health and in motor neuron disease. *Neuropathol. Appl. Neurobiol.*, **16**, 461–75.

Kuncl, R.W., Crawford, T.O., Rothstein, J.D. *et al.* (1992) Motor neuron diseases, in *Diseases of the Nervous System. Clinical Neurobiology*, Vol. II (eds A.K. Asbury, G.M. McKhann and W.I. McDonald), W.B. Saunders, Philadelphia, pp. 1179–208.

Kusaka, H. and Hirano, A. (1985) Fine structure of anterior horns in patients without amyotrophic lateral sclerosis. *J. Neuropathol. Exp. Neurol.*, **44**, 430–8.

Kusaka, H., Matsumato, S. and Imai, T. (1990) An adult-onset case of sporadic motor neuron disease with basophilic inclusions. *Acta Neuropathol.*, **80**, 660–5.

Kushner, M.J., Parrish, M., Burke, A. *et al.* (1984) Nystagmus in motor neuron disease: clinico-pathologic study of two cases. *Ann. Neurol.*, **16**, 71–7.

Kushner, P.D., Stephenson, B.A. and Wright, S. (1991) Reactive astrogliosis is widespread in the subcortical white matter of amyotrophic lateral sclerosis brain. *J. Neuropathol. Exp. Neurol.*, **50**, 263–77.

Lafuente, J.V., Rossi, M.L., Pugh, B.C. *et al.* (1992) Quantitative observations of

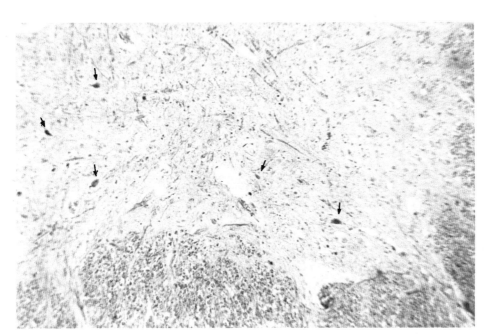

Plate 1 **MND**: Cervical cord anterior horn showing only very occasional remaining shrunken motor neurones (arrows) (Kluver–Barrera, ×150).

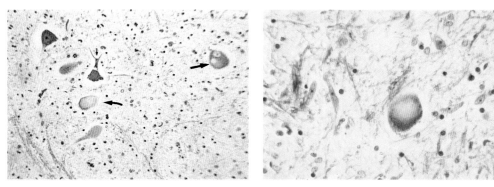

Plate 2(a) and (b) **MND**: Lumbar cord anterior horn showing swollen (one vacuolated), chromatolytic (arrows) and degenerating neurones (Kluver–Barrera, a ×250; b ×400).

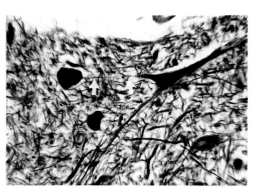

Plate 2(c) **MND**: spheroid (dark). Note connection with parent neurone (arrows) (Glees–Marsland, ×500).

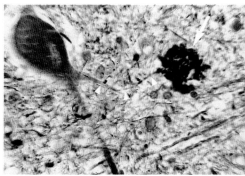

Plate 2(d) **MND**: Pericapillary rosette (arrow) with neuronal process reaching it (arrowheads) (anti-neurofilament antibody 2F11, Bradsure Biologicals, ×500).

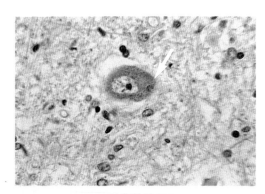

Plate 2(e) **MND**: Bunina body (arrow) in the cytoplasm of a lower motor neurone in the lumbar cord (haematoxylin and eosin, × 500).

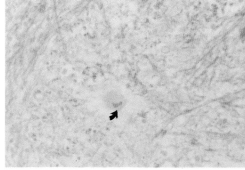

Plate 2(f) **MND**: Bunina body (arrow) in the cytoplasm of a lower motor neurone in the lumbar cord (luxol, ×250).

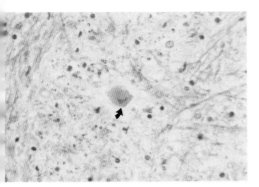

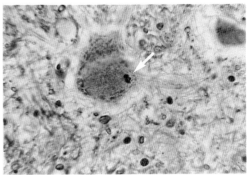

Plate 2(g) **MND**: Bunina body (arrow) in the cytoplasm of a lower motor neurone in the lumbar cord [luxol fast blue (see Plate 2(f), same section) and cresyl violet (Kluver–Barrera)] (×250).

Plate 2(h) **MND**: Bunina body (arrow) in the cytoplasm of a lower motor neurone in the lumbar cord (Kluver–Barrera, ×500).

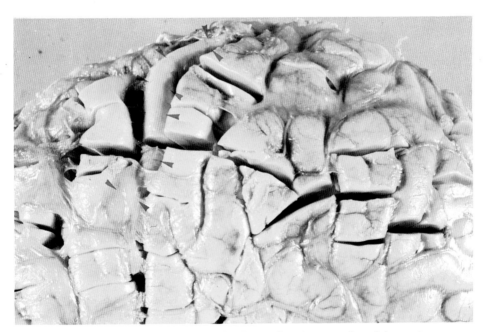

Plate 3 **MND**: Golgi–Cox impregnated forebrain showing atrophy of the motor strip (arrowheads), normal sensory cortex (on the right) and premotor area (on the left). The cuts were made at autopsy to facilitate impregnation.

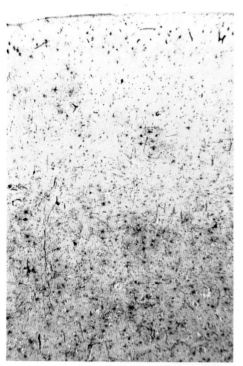

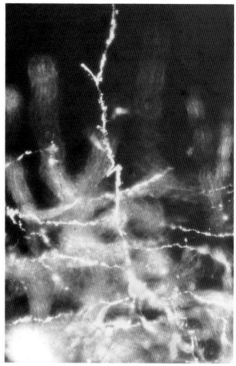

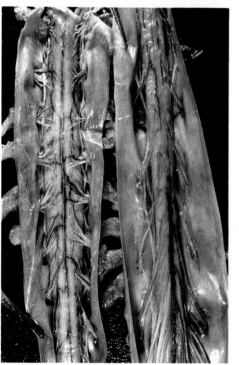

Plate 4 **MND**: motor cortex. Note foci of astrocytosis and diffuse astrocytosis (in deep cortical layers) (10-μm Golgi–Cox-impregnated paraffin section counter-stained with Nissl and Glial Fibrillary Acidic Protein (GFAP), ×71.

Plate 5 **Normal** motor cortex. Polarized image of a pyramidal cell to demonstrate dendritic spines (Golgi–Cox, paraffin section, 30 μm, ×400).

Plate 6 **MND**: spinal cord anterior surface: upper (left) and lower (right) cord showing atrophic and greyish anterior roots.

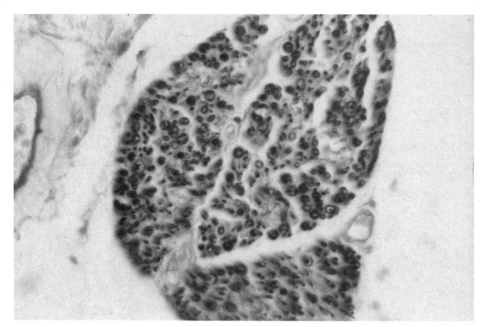

Plate 7 **Normal** anterior root (luxol, same magnification as Plate 8).

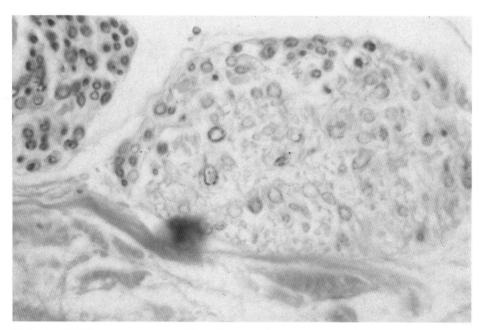

Plate 8 **MND**: anterior root. Note the poorly staining myelinated fibres, reduction in their number and their irregular outline. Compare with Plate 7 (luxol, same magnification as Plate 7).

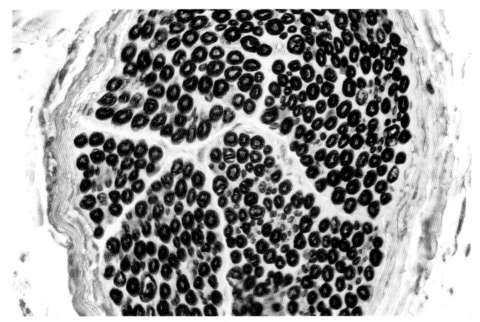

Plate 9 **Normal** femoral nerve (osmium impregnation, paraffin section, counterstained with monoclonal anti-neurofilament antibody, Monosan 2F11, ×400).

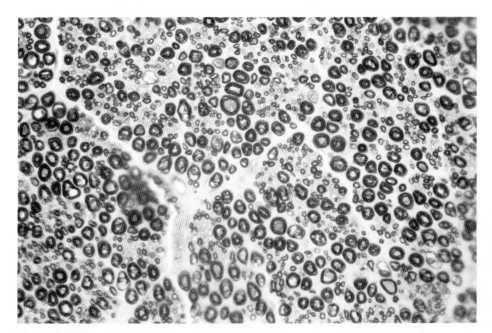

Plate 10 **MND**: femoral nerve. Note reduction in myelinated fibres, myelin abnormalities and paler staining axons in comparison with Plate 9 (osmium impregnation, paraffin section, counterstained with monoclonal anti-neurofilament antibody, Monosan 2F11, ×400).

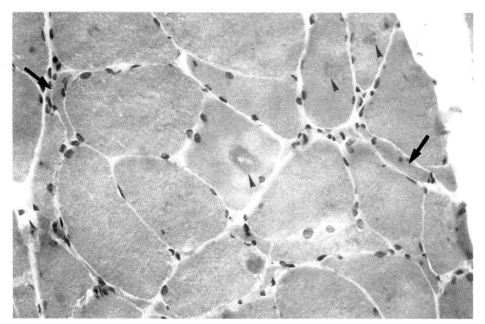

Plate 11 **MND** (post-mortem, muscle): atrophic angular fibres (arrows) and target hypertrophic fibres (arrowheads) (frozen section, haematoxylin and eosin, ×400).

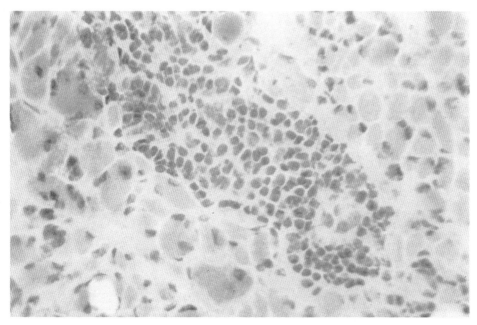

Plate 12 **MND** (post-mortem, muscle): focus of inflammation (frozen section, haematoxylin and eosin, ×250).

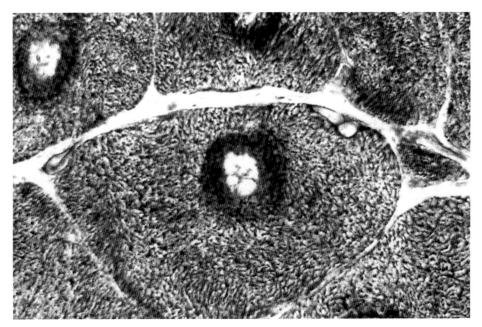

Plate 13(a)   **MND** (post-mortem, muscle): target fibre (frozen section, NADH-TR, ×650).

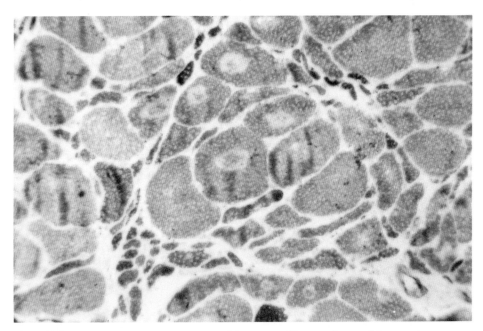

Plate 13(b)   **MND** (post-mortem, muscle): target fibre and atrophic angular fibres (frozen section, ATPase pH 9.4, ×250).

the Golgi impregnate in the motor cortex representing the hand in motor neuron disease (abstract). *Neuropathol. Appl. Neurobiol.*, **18**, 309.

Lampson, L.A., Kushner, P.D. and Sobel, R.A. (1990) Major histocompatibility complex antigen expression in the affected tissues in amyotrophic lateral sclerosis. *Ann. Neurol.*, **28**, 365–72.

Lawyer, T. and Netsky, M.G. (1953) Amyotrophic lateral sclerosis: a clinico-anatomic study of 53 cases. *Arch. Neurol. Psychiat.*, **69**, 171–92.

Leigh, P.N., Swash, A.D., Brion, J.P. *et al.* (1989) Cytoskeletal abnormalities in motor neuron disease. An immunocytochemical study. *Brain*, **112**, 521–35.

Lowe, J., Lennox, G., Jefferson, D. *et al.* (1988) A filamentous inclusion body within anterior horn neurons in motor neuron disease defined by immunocytochemical localisation to ubiquitin. *Neurosci. Lett.*, **94**, 203–10.

Malamud, N. (1968) Neuromuscular disease, in *Pathology of the Nervous System*, Vol. I (ed. J. Minckler), McGraw Hill, New York, pp. 712–25.

Manetto, V., Sternberger, N.H., Perry, G. *et al.* (1988) Phosphorylation of neurofilaments is altered in amyotrophic lateral sclerosis. *J. Neuropathol. Exp. Neurol.*, **47**, 642–53.

Mannen, T., Inata, M. and Tokoyura, Y. (1977) Preservation of a certain motor neuron group of the sacral cord in amyotrophic lateral sclerosis: its clinical significance. *J. Neurol. Neurosurg. Psychiat.*, **40**, 464–9.

Mannen, T., Iwata, M. and Toyokura, Y. (1982) The Onuf's nucleus and the external and sphincter muscles in amyotrophic lateral sclerosis and Shy-Drager syndrome. *Acta Neuropathol.*, **58**, 255–60.

Matsumoto, S., Hirano, A. and Goto, S. (1990) Ubiquitin-immunoreactive filamentous inclusions in anterior horn cells of Guamanian and non-Guamanian amyotrophic lateral sclerosis. *Acta Neuropathol.*, **80**, 233–8.

Matsumoto, S., Mizusawa, H., Hirano, A. *et al.* (1989) Immunocytochemical study of phosphorylated neurofilaments in the anterior horn cells of amyotrophic lateral sclerosis. *Neurol. Med.*, **30**, 370–7.

Matsumoto, S., Kusaka, H., Murakami, N. *et al.* (1992) Basophilic inclusions in sporadic juvenile amyotrophic lateral sclerosis: and immunocytochemical and ultrastructural study. *Acta Neuropathol.*, **83**, 579–83.

Migheli, A., Autilio-Gambetti, L., Gambetti, P. *et al.* (1990) Ubiquitinated filamentous inclusions in spinal cord of patients with motor neuron disease. *Neurosci. Lett.*, **114**, 5–10.

Mitsumoto, H. and Boggs, A.L. (1987) Vacuolated anterior horn cells in wobbler mouse motor neuron disease: peripheral axons and regenerative capacity. *J. Neuropathol. Exp. Neurol.*, **46**, 214–22.

Mitsumoto, H. and Bradley, W.G. (1982) Murine motor neuron disease (the Wobbler mouse). Degeneration and regeneration in the lower motor neuron. *Brain*, **105**, 811–34.

Miyata, Y. (1983) A new mutant mouse with motor neuron disease. *Exp. Brain Res.*, **10**, 139–42.

Mortara, P., Chio, A., Rossa, M.G. *et al.* (1984) Motor neuron disease in the province of Turin, Italy, 1966–1980. *J. Neurol. Sci.*, **66**, 165–73.

Classical pathology

Munoz, D.G., Greene, C., Perl, D.P. *et al.* (1988) Accumulation of phosphory-lated neurofilaments in anterior horns of amyotrophic lateral sclerosis patients. *J. Neuropathol. Exp. Neurol.*, **47**, 9–18.

Murayama, S., Bouldin, T.W. and Suzuki, K. (1992) Immunocytochemical and ultrastructural studies of upper motor neurons in amyotrophic lateral sclerosis. *Acta Neuropathol.*, **83**, 518–24.

Murayama, S., Mori, H., Ihara, Y. *et al.* (1990) Immunocytochemical and ultrastructural studies of lower motor neurons in amyotrophic lateral sclerosis. *Ann. Neurol.*, **27**, 137–48.

Nakano, I. and Hirano, A. (1987) Atrophic cell processes in large motor neurons in the anterior horn in amyotrophic lateral sclerosis: observation with silver impregnation method. *J. Neuropathol. Exp. Neurol.*, **46**, 40–9.

Nakano, I., Hashizume, Y. and Tomonaga, G. (1990) Bunina bodies in neurons of the medullary reticular formation in a case of amyotrophic lateral sclerosis. *Acta Neuropathol.*, **79**, 689–91.

Nakano, Y., Hirayama, K. and Terao, K. (1987) Hepatic ultrastructural changes and liver dysfunction in amyotrophic lateral sclerosis. *Arch Neurol.*, **44**, 103–6.

Neary, D., Snowden, J.S., Mann, D.M.A. *et al.* (1990) Frontal lobe dementia and motor neuron disease. *J. Neurol. Neurosurg. Psychiat.*, **53**, 23–32.

Norris, F.H. (1991) Epidemiology of amyotrophic lateral sclerosis, in *Human Motor Neuron Disease* (ed. L.P. Rowland), Raven Press, New York.

Okazaki, H. (1983) *Fundamentals of Neuropathology.* Igaku-Shoin, New York, Tokyo, p. 164.

Ono, S. and Yamauchi, M. (1992) Collagen cross linking of skin in patients with amyotrophic lateral sclerosis. *Ann. Neurol.*, **31**, 305–10.

Ono, S., Toyokura, Y., Mannen, T. *et al.* (1986) Amyotrophic lateral sclerosis: histologic, histochemical and ultrastructural abnormalities of skin. *Neurology*, **36**, 948–56.

Oppenheimer, D.R. (1984) Diseases of the basal ganglia, cerebellum and motor neurons, in *Greenfield's Neuropathology*, 4th edn (eds J.H. Adams, J.A.N. Corsellis and L.W. Duchen), Edward Arnold, London, p. 730.

Oyanagi, K., Makifuchi, T., Horikawa, Y. *et al.* (1991) Nucleocytoplasmic progression in the neurons and anteroposterior extension in the spinal gray matter of lesions in amyotrophic lateral sclerosis, in *Neuropathology in Brain Research* (ed. F. Ikuta), Elsevier, Amsterdam, pp. 115–26.

Patten, B.M., Zito, G. and Harati, Y. (1979) Histological findings in motor neuron disease. Relation to clinically determined activity, duration and severity of disease. *Arch. Neurol.*, **36**, 560–4.

Perrie, W.T., Lee, G.T., Buller, J.R. *et al.* (1991) Axonal degeneration and demyelination of peripheral nerves in motor neuron disease (abstract). *Neuropathol. Appl. Neurobiol.*, **17**, 249.

Perrie, W.T., Lee, G.T., Curtis, L. *et al.* Changes in the myelinated axons of femoral nerve in amyotrophic lateral sclerosis. *J. Neural Transmission*, **39**, 223–33.

Pestronk, A., Cornblath, D., Ilyas, A.A. *et al.* (1988) A treatable multifocal motor neuropathy with antibodies to GM1 ganglioside. *Ann. Neurol.*, **24**, 73–8.

Pestronk, A., Adams, R., Cornblath, D. *et al.* (1989) Patterns of serum IgM antibodies to GM1a gangliosides in amyotrophic lateral sclerosis. *Ann. Neurol.*, **25**, 98–102.

Pestronk, A., Shaudry, V., Feldman, E.L. *et al.* (1990) Lower motor neuron syndromes defined by patterns of weakness, nerve conduction abnormalities, and high titer of antiglycolipid antibodies. *Ann. Neurol.*, **27**, 316–26.

Poloni, M., Mascherpa, C., Faggi, L. *et al.* (1982) Cerebral atrophy in motor neuron disease evaluated by computed tomography. *J. Neurol. Neurosurg. Psychiatr.*, **45**, 1102–5.

Poulton, K.R. and Rossi, M.L. (1991) Fructose metabolism in neuromuscular disease (abstract). *Neuropathol. Appl. Neurobiol.*, **17**, 529.

Pugh, B.C. and Rossi, M.L. (1991) Motor neuron disease and the Golgi Cox technique, in *New Evidence in Motor Neuron Disease/Amyotrophic Lateral Sclerosis Research* (ed. F. Clifford Rose), Smith-Gordon, London, pp. 157–62.

Pugh, B.C. and Rossi, M.L. (1992) A paraffin wax technique of Golgi-Cox impregnated neocortex that permits the joint application of other histological and immunocytochemical techniques. *J. Neural Transmission*, **39**, 97–105.

Rosen, A.D. (1978) Amyotrophic lateral sclerosis. Clinical features and prognosis. *Arch. Neurol.*, **35**, 638–42.

Rosenfeld, M.R. and Posner, J.B. (1991) Paraneoplastic motor neuron disease, in *Human Motor Neuron Disease* (ed. L.P. Rowland), Raven Press, New York.

Rossi, M.L., Pugh, B.C. and Buller, J.R. (1991) A modified Golgi-Cox technique applied to paraffin and gelatin section of CNS in combination with other histological techniques with particular reference to motor neuron disease (abstract). *Ital. J. Neurol. Sci.*, **5** (Suppl.), 98.

Rossi, M.L., Pugh, B.C., Perrie, W.T. *et al.* (1990) A preliminary investigation of Motor Neuron Disease using a modified Golgi sublimate method (abstract). *Neuropathol. Appl. Neurobiol.*, **16**, 532–3.

Rossi, M.L., Pugh, B.C., Perrie, W.T. *et al.* (1991) A preliminary investigation of motor neuron disease using a modified Golgi sublimate method (abstract). *Clin. Neuropathol.*, **10**, 162.

Rossi, M.L., Pugh, B.C., Lafuente, J.V. *et al.* (1992) Neocortical changes in motor neuron disease: a Golgi/immunohistochemical study (abstract). *Neuropathol. Appl. Neurobiol.*, **18**, 309.

Santero, M., Thomas, F.P., Fink, M.E. *et al.* (1990) IgM deposits at nodes of Ranvier in a patient with amyotrophic lateral sclerosis, anti GM1 antibodies, and multifocal motor conduction block. *Ann. Neurol.*, **28**, 373–7.

Sasaki, S. and Maruyama, S. (1992) Pericapillary rosettes in the human spinal cord. *Act Neuropathol.*, **83**, 598–604.

Sasaki, S., Yamane, K., Sakuma, H. *et al.* (1989) Case report. Sporadic motor neuron disease with Lewy body-like hyaline inclusions. *Acta Neuropathol.*, **78**, 555–60.

Classical pathology

Schochet Jr S.S., Hardman, J.M., Ladewig, P.P. *et al.* (1969) Intraneuronal conglomerates in sporadic motor neuron disease. *Arch. Neurol.*, **20**, 548–53.

Schoene, W.G. (1985) Degenerative diseases of the CNS, in *Textbook of Neuropathology* (eds R.L. Davis and D.M. Roberston), Williams & Wilkins, Baltimore, p. 185.

Schroder, H.D. and Reske-Nielsen, E. (1984) Preservation of the nucleus X-pelvic floor motor system in amyotrophic lateral sclerosis. *Clin. Neuropathol.*, **3**, 210–16.

Shy, M.E., Rowland, L.P., Smith, T.S. *et al.* (1986) Motor neuron disease and plasma cell dyscrasia. *Neurology*, **36**, 1429–36.

Smith, B.H. and Arnason, B. (1977) Pathology of neuron–target cell interactions. *Neurosci. Res. Progr. Bull.*, **14**, 360–6.

Smith, M.C. (1956) The recognition and prevention of artefacts of the Marchi method. *J. Neurol. Neurosurg. Psychiat.*, **19**, 74–83.

Smith, M.C. (1960) Nerve fibre degeneration in the brain in amyotrophic lateral sclerosis. *J. Neurol. Neurosurg. Psychiat.*, **23**, 269–82.

Smith, M.C., Strich, S.J. and Sharp, P. (1956) The value of the Marchi method for staining tissue stored in formalin for prolonged periods. *J. Neurol. Neurosurg. Psychiat.*, **19**, 62–4.

Steiner, T.J., Sethi, K.D. and Rose, F.C. (1984) Autonomic function in motor neuron disease, in *Research Progress in Motor Neuron Disease* (ed. F. Clifford Rose), Pitman, London, pp. 180–8.

Swash, M., Leader, M., Brown, A. *et al.* (1986) Focal loss of anterior horn cells in the cervical cord in motor neuron disease. *Brain*, **109**, 939–52.

Swash, M., Scholtz, C.L., Vowles, G. *et al.* (1988) Selective and asymmetric vulnerability of corticospinal and spinocerebellar tracts in motor neuron disease. *J. Neurol. Neurosurg. Psychiat.*, **51**, 785–9.

Tomonaga, M., Saito, M. and Yoshimura, M. (1978) Ultrastructure of the Bunina bodies in anterior horn cells in amyotrophic lateral sclerosis. *Acta Neuropathol.*, **42**, 81–6.

Troost, D., Van Den Ord, J.J. and De Jong, J.M.B.V. (1990) Immunohistochemical characterization of the inflammatory infiltrate in amyotrophic lateral sclerosis. *Neuropathol. Appl. Neurobiol.*, **16**, 401–10.

Troost, D., Van Den Ord, J.J., De Jong, J.M.B.V. *et al.* (1989) Lymphocytic infiltration in the spinal cord of patients with amyotrophic lateral sclerosis. *Clin. Neuropathol.*, **8**, 289–94.

Tsukagoshi, H., Yanigasawa, N., Oguchi, K. *et al.* (1979) Morphometric quantification of the cervical limb motor cells in controls and in amyotrophic lateral sclerosis. *J. Neurol. Sci.*, **41**, 287–97.

Udaka, F., Kameyama, M. and Tomonaga, M. (1986) Degeneration of Betz cells in motor neuron disease. A Golgi study. *Acta Neuropathol.*, **70**, 289–95.

Virk, P.K., Sturman, S.G., Karim, A.R. *et al.* (1991) Interaction with MND plasma with glucose transport (abstract). *Ital. J. Neurol. Sci.*, **5** (Suppl.), 80.

Woolf, A.L., Serrano, R.A. and Johnson, A.G. (1969) The intramuscular nerve endings and muscle fibres in amyotrophic lateral sclerosis: a biopsy study, in *Motor Neuron Disease* (eds F.H. Norris and L.T. Kurland), Grune & Stratton, New York, pp. 166–74.

Younger, D.S., Rowland, L.P., Latov, N. *et al.* (1991) Lymphoma, motor neuron diseases and amyotrophic lateral sclerosis. *Ann. Neurol.*, **29**, 78–86.

Yuasa, R., Mizushima, S. and Oyanagi, S. (1980) A case of amyotrophic lateral sclerosis with severe motor cortex lesions. *Adv. Neurol. Sci.*, **24**, 293–303.

16   *Ubiquitin*

P.N. LEIGH

16.1   INTRODUCTION

In many neurodegenerative disorders, altered or abnormal proteins accumulate in neurones, glia or the extracellular matrix (Table 16.1). Ubiquitin, a highly conserved cellular protein which (as its name suggests) is ubiquitous in eukaryotes, is a component of many of the intracellular inclusions associated with these diverse disorders. In that sense the presence of ubiquitin is non-specific. The biology of ubiquitin, however, is of great interest, and abnormalities of the cellular processes in which ubiquitin participates could contribute to neuronal degeneration. Ubiquitin and other heat-shock proteins may participate in 'protective responses' of cells to injury and may thus be important in limiting damage caused by many types of injury. At a descriptive level, ubiquitin immunocytochemistry often reveals new aspects of cellular pathology. This has been particularly important in motor neurone disease (MND; amyotrophic lateral sclerosis, ALS), in which, in comparison with Alzheimer's disease, Parkinson's disease and several other neurodegenerative disorders, traditional stains and immunocytochemical approaches revealed few really characteristic or specific aspects of the cellular and molecular pathology. In contrast, ubiquitin antibodies have revealed entirely new aspects of the molecular pathology of MND, and have also revealed important similarities and differences between MND and other neurodegenerative conditions. At the level of cellular pathology MND differs from other neurodegenerative disorders because the characteristic intracellular inclusions usually do not contain cytoskeletal elements that can be identified with appropriate antibodies. Of course, cytoskeletal proteins and their epitopes may be altered or hidden, and thus undetectable with the antibodies currently available. Nonetheless, ubiquitin remains the only identifiable component of the most characteristic form of intraneuronal inclusions in MND.

   This chapter discusses the biology of ubiquitin in relation to

Table 16.1 Cytoskeletal changes observed in chronic neurodegenerative conditions

Inclusion	Disease	Protein	Ubiquitin
NFT	AD PSNP Dementia pugilistica Post-encephalitic PD PDC (Guam)	PNF fragments MAP-2 fragments MAP-1B fragments A68 Tropomyosin	++++
Plaque neurites	AD Cortical LB disease	Tau PNF	++
Brainstem LB	Parkinson's disease Diffuse LB disease	PNF Tau −ve MAP-2 MAP-1 Tubulin Tropomyosin −ve Gelsolin	++
Cortical LB	Cortical LB disease AD?	PNF Tropomyosin (some) MAP-2	++
Spheroids	MND Neuroaxonal dystrophies PSNP	PNF MAP-2 − ve	++
Hirano bodies	AD CJD Hallervorden–Spatz	Actin Tropomyosin Tau?	−
Granulovacuoles	AD Pick's disease	Tau PNF	Some +ve
MND inclusions (anterior horn)	MND	−	+++
Dentate granule cell inclusions Neocortical layer II and III inclusions	MND dementia Some frontal lobe dementias	−	++
Pick bodies	Pick's disease	Tau PNF MAP-2 Tropomyosin Chromogranin A	+++
Ballooned neurones	Pick's disease Corticobasal degeneration CJD AD	PNF Tau α-B-Crystallin	+
Glial cell inclusions	MSA (SND/OPCA)	Tau Tubulin	++

Abbreviations: AD, Alzheimer's disease; CJD, Creutzfeld–Jakob disease; LB, Lewy body; MAP, microtubule-associated protein; MND, motor neurone disease; MSA, multiple system atrophy; OPCA, olivopontocerebellar atrophy; PD, Parkinson's disease; PDC, parkinsonism–dementia complex; PNF, phosphorylated neurofilaments; PSNP, progressive supranuclear palsy (Steele–Richardson–Olzewski syndrome); SND, strionigral degeneration.

neurodegeneration, describes the morphology of ubiquitin-immunoreactive inclusions and considers their significance in MND and related neurodegenerative disorders.

16.2 UBIQUITIN AND NEURODEGENERATIVE DISORDERS

Ubiquitin was identified as a component of neurofibrillary tangles in 1986 by Mori, Kondo and Ihara (1986), and subsequently many other groups have confirmed this observation. Ubiquitin is now known to be a component of Lewy bodies, Pick bodies, neurofibrillary tangles in many disorders, glial cell inclusions in multiple system atrophy, and inclusions in some muscle diseases (Table 16.1; Cole and Timiras, 1987; Perry et al., 1987; Kuzahara et al., 1988; Love et al., 1988; Lowe et al., 1988a; Bancher et al., 1989; Manetto et al., 1989; Leigh et al., 1989a; Papp, Kahn and Lantos, 1989; Nakazato et al., 1990; Dale et al., 1992; Papp and Lantos, 1992). The immunocytochemical localization of ubiquitin has become a useful tool in neuropathological diagnosis because it reveals new aspects of the molecular pathology of these disorders (Leigh et al., 1989a; Lennox et al., 1989), and its presence has fostered speculation that it may represent a crucially important clue to the pathogenesis of neurodegenerative disorders. Thus it is relevant to survey some aspects of the biochemistry of this highly conserved protein.

16.3 THE FUNCTIONS OF UBIQUITIN

Ubiquitin is a 76 amino acid polypeptide with a relative molecular mass (M_r) of 8500. It is the most highly conserved of known proteins, such that the sequence (Figure 16.1) is identical in insects, amphibians, fish, and mammals such as cattle and man, although in yeast the sequence differs by three residues from the human (Rechsteiner, 1987; Wilkinson, 1988). It was first identified as a protein that could induce the differentiation of B lymphocytes and which was present in all eukaryotic cells – hence its name (Goldstein et al., 1975). It is identifiable free within the cytosol and in the form of ubiquitin–protein conjugates. Ubiquitin is now known to participate in many cellular processes (Ciechanover, 1993). The function that has received most attention is the non-lysosomal degradation of short-lived or abnormal proteins (Hershko et al., 1980; Rechsteiner, 1987; Wilkinson, 1987; Hough, Pratt and Rechsteiner, 1988; Ciechanover, 1993). In addition ubiquitin is covalently bound to nuclear histones H2A and H2B (Thorne et al., 1987; Nickel and Davie, 1989) and is implicated in the regulation of gene expression and in the regulation of the cell cycle by degrading cyclin (Glotzer, Murray and Kirschner, 1991; Hershko et al., 1991; Ciechanover,

Ubiquitin

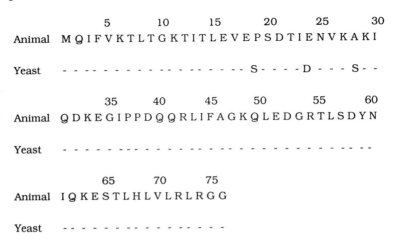

Figure 16.1 The amino acid sequences of ubiquitin. The sequence common to animals is shown above the yeast sequence; dashes represent identity with the animal sequence. Letters are standard symbols for amino acids. (Modified from Wilkinson, 1988, with permission of the author and publishers.)

1993). Ubiquitin is also involved in the degradation of oncoproteins such as N-*myc*, c-*myc*, c-*fos* and p53, and removal of p53 by ubiquitin may be involved in cell transformation (Ciechanover *et al.*, 1991; Ciechanover, 1993). The function of membrane receptors may be modified by ubiquitination. Thus the lymphocyte B homing receptor and the receptor for platelet-derived growth factor involved in specific cell–cell recognition are ubiquitinated (Siegelman *et al.*, 1986; Yarden *et al.*, 1986; Leung *et al.*, 1987). The insertion of monoamine oxidase B into mitochondrial outer membranes may be mediated through a process involving ubiquitin (Zhaung and McCauley, 1989). Ubiquitin is also a member of the heat-shock family of proteins (Bond and Schlesinger, 1985; Lindquist, 1986; Lindquist and Craig, 1988).

16.4 UBIQUITIN AND THE NON-LYSOSOMAL DEGRADATION OF PROTEINS

While studying an ATP-dependent proteolytic system from reticulocytes, Hershko *et al.* (1980) isolated a small heat-stable polypeptide that determined the ATP-dependent proteolytic activity of the reticulocyte lysates. When purified, this polypeptide was identified as ubiquitin. Ubiquitin was then shown to be covalently conjugated to protein substrates, and it became clear that conjugation is an indispensable process in protein breakdown (Ciechanover *et al.*, 1980; Hershko and Ciechanover, 1986). Conjugated proteins are then degraded by specific proteases (Ciechanover *et al.*, 1980; Hershko *et al.*, 1980). However, Fried *et al.* (1987) have suggested that ubiquitin has intrinsic proteolytic activity and that its conjugation to target proteins can convert these conjugates into *ad hoc* proteolytic enzymes.

Recent reviews of this topic, and wider aspects of proteolysis including the role of ubiquitin in the lysosomal system, are those of Finley and Chau (1991), Hershko (1991), Hershko and Ciechanover (1992), Mayer *et al.* (1992) and Ciechanover (1993).

16.4.1 The ubiquitin conjugation pathway

The pathways involved in the conjugation of ubiquitin to target proteins are shown in Figure 16.2.

The first step involves the activation of ubiquitin by a specific activating enzyme (E1), which catalyses a two-step reaction in which ubiquitin adenylate is first formed in an ATP-dependent reaction; the activated ubiquitin is then transferred to a thiol site of the enzyme, with the release of AMP (Ciechanover *et al.*, 1981; Haas *et al.*, 1982). The activated amino acid residue of ubiquitin is the carboxy-terminal glycine (Hershko, Ciechanover and Rose, 1981). The E1–ubiquitin thiol ester then acts as a 'donor' for the formation of ubiquitin conjugates with proteins (Haas *et al.*, 1982; Hershko *et al.*, 1983). The genes for E1 have been cloned and are highly conserved, showing 53% homology between the yeast and human E1 sequences (Hershko, 1991).

E2 has a ubiquitin-carrier function and is the acceptor of activated ubiquitin from E1, transferring it to amino groups of proteins (Hershko *et al.*, 1983). There are at least seven E2 proteins, which range in native molecular weight from 14 to 55 kDa, most of them being homodimers (Pickart and Rose, 1985; Hershko, 1991; Ciechanover, 1993). Some E2s transfer ubiquitin to histones, without the participation of E3, but the smallest of the E2 carrier proteins is involved in E3-dependent ligation to substrates of the ubiquitin proteolytic pathway. In this reaction, many ubiquitin molecules are conjugated to each molecule of the substrate protein, which is then targeted for degradation.

Ubiquitin–protein ligase (E3) catalyses the formation of isopeptide bonds between the activated carboxy terminus of ubiquitin and the ε-amino groups of lysine residues in target proteins, producing conjugates that usually have one molecule of ubiquitin for each molecule of protein (Pickart and Rose, 1985; Pickart and Vella, 1988; Haas, Bright and Jackson, 1988). E3 has a central role in selecting proteins suitable for degradation (Ciechanover, 1993).

Ubiquitin

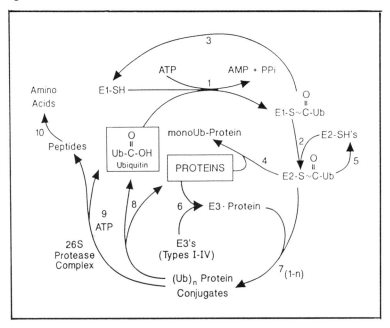

Figure 16.2 Proposed sequence of events in conjugation and degradation of proteins by the ubiquitin system. 1, Activation of ubiquitin by E1 (ubiquitin-activating enzyme); 2, transfer of high-energy ubiquitin intermediate to E2 (ubiquitin carrier protein); 3, recycling of E1; 4, conjugation of protein to ubiquitin by E2; 5, recycling of E2; 6, formation of E3 (ubiquitin–protein ligase)–protein complex; 7, conjugation of multiple molecules of ubiquitin to the protein substrate; 8, recycling of an intact substrate and ubiquitin [mediated by isopeptidase(s)]; 9, ATP-dependent degradation of conjugates into peptides by the 26S protease complex; 10, release of amino acids from peptides. (Reproduced from Ciechanover, 1993, with permission.)

16.4.2 Selection of substrates for conjugation and degradation

Ubiquitin ligase (E3) recognizes structural determinants of proteins that render them susceptible to the ubiquitin proteolytic system. Selective modification of the beta-amino group of proteins inhibits their degradation in a ubiquitin-dependent system, indicating that a free and exposed terminal amino group is an important signal for protein degradation by the ubiquitin system. Conversely, the addition of new beta-amino groups can convert the proteins with blocked N-termini into good substrates (Hershko *et al.*, 1984a; Chin *et al.*, 1986; Bachmair, Finley and Varshavsky, 1986). This principle has been termed the 'N-end rule' (Finley and Chau, 1991; Varshavsky, 1992).

Four different types of substrates can be distinguished. Type I substrates have a basic N-terminal residue (His, Arg and Lys). Type II substrates have bulky hydrophobic N-termini (Leu, Trp, Phe and Tyr). A third group of substrates display a Ser, Ala or Thr residue in the N-terminal position (Gonda *et al.*, 1989). Finally, proteins with N-terminal residues other than those cited above are recognized by a fourth type of protein binding site on E3 (Reiss, Kaim and Hershko, 1988). Substrates with acidic N-terminal residues (such as Asn, Gln, Cys) require the participation of arginyl-tRNA-protein transferase, which catalyses the transfer of arginine to the acidic N-termini (Ciechanover *et al.*, 1985; Ferber and Ciechanover, 1986, 1987; Ciechanover, 1993). Acidic residues at the N-terminus probably cannot bind to type 1 E3 alpha (Figure 16.2), but conversion of the acidic residue into a basic residue permits binding between ligase and substrate.

Lysine residues proximal to the free N-terminal residue may also determine binding between ubiquitin and substrate and susceptibility to degradation. Dihydrofolate reductase molecules with different N-terminal residues are metabolically stable, but insertion of 43 amino acid residues derived from the N-terminal region of β-galactosidase at the original N-terminus of the dihydrofolate reductase molecule renders the chimeric molecule susceptible to degradation (Bachmair and Varshavsky, 1989). The β-galactosidase fragment contains two internal lysine residues proximal to the N-terminus, and these confer lability.

These lysine residues bind to multiple ubiquitin residues, which form polyubiquitin chains, labilizing the whole molecule (Chau *et al.*, 1989). These chains are thought to be recognized by the ATP-dependent 26S protease complex, of which the multicatalytic protease (MCP) or proteosome is a component (see below).

In summary, E3 isoenzymes have appropriate protein binding sites, distinguish with a high degree of specificity between different N-terminal residues of proteolytic substrates, and catalyse the conjugation of many ubiquitin molecules linked by the carboxy-terminal glycine residues to ϵ-NH$_2$ groups of lysine residues of the substrate proteins through isopeptide bonds (Ciechanover *et al.*, 1980; Hershko *et al.*, 1986; Reiss, Kaim and Hershko, 1988). Much remains to be learned about the mechanisms by which proteins are targeted for degradation through the ubiquitin system (Ciechanover, 1993).

16.4.3 Protein degradation and regeneration of free ubiquitin

Proteins conjugated to ubiquitin chains through E3 are marked for degradation by an ATP-dependent large protease complex (M_r 1300 kDa, S value 26), which has been identified and purified from reticulocytes (Hershko *et al.*, 1984b; Hough, Pratt and Rechsteiner, 1986, 1987; Ganoth *et al.*, 1988; Rivett *et al.*, 1991). Three different factors, all of which are required for conjugate breakdown, combine to form a multienzyme complex whose exact mode of action is still not known. The largest component of the 26S complex is a 20S, 700-kDa enzyme complex, known variously as macropain, the multicatalytic protease (MCP) or the proteosome (Hershko, 1991; Rivett *et al.*, 1991; Ciechanover, 1993). The 26S complex consists of several subunits, the largest having molecular weights of 100 kDa and 110 kDa, and a number of smaller subunits with molecular weights ranging from about 20 to 64 kDa. Three conjugate-degrading factors (CF-1, CF-2 and CF-3) were isolated fron reticulocytes, and CF-3 was identified as the 20S multicatalytic protease (Eytan *et al.*, 1989). The presence of the three factors is thought to confer specificity on the complex, so that only ubiquitin conjugates are degraded (Ciechanover, 1993). Ultrastructurally, MCP from rat liver consists of at least 24 subunits arranged as a hollow cylindrical structure consisting of four hexagonal rings. The polypeptides of rat MCP are encoded by at least nine genes, some of which belong to the same family. The complex also contains RNA, which is protected from nucleases by the proteins (Rivett *et al.*, 1991). An important physiological role for the proteosome is implied by the observation that mutations of genes encoding for the proteosome subunits are lethal for yeast cells (Fujiwara *et al.*, 1990; Heinemeyer *et al.*, 1991).

Free ubiquitin is finally recycled by the action of specific hydrolases that cleave the peptide bond at its carboxy-terminal glycine (Hershko *et al.*, 1980). A family of such enzymes has been characterized from bovine thymus (Mayer and Wilkinson, 1989). All of them appear to be thiol proteases. A cDNA for the isozyme that is predominant in bovine thymus has recently been cloned (Wilkinson *et al.*, 1989) and analysis of its amino acid sequence has revealed a 54% homology with the neurone-specific protein PGP 9.5. Wilkinson *et al.* (1989) showed that PGP 9.5 actually possesses ubiquitin terminal hydrolase activity.

16.5 UBIQUITIN AND LYSOSOMES

It has recently been suggested that the amyloid precursor protein (APP) and prion protein, which are implicated in the pathogenesis of Alzheimer's disease and spongiform encephalopathies, are processed via the endosomal–lysosomal system (Lowe *et al.*, 1990; Mayer *et al.*, 1992; Golde *et al.*, 1992; Haas *et al.*, 1992). Indeed, it has been suggested that the generation of amyloidogenic fragments from APP may take place in the lysosome (Golde *et al.*, 1992). Ubiquitin immunoreactivity and APP immunoreactivity are both localized in lysosomal dense bodies in animals that have received prolonged intraventricular infusions of the protease inhibitor leupeptin, and this treatment increases the number of potentially amyloidogenic APP fragments (Hajimohammadreza et al., 1992). Ubiquitin–protein conjugates accumulate when lysosomal function is disturbed by drugs (Doherty et al., 1989; Anderson et al., 1992), and ubiquitin-IR immunoreactive material corresponding to lysosomal dense bodies accumulates in the ageing brain (Dickson et al., 1990; Migheli et al., 1992). Lysosomes contain both free and conjugated ubiquitin (Shwartz et al., 1988; Laszlo et al., 1990). It is not yet clear what part ubiquitin plays in lysosomal functions, but cells carrying a mutation of the ubiquitin-activating enzyme E1 cannot degrade proteins in lysosomes, suggesting that ubiquitin has a significant role in lysosomal protein processing (Gropper et al., 1991). Nevertheless, anti-ubiquitin antibodies do not usually label membrane-bound inclusions in typical lysosomal storage disorders such as GM2 gangliosidosis or mucopoly-saccharidosis type II (Manetto et al., 1989; Zhan, Beyreuther and Schmitt, 1992).

In summary, the ubiquitin proteolytic system is a complex pathway for degrading and modifying proteins (Wilkinson, 1987). The rapid degradation of proteins such as cyclin and p53 suggests that ubiquitin is important in modifying key cellular functions, as well as in removing damaged and potentially damaging proteins. Induction of ubiquitin synthesis occurs as a result of cell stress, including accumulation of damaged proteins and heat shock and, in some situations, the ability to synthesize ubiquitin determines cell survival after heat shock. Failure to degrade abnormal proteins produced as a result of toxic damage by an environmental agent, or as the result of genetic defects, could lead to progressive cellular damage and the accumulation of insoluble, damaging material in the form of inclusions. While this is an attractive hypothesis, there is no direct evidence that neuronal inclusions are more than markers of cell damage. Nor is there evidence to suggest that a primary abnormality of the ubiquitin proteolytic system is responsible for any neurodegenerative process or disease. The association between ubiquitin and a wide range of morphologically different inclusions in many diverse diseases (neurological and non-neurological) argues against a primary pathogenic role for ubiquitin in neurodegeneration. There is a close but not invariable association between ubiquitin and altered intermediate filaments (Manetto et al., 1989; Lowe and Mayer, 1990), but this by itself need not imply a defect in the ubiquitin system. Nevertheless, further investigation of the neurobiology of the ubiquitin and other cell stress systems may clarify aspects of the neurodegenerative process, and there can be no question that antibodies against

351

ubiquitin have provided a powerful new tool in the pathological analysis of MND.

16.6 MORPHOLOGICAL FEATURES OF UBIQUITIN-IMMUNOREACTIVE INCLUSIONS IN MND

Following the discoveries discussed in the preceding section, it was natural to ask whether ubiquitin immunocytochemisty might reveal new aspects of the cellular pathology of MND, on the basis that antibodies might bind to ubiquitin conjugated to unknown or hitherto undetectable cellular proteins. This turned out to be the case, and Leigh *et al.* (1988) and Lowe *et al.* (1988b) independently reported the presence of characteristic ubiquitin-immunoreactive (IR) inclusions within anterior horn cells. These observations have since been confirmed and extended in many studies from the USA, Europe and Japan.

Ubiquitin-IR inclusions in MND take several forms, and are present in anterior horn motor neurones, in brainstem motor neurones and rarely in cortical motor neurones in patients dying from typical sporadic MND of Charcot type (ALS), in patients who have only lower motor neurone signs (progressive muscular atrophy), in patients with familial MND/ALS, and in patients with MND and dementia (Leigh *et al.*, 1988; Lowe *et al.*, 1988b, 1989; Murayama *et al.*, 1989; Kato *et al.*, 1989; Sasaki *et al.*, 1989; Murayama *et al.*, 1990a; Migheli *et al.*, 1990; Mizusawa *et al.*, 1991; Schiffer *et al.*, 1991; Leigh *et al.*, 1991). Filamentous inclusions (Figure 16.3), originally described as 'skein-like' inclusions (Leigh *et al.*, 1988), represent the most abundant type. These often form delicate interlacing bundles in the perikarya and sometimes in the dendrites of anterior horn cells or brain'stem motor neurones (Leigh *et al.*, 1991). Ultrastructurally they consist of bundles of filaments measuring 10–25 nm (and thus thicker than typical neurofilaments) arranged in the form of tubular structures, and associated with granular material (Lowe *et al.*, 1988b; Mizusawa *et al.*, 1991; Schiffer *et al.*, 1991). Murayama *et al.* (1990a) considered that 12-nm coated filaments were associated with Bunina bodies and suggested that these ubiquitinated structures might represent the precursors of true Bunina bodies.

The second most common type of ubiquitin-IR inclusion is the dense accumulation or dense body (Figure 16.4). In sections stained with haematoxylin and eosin or other routine stains, dense bodies sometimes correspond to Lewy body-like inclusions or to poorly defined hyaline or vacuolar areas that are neither eosinophilic nor basophilic (Leigh *et al.*, 1991; Mather *et al.*, in press). Ultrastructurally, dense bodies of Lewy body-like type are composed of radially arranged filaments with a granulofilamentous core, often containing lipofuscin granules (Kusaka

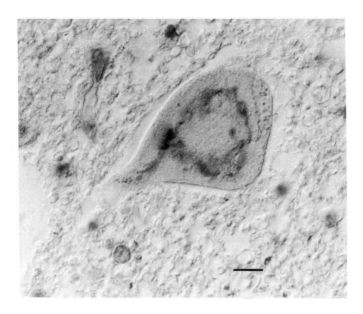

Figure 16.3 MND. Spinal motor neurone containing skein-like ubiquitin-IR inclusion which is extending into the dendrite. Nomarski interference optics. Bar = 15 μm.

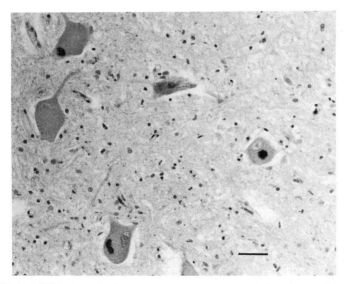

Figure 16.4 MND. Anterior horn motor neurones containing dense ubiquitin-IR inclusions. Bar = 50 μm.

Ubiquitin

et al., 1988; Lowe *et al.*, 1988b; Murayama *et al.*, 1989, 1990a; Schiffer *et al.*, 1991; Kusaka *et al.*, 1992). Some of the filaments are 10–15 nm in diameter (and thus may represent neurofilaments), while some are 15–25 nm in diameter and are thus slightly larger than typical neurofilaments. Some of the structures described in anterior horn cells (Kusaka *et al.*, 1992) are similar to those that have been observed in the dentate granule cells of the hippocampus.

While Lewy body-like inclusions are often ubiquitin positive, Bunina bodies are not usually labelled by antibodies against ubiquitin (Matsumoto, Hirano and Goto, 1990; Leigh *et al.*, 1991) although they are often associated with ubiquitin-IR structures (Murayama *et al.*, 1990a).

Skeins are usually more abundant than ubiquitin-IR dense bodies, but in some patients one may see only skeins or only dense bodies (Leigh *et al.*, 1988, 1991). Between 1 and 40% of surviving motor neurones contain ubiquitin-IR inclusions. The inclusions are least abundant in patients with severe cell loss, and most abundant when the disease is of short duration, probably because there are more motor neurones surviving (Schiffer *et al.*, 1991). In some cases a careful search must be made of motor neurones in 10 or more sections before any inclusions can be identified.

The diagnostic specificity and sensitivity of these inclusions has not been rigorously tested, and relatively few neurologically abnormal controls have been examined in detail. Nevertheless, inclusions are found in virtually all MND patients, but only very rarely in neurologically normal controls or in patients with other neurological disorders (Leigh *et al.*, 1991). Intraneuronal skein-like inclusions have recently been described in multiple system atrophy (MSA), although the ubiquitin-IR inclusions were present in neurones of the pontine nuclei rather than motor neurones (Papp and Lantos, 1992). Similar inclusions are not seen in spinal motor neurones following poliomyelitis (Lowe *et al.*, 1989; Leigh *et al.*, 1991) or in patients with spinal muscular atrophy (SMA) (Murayama, Bouldin and Suzuki, 1991; Garofalo *et al.*, 1991a) in which swollen neurones often show diffuse or concentric immunolabelling with ubiquitin antibodies.

Spinal motor neurones in the Western Pacific form of MND (the ALS–parkinsonism–dementia complex) contain ubiquitin-IR inclusions identical to those seen in typical MND (Matsumoto, Hirano and Goto, 1990), which perhaps is not surprising since the pathology of motor system degeneration in Western Pacific ALS is very similar to that of typical MND. It is interesting that even in Guam ALS/MND, the ubiquitin-IR inclusions in lower motor neurones are not associated with tau or other altered cytoskeletal proteins. Thus the typical molecular pathology of MND (i.e. ubiquitin-IR inclusions that are not identified by other

Table 16.2 Molecular pathology of cortical inclusions in MND with dementia

		Molecular marker							
Inclusion	*Distribution*	*UB*	*Ag*	*PNF*	*Tau*	*CG-A*	*αBC*	*GS*	*EM*
Pick body	FT NC, DGCs HC-PCs	+	++	++	++	++	−	−	15-nm filaments
Cortical LBs	TP NC, PHG	++	+/−	+/−	−	?	++	+	10–15-nm filaments, granular material
MND	FT NC, DGCs	++	−	−	−	+/−	−[a]	−[b]	20-nm filaments, granular material

Modified, with permission, from Kew and Leigh, 1992.
[a] Courtesy of Dr James Lowe.
[b] Courtesy of Professor M. Haltia.
Abbreviations: αBC, α-B-Crystallin; Ag, silver stains; CG-A, chromogranin A; DGCs, dentate granule cells; EM, electron microscope appearance; FT, frontotemporal; GS, gelsolin; HC-PC, hippocampal pyramidal cells; LB, Lewy bodies; MND, neocortical inclusions in motor neurone disease; NC, neocortex; PHG, parahippocampal gyrus; PNF, phosphorylated neurofilaments; TP, temporoparietal.

antibodies or stains) may exist alongside the widespread accumulation of altered tau in other brain regions.

It is also interesting that, outside the endemic foci in the Western Pacific, MND is occasionally associated with dementia, which is often of frontal lobe type (Hudson, 1981; Neary *et al.*, 1990; Kew and Leigh, 1992) and frequently familial (Hudson, 1981; Gunnarsson, Dahlbom and Strandman, 1992). In the MND–dementia syndrome, spinal cord and brainstem motor neurones contain ubiquitin-IR inclusions identical to those in typical MND, but the cerebral pathology is distinctive, and differs from that of Alzheimer's disease, the ALS–parkinsonism–dementia complex and typical Pick's disease (Table 16.2). A characteristic feature of MND–dementia is the presence of round, elliptical or elongated ubiquitin-IR inclusions in hippocampal dentate granule cells (Figure 16.5). Although these inclusions are particularly striking in patients with MND–dementia (Okamoto *et al.*, 1992; Wightman *et al.*, 1992), they have also been noted in MND patients who are not demented (Okamoto *et al.*, 1991a; Wightman *et al.*, 1992). At the ultrastructural level, the inclusions differ from Pick bodies (Figure 16.6), which typically consist of randomly orientated straight filaments of

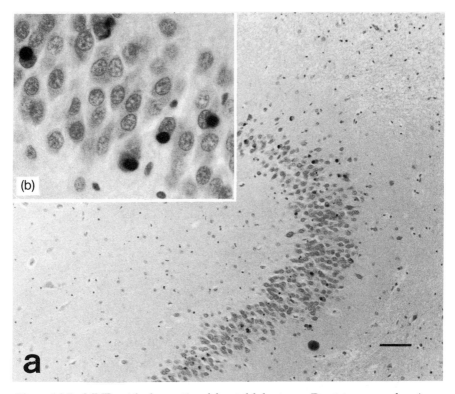

Figure 16.5 MND with dementia of frontal lobe type. Dentate gyrus showing ubiquitin-IR inclusions at low (a) and high (b) magnification. Bar = 150 μm (a) and 20 μm (b).

about 15 nm diameter, associated with paired twisted profiles with a minimum diameter of 13 nm and a maximum diameter of 26 nm, and a twist periodicity of 120 nm (Murayama *et al.*, 1990b). The dentate granule cell inclusions in MND, in contrast, are composed of two main structures (Figure 16.7). Firstly, there are rounded granular deposits with a diameter of 40–80 nm. Sometimes these appear tubular, or have a denser outer ring and less dense centre. Secondly, there are randomly orientated 'fuzzy' or coated, straight or slightly curved filaments that measure 20 nm in diameter. Both Pick bodies and MND-dentate granule cell inclusions may be associated with lipofuscin granules (Figure 16.6 and 16.7). Immunocytochemically, Pick bodies and the MND inclusions are distinctive, since the former are strongly labelled with antibodies against tau and neurofilaments, whereas the latter are only identified by anti-ubiquitin antibodies (Table 16.2).

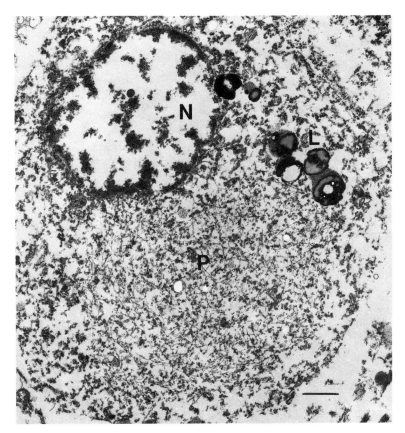

Figure 16.6 Pick's disease; dentate granule cell viewed in the electron microscope. A typical Pick body (P) occupies the lower part of the neurone. Fine 15-nm filaments are associated with granular material and lipofuscin (L). N, nucleus. Bar = 1 μm. (By courtesy of Ms Gillian Wightman.)

Filamentous or rounded ubiquitin-IR inclusions are also seen in neurones of the frontal and temporal neocortex, particularly in layers II and III, where cell loss is most marked in such cases (Figure 16.8). Like the hippocampal inclusions, neocortical inclusions are not argyrophilic, nor are they labelled by antibodies against neurofilaments or the microtubule-associated protein tau (Okamoto *et al.*, 1992; Wightman *et al.*, 1992). Again, this contrasts with Pick bodies, which are strongly argyrophilic, and immunoreactive with antibodies against neurofilaments and tau (Murayama *et al.*, 1990b; Wightman *et al.*, 1992).

Identical inclusions have been reported (Okamoto *et al.*, 1991a; Wightman *et al.*, 1992) in MND patients without significant cognitive

357

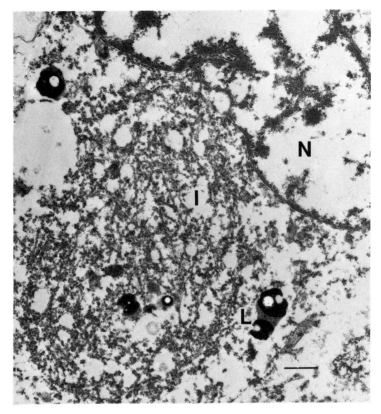

Figure 16.7 MND with dementia of frontal lobe type. Dentate granule cell inclusion (I) showing 20-nm filaments and granular material, associated with lipofuscin (L). Bar = 1 μm. (By courtesy of Ms Gillian Wightman.)

impairment, suggesting that individuals with extra motor cortex involvement may represent a subgroup of MND patients. It remains to be seen whether the hippocampal inclusions are associated with cell loss, or with cognitive abnormalities. Our own preliminary studies do not indicate that there is any loss of dentate granule neurones in MND with dementia. It is, however, known that a significant proportion of MND patients who do not have clinically apparent dementia nevertheless show subtle cognitive impairments, typically when performing tasks that test frontal lobe functions (David and Gilham, 1986; Gallassi *et al.*, 1989). We have recently shown abnormalities of regional cerebral blood flow in the medial frontal lobe, parahippocampal gyrus and retrosplenial cortex using positron emission tomographic (PET) activation techniques (Kew *et al.*, in press). Thus, the pathological findings

358

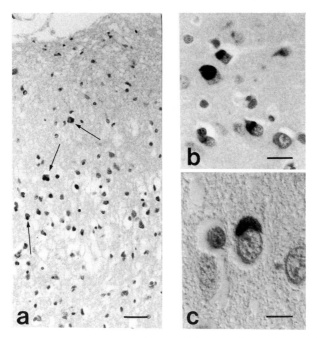

Figure 16.8 MND with dementia of frontal lobe type. Frontal cortex (a) showing pial surface and layers I, II and III, with ubiquitin-IR inclusions in layers II and III (arrows). Bar = 150 μm. Ubiquitin-IR inclusions in the neocortex may be round or 'tangle' shaped (b; bar = 20 μm) or banana-shaped (c; bar = 10 μm).

and changes on functional brain imaging suggest that involvement of the extra motor cortex may be more common than has been appreciated, and any cognitive changes are more likely to be related to neocortical pathology than damage to the dentate granule cells. The foregoing discussion raises the question of whether MND should now be regarded as a multisystem disorder with predilection for the motor system. This certainly seems to be the case with familial MND (Trevor-Hughes and Jerrome, 1971; Kato, Hirano and Kurland, 1987; Wolf, Crain and Siddique, 1991; Kato and Hirano, 1992; Tranchant *et al.*, 1992). It will be interesting to know whether ubiquitin-IR inclusions accumulate in areas of the brain not usually involved in MND, but which degenerate in patients with unusually prolonged survival (Hayashi and Kato, 1989; Mizutani *et al.*, 1992). Such patients show much in common pathologically with the familial patients who show quite widespread neuronal degeneration.

Generally, clinical features of the disease do not correlate closely with the distribution and type of ubiquitin-IR inclusions. It is rare to find

359

ubiquitin-IR inclusions in the motor cortex (Leigh *et al.*, 1991). When they are present they take the form of dense bodies or skeins (Lowe *et al.*, 1989; Leigh *et al.*, 1991), although occasionally small ubiquitin-IR inclusions identical to those seen in the frontotemporal cortex in MND with dementia have been noted in layers II and V of the motor cortex (Nihei, McKee and Kowall, 1991). These motor cortex inclusions may be more common in patients with predominantly upper motor neurone signs (Lowe *et al.*, 1989).

Rarely, Bunina bodies and ubiquitin-IR inclusions in the neurones of Onuf's nucleus in the sacral spinal cord may be associated with urinary incontinence (Lowe *et al.*, 1989). This suggests that selective sparing of this nucleus is a relative phenomenon (Kihira *et al.*, 1991; Okamoto *et al.*, 1991b). Similarly, inclusions are occasionally present in the oculomotor nuclei, although they are typically spared by the disease process (Leigh *et al.*, 1991). Anterior horn cell ubiquitin-IR inclusions may be more abundant in patients with a relatively short clinical course (Schiffer *et al.*, 1991), perhaps because there are more surviving neurones in such cases. Skein-like (ubiquitin-IR) inclusions are often present in anterior horn cells looking relatively normal, although more frequently they are seen in shrunken hyaline or achromasic neurones. The inclusions are more commonly found in neurones that lack Nissl substance (Leigh *et al.*, 1991).

Antibodies against the ubiquitin terminal hydrolase PGP 9.5 label Lewy bodies, but not inclusions in MND, although some motor neurones are more intensely labelled than others, leading to speculation that some cells may be responding to the accumulation of ubiquitin–protein conjugates by increasing attempts to liberate free ubiquitin.

Thus ubiquitin-IR inclusions represent a characteristic and possibly specific feature of the cellular pathology of MND in its various forms, and represent an important pathological marker. Because they are more easily detected and more common than Bunina bodies or Lewy body-like inclusions, they can be regarded as the cellular hallmark of MND. Further work, however, is necessary to establish the precise sensitivity and specificity of the presence of ubiquitin-IR inclusions in anterior horn motor neurones.

16.7 UBIQUITIN-IR INCLUSIONS AND THE PATHOGENESIS OF MND

The presence of ubiquitin-IR material in motor and non-motor neurones in MND probably indicates that ubiquitin–protein conjugates which are resistant to degradation via the ubiquitin proteolytic pathway accumulate in vulnerable neurones. Intermediate filaments may be targeted for ubiquitination, but there is little direct biochemical evidence for this

(Manetto *et al.*, 1989; Lowe, Mayer and Landon, 1993). Although fila-mentous structures are present in skeins and in Lewy body-like inclusions in MND, there is little evidence from many immunocyto-chemical studies that neurofilaments are the target for ubiquitin conjugation. Furthermore, antibodies against a wide range of cyto-skeletal proteins (Leigh *et al.*, 1989a) have not identified other components of the ubiquitin-IR inclusions in MND.

Ubiquitin-IR inclusions in MND so far have not been analysed biochemically, although attempts have been made to do so (Garofalo *et al.*, 1991b). The inclusions are scarce in comparison with neurofibrill-ary tangles, which can be isolated from post-mortem tissue. It seems unlikely that protein chemistry and microsequencing will be applicable to the molecular dissection of the MND inclusions, although affinity techniques such as the use of magnetic beads coated with anti-ubiquitin antibody may eventually prove successful.

The presence of ubiquitin in injured cells may reflect a heat-shock response; Heggie *et al.* (1989) examined ubiquitin gene expression and found increased expression of the ubiquitin C gene (which is under the control of a heat-shock promoter) in MND spinal cord compared with controls. Ubiquitin could be overexpressed as a result of increased turnover, or ubiquitin may be involved in a non-specific response of the damaged neurone. Is the increased expression of ubiquitin cytoprotec-tive, a form of 'cell sanitization', as suggested by Mayer *et al.* (1989)? Ubiquitin expression is increased in damaged or stressed cells, as is heat-shock protein 72 (hsp 72). Heat-shock proteins are synthesized in response to cell damage of various kinds and can indeed be cytoprotec-tive, (Lindquist, 1986; Pelham, 1986; Riabowol, Mizzen and Welch, 1988; Lowe, Mayer and Landon, 1993). Surviving neurones in MND do not, however, express hsp 72 at a high level judged by immunocyto-chemistry (Garofalo *et al.*, 1991a). At present there is no evidence that the presence of ubiquitin in inclusions represents a non-specific expression of a stress response.

Fundamental questions about ubiquitin-IR inclusions in MND remain unanswered. What proteins, if any, are associated with the ubiquitin? If ubiquitin is associated with altered neurofilaments or other cytoskeletal proteins, why are the inclusions not identified by appropriate anti-bodies? What is the relationship between MND and other disorders in which Lewy bodies or similar structures are found? Ultimately it may be possible to identify key molecular events that trigger cytoskeletal degeneration and ubiquitination of cellular proteins – although at present there is no direct evidence that the presence of immunoreactive ubiquitin represents ubiquitin–protein conjugates, or indeed is related to this particular function of ubiquitin. The finding of point mutations in the gene encoding the cytosolic enzyme superoxide dismutase 1 (SOD 1) in familial MND (Rosen *et al.*, 1993) raises the possibility that free radical-related damage could lead to cross-linking of cellular proteins. Cross-linked proteins are not good substrates for degradation, and can form insoluble aggregates. In addition, damaged or abnormal proteins can induce a heat-shock response, as can free radicals directly (Ananthan, Goldberg and Voelly, 1986). On balance, the evidence suggests that ubiquitin-IR deposits in neurones probably do represent aggregated proteins that are resistant to the normal proteolytic processes.

16.8 SUMMARY AND CONCLUSIONS

The discovery of characteristic ubiquitin-immunoreactive inclusions in vulnerable neurones in MND has provided a new basis for investigating the molecular consequences and possibly the pathogenic mechanisms of cell damage. New insights into the biology of ubiquitin and the heat-shock response may explain why ubiquitin accumulates in degenerating motor neurones, although its presence may yet turn out to be a non-specific response. The presence of filamentous structures within these inclusions probably indicates that ubiquitin is associated with altered cytoskeletal components of some sort, but MND is strikingly different from other neurodegenerative diseases in that antibodies against cytoskeletal proteins do not identify the skein-like inclusions, although occasionally hyaline bodies or Lewy body-like inclusions are labelled by anti-neurofilament antibodies. At present there is no evidence that abnormalities of neurofilament phosphorylation or processing play a pathogenic role in MND, although this possibility has not been absolutely discounted.

The next few years of research are likely to bring important new information on the clinical, pathological and molecular significance of the findings described in this chapter, particularly as the implications of the mutations identified in familial MND are explored. The study of molecular pathology has been decisive in locating genetic abnormalities in Alzheimer's disease and the prion disorders, and there is hope that this approach will also be fruitful in MND, particularly since not all familial cases can be explained on the basis of SOD 1 mutations, and in the majority of sporadic cases the pathogenic role of SOD 1 and related enzymes remains wholly conjectural. Identification of abnormal proteins in MND motor neurones may enable us to move closer to the biochemical processes associated with cell death, and thus to the pathogenic mechanisms of the disease. It should soon be possible to model MND through transgenic approaches, and ultimately to bring together the molecular pathology and biochemical pathology.

REFERENCES

Ananthan, J., Goldberg, A.L. and Voelly, R. (1986) Abnormal proteins serve as eukaryotic stress signals and trigger activation of heat shock genes. *Science*, **232**, 522–4.

Askanas, V., Serdaroglu, P.K., Engel, W. and Alvarez, R.B. (1991) Immunolocalization of ubiquitin in muscle biopsies of patients with inclusion body myositis and oculopharyngeal muscular dystrophy. *Neurosci. Lett.*, **130**, 73–6.

Bachmair, A. and Varshavsky, A. (1989) The degradation signal in a short-lived protein. *Cell*, **56**, 1019–32.

Bachmair, A., Finley, D. and Varshavsky, A. (1986) *In vivo* half-life of a protein is a function of its amino-terminal residue. *Science*, **234**, 179–86.

Bancher, C., Lassmann, H., Budka, H. *et al.* (1989) An antigenic profile of Lewy bodies: immunocytochemical indication for protein phosphorylation and ubiquitination. *J. Neuropathol. Exp. Neurol.*, **48**, 81–93.

Bond, U. and Schlesinger, M.J. (1985) Ubiquitin is a heat shock protein in chicken embryo fibroblasts. *Mol. Cell. Biol.*, **5**, 949–56.

Chau, V., Tobias, J.W., Bachmair, A. *et al.* (1989) A multiubiquitin chain is confined to specific lysine in a targeted short-lived protein. *Science*, **243**, 1576–83.

Chin, D.T., Carlson, N., Kuehl, L. and Rechsteiner, M. (1986) The degradation of guanidinated lysozyme in reticulocyte lysate. *J. Biol. Chem.*, **261**, 3883–90.

Ciechanover, A. (1993) The ubiquitin-mediated proteolytic pathway. *Brain Pathol.*, **3**, 67–75.

Ciechanover, A., Finley, D. and Varshavsky, A. (1984) Ubiquitin dependence of selective protein degradation demonstrated in the mammalian cell cycle mutant ts85. *Cell*, **37**, 57–66.

Ciechanover, A., Heller, H., Elias, S. *et al.* (1980) ATP-dependent conjugation of reticulocyte proteins with the polypeptide required for protein degradation. *Proc. Natl. Acad. Sci. USA*, **77**, 1365–8.

Ciechanover, A., Heller, H., Katz-Etzion, R. and Hershko, A. (1981) Activation of the heat stable polypeptide of the ATP-dependent proteolytic system. *Proc. Natl. Acad. Sci. USA*, **78**, 761–5.

Ciechanover, A., Wolin, S.L., Steitz, J.A. and Lodish, H.F. (1985) Transfer RNA is an essential component of the ubiquitin- and ATP-dependent proteolytic system. *Proc. Natl. Acad. Sci. USA*, **82**, 1341–5.

Ciechanover, A., DiGiuseppe, J., Bercovich, B. *et al.* (1991) Degradation of nuclear oncoproteins by the ubiquitin system *in vitro*. *Proc. Natl. Acad. Sci. USA*, **88**, 139–43.

Cole, G.M. and Timiras, P.S. (1987) Ubiquitin–protein conjugates in Alzheimer's lesions. *Neurosci. Lett.*, **79**, 207–12.

Ubiquitin

David, A.S. and Gilham, R.A. (1986) Neuropsychological study of motor neuron disease. *Psychosomatics*, **27**, 441–5.

Dickson, D.W., Wertkin, A., Kress, Y. *et al.* (1990) Ubiquitin immunoreactive structures in normal human brains. *Lab. Invest.*, **63**, 87–99.

Doherty, F.J., Osborn, N.U., Wassall, J.A. *et al.* (1989) Ubiquitin–protein conjugates accumulate in the lysosomal system of fibroblasts treated with cysteine proteinase inhibitors. *Biochem. J.*, **263**, 47–55.

Eytan, E., Ganoth, D., Armon, T. and Hershko, A. (1989) ATP-dependent incorporation of 20S complex that degrades proteins conjugated to ubiquitin. *Proc. Natl. Acad. Sci. USA*, **86**, 7751–5.

Ferber, S. and Ciechanover, A. (1986) Transfer RNA is required for conjugation of ubiquitin to selective substrates of the ubiquitin- and ATP-dependent proteolytic system. *J. Biol. Chem.*, **261**, 3128–34.

Ferber, S. and Ciechanover, A. (1987) Role of arginine-tRNA in protein degradation by the ubiquitin pathway. *Nature*, **326**, 808–11.

Finley, D. and Chau, V. (1991) Ubiquitination. *Annu. Rev. Cell. Biol.*, **7**, 25–69.

Fried, V.A., Smith, H.T., Hildebrandt, E. and Weiner, K. (1987) Ubiquitin has intrinsic proteolytic activity: implications for cellular regulation. *Proc. Natl. Acad. Sci. USA*, **84**, 3685–9.

Fujiwara, T., Tanaka, K., Orino, E. *et al.* (1990) Proteosomes are essential for yeast proliferation: cDNA cloning and gene disruption of two major subunits. *J. Biol. Chem.*, **265**, 16604–13.

Galassi, R., Montagna, P., Morreale, A. *et al.* (1989) Neuropsychological, electroencephalogram, and brain-computed tomographic findings in motor neurone disease. *Eur. Neurol.*, **29**, 115–20.

Ganoth, D., Leshinsky, E., Eytan, E. and Hershko, A. (1988) A multicomponent system that degrades proteins conjugated to ubiquitin. *J. Biol. Chem.*, **263**, 12412–19.

Garofalo, O., Leigh, N., Martin, J. *et al.* (1991) An immunocytochemical study of spinal muscular atrophy, in *New Evidence in MND/ALS Research*, vol. 2, *Advances in ALS/MND* (ed. F. Clifford Rose), Smith-Gordon, London, pp. 225–8.

Garofalo, O., Kennedy, P.G.E., Swash, M. *et al.* (1991b) Ubiquitin and heat shock expression in amyotrophic lateral sclerosis. *Neuropathol. Appl. Neurobiol.*, **17**, 39–46.

Garofalo, O., Hajimohammadreza, I., Leigh, P.N. *et al.* (1991a) Development of methods for the identification of abnormal proteins in ALS, in *New Evidence in MND/ALS Research*, vol. 2, *Advances in ALS/MND* (ed. F. Clifford Rose), Smith-Gordon, London, pp. 139–41.

Glotzer, M., Murray, A.W. and Kirschner, M.W. (1991) Cyclin is degraded by the ubiquitin pathway. *Nature*, **349**, 132–8.

Golde, T.E., Estus, S., Younkin, L.H. *et al.* (1992) Processing of the amyloid protein precursor to potentially amyloidogenic derivatives. *Science*, **255**, 728–30.

Goldstein, G., Scheid, M., Hammmerling, U. *et al.* (1975) Isolation of a polypeptide that has lymphocyte-differentiating properties and is probably represented universally in living cells. *Proc. Natl. Acad. Sci. USA*, **72**, 11–15.

Gonda, D.K., Bachmair, A., Wunning, I. *et al.* (1989) Universality and structure of the N-end rule. *J. Biol. Chem.*, **264**, 16700–12.

Gropper, R., Brandt, R.A., Elias, S. *et al.* (1989) The ubiquitin-activating enzyme, E1, is required for stress-induced lysosomal degradation of cellular proteins. *J. Biol. Chem.*, **266**, 3602–10.

Gunnarsson, L.-C., Dahlbom, K. and Strandman, E. (1991) Motor neuron disease and dementia reported among 13 members of a single family. *Acta Neurol. Scand.*, **84**, 429–33.

Haas, A.L., Bright, P.M. and Jackson, V.E. (1988) Functional diversity among putative E2 isozymes in the mechanism of ubiquitin–histone ligation. *J. Biol. Chem.*, **263**, 13268–75.

Haas, A.L., Warms, J.V.B., Hershko, A. and Rose, I.A. (1982) Ubiquitin-activating enzyme. *J. Biol. Chem.*, **257**, 2543–8.

Haas, C., Koo, E.H., Mellon, A. *et al.* (1992) Targeting of cell surface β-amyloid precursor protein to lysosomes: alternative processing into amyloid-bearing fragments. *Nature*, **357**, 500–3.

Hajimohammadreza, I., Anderson, V.E.R., Cavanagh, J.B. *et al.* (1992) Leupeptin induces an accumulation of ubiquitin-conjugated proteins and amyloid precursor protein (APP) fragment in rat brain. *Society for Neuroscience Abstracts*, 22nd Annual Meeting, Anaheim, California, October 1992, **18**, 565.

Hayashi, H. and Kato, S. (1989) Total manifestations of ALS. ALS in the totally locked-in state. *J. Neurol. Sci.*, **93**, 19–35.

Heggie, P., Burdon, T., Lowe, J. *et al.* (1989) Ubiquitin gene expression in brain and spinal cord in motor neurone disease. *Neurosci. Lett.*, **102**, 343–8.

Heinemeyer, W., Kleinschmidt, J.A., Saidowsky, J. *et al.* (1991) Proteinase yscE, the yeast protosome/multicatalytic-multifunctional proteinase: mutants unravel its function in stress induced proteolysis and uncover its necessity for cell survival. *EMBO J.*, **10**, 555–62.

Hershko, A. (1991) The ubiquitin pathway for protein degradation. *Trends Biochem. Sci.*, **16**, 265–8.

Hershko, A. and Ciechanover, A. (1992) The ubiquitin system for protein degradation. *Annu. Rev. Biochem.*, **61**, 761–807.

Hershko, A., Ciechanover, A. and Rose, I.A. (1981) Identification of the active aminoacid residue of the polypeptide of ATP-dependent protein breakdown. *J. Biol. Chem.*, **256**, 1525–8.

Hershko, A., Ciechanover, A., Heller, H. *et al.* (1980) Proposed role of ATP in protein breakdown: conjugation of proteins with multiple chains of the polypeptide of ATP-dependent proteolysis. *Proc. Natl. Acad. Sci. USA*, **77**, 1783–6.

Hershko, A., Eytan, E., Ciechanover, A. and Haas, A.L. (1982) Immunochemical analysis of the turnover of ubiquitin–protein conjugates in intact cells. *J. Biol. Chem.*, **257**, 13964–70.

Ubiquitin

Hershko, A., Heller, H., Elias, S. and Ciechanover, A. (1983) Components of ubiquitin–protein ligase system. *J. Biol. Chem.*, **258**, 8206–14.

Hershko, A., Heller, H., Eytan, E. *et al.* (1984a) Role of the alpha-amino group of protein in ubiquitin-mediated protein breakdown. *Proc. Natl. Acad. Sci. USA*, **81**, 7021–5.

Hershko, A., Leshinsky, E., Ganoth, D. and Heller, H. (1984b) ATP-dependent degradation of ubiquitin–protein conjugates. *Proc. Natl. Acad. Sci. USA*, **81**, 1619–23.

Hershko, A., Heller, H., Eytan, E. and Reiss, Y. (1986) The protein substrate binding site of the ubiquitin–protein ligase system. *J. Biol. Chem.*, **261**, 11992–9.

Hershko, A., Ganoth, D., Pehrson, J. *et al.* (1991) Methylated ubiquitin inhibits cyclin degradation in clam embryo extracts. *J. Biol. Chem.*, **255**, 376–9.

Hough, R., Pratt, G. and Rechsteiner, M. (1986) Ubiquitin–lysozyme conjugates. Identification and characterization of an ATP-dependent protease from rabbit reticulocyte lysates. *J. Biol. Chem.*, **261**, 2400–8.

Hough, R., Pratt, G. and Rechsteiner, M. (1987). Purification of two high molecular weight proteases from rabbit reticulocyte lysate. *J. Biol. Chem.*, **262**, 8303–13.

Hough, R.F., Pratt, G.W. and Rechtsteiner, M. (1988) Ubiquitin/ATP-dependent protease, in *Ubiquitin* (ed. M. Rechsteiner), Plenum Press, New York, pp. 101–34.

Hudson, A.J. (1981) Amyotrophic lateral sclerosis and its association with dementia, parkinsonism, and other neurological disorders. *Brain*, **104**, 217–47.

Kato, S. and Hirano, A. (1992) Involvement of the brain stem reticular formation in familial amyotrophic lateral sclerosis. *Clin. Neuropathol.*, **11**, 41–4.

Kato, T., Hirano, A. and Kurland, L.T. (1987) Asymmetric involvement of the spinal cord involving both large and small anterior horn cells in a case of familial amyotrophic lateral sclerosis. *Clin. Neuropathol.*, **6**, 67–70.

Kato, T., Katagiri, T., Hirano, A. *et al.* (1989) Lewy body-like hyaline inclusions in sporadic motor neuron disease are ubiquitinated. *Acta Neuropathol.*, **77**, 391–6.

Kew, J.J.M. and Leigh, P.N. (1992) Dementia with motor neurone disease, in *Clinical Neurology. International Practice and Research*. Vol. 1, no. 3. *Unusual Dementias* (ed. M.N. Rossor), Bailliere Tindall, London, pp. 611–26.

Kew, J.J.M., Leigh, P.N., Playford, E.D. *et al.*, Cortical function in amyotrophic lateral sclerosis. *Brain* (in press).

Kihira, T., Yoshida, S., Uebayashi, Y. *et al.* (1991) Involvement of Onuf's nucleus in ALS. Demonstration of intraneuronal conglomerate inclusions and Bunina bodies. *J. Neurol. Sci.*, **104**, 119–28.

Kuncl, R.W., Jin, L. and Rothstein, J.D. (1992) Chronic glutamate toxicity in motor neurons from organotypic spinal cord cultures. *Society for Neuroscience Abstracts*, 22nd Annual Meeting, Anaheim, California, October 1992, **18**, 756.

Kusaka, H., Imai, T., Hashimoto, S. *et al.* (1988) Ultrastructural study of chromatolytic neurons in an adult-onset sporadic case of amyotrophic lateral sclerosis. *Acta Neuropathol.*, **75**, 523–8.

Kuzuhara, S., Mori, H., Izumiyama, N. *et al.* (1988) Lewy bodies are ubiquitinated. A light and electron microscopic immunocytochemical study. *Acta Neuropathol.*, **75**, 345–53.

Laszlo, L., Doherty, F.J., Osborn, N.U. *et al.* (1990) Ubiquitinated protein conjugates are specifically enriched in the lysosomal system of fibroblasts. *FEBS Lett.*, **261**, 365–8.

Leigh, P.N., Anderton, B.H., Dodson, A. *et al.* (1988) Ubiquitin deposits in anterior horn cells in motor neurone disease. *Neurosci Lett.*, **93**, 197–203.

Leigh, P.N., Probst, A., Dale, G.E. *et al.* (1989a) New aspects of the pathology of neurodegenerative disorders as revealed by ubiquitin antibodies. *Acta Neuropathol.*, **79**, 61–72.

Leigh, P.N., Dodson, A., Swash, M. *et al.* (1989b) Cytoskeletal abnormalities in motor neuron disease: an immunocytochemical study. *Brain*, **112**, 521–35.

Leigh, P.N., Whitwell, H., Garofalo, Q. *et al.* (1991) Ubiquitin-immunoreactive intraneuronal inclusions in amyotrophic lateral sclerosis: morphology, distribution, and specificity. *Brain*, **114**, 775–88.

Lennox, G., Lowe, J., Landon, M. and Mayer, R.J. (1989) Anti-ubiquitin immunocytochemistry is more sensitive than conventional techniques in the detection of diffuse Lewy body disease. *J. Neurol. Neurosurg. Psychiatry*, **52**, 67–71.

Leung, D.W., Spencer, S.A., Cachianes, G. *et al.* (1987) Growth hormone receptor and serum binding protein: purification, cloning and expression. *Nature*, **330**, 537–43.

Lindquist, S. (1986) The heat-shock response. *Annu. Rev. Biochem.*, **55**, 1151–91.

Lindquist, S. and Craig, E.A. (1988) The heat-shock proteins. *Annu. Rev. Genet.*, **22**, 631–77

Love, S., Saitoh, T., Quijada, S. *et al.* (1988) Alz-50, ubiquitin and tau immunoreactivity of neurofibrillary tangles, Pick bodies and Lewy bodies. *J. Neuropathol. Exp. Neurol.*, **47**, 393–405.

Lowe, J. and Mayer, R.J. (1990) Ubiquitin, cell stress and diseases of the nervous system. *Neuropathol. Appl. Neurobiol.*, **16**, 281–92.

Lowe, J., Mayer, R.J. and Landon, M. (1993) Ubiquitin in neurodegenerative diseases. *Brain Pathol.*, **3**, 55–65.

Lowe, J., Blanchard, A., Morrell, K. *et al.* (1988a) Ubiquitin is a common factor in intermediate filament inclusion bodies of diverse type in man, including those of Parkinson's disease, Pick's disease, and Alzheimer's disease, as well as Rosenthal fibres in cerebellar astrocytomas, cytoplasmic bodies in muscle, and Mallory bodies in alcoholic liver disease. *J. Pathol.*, **155**, 9–15.

Lowe, J., Lennox, G., Jefferson, D. *et al.* (1988b) A filamentous inclusion body within anterior horn neurones in motorneurone disease defined by immunocytochemical localisation of ubiquitin. *Neurosci. Lett.*, **94**, 203–10.

Ubiquitin

Lowe, J., Aldridge, F., Lennox, G. *et al.* (1989) Inclusion bodies in motor cortex and brainstem of patients with motor neurone disease are detected by immunocytochemical localisation of ubiquitin. *Neurosci. Lett.*, **105**, 7–13.

Lowe, J., McDermott, H., Kenward, N. *et al.* (1990) Ubiquitin conjugate immunoreactivity in the brains of scrapie infected mice. *J. Pathol.*, **162**, 61–6.

Manetto, V., Abdul-Karim, F.W., Perry, G. *et al.* (1989) Selective presence of ubiquitin in intracellular inclusions. *Am. J. Pathol.*, **134**, 505–13.

Mather, K., Martin, J., Swash, M. *et al.*, Histochemical and immunocytochemical study of ubiquitinated inclusions in amyotrophic lateral sclerosis. *Neuropathol. Appl. Neurobiol.* (in press).

Matsumoto, S., Hirano, A. and Goto, S. (1990) Ubiquitin-immunoreactive filamentous inclusions in anterior horn cells of Guamanian and non-Guamanian amyotrophic lateral sclerosis. *Acta Neuropathol.*, **80**, 233–8.

Mayer, A.N., and Wilkinson, K.D. (1989) Detection, resolution and nomenclature of multiple ubiquitin carboxyl-terminal esterases from bovine calf thymus. *Biochemistry*, **28**, 166–72.

Mayer, R.J. Landon, M., Laszlo, L. *et al.* (1992) Protein processing in lysosomes: the new therapeutic target in neurodegenerative disease. *Lancet*, **340**, 156–9.

Migheli, A., Autilio-Gambetti, L., Gambetti, P. *et al.* (1990) Ubiquitinated filamentous inclusions in spinal cord of patients with amyotrophic lateral sclerosis. *Neurosci. Lett.*, **114**, 5–10.

Migheli, A., Attanasio, A., Pezzulo, T. *et al.* (1992) Age-related deposits in dystrophic neurites: an immunoelectron microscopic study. *Neuropathol. Appl. Neurobiol.*, **18**, 3–11.

Mizusawa, H., Nakamura, H., Wakayama, I. *et al.* (1991) Skein-like inclusions in the anterior horn cells in motor neuron disease. *J. Neurol. Sci.*, **105**, 14–21.

Mizutani, T., Sakamaki, S., Tsuchiya, N. *et al.* (1992) Amyotrophic lateral sclerosis with ophthalmoplegia and multisystem degeneration in patients on long-term use of respirators. *Acta Neuropathol.*, **84**, 372–7.

Mori, H., Kondo, J. and Ihara, Y. (1986) Ubiquitin is a component of paired helical filaments in Alzheimer's disease. *Science*, **235**, 1641–6.

Murayama, S., Bouldin, T.W. and Suzuki, K. (1991) Immunocytochemical and ultrastructural studies of Werdnig–Hoffmann disease. *Acta Neuropathol.*, **81**, 408–17.

Murayama, S., Mori, H., Ihara, Y. *et al.* (1990a) Immunocytochemical and ultrastructural studies of lower motor neurons in ALS. *Ann. Neurol.*, **27**, 137–48.

Murayama, S., Mori, H., Ihara, Y. and Tomonaga, M. (1990b) Immunocytochemical and ultrastructural studies of Pick's disease. *Ann. Neurol.*, **27**, 394–405.

Nakazato, Y., Yamazaki, H., Hirato, J. *et al.* (1990) Oligodendroglial microtubular tangles in olivopontocerebellar atrophy. *J. Neuropathol. Exp. Neurol.*, **49**, 521–30.

Neary, D., Snowden, J.S., Mann, D.M.A. *et al.* (1990) Frontal lobe dementia and motor neuron disease. *J. Neurol. Neurosurg. Psychiatr.*, **53**, 23–32.

Nickel, B.E. and Davie, J.R. (1989) Structure of polyubiquitinated histone H2A. *Biochemistry*, **28**, 964–8.

References

Nihei, K., McKee, A.C., and Kowall, N.W. (1991) Ubiquitin immunoreactivity in the Rolandic cortex of patients with sporadic and familial amyotrophic lateral sclerosis (abstract). *J. Neuropathol. Exp. Neurol.*, **50**, 310.

Nihei, K., McKee, A. C., and Kowall, N. W. (1992) GABAergic local circuit neurons degenerate in the motor cortex of amyotrophic lateral sclerosis patients. *Society for Neuroscience Abstracts*, 22nd Annual Meeting, Anaheim, California, October 1992, **18**, 1249.

Okamato, K., Hirai, S., Yamazaki, T. *et al.* (1991a) New ubiquitin-positive intraneuronal inclusions in the extra-motor cortices in patients with amyotrophic lateral sclerosis. *Neurosci. Lett.*, **129**, 233–6.

Okamoto, K., Hirai, S., Ishiguro, K. *et al.* (1991b) Light and electron microscopic and immunohistochemical observations of the Onuf's nucleus of amyotrophic lateral sclerosis. *Acta Neuropathol.*, **81**, 610–14.

Okamoto, K., Murakami, N., Kusaka, H. *et al.* (1992) Ubiquitin-positive intraneuronal inclusions in the extra-motor cortices of presenile dementia patients with motor neuron disease. *J. Neurol.*, **239**, 426–30.

Papp, M.I. and Lantos, P.L. (1992) Accumulation of tubular structures in oligodendroglial and neuronal cells as the basic alteration in multiple system atrophy. *J. Neurol. Sci.*, **107**, 172–82.

Papp, M.I., Kahn, J.E. and Lantos, P.L. (1989) Glial cytoplasmic inclusions in the CNS of patients with multiple system atrophy (striatonigral degeneration, olivopontocerebellar atrophy and Shy–Drager syndrome). *J. Neurol. Sci.*, **94**, 79–100.

Pelham, H.R.B. (1986) Speculations on the functions of the major heat shock and glucose-regulated proteins. *Cell*, **46**, 959–61.

Perry, G., Friedman, R., Shaw, G. and Chau, V. (1987) Ubiquitin is detected in neurofibrillary tangles and senile plaque neurites of Alzheimer disease brains. *Proc. Natl. Acad. Sci. USA*, **84**, 3033–6.

Pickart, C.M. and Rose, I.A. (1985) Functional heterogeneity of ubiquitin-carrier proteins. *J. Biol. Chem.*, **260**, 1573–81.

Pickart, C.M. and Vella, A.T. (1988) Levels of active ubiquitin carrier proteins decline during erythroid maturation. *J. Biol. Chem.*, **263**, 12028–35.

Rechsteiner, M. (1987) Ubiquitin-mediated pathways for intracellular proteolysis. *Annu. Rev. Cell. Biol.* **3**, 1–30.

Reiss, Y., Kaim, D. and Hershko, A. (1988) Specificity of binding of NH_2-terminal residue of proteins to ubiquitin–protein ligase. *J. Biol. Chem.*, **263**, 2693–8.

Riabowol, K.T., Mizzen, L.A. and Welch, W.J. (1988) Heat shock is lethal to fibroblasts microinjected with antibodies against hsp 70. *Science*, **242**, 433–6.

Rivett, A.J., Skilton, H.E., Rowe, A.J. *et al.* (1991) Components of the multicatalytic proteinase complex. *Biomed. Biochim. Acta*, **50**, 447–50.

Rosen, D.R., Siddique, T., Patterson, D. *et al.* (1993) Mutations in Cu/Zn superoxide dismutase gene are associated with familial amyotrophic lateral sclerosis. *Nature*, **362**, 59–62.

Sasaki, S., Yamane, K., Sakuma, H. and Murayama, S. (1989) Sporadic motor neuron disease with Lewy body-like hyaline inclusions. *Acta Neuropathol.*, **78**, 555–60.

Ubiquitin

Schiffer, D., Autilio-Gambetti, L., Chio, A. et al. (1991) Ubiquitin in motor neuron disease; a study at the light and electron microscope level. *J. Neuropathol. Exp. Neurol.*, **50**, 463–73.

Schwartz, A.L., Ciechanover, A., Brandt, R.A. et al. (1988) Immunoelectron microscopic localization of ubiquitin in hepatoma cells. *EMBO J.*, **7**, 2961–6.

Siegelman, M., Bond, M.W., Gallatin, W.M., et al. (1986) Cell surface molecule associated with lymphocyte homing is a ubiquitinated branched-chain glycoprotein. *Science*, **231**, 823–9.

Thorne, A.W., Sautier, P., Briand, G. and Crane-Robinson, C. (1987) The structure of ubiquitinated histone H2B. *EMBO J.*, **6**, 1005–10.

Tranchant, C., Dugay, M.-H., Mohr, M. et al. (1992) Familial motor neuron disease with Lewy body-like inclusions in the substantia nigra, the subthalamic nucleus, and the globus pallidus. *J. Neurol. Sci.*, **108**, 18–23.

Trevor-Hughes, J. and Jerrome, D. (1971) Ultrastructure of anterior horn motor neurones in the Hirano–Kurland–Sayre type of combined neurological system degeneration. *J. Neurol. Sci.*, **13**, 389–99.

Varshavsky, A. (1992) The N-end rule. *Cell*, **69**, 725–35.

Wightman, G., Anderson, V.E.R., Martin, J. et al. (1992) Hippocampal and neocortical ubiquitin-immunoreactive inclusions in amyotrophic lateral sclerosis with dementia. *Neurosci. Lett.*, **139**, 269–74.

Wilkinson, K.D. (1987) Protein ubiquitination: a regulatory post-translational modification. *Anti-Cancer Drug Design*, **2**, 211–29.

Wilkinson, K.D. (1988) Purification and structural properties of ubiquitin, in *Ubiquitin* (ed. M. Rechsteiner), Plenum Press, New York, pp. 5–38.

Wilkinson, K.D., Keunmyoung, L., Deshpande, S. et al. (1989) The neuron-specific protein PGP 9.5 is a ubiquitin carboxyl-terminal hydrolase. *Science*, **246**, 670–73.

Wolf, H.K., Crain, B.J. and Siddique, T. (1991) Degeneration of the substantia nigra in familial amyotrophic lateral sclerosis. *Clin. Neuropathol.*, **10**, 291–6.

Yarden, Y., Escobedo, J.A., Kuang, W.J. et al. (1986) Structure of the receptor for platelet-derived growth factor helps define a family of closely related growth factor receptors. *Nature*, **32**, 226–32.

Zhan, S.-S., Beyreuther, K. and Schmitt, H.P. (1992) Neuronal ubiquitin and neurofilament expression in different lysosomal storage disorders. *Clin. Neuropathol.*, **11**, 251–5.

Zhaung, Z. and McCauley, R. (1989) Ubiquitin is involved in the *in vitro* insertion of monoamine oxidase B into mitochondrial outer membranes. *J. Biol. Chem.*, **264**, 14594–6.

17 Neurofilamentous pathology

DANNY F. WATSON

17. INTRODUCTION

Clinical and pathologic evidence indicates that lower motor neurons in ALS patients persist for days or weeks in a state between normal health and cell death. We still have little information about the cellular processes that occur during this time, processes that link the etiologic agent to cell death. One clue to these processes is the disturbance of neurofilament transport and phosphorylation that occurs during neuronal degeneration in ALS.

Study of the pathogenesis of the neuronal degeneration, the steps by which primary neuronal injury becomes irreversible, seems a valuable avenue for investigation in ALS. As an example, neuronal cell death after hypoxia was once viewed as a straightforward process: ATP stores were depleted, and a variety of endothermic reactions required for cellular homeostasis simply proceeded down their free-energy gradients in the absence of coupling to ATP hydrolysis. Now it has become clear that post-hypoxic neuronal death in fact involves activation of a variety of pathways, such as calcium-activated proteolysis and lipid peroxidation, that lead to catalyzed disintegration of cellular structures. This understanding has led in turn to a variety of investigations into the possibility of intervention to ameliorate the effects of hypoxia.

The study of the process of degeneration in cellular terms, even if it does not address the primary etiology of ALS, could have importance in several ways. For example, the aberrant distribution and modification of NF may directly convert the effects of the primary etiologic agent into irreversible neuronal damage and cellular death. The abnormal distribution and phosphorylation of neurofilaments might also be important as a marker for other intracellular regulatory pathways that have gone awry. Some of the candidate etiologies for ALS include ongoing immune attack on motor neurons or neurotoxins that accumulate in tissue. These etiologies may prove impractical to reverse completely. Hence another

371

potential role for the study of intracellular functions such as transport and phosphorylation of cytoskeletal proteins is to identify potential avenues for therapeutic intervention, areas where the function of damaged motor neurons may be rendered more nearly normal.

This chapter will first review the current data concerning neurofilamentous pathology in ALS, and the few observations in ALS of abnormalities of other cytoskeletal proteins. Next the basic biology of neurofilaments will be reviewed with emphasis on those features especially likely to relate to diseases. Animal models of neurofilamentous pathology will be discussed in light of the recent basic information they have provided about the pathology of neurofilaments.

17.2 NEUROFILAMENTOUS PATHOLOGY IN HUMAN DISEASE

The first modern analysis of the axonal swellings in ALS was performed by Carpenter (1968), who demonstrated that the argyrophilic swellings occasionally mentioned by earlier authors were in fact expansions of proximal axons of lower motor neurons, and further demonstrated that the swellings consisted of massive accumulations of 10-nm neurofilaments. Although small neurofilamentous axonal swellings are a non-specific feature of post-mortem spinal cords (Clark et al., 1984), the axonal swellings in ALS are distinctive in their size and their abundance relative to motor neuron numbers (Delisle and Carpenter, 1984). Some axonal swellings with neurofilamentous accumulations are also seen in the lateral corticospinal tracts of ALS patients (Okamoto et al., 1990).

This proximal distribution of neurofilamentous swellings is characteristic of motor neuron diseases. Distal motor axons in ALS do not exhibit swellings; if any abnormality is apparent among surviving distal motor axons, it is atrophy (Bradley et al., 1983). The two other human disorders with prominent neurofilamentous swellings exhibit them distally: hexacarbon neuropathy (Spencer and Schaumburg, 1977; Ferri et al., 1988) and giant axonal neuropathy (Asbury et al., 1972; Pena, 1982; Donaghy et al., 1988). In these instances, the abnormalities are not specific for motor neurons and the illnesses have little clinical similarity to ALS.

In spinal cords from patients with ALS, the neurofilaments (NF) in the axonal swellings are not simply in the wrong place. They also show abnormal immunohistochemical reactions that identify them as inappropriately highly phosphorylated for their location (Schmidt et al., 1987; Manetto et al., 1988; Munoz et al., 1988; Sasaki et al., 1989; Toyoshima et al., 1989; Matsumoto, Hirano and Goto, 1990a; Murayama et al., 1990; Sobue et al., 1990; Itoh et al., 1992). This pattern has a degree of specificity for disorders with degeneration of cell bodies, for injuries to the motor axon produce little change in phosphorylation (Mansour *et al.*, 1989) and the distal NF accumulations in experimental hexacarbon neuropathy (Watson *et al.*, 1991) and in giant axonal neuropathy (Donaghy *et al.*, 1988; and D.F. Watson, unpublished observations) do not exhibit any striking abnormality of reaction with antibodies to phosphorylated NF epitopes.

The NF swellings are quite unlikely to come from excessive production of NF proteins. Analysis of the mRNA abundance in ALS spinal cords (Clark *et al.*, 1990) showed no significant increase in NF mRNA. Further, as discussed below, the neuronal reaction to a variety of injuries is down-regulation of the synthesis of NF, with the possible complication of some increase in peripherin synthesis (Shelanski, 1991). Hence the focus of understanding the NF swellings has been on the process of active transport that normally distributes NF from their sites of synthesis in the cell bodies to the axon and dendrites.

It is currently equally plausible that aberrant phosphorylation leads to NF accumulation or that it results from NF accumulation induced by another mechanism. There is an abnormal segregation of NF away from the other elements of the axonal cytoskeleton in the regions of NF accumulation. This raises the issue that another cytoskeletal abnormality may underlie the NF accumulation. In this regard, changes in the isotypes of alpha- and beta-tubulin (the chief constituent proteins of microtubules) have been noted in ALS (Binet and Meininger, 1988). In ALS there are apparently also abnormalities in ALS of the fast axonal transport process (Breuer and Atkinson, 1988), which is dependent on microtubules and accomplished by specialized microtubule-associated proteins.

Motor neurons of ALS patients also contain inclusions that are strongly reactive with *ubiquitin* (Matsumoto, Hirano and Goto, 1990b; Migheli *et al.*, 1990; Garofalo *et al.*, 1991; Leigh *et al.*, 1991; Schiffer *et al.*, 1991). The distribution of ubiquitin immunoreactivity overlaps with, but is not identical to, the NF accumulation. Although ubiquitin is not viewed as a true cytoskeletal structure, it is thought to play an important regulatory role in the degradation of cytoplasmic proteins such as neurofilaments. The abnormalities of ubiquitin distribution therefore raise the issue that NF degradation may be altered in ALS, in addition to altered NF transport and phosphorylation.

17.3 BIOLOGY OF NEUROFILAMENTS

The mechanisms that produce abnormal distribution and phosphorylation of NF are not readily studied in human material. Hence, hypotheses concerning the mechanisms of the pathological change rely on the concepts of the chemistry and cell biology of NF obtained largely from experimental data.

17.3.1 NF structure

Neurofilaments are the chief neuronal intermediate filament, the class of intracellular polymer that includes cytokeratins, vimentin, desmin and nuclear lamins. Native NF are usually heteropolymers assembled from three individual subunit proteins. The protein of lowest mass, termed NF-L, is capable of assembly into 10-nm filaments in the absence of the middle (NF-M) and high (NF-H) molecular weight subunits (Geisler and Weber, 1981; Liem and Hutchinson, 1982). The converse is not true – NF-M and NF-H (or a mixture of the two) aggregate into short linear structures that do not closely resemble native neurofilaments.

The amino acid sequence of the NF triplet subunits is known in several vertebrate species (Geisler *et al.*, 1983, 1985; Julien *et al.*, 1987; Levy *et al.*, 1987; Myers *et al.*, 1987; Napolitano *et al.*, 1987; Zopf *et al.*, 1987; Dautigny *et al.*, 1988). The general similarity in architecture is striking, but some variation is found in the number and arrangement of the domains in the carboxy-terminal extensions of NF-M and NF-H, variations that are probably of biological relevance. Each of the three subunits contains polypeptide domains that closely resemble other intermediate filaments in sequence and structure. These regions apparently co-assemble into the backbone of the filament. The long carboxy-terminal extensions of NF-M and NF-H, which are unique among the intermediate filaments, project as side arms (Willard and Simon, 1981). These projections contain the main phosphorylation sites (Geisler *et al.*, 1985; Carden, Schlaepfer and Lee, 1985) and probably mediate most of the interaction of NF with the rest of the structures in the axoplasm.

Lower motor neurons also contain modest amounts of yet another intermediate filament protein, *peripherin* (Portier, de Nechaud and Gros, 1983; Parysek and Goldman, 1987; Landon *et al.*, 1989; Escurat *et al.*, 1990). Other PNS axons also contain peripherin, which has been identified as being related to NF by amino acid sequence and genomic cloning. Some immunocytochemical evidence suggests peripherin may co-assemble with triplet NF proteins *in situ*. So far, much less is known about the biology and pathology of peripherin than the classic NF triplets. *Alpha-internexin*, or NF 66 kDa, is yet another neuronal intermediate filament protein (Pachter, 1985; Chiu *et al.*, 1989). It is absent or perhaps very sparse in lower motor neurons. The possibility that either of these two proteins contributes to the neurofilamentous swellings of ALS has not yet been satisfactorily addressed.

17.3.2 NF phosphorylation

The side arms projecting from the surface of NF contain the Lys–Ser–Pro sites and other serine-rich motifs that form the major multiphosphorylation region (Carden, Schlaepfer and Lee, 1985; Geisler, Vanderkerchove and Weber, 1987). Circular dichroism measurements of synthetic peptides of the sequence of this region from rat NF-M show that phosphorylation induces a marked conformational change from a flexible random coil structure to a more rigid conformation (Otvos et al., 1988). The presence of calcium or aluminum ions markedly affects the conformational change (Hollosi et al., 1992). These are likely to be relevant to the conformation in vivo; a variety of antibodies that recognize phosphorylated NF in vivo also recognize the phosphorylation-induced conformational change in the synthetic peptides.

The number of serine phosphorylation sites in human NF-H (which seems representative of mammalian NF) is 43. Obviously, if all potential phosphorylation events were independent and biologically significant, there would be the possibility of 2^{43} different states of a single human NF-H molecule. Since a structural NF could contain NF-H subunits with different degrees of phosphorylation, the potential complexity of 'phosphorylation state' of a neurofilament is enormous. It is this complexity that has rendered impractical any complete physiochemical characterization of phosphorylation of native NF and led to immunological approaches to all except gross changes in NF phosphorylation.

At least five separable kinases are capable of phosphorylating NF in vivo (Vallano et al., 1986; Caputo et al., 1989). It remains most uncertain which of these accomplishes the in situ phosphorylation of NF; however, some degree of phosphorylation is found in virtually all neurons. Phosphorylation may proceed for long periods after NF synthesis (Black and Lee, 1988; Nixon and Logvinenko, 1986). Very little is known about the phosphatases that might act on NF in situ; however, NF do exhibit turnover of their phosphoryl groups (Nixon and Lewis, 1986; Nixon, Lewis and Marotta, 1987).

The one NF phosphorylation event that is reasonably well understood does not relate to the NF-H and NF-M side arms, but rather to a serine in the amino-terminal 'head' region of the NF-L subunit. This site is phosphorylated (in vitro and probably in vivo) by a protein kinase C (Sihag and Nixon, 1989, 1990). Phosphorylation at a homologous site regulates intermediate filament assembly in other cell types (assembly inhibited while the serine is phosphorylated and favored once the phosphoryl residue is cleaved). Phosphorylation at this site in neurons can be demonstrated for a proportion of newly synthesized NF-L in a readily soluble form, but assembled NF-L is dephosphorylated, suggesting the operation of a similar regulatory mechanism in neurons.

NF phosphorylation normally increases during development, and it differs substantially from site to site within the nervous system (Dahl and Bignami, 1986; Lee et al., 1987; Dahl, Labkovsky and Bignami, 1988; Watson et al., 1989a). The large myelinated axons of alpha-motor neurons have relatively high immunochemical indices of phosphorylation compared with unmyelinated fibers or with most axons of the central nervous system (Watson, 1991). No examples of large myelinated axons with a low index of NF phosphorylation are known, but among small myelinated fibers systems with similar axonal diameters may show different abundance and phosphorylation of NF (Szaro, Lee and Gainer, 1989; Watson, 1991). NF phosphorylation even varies markedly from site to site within a single cell, with gradually increasing phosphorylation at a distance from the cell bodies and with markedly greater phosphorylation of the centrally directed than the peripherally directed process of neurons of the sensory ganglia (Sloan and Stevenson, 1987; Watson et al., 1989a, 1991).

17.3.3 Transport of NF

Although NF synthesis occurs in the cell body and proximal dendrites, most of the NF in a motor neuron reside in the axon. Active mechanisms transport NF proteins along the axon (Hoffman and Lasek, 1975) probably in the form of assembled filaments. This process requires months to years for completion, depending on the length of the axon. The mechanoenzyme responsible for this phase of transport has not yet been clearly identified, in contrast to the molecular motors of 'fast' axonal transport of membranous organelles (Vale, 1987).

NF transport rates vary somewhat from site to site within the nervous system, with proximal motor axons among the more rapid sites (Hoffman et al., 1985a; Watson et al., 1989b). By analogy to models discussed below, it seems plausible that a net slowing of transport rate in the proximal axon is the immediate cause of NF accumulation in the axonal swellings. This would also potentially account for distal axonal atrophy, as the retention of NF proximally would be expected to lead to a deficit distally.

As developed below, there are suggestive correlations among the transport rate of NF and the phosphorylation of NF-H and NF-M subunits. For those systems where most other biological variables are

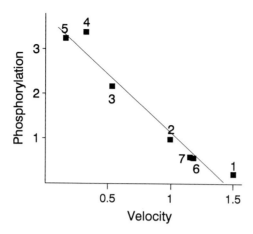

Figure 17.1 Relationship of phosphorylation of neurofilaments to velocity of neurofilament transport in rat peripheral motor and sensory axons (at the L5 level). Data from Watson *et al.* (1989a,b) and Watson *et al.* (1991) are summarized and replotted. Points 1–4 are from normal rats, where the phosphorylation and transport rates in the proximal L5 ventral roots at age 12 weeks were chosen as the reference values. Points 5–7 are from experimental intoxications, and the ratio of phosphorylation index and transport velocity to untreated controls (same age and site) are indicated. The least squares regression line is shown. The transport rates were determined by advance of radiolabeled neurofilament proteins. The phosphorylation index was determined by the ratio of binding of antibodies to phosphorylated and non-phosphorylated epitopes of NF-H (with a lesser reaction to similar epitopes on NF-M) in solubilized neurofilaments (Watson *et al.*, 1989a,b). The structure of axoplasm and the relative abundance of transported cytoskeletal proteins are normally similar at all these sites, and large myelinated axons contain the bulk of the neurofilaments. Hence many unmeasured biologic variables are probably similar among the different groups. In each case, a higher degree of neurofilament phosphorylation is associated with a slower net rate of transport. This relationship even holds for the experimental acceleration of transport by chronic 2,5-hexanedione, where the phosphorylation index is decreased. 1, Ventral root, age 3 weeks; 2, ventral root, age 12 weeks; 3, ventral root, age 18 weeks; 4, dorsal root, age 12 weeks; 5, ventral root, IDPN, age 6 weeks; 6, peripheral sensory axons, 2,5-hexanedione, age 20 weeks; 7, dorsal root, 2,5-hexanedione, age 20 weeks.

constant, increasing degrees of neurofilament phosphorylation (immunochemically determined) correlate with a slower rate of transport of NF (Figure 17.1) (Watson *et al.*, 1989a, 1991). This should not be construed as indicating a universal constant relating NF transport rates and phosphorylation, since when comparisons are made across structurally and biologically dissimilar axons the correlation is slight. Rather, it seems that a variety of factors is likely to influence the rate of axonal transport of NF, and phosphorylation is one factor. It should also be noted that the time resolution of transport experiments dealing with NF is poor with regard to potentially rapid events such as protein phosphorylation. Hence it is not at all possible to ascertain whether phosphorylation of NF alters their transport rates, or whether NF that slow down with regard to transport secondarily become more highly phosphorylated.

Few details are understood of the regulation of the proteolysis of NF. It seems that calcium-activated proteases are the best candidates to accomplish *in situ* NF degradation, and it is likely that a significant portion of degradation occurs at axon terminals. The amount of NF degradation that normally might occur along the length of the axon is a point of controversy (reviewed in Schlaepfer, 1987).

17.3.4 Focal regulation of NF phosphorylation

Although it has been known for a long time that the total number of NF in a cross-section of a myelinated internode greatly exceeds the number of NF in a cross-section of a node, the mechanisms of this focal control of NF distribution have been poorly understood. There have been several recent lines of evidence that indicate that the myelinating Schwann cell directly exerts an influence on the arrangement and phosphorylation of NF in the internodal axoplasm. Nerve trunks composed of unmyelinated axons have much less phosphorylation of NF than mixed or predominantly myelinated trunks (Watson, 1991). NF in the region of the node are much less phosphorylated by immunological criteria than in the internode, with a rather abrupt transition in the paranodal region adjacent to the node (Mata, Kupina and Fink, 1992). When the abnormal Schwann cells of the trembler mouse are transplanted into a normal mouse sciatic nerve, the regenerated axons in contact with the trembler Schwann cells (which are incapable of normal myelination) demonstrate aberrant close spacing of NF and hypophosphorylation of NF (de Waegh, Lee and Brady, 1992). The same axons proximal and distal to this region, in contact with normal Schwann cells, exhibit normal NF spacing and phosphorylation. In sum, these observations all seem to indicate that there is an influence of the myelinating Schwann cell to produce in the internode the accumulation of highly phosphorylated NF that serve to expand the volume of internodal axoplasm. Many experiments have indicated that axonal contact promotes the myelinating phenotype of the Schwann cell; apparently there is a positive feedback mechanism by which the Schwann cell promotes internodal axonal enlargement that further facilitates rapid saltatory conduction.

17.4 EXPERIMENTAL MODELS OF NF PATHOLOGY

The rate of axonal transport of NF, phosphorylation of NF and abundance of NF all can be altered in experimental pathology. A brief account will be given of several models, starting with those most structurally similar to human ALS pathology. As will become apparent, none of the models yet can directly address the mechanistic issues relevant to ALS pathology, but they suggest hypotheses that soon may be testable. A few models are instructive in the sense that they demonstrate some of the converse findings of those in ALS.

17.4.1 Hereditary canine spinal muscular atrophy

This genetically determined model (recently reviewed in Cork, 1991) lacks clear upper motor neuron pathology, and so is clinically more akin to a spinal muscular atrophy than to ALS. Nonetheless, the degeneration of the lower motor neurons has pathological similarities to human ALS. In the acutely developing disease marked proximal axonal accumulations of NF develop. These NF are highly phosphorylated by immunochemical reaction. There is a decrease in the net flux of radiolabeled NF along the ventral roots (Griffin, Cork and Adams, 1982) and apparently a slowing of the rate of transport of NF (although it is possible that the transport rates were underestimated because the amount of labeling was low).

17.4.2 Acute β,β^1–iminodipropionitrile

The toxin β,β^1–iminodipropionitrile (IDPN), given in acute high doses, rapidly causes proximal neurofilamentous swellings. These are associated with a profound defect of axonal transport of NF in proximal motor axons (Griffin et al., 1978). Acute IDPN in young rats (normally with a low phosphorylation index compared with adults) causes a marked increase in reactivity of the NF with antibodies to the phosphorylated conformation (Watson et al., 1989a). This antibody reaction is largely abolished by phosphatase digestion of the NF, suggesting that actual phosphorylation, rather than (or in addition to) any covalent binding of IDPN to NF, accounts for the change. The reactivity of NF from IDPN-intoxicated rats differs with regard to one antibody that normally is 'phosphorylation independent', suggesting that phosphorylation may occur at a site not normally occupied by phosphoryl groups. These observations suggest, but certainly do not prove, the sequence in which IDPN leads to aberrant NF phosphorylation, secondary slowing of axonal transport of NF and consequently NF accumulation in proximal axons.

Neurofilamentous pathology

IDPN clearly is not a simple model. Low-dose chronic intoxication very gradually may produce NF accumulations without clear change in phosphorylation of the bulk of NF (Carden et al., 1987). On the other hand, acute high-dose, followed by chronic low-dose, IDPN intoxication causes lasting change in the immunohistochemical reaction of NF in sensory neurons and proximal axonal swellings in sensory ganglia (Gold and Austin, 1991). Of course, very chronic intoxications cannot be studied in very young rats, so it remains unresolved whether the rate of intoxication, the age of the rat or both are important for accounting for the reported differences between acute and chronic intoxication. A potent hexacarbon neurotoxin, 3,4-dimethyl-2,5-hexanedione (DMHD), also can produce proximal NF accumulations associated with marked impairment of NF transport in proximal motor neurons (Griffin et al., 1984). The status of NF phosphorylation in this circumstance is not yet known.

17.4.3 Aluminum

Intracisternal injection of aluminum salts in rabbits produces accumulation of neurofilaments in motor neuron cell bodies and proximal axons. There is an associated defect of transport of labeled NF and an associated increase in the immunochemical degree of phosphorylation of NF (Bizzi and Gambetti, 1986; Troncoso et al., 1985, 1986). There is degeneration of some of the lower motor neurons. Because of the relatively large doses of aluminum employed, this model is not thought to resemble environmental exposure to aluminum, but rather it is an artificial model of neurofilamentous pathology.

More recently, effects of chronic aluminum intoxication in other species have been investigated. Monkeys fed a diet that was simultaneously calcium deficient and aluminum enriched developed axonal swellings and some increase in neurofilament phosphorylation in their motor neurons (Garruto et al., 1989). Chronic oral aluminum intoxication of rats has been investigated with regard to in vitro and in vivo phosphorylation of NF and the cytoskeletal protein MAP-2 (which has a phosphorylation domain of related but not identical sequence). In this model, incorporation of tracer amounts of ^{32}P into NF-H and MAP-2 was increased in vivo, under conditions in which the incorporation was believed to be proportional to endogenous enzyme activity. Because cAMP levels are known to increase in whole brain under these conditions, the activity of a cAMP kinase was suggested. Other studies of the cAMP-stimulated phosphorylation of NF and MAP-2 in brain homogenates from aluminum-intoxicated rats again demonstrated an increase in basal ^{32}P incorporation and in cAMP-stimulatable incorporation into NF and MAP-2 proteins (Johnson, Cogdill and Jope, 1990). Under these same conditions calcium–calmodulin kinase and protein kinase C activities were not altered. Unfortunately, the precise pathologic and immunohistochemical correlates of the enzymatic change are not yet well established in this particular model of chronic aluminum intoxication in rats.

17.4.4 Tri-*o*-cresyl phosphate

Early after exposure of hens to tri-*o*-cresyl phosphate (TOCP), the activity of calcium–calmodulin kinase toward the NF proteins, tubulin and MAP-2, is increased (Lapadula, Lapadula and Abou-Donia, 1992). This alteration precedes the major structural disintegration of axons that occurs in delayed fashion after exposure to this toxin. Hence the possibility exists that direct activation of the kinase by the toxin might be a central event in pathogenesis of the subsequent neuropathy. The precise relationships among this enzymatic change, immunohistochemical pathology and axonal transport of cytoskeletal proteins remain to be better defined.

17.4.5 Chronic 2,5-hexanedione

In many respects, this model is a mirror image of the pathology of ALS and of acute IDPN. A moderate acceleration of NF transport in proximal axons occurs in rats intoxicated for many weeks with this compound (Monaco *et al.*, 1989a,b; Watson *et al.*, 1991). There is associated axonal atrophy and hypophosphorylation of NF in proximal motor axons (Lapadula, Suwita and Abou-Donia, 1988; Watson *et al.*, 1991). Analysis of the abundance of mRNA for NF-L suggests that there is no change in actual synthesis rate. Distal axons develop some NF accumulations, although the protocol employed produces only a few of these in any given section. Analysis of nerves from the region containing these sparse swellings shows no net change in NF content or phosphorylation (Watson *et al.*, 1991). Electron microscopic immunocytochemistry to define the exact status of NF phosphorylation within the swellings has not yet been accomplished.

17.4.6 Axotomy

Changes in NF during axonal regeneration are naturally of interest in ALS, as some motor neurons may be acutely disconnected from their targets in muscle shortly before pathological examination. However, there are many points of distinction of the ALS pathology from simple axotomy effects, clearly indicating that ALS NF pathology does not simply reflect disconnection of cell bodies from targets by terminal axonal degeneration.

The abundance of mRNA for NF proteins and/or the incorporation of amino acids into NF and/or the abundance of NF proteins is decreased after axotomy (Hoffman, Griffin and Price, 1984; Hoffman *et al.*, 1985b, 1987; Wong and Oblinger, 1987; Goldstein *et al.*, 1988). Proximal axons undergo atrophy (Hoffman *et al.*, 1985b) as the supply of NF to the axon dwindles. No clear examples of proximal axonal swellings in response to axotomy are known.

However, some alteration of NF phosphorylation does seem to follow axotomy. This point is least clear in motor neurons (Mansour *et al.*, 1989), but increased abundance of phosphorylated NF epitopes in sensory ganglion cells (Goldstein *et al.*, 1987; Rosenfeld *et al.*, 1987; Mansour *et al.*, 1989) and septal cholinergic neurons (Koliatsos *et al.*, 1989) is striking. The more proximal increase in NF phosphorylation does not extend into the fresh regenerating axonal sprouts, which have a markedly lower degree of phosphorylation than their parent axons (Bignami, Chi and Dahl, 1986; Pestronk, Watson and Yuan, 1990).

17.5 INTERPRETATION OF EXPERIMENTAL MODELS: IS NF PHOSPHORYLATION A BIOLOGIC 'STOP SIGN'?

A common theme in the situations discussed above is that whenever NF accumulate there is an increase in phosphorylation. (The chief exception is the trembler transplants, but this special case seems to be dominated by abnormal spacing of NF more than by net NF accumulation.) None of the observations can completely resolve whether NF phosphorylation is itself the signal by which axonal transport of NF is reduced, with secondary NF accumulation, or whether the increase in NF phosphorylation happens secondarily after another event reduces net NF transport. Given the clear evidence that the phosphorylation of NF leads to marked conformational change on the exposed side arms, and given the multiple examples of protein phosphorylation as a regulatory event in other systems, it seems more likely that the NF phosphorylation itself is a signal that leads to longer residence of the phosphorylated NF in the axoplasm.

At least two different allosterically regulated kinase systems, protein kinase A (Johnson, Cogdill and Jope, 1990), and calcium–calmodulin kinase (Lapadula, Lapadula and Abou-Donia, 1992), are implicated in different toxic models as potentially important for *in situ* NF phosphorylation. Myelinating Schwann cells are one important source of a signal that may activate NF phosphorylation (de Waegh, Lee and Brady, 1992) via these kinases or via pathways yet to be defined.

17.6 NF PHOSPHORYLATION ABNORMALITIES IN THE PATHOGENESIS OF ALS

The foregoing information still cannot place the observations of neurofilamentous pathology along the continuum of importance in ALS from 'unimportant epiphenomenon' to 'central event in neuronal degeneration'. A consideration of the possible levels of involvement of NF phosphorylation and transport in ALS pathogenesis may at least serve to refine our current hypotheses.

The proximal neurofilamentous swellings filled with highly phosphorylated NF in motor neurons of ALS may be a marker for abnormal activation of a protein kinase (or inhibition of a protein phosphatase). This might be a proxy for yet another event in cell degeneration. It is not hard to imagine toxic or immune-mediated damage to the motor neuron plasmalemma leading to abnormal calcium entry, activation of proteases (and other deleterious processes) that lead to cell death, with activation of a calcium–calmodulin kinase phosphorylating neurofilaments as an innocuous epiphenomenon. (It is not hard to imagine, only hard to accumulate solid evidence relating to this point.)

It is also plausible that increased NF phosphorylation in proximal motor axons is a marker for a particular event that is central to cell death. Several of the kinases known to act on NF are multifunctional and act on multiple substrates. It is possible that pathologic activation of a kinase, whose activity is detectable by its action on NF, leads to concurrent phosphorylation of other regulatory proteins that cause the degeneration and death of the motor neuron.

Neurofilamentous pathology may be more than a marker; it potentially may contribute to neuronal degeneration. Because the retention of NF in the proximal axon normally equates with NF loss and axonal atrophy distally, the process of proximal NF accumulation may contribute to distal axonal pathology before the loss of the motor neuron cell body is complete. Such distal axonal pathology is not of itself sufficient to cause motor neuronal degeneration, but the loss of normal connection to muscle may deprive the motor neuron of trophic support and further tip the balance of an injured neuron toward irreversible degeneration rather than recovery.

Finally, aberrant NF phosphorylation and NF accumulation may potentially interfere with intracellular transport of other materials. At a certain critical level of metabolic disconnection of the cell bodies from their axons and trophic support of targets, this could be a key event in death of the motor neuron.

The experimental models known to date encourage the speculation that specific interventions into the process of NF transport and phosphorylation will eventually become possible. Although the gap between such experimental manipulations and any practical intervention in human disease still seems large, further developments in understanding the biology of neurofilaments promise to reduce the gap.

REFERENCES

Asbury, A.K., Gale, M.K., Cox, S.C. *et al* (1972) Giant axonal neuropathy. A unique case with segmental neurofilamentous masses. *Acta Neuropathol.*, **20**, 237–47.

Bignami, A., Chi, N.H. and Dahl, D. (1986) Neurofilament phosphorylation in peripheral nerve regeneration. *Brain Res.*, **375**, 73–82.

Binet, S. and Meininger, V. (1988) Modifications of microtubule proteins in ALS nerve precede detectable histologic and ultrastructural changes. *Neurology*, **38**, 1596–600.

Bizzi, A. and Gambetti, P. (1986) Phosphorylation of neurofilaments is altered in aluminium intoxication. *Acta Neuropathol.*, **71**, 154–8.

Black, M.M. and Lee, V.M.-Y. (1988) Phosphorylation of neurofilament proteins in intact neurons: demonstration of phosphorylation in cell bodies and axons. *J. Neurosci.*, **8**, 3296–305.

Bradley, S.G., Good, P., Rasool, C.G. and Adelman, L.S. (1983) Morphometric and biochemical studies of peripheral nerves in amyotrophic lateral sclerosis. *Ann. Neurol.*, **14**, 267–77.

Breuer, A.C. and Atkinson, M.B. (1988) Fast axonal transport alterations in amyotrophic lateral sclerosis (ALS) and in parathyroid hormone (PTH)-treated axons. *Cell Motil. Cytoskeleton*, **10**, 321–30.

Caputo, C.B., Sygowski, L.A., Brunner, W.F. *et al.* (1989) Properties of several protein kinases that copurify with rat spinal cord neurofilaments. *Biochim. Biophys. Acta*, **1012**, 299–307.

Carden, M.J., Schlaepfer, W.W. and Lee, V.M.-Y. (1985) The structure, biochemical properties, and immunogenicity of neurofilament peripheral regions are determined by phosphorylation state. *J. Biol. Chem.*, **260**, 9805–17.

Carden, M.M., Goldstein, M.E., Bruce, J. *et al.* (1987) Studies of neurofilaments that accumulate in proximal axons of rats intoxicated with beta, beta'-iminodipropionitrile. *Neurochem. Pathol.*, **7**, 189.

Carpenter, S. (1968) Proximal axonal enlargement in motor neuron disease. *Neurology*, **18**, 841–51.

Chiu, F.C., Barnes, E.A., Das, K. *et al.* (1989) Characterization of a novel 66 kd subunit of mammalian neurofilaments. *Neuron*, **2**, 1435–45.

Clark, A.W., Parhad, I.M., Griffin, J.W. and Price, D.L. (1984) Neurofilamentous swellings as a normal finding in the spinal anterior horn of man and other primates. *J. Neuropath. Exp. Neurol.*, **43**, 253–62.

Clark, A.W., Tran, P.M., Parhad, I.M. *et al.* (1990) Neuronal gene expression in amyotrophic lateral sclerosis. *Mol. Brain Res.*, **7**, 75–83.

Cork, L.C. (1991) Hereditary canine spinal muscular atrophy: an animal model of motor neuron disease. *Can. J. Neurol. Sci.*, **18**(3 Suppl), 432–4.

Dahl, D. and Bignami, A. (1986) Neurofilament phosphorylation in development. A sign of axonal maturation? *Exp. Cell Res.*, **162**, 220–30.

Dahl, D., Labkovsky, B. and Bignami, A. (1988) Neurofilament phosphorylation in axons and perikarya: immunofluorescence study of the rat spinal cord and dorsal root ganglia with monoclonal antibodies. *J. Comp. Neurol.*, **271**, 445.

Dautigny, A., Pham-Dinh, D., Roussel, C. *et al.* (1988) The large neurofilament subunit (NF-H) of the rat: cDNA cloning and in situ detection. *Biochem. Biophys. Res. Commun.*, **154**, 1099–106.

Delisle, M.B. and Carpenter, S. (1984) Neurofibrillary axonal swellings and amyotrophic lateral sclerosis. *J. Neurol. Sci.*, **63**, 241–50.

de Waegh, S.M., Lee, V.M.-Y. and Brady, S.T. (1992) Local modulation of neurofilament phosphorylation, axonal caliber and slow axonal transport by myelinating Schwann cells. *Cell*, **68**, 451–63.

Donaghy, M., King, R.H., Thomas, P.K. and Workman, J.M. (1988) Abnormalities of the axonal cytoskeleton in giant axonal neuropathy. *J. Neurocytol.*, **17**, 197–200.

Escurat, M., Djabali, M., Gumpel, M. *et al.* (1990) Differential expression of two neuronal intermediate-filament proteins, peripherin and the low-molecular-mass neurofilament protein (NF-L), during the development of the rat. *J. Neurosci.*, **10**, 764–84.

Ferri, G.-L., Zareh, S., Amadori, A. *et al.* (1988) 2,5-Hexanedione-induced accumulations of neurofilament-immunoreactive material throughout the rat autonomic nervous system. *Brain Res.*, **444**, 383.

Garofalo, O., Kennedy, P.G., Swash, M. *et al.* (1991) Ubiquitin and heat shock protein expression in amyotrophic lateral sclerosis. *Neuropathol. Appl. Neurobiol.*, **17**, 39–45.

Garruto, R.M., Shankar, S.K., Yanagihara, R. *et al.* (1989) Low-calcium, high-aluminum diet-induced motor neuron pathology in cynomolgus monkeys. *Acta Neuropathol.*, **78**, 210–19.

Geisler, N. and Weber, K. (1981) Self-assembly *in vitro* of the 68,000 molecular weight component of the mammalian neurofilament triplet proteins into intermediate sized filaments. *J. Mol. Biol.*, **151**, 565–71.

Geisler, N., Vanderkerchove, J. and Weber, K. (1987) Location and sequence characterization of the major phosphorylation sites of the high molecular mass neurofilament proteins M and H. *FEBS Lett.*, **221**, 403–7.

Geisler, N., Kaufmann, E., Fischer, S. *et al.* (1983) Neurofilament architecture combines structural principles of intermediate filaments with carboxy-terminal extensions increasing in size between triplet proteins. *EMBO J.*, **2**, 1295–302.

Neurofilamentous pathology

Geisler, N., Fischer, S., Vanderkerchove, J. *et al.* (1985) Protein-chemical characterization of NF-H, the largest mammalian meurofilament component; intermediate filament-type sequences followed by a unique carboxy-terminal extension. *EMBO J.*, **4**, 57–63.

Gold, B.G. and Austin, D.R. (1991) Regulation of aberrant neurofilament phosphorylation in neuronal perikarya. 3. Alterations following single and continuous beta,beta[1]-iminodipropionitrile administrations. *Brain. Res.*, **563**, 151–62.

Goldstein, M.E., Cooper, H.S., Bruce, J. *et al.* (1987) Phosphorylation of neurofilament proteins and chromatolysis following transection of rat sciatic nerve. *J. Neurosci.*, **7**, 1586–94.

Goldstein, M.E., Weiss, S.R., Lazzarini, R.A. *et al.* (1988) mRNA levels of all three neurofilament proteins decline following nerve transection. *Mol. Brain. Res.*, **3**, 287.

Griffin, J.W., Cork, L.C. and Adams, R.J. (1982) Axonal transport in hereditary canine spinal muscular atrophy. *J. Neuropathol. Exp. Neurol.*, **42**, 370.

Griffin, J.W., Hoffman, P.N., Clark, A.W. *et al.* (1978) Slow axonal transport of neurofilament proteins: impairment by beta,beta[1]-iminodipropionitrile administration. *Science*, **202**, 633–5.

Griffin, J.W., Anthony, D.C., Fahnestock, K.E. *et al.* (1984) 3,4-Dimethyl-2,5-hexanedione impairs the axonal transport of neurofilament proteins. *J. Neurosci.*, **4** 1516–26.

Hoffman, P.N. and Lasek, R.J. (1975) The slow component of axonal transport: identification of the major structural polypeptides of the axon and their generality among mammalian neurons. *J. Cell Biol.*, **66**, 351–66.

Hoffman, P.N., Griffin, J.W. and Price, D.L. (1984) Control of axonal caliber by neurofilament transport. *J. Cell Biol.*, **99**, 705–14.

Hoffman, P.N., Griffin, J.W., Gold, B.G. and Price, D.L. (1985) Slowing of neurofilament transport and the radial growth of developing nerve fibers. *J. Neurosci.*, **5**, 2920–9.

Hoffman, P.N., Thompson, G.W., Griffin, J.W. and Price, D.L. (1985) Changes in neurofilament transport coincide temporally with alterations in the caliber of axons in regenerating motor fibers. *J. Cell Biol.*, **101**, 1332–40.

Hoffman, P.N., Cleveland, D.W., Griffin, J.W. *et al.* (1987) Neurofilament gene expression: a major determinant of axonal caliber. *Proc. Natl. Acad. Sci. USA*, **84**, 3472–6.

Hollosi, M., Urge, L., Perczel, A. *et al.* (1992) Metal ion-induced conformational changes of phosphorylated fragments of human neurofilament (NF-M) protein. *J. Mol. Biol.*, **223**, 673–82.

Itoh, T., Sobue, G., Ken, E. *et al.* (1992) Phosphorylated high molecular weight neurofilament protein in the peripheral motor, sensory and sympathetic neuronal perikarya – system-dependent normal variations and changes in amyotrophic lateral sclerosis and multiple system atrophy. *Acta Neuropathol.*, **83**, 240–5.

Johnson, G.V.W., Cogdill, K.W. and Jope, R.S. (1990) Oral aluminum alters invitro protein phosphorylation and kinase activities in rat brain. *Neurobiol. Aging*, **11**, 209–16.

Julien, J.-P., Grosfeld, F., Yazdanbaksh, K. *et al.* (1987) The structure of a human neurofilament gene (NF-L): a unique exon–intron organization in the intermediate filament gene family. *Biochim. Biophys. Acta*, **909**, 10–20.

Koliatsos, V.E., Applegate, M.D., Kitt, C.A. *et al.* (1989) Aberrant phosphorylation of neurofilaments accompanies transmitter-related changes in rat septal neurons following transection of the fimbria–fornix. *Brain Res.*, **482**, 205–18.

Landon, F., Lemonnier, M., Benarous, R. *et al.* (1989) Multiple mRNAs encode peripherin, a neuronal intermediate filament protein. *EMBO J.*, **8**, 1719–26.

Lapadula, D.M., Suwita, E. and Abou-Donia, M.B. (1988) Evidence for multiple mechanisms responsible for 2,5-hexanedione-induced neuropathy. *Brain Res.*, **131**, 123–31.

Lapadula, E.S., Lapadula, D.M. and Abou-Donia, M.B. (1992) Biochemical changes in sciatic nerve of hens treated with tri-omicron-cresyl phosphate – increased phosphorylation of cytoskeletal proteins. *Neurochem. Int.*, **20**, 247–55.

Lee, V.M.-Y., Carden, M.J., Schlaepfer, W.W. and Trojanowski, J.Q. (1987) Monoclonal antibodies distinguish several differentially phosphorylated states of the two largest rat neurofilament subunits (NF-H and NF-M) and demonstrate their existence in the normal nervous system of adult rats. *J. Neurosci.*, **7**, 3474–88.

Leigh, P.N., Whitwell, H., Garofalo, O. *et al.* (1991) Ubiquitin–immunoreactive intraneuronal inclusions in amyotrophic lateral sclerosis. Morphology, distribution, and specificity. *Brain*, **114**, 775–88.

Levy, E., Liem, R.K.H., D'Eustachio, P. and Cowan, N.J. (1987) Structure and evolutionary origin of the gene encoding mouse NF-M, the middle-molecular-mass neurofilament protein. *Eur. J. Biochem*, **166**, 71–7.

Liem, R.K.H. and Hutchinson, S.B. (1982) Purification of individual components of the neurofilament triplet: filament assembly from the 70,000-Dalton subunit. *Biochemistry*, **21**, 3221–6.

Manetto, V., Sternberger, N.H., Perry, G. *et al.* (1988) Phosphorylation of neurofilaments is altered in amyotrophic lateral sclerosis. *J. Neuropathol. Exp. Neurol.*, **47**, 642–53.

Mansour, H., Bignami, A., Labkovsky, B. and Dahl, D. (1989) Neurofilament phosphorylation in neuronal perikarya following axotomy – a study of rat spinal cord with ventral and dorsal root transection. *J. Comp. Neur.*, **283**, 481–5.

Mata, M., Kupina, N. and Fink, D.J. (1992) Phosphorylation-dependent neurofilament epitopes are reduced at the node of ranvier. *J. Neurocytol.*, **21**, 199–210.

Matsumoto, S., Hirano, A. and Goto, S. (1990a) Spinal cord neurofibrillary tangles of guamanian amyotrophic lateral sclerosis and parkinsonism–dementia complex – an immunohistochemical study. *Neurology*, **40**, 975–9.

Matsumoto, S., Hirano, A. and Goto, S. (1990b) Ubiquitin-immunoreactive filamentous inclusions in anterior horn cells of Guamanian and non-Guamanian amyotrophic lateral sclerosis. *Acta Neuropathol*, **80**, 233–8.

Migheli, A., Autilio-Gambetti, L., Gambetti, P. *et al.* (1990) Ubiquitinated filamentous inclusions in spinal cord of patients with motor neuron disease. *Neurosci. Lett.*, **114**, 5–10.

Monaco, S., Autilio-Gambetti, L., Lasek, R.J. *et al.* (1989a) Experimental increase of neurofilament transport rate: decreases in neurofilament number and in axon diameter. *J. Neuropathol. Exp. Neurol.*, **48**, 23–32.

Monaco, S., Jacob, J., Jenich, H. *et al.* (1989b) Axonal transport of neurofilament is accelerated in peripheral nerve during 2,5-hexanedione intoxication. *Brain Res.*, **491**, 328–34.

Munoz, D.G., Greene, C., Perl, D.P. and Selkoe, D.J. (1988) Accumulation of phosphorylated neurofilaments in anterior horn motorneurons of amyotrophic lateral sclerosis patients. *J. Neuropathol. Exp. Neurol.*, **47**, 9–18.

Murayama, S., Mori, H., Ihara, V. *et al.* (1990) Immunocytochemical and ultrastructural studies of lower motor neurons in amyotrophic lateral sclerosis. *Ann. Neurol.*, **27**, 137–48.

Myers, M.W., Lazzarini, R.A., Lee, V.M.-Y. *et al.* (1987) The human mid-size neurofilament subunit: a repeated protein sequence and the relationship of its gene to the intermediate gene family. *EMBO J.*, **6**, 1617–26.

Napolitano, E.W., Chin, S.S.M., Colman, D.R. and Liem, R.K.H. (1987) Complete amino acid sequence and invitro expression of rat NF-M, the middle molecular weight neurofilament protein. *J. Neurosci.*, **7**, 2590–9.

Nixon, R.A. and Lewis, S.E. (1986) Differential turnover of phosphate groups on neurofilament subunits in mammalian neurons in vivo. *J. Biol. Chem.*, **261**, 16298–301.

Nixon, R.A. and Logvinenko, K.B. (1986) Multiple fates of newly synthesized neurofilament proteins: evidence for a stationary neurofilament network distributed nonuniformly along axons of retinal ganglion cell neurons. *J. Cell Biol.*, **102**, 647–59.

Nixon, R.A., Lewis, S.A. and Marotta, C.A. (1987) Posttranslational modification of neurofilament proteins by phosphate during axoplasmic transport in retinal ganglion cell neurons. *J. Neurosci.*, **7**, 1145–58.

Okamoto, K., Hirai, S., Shoji, M. *et al.* (1990) Axonal swellings in the corticospinal tracts in amyotrophic lateral sclerosis. *Acta Neuropathol.*, **80**, 222–6.

Otvos, L., Hollosi, M., Perczel, A., Dietzschold, B. and Fasman, G.D. (1988) Phosphorylation loops in synthetic peptides of the human neurofilament protein middle-sized subunit. *J. Protein Chem.*, **7**, 365–76.

Pachter, J.S. (1985) Alpha-internexin, a 66kDa intermediate filament-binding protein from mammalian central nervous tissues. *J. Cell. Biol.*, **101**, 1316–22.

Parysek, L.M. and Goldman, R.D. (1987) Characterization of intermediate filaments in PC12 cells. *J. Neurosci.*, **7**, 781–91.

Pena, S.D.J. (1982) Giant axonal neuropathy: an inborn error of organization of intermediate filaments. *Muscle Nerve*, **5**, 166–72.

Pestronk, A., Watson, D.F. and Yuan, C.M. (1990) Neurofilament phosphorylation in peripheral nerve – changes with axonal length and growth state. *J. Neurochem.*, **54**, 977–82.

Portier, M.M., de Nechaud, B. and Gros, F. (1983) Peripherin, a new member of the intermediate filament protein family. *Dev. Neurosci.*, **6**, 335–44.

Rosenfeld, J., Dorman, M.E., Griffin, J.W. *et al.* (1987) Distribution of neurofilament antigens after axonal injury. *J. Neuropathol. Exp. Neurol.*, **46**, 269–82.

Sasaki, S., Maruyama, S., Yamane, K. *et al.* (1989) Swellings of proximal axons in a case of motor neuron disease. *Ann. Neurol.*, **25**, 520–2.

Schiffer, D., Autilio-Gambetti, L., Chi'o, A. *et al.* (1991) Ubiquitin in motor neuron disease: study at the light and electron microscope. *J. Neuropathol. Exp. Neurol.*, **50**, 463–73.

Schlaepfer, W.W. (1987) Neurofilaments: structure, metabolism and implications in disease. *J. Neuropathol. Exp. Neurol.*, **46**, 117–29.

Schmidt, M.L., Carden, M.J., Lee, V.M.-Y. and Trojanowski, J.Q. (1987) Phosphate dependent and independent neurofilament epitopes in the axonas swellings of patients with motor neuron disease and controls. *Lab. Invest.*, **56**, 282–94.

Shelanski, M.L. (1991) Neurofibrillary proliferation revisited. *Adv. Neurol.*, **56**, 75–9.

Sihag, R.K. and Nixon, R.A. (1989) In vivo phosphorylation of distinct domains of the 70-kilodalton neurofilament subunit involves different protein kinases. *J. Biol. Chem.*, **264**, 457–64.

Sihag, R.K. and Nixon, R.A. (1990) Phosphorylation of the amino-terminal head domain of the middle molecular mass 145-kDa subunit of neurofilaments – evidence for regulation by 2nd messenger-dependent protein kinases. *J. Biol. Chem.*, **265**, 4166–71.

Sloan, K.E. and Stevenson, J.A. (1987) Differential distribution of phosphorylated and non-phosphorylated neurofilaments within the retina and optic nerve of hamsters. *Brain Res.*, **437**, 365.

Sobue, G., Hashizume, Y., Yasuda, T. *et al.* (1990) Phosphorylated high molecular weight neurofilament protein in lower motor neurons in amyotrophic lateral sclerosis and other neurodegenerative diseases involving ventral horn cells. *Acta Neuropathol.*, **79**, 402–8.

Spencer, P.S. and Schaumburg, H.H. (1977) Ultrastructural studies on the dying-back process. III. The evolution of experimental peripheral giant axonal degeneration. *J. Neuropathol. Exp. Neurol.*, **36**, 276–99.

Szaro, B.G., Lee, V.M.-Y. and Gainer, H. (1989) Spatial and temporal expression of phosphorylated and non-phosphorylated forms of neurofilament proteins in the developing nervous system of Xenopus-Laevis. *Develop. Brain Res.*, **48**, 87–103.

Toyoshima, I., Yamamoto, A., Masamune, O. and Satake, M. (1989) Phosphorylation of neurofilament proteins and localization of axonal swellings in motor neuron disease. *J. Neurol. Sci.*, **89**, 269–77.

Troncoso, J.C., Hoffman, P.N., Griffin, J.W. *et al.* (1985) Aluminum intoxication:

a disorder of neurofilament transport in motor neurons. *Brain Res.*, **342**, 172–5.

Troncoso, J.C., Sternberger, N.H., Sternberger, L.A. *et al.* (1986) Immunocytochemical studies of neurofilament antigens in the neurofibrillary pathology induced by aluminum. *Brain Res.*, **364**, 295–300.

Vale, R.D. (1987) Intracellular transport using microtubule-based motors. *Annu. Rev. Cell. Biol.*, **3**, 347–78.

Vallano, M.L., Goldenring, J.R., Lasher, R.S. and DeLorenzo, R.J. (1986) Association of calcium/calmodulin-dependent kinase with cytoskeletal preparations: phosphorylation of tubulin, neurofilament and microtubule-associated proteins. *Ann. NY Acad. Sci.*, **466**, 357–74.

Watson, D.F. (1991) Regional variation in the abundance of axonal cytoskeletal proteins. *J. Neurosci. Res.*, **300**, 226–31.

Watson, D.F., Fittro, K.P., Griffin, J.W. and Hoffman, P.N. (1989) Phosphorylation-dependent immunoreactivity of neurofilaments increases during axonal maturation and IDPN intoxication. *J. Neurochem.*, **53**, 1818–29.

Watson, D.F., Hoffman, P.N., Fittro, K.P. and Griffin, J.W. (1989) Neurofilament and tubulin transport slows along the course of mature motor axons. *Brain Res.*, **447**, 225–32.

Watson, D.F., Fittro, K.P., Hoffman, P.N. and Griffin, J.W. (1991) Phosphorylation-related immunoreactivity and the rate of transport of neurofilaments in chronic 2,5-hexanedione intoxication. *Brain Res.*, **539**, 103–9.

Willard, M. and Simon, C. (1981) Antibody decoration of neurofilaments. *J. Cell Biol.*, **89**, 198–205.

Wong, J. and Oblinger, M.M. (1987) Changes in neurofilament gene expression occur after axotomy of dorsal root ganglion neurons: an in situ hybridization study. *Metab. Brain. Dis.*, **2**, 291.

Zopf, D., Hermans-Borgmeyer, I., Gundelfinger, E.D. and Betz, H. (1987) Identification of gene products expressed in the developing chick visual system: characterization of a middle-molecular-weight neurofilament cDNA. *Genes Dev.*, **1**, 699–708.

PART FOUR

18 *Epidemiology*

CHRISTOPHER N. MARTYN

18.1 INTRODUCTION

Our knowledge of the descriptive epidemiology of motor neurone disease is far from complete. In many parts of the world the occurrence of the disease has hardly been studied at all, and even in Europe, Scandinavia and North America, where a number of surveys have been undertaken, differences in the way that they have been conducted constrain comparison of the results. Information about time trends of the disease depends almost entirely on routinely collected mortality data. While these data may be remarkably reliable for conditions with as high a case fatality as motor neurone disease, it is hard to be sure that changes in mortality over time truly reflect trends in the incidence of the disease rather than changes in diagnostic and certification practices.

It is a paradox that, with these deficiencies in the epidemiological data, interpretations are offered with such certainty. Enshrined in the literature is the view that, with the notorious exception of the foci of the disease in the Western Pacific, the incidence of motor neurone disease is similar worldwide (Kurtzke, 1982). This belief is so widely accepted that local rates of motor neurone disease have sometimes been used as a yardstick against which to measure the frequency of other neurological diseases when no reliable population denominator was available (Kurtzke, 1975a,b). But, as a recent editorial in the *Lancet* (Anon., 1990) pointed out, if one stops to consider the variety of conditions in which people live (and therefore the range of environmental agents to which they are exposed) and the diversity of their genetic inheritance, the idea that any disease – whatever its aetiology – could be evenly distributed throughout the world seems scarcely credible.

The main purpose of studying the epidemiology of a disease is to identify the causes of that disease. By investigating the geographical distribution of a disease both on a global scale and within smaller areas, changes in the frequency with which the disease occurs over time and

393

the characteristics of the people who suffer from it, epidemiologists seek patterns that they hope will provide clues about its aetiology. Incompleteness of data need not induce paralysis. We can attempt a critical appraisal of the information available, quantify the uncertainty and try to set bounds on our ignorance. At the very least, this should begin to provide us with some sort of framework in which we can consider hypotheses about aetiology. Ideas about the causes of a disease must, after all, be compatible with what is known about the descriptive epidemiology of the condition. Further, the exercise will focus attention on areas where information is lacking and it should help to clarify priorities for future epidemiological research.

18.2 CONSIDERATIONS OF METHODOLOGY

An account of epidemiological methods would be out of place here but, because the results of surveys of incidence are so strongly influenced by them, two aspects of survey design – definition of cases and methods of case ascertainment – require discussion. Also, because mortality rates have been used quite extensively to investigate both the geography and secular trends of motor neurone disease, it may be worthwhile briefly to consider the strengths and limitations of the data from which these rates are derived.

18.2.1 Definition of the disease – diagnostic criteria

In the absence of a sensitive and specific test, the diagnosis of motor neurone disease depends very largely on the clinical features manifested by the patient. It is, perhaps, unfair to criticize the recent attempt by a subcommittee of the World Federation of Neurology to produce a set of diagnostic criteria for amyotrophic lateral sclerosis (World Federation of Neurology, 1991) from an epidemiological viewpoint since the averred aim was to develop criteria that would be useful in clinical trials of treatment and investigations of the molecular genetics of the disease. But it is hard to see how it would be feasible to implement the proposed scheme in population-based research. The recommended criteria and system whereby cases are classified into proven, definite, probable, possible and suspected categories of diagnostic certainty require quite extensive laboratory and electrophysiological investigations. Many of the criteria for exclusion of the diagnosis are not fully described, and no help is given in how to classify patients in whom the required electrophysiological, laboratory and pathological tests were not carried out.

Without generally agreed criteria for diagnosis, investigators have been forced to construct their own operational definition of the disease. Inevitably, these have varied between studies and often, in published accounts, only incomplete descriptions are given. All published surveys to date have been retrospective and, even when case records have been reviewed independently, accuracy of diagnosis is bound to rely heavily on the competence of the physician whose care the patient was under. The difficulties of obtaining a uniform standard of diagnosis internationally are revealed by the results of a study specifically designed to examine agreement between neurologists in the weight they attached to particular symptoms, signs and clinical investigations in the diagnosis of motor neurone disease (Li *et al.*, 1991). Summaries of the medical histories and findings on neurological examination of pathologically confirmed cases of motor neurone disease were sent to neurologists in the UK, Germany and China. Significant differences in the way this information was interpreted were found. One important conclusion from this study is that any international agreement concerning a set of criteria for the diagnosis of motor neurone disease must be followed by a cooperative international effort to establish their validity.

18.2.2 Case ascertainment

The accuracy of any estimate of frequency of disease, whether incidence, prevalence or mortality, depends upon how completely cases of that disease are identified. The problem of ensuring complete ascertainment of cases is most severe in incidence surveys of rare diseases where, unless a large population has been studied over a long period, the number of cases is inevitably small. The omission of even a few cases of the disease or, conversely, the inclusion of a few misclassified patients who do not have the disease is bound to have large effects on the estimated rate. In surveys of motor neurone disease there is a definite tendency for those that employ several different methods to identify all possible cases to produce higher estimates of incidence than those that use a single source of information. A much greater degree of reliance should be placed on estimates of incidence from surveys in which the investigators used sources of information in addition to the records of neurologists. These sources include records of investigation by neurophysiology departments, data from hospital discharges, information from doctors working in primary care, records of organizations involved in community care and patient welfare and death certificates that include a mention of motor neurone disease. The proviso must, of course, be made that possible cases detected from these sources are subsequently scrutinized to be sure that they fulfil the diagnostic criteria for the disease.

Epidemiology

18.2.3 Mortality data

Mortality data ultimately depend on what was written on the death certificate by the medical practitioner certifying death. In most countries, the information recorded on the death certificate is passed to a central office of health statistics, which uses it to identify and code, using the International Classification of Diseases, the underlying cause of death. In only a few countries are other medical conditions mentioned on the death certificate also coded. For many chronic diseases, data based on the underlying cause of death are a poor indicator of their frequency because many patients die of an unrelated illness. But for conditions as rapidly and universally fatal as motor neurone disease this problem is likely to be small. There is, however, a potential difficulty in relation to the application of WHO rule 3. This rule concerns how the underlying cause of death is established from the entries in Parts 1 and 2 of the death certificate. It will be recalled that morbid events leading to death are recorded in Part 1, while diseases that contributed to the death but were not considered part of the direct sequence that led to death are recorded in Part 2. The way in which this rule should be interpreted was clarified in 1984. Since 1984, in cases in which bronchopneumonia, pulmonary embolism, heart failure or cardiac arrest is the only entry under Part 1, information recorded under Part 2 of the death certificate is always used to determine the underlying cause of death. Prior to 1984, information in Part 2 was sometimes disregarded and the underlying cause of death identified only from causes of death listed under Part 1. This change in coding practice has apparently produced a striking increase in mortality rates for some chronic neurological diseases (Martyn and Pippard, 1988).

Unfortunately, it is hard to be certain about the size of the effect on the apparent mortality from motor neurone disease. The Office of Population Censuses and Surveys for England and Wales coded all deaths registered in 1984 by both methods and was therefore able to measure directly the effect of the change in the application of WHO rule 3 on mortality from specific diseases. They estimated that mortality from motor neurone disease increased by only 6.3% as a result of the change. But inspection of the numbers of deaths from motor neurone disease for the years surrounding 1984 strongly suggests that this figure is an underestimate. In 1982 and 1983, there were 1766 deaths from motor neurone disease; in 1984 and 1985, the corresponding figure was 2108. This represents an increase of nearly 20%.

A number of studies from different countries (Hoffman and Brody, 1971; Kondo and Tsubaki, 1977; Buckley et al., 1983; O'Malley, Dean and

396

Elian, 1987; Chio *et al.*, 1992) have been carried out to validate mortality data as a measure of the occurrence of motor neurone disease. They have shown that a high proportion, between 72 and 96%, of patients diagnosed during life as having motor neurone disease have this disease coded as the underlying cause of death. The rate of false negatives is therefore fairly low. Only two studies, one from Japan, the other from Scotland (Kondo and Tsubaki, 1977; Chancellor, Swingler and Fraser, 1993), have attempted to quantify the number of false positives contained in death certificate data for motor neurone disease. In the Japanese study, 28% of deaths coded as motor neurone disease had this diagnosis rejected after re-evaluation of clinical information obtained directly from the physician certifying death and from the families of the patients. In the study from Scotland, 10% of deaths from motor neurone disease were found to be wrongly coded. The largest single source of error leading to a false-positive coding was the misclassification of cases of pseudobulbar palsy of vascular origin. These two types of error, under-recording of true cases of motor neurone disease and the inclusion of patients who did not actually have the disease, tend to cancel each other out, and reported figures may approximate quite closely to the true mortality.

It is very much harder to judge how much the accuracy of death certificate data has changed over time. Cross-sectional studies in the USA, England and Wales and Norway that have compared geographical patterns of mortality from motor neurone disease with the distribution of neurologists or with the local ratio of physicians to population found no strong correlation (Bharucha *et al.*, 1983; Buckley *et al.*, 1983; Gunnarsson *et al.*, 1990). Although this suggests that the current diagnostic rate of motor neurone disease is not much influenced by differences in the provision of medical care within the range found in these three countries, the possibility remains that changing levels of awareness of the disease amongst physicians or increased availability of specialized medical services have influenced the frequency with which the diagnosis is made. One documented example of this is a transient local increase in numbers of cases of motor neurone disease that occurred after neurological services to a community were improved (Zack, Levitt and Schoenberg, 1977).

The great advantage of studies of mortality over most surveys of incidence is that, because all deaths within a country are monitored, the number of cases from which rates can be calculated is very much larger. Rates based on large numbers are, of course, less susceptible to random variation in the occurrence of disease and therefore give a more stable estimate of disease frequency.

18.3 GEOGRAPHICAL DISTRIBUTION

18.3.1 Surveys of incidence

The task of summarizing the geographical distribution of motor neurone disease has been greatly facilitated by a recent review by Chancellor and Warlow (1992) of population-based surveys of the disease carried out since 1950. Their review is especially valuable because of the efforts that they made to ensure that it was comprehensive. A systematic search strategy minimized the likelihood that any survey whose results had been published in the English language was overlooked. Also, the methodology employed by the investigators who had carried out the surveys was carefully considered. Particular attention was paid to completeness of case ascertainment, the need for a well-defined population denominator and, so that comparisons could be made between surveys, the requirement for age standardization of crude rates and calculation of confidence intervals for point estimates of incidence.

Only nine surveys of incidence of motor neurone disease were judged by Chancellor and Warlow to have achieved complete or nearly complete ascertainment of cases (see Table 18.1). Estimates of crude incidence rates from these surveys ranged from 0.6 cases per 100 000 population per year in Sardinia to 2.6 cases per 100 000 population per year in Sweden. Statistically significant differences in incidence rates between these surveys remained after direct age standardization of these rates to a single population. This is clear evidence of geographical variation in the occurrence of motor neurone disease.

Many other incidence surveys have been published but, because they have largely or exclusively relied upon the records of a neurological centre to identify cases, there are reasons to doubt whether the investigators discovered all the cases of motor neurone disease in the population that they intended to survey. This doubt is reinforced by the finding that the reported incidence in these surveys tended to be lower than from those surveys that employed multiple methods of case ascertainment. There is, unfortunately, no way of accurately assessing the size of the underestimate of the true incidence of motor neurone disease in most of these surveys. Any inferences about geographical variation in rates drawn from them are likely to be too fragile to be useful.

Nonetheless, one of these surveys deserves special mention (Olivares, Esteban and Alter, 1972). This was a study of the incidence of motor neurone disease over an 8-year period in Mexico City amongst government workers and their dependants enrolled in a government-sponsored comprehensive health programme. The methods of case

Table 18.1   Incidence studies of motor neurone disease

Reference	Location	Years included in survey	Cases (n)	Incidence 100 000/year (95% CI)
Rosati *et al.*, 1977	Sardinia, Italy	1965–74	96	0.6 (0.5–0.7)
Forsgren *et al.*, 1983	North Sweden	1969–80	128	1.7 (1.4–2.0)
Murros and Fogelholm, 1983	Middle Finland	1976–81	36	2.4 (1.7–3.3)
Gunnarsson and Palm, 1984	West Sweden	1970–81	89	2.6 (2.1–3.2)
Kahana and Zilber, 1984	Israel	1959–74	246	0.7 (0.6–0.8)
Hudson, Davenport and Hader, 1986	Ontario, Canada	1978–82	139	1.6 (1.3–1.9)
Yoshida *et al.*, 1986	Rochester, USA	1925–84	44	2.0 (1.4–2.7)
Højer-Pederson, Christensen and Jensen, 1989	Denmark	1974–86	186	1.4 (1.2–1.6)
Mitchell, Gibson and Gatrell, 1990	NW England	1976–86	173	1.9 (1.6–2.2)

ascertainment described by the investigators included personal contact with physicians and staff at peripheral clinics, scrutiny of hospital discharge summaries and inspection of records of neurological and psychiatric clinics and the records of the pathology department of the central hospital, though no monitoring of death certificates was attempted. Sixteen patients with possible motor neurone disease were identified. The clinical information in the published report of this survey suggests that in five of these cases the diagnosis was doubtful. However, even when these doubtful cases were included, the mean annual incidence rate was very low (0.4 per 100 000 population). This estimate of incidence was not changed by age adjustment to the US population.

The results of this survey are sometimes set aside on the grounds that identification of cases in Mexico, where specialized medical services are not readily available to the whole population, was likely to have been very incomplete. But this criticism ignores the fact that the investigators restricted their attention to a subpopulation enrolled in a government health programme. As far as can be judged, standards of medical care for this group were high. And the methods used to ascertain cases within this subpopulation were at least as good as those used in surveys that have produced estimates of incidence two- or threefold higher elsewhere.

18.3.2 Studies using mortality data

Goldberg and Kurland (1962) collected mortality data for, amongst other conditions, motor neurone disease and muscular atrophy (ICD code 356, 6th revision) from 26 countries for periods of up to 5 years between 1951 and 1958. To avoid distortion introduced by differences in the demographic characteristics of these countries, rates were directly age adjusted to the 1950 census population of the USA. Mean annual adjusted rates varied over an order of magnitude – from 0.3 or less per 100 000 population for Mexico, Chile, Czechoslovakia and the White population of South Africa to 1.1 or higher per 100 000 population for Iceland, New Zealand, Norway, Switzerland and the Netherlands. Goldberg and Kurland commented that the high fatality and general ease of diagnosis of conditions under this ICD classification made it unlikely that this variation merely reflected errors in diagnosis and certification. Others since have preferred to ascribe it to vagaries in the quality of data resources and death certification (Kondo, 1978; Kurtzke, 1991).

Suspicion that low mortality rates of uncommon diseases in countries with relatively poor medical resources are a consequence of low rates of diagnosis is justified. But it is surely a mistake to disregard all geographical variation in mortality without positive evidence that it can be accounted for by incomplete diagnosis or errors in death certification. It seems particularly implausible that the low mortality from motor neurone disease among White South Africans, a population with access to excellent medical facilities, can be explained in this way.

More recently, geographical differences in patterns of mortality have been found within countries. In the USA mortality is higher in counties to the west of the Mississippi than it is to the east (Bharucha *et al.*, 1983). In England and Wales mortality is higher in the south and east of the country than it is in the north and west (Martyn, Barker and Osmond, 1988). In Finland, higher rates are found in the south-eastern counties than in the rest of the country (Jokelainen, 1976).

18.3.3 Evidence of clustering of motor neurone disease

Reports of clusters of disease are invariably fascinating to clinicians. They feel intuitively that the cluster must hold an important clue to the causation of the disease. Epidemiologists are more sceptical; they are aware of the poor track record of cluster analysis in giving insights into the aetiology of chronic disease and have a livelier appreciation of the fact that, in small populations, large fluctuations in the frequency of uncommon diseases may occur by chance.

Rothman (1990) has argued convincingly that there is little scientific point in investigating individual disease clusters at all. He has pointed out that many clusters arise because of the way in which the boundaries of space and time that encompass the cases of disease are chosen – a process dubbed the Texas sharpshooter's procedure. (The sharpshooter first fires at the side of the barn and then paints a target centred on the bullet hole.) The impact of many, if not all, of the reported clusters of motor neurone disease (Hochberg, Bryan and Whelan, 1974; Kilnes and Hochberg, 1977; Sanders, 1980; Melmed and Krieger, 1982; Hyser, Kissel and Mendell, 1987; Sienko et al., 1990) depends upon the implicit use of this procedure to define an extremely restricted population that has experienced a high rate of motor neurone disease.

The problems of evaluating reports of an apparent excess of cases of neurological disease have also been helpfully discussed by Armon et al. (1991a). They showed how an apparent cluster of 12 patients from a small community (population 20 500) diagnosed as having motor neurone disease in a 5-year period evaporated when it was investigated systematically.

Mitchell, Gibson and Gatrell (1990) investigated clustering of place of residence in cases of motor neurone disease in Lancashire and south Cumbria. They identified 171 patients seen at the regional neurological centre or discharged from district general hospitals with a diagnosis of motor neurone disease between 1976 and 1986. Medical records were scrutinized, and only those patients with a definite diagnosis of motor neurone disease were included. A significant excess of cases was reported to have occurred in 2 out of the 15 county districts within the study area. However, the authors appear to have used one-tailed tests in assessing statistical significance. They have effectively disregarded the possibility that an area might show a significant deficit of cases. My own calculations of the statistical significance of these findings, using data provided in the published report, do not indicate that the excess is significant at the 5% level when a conventional two-tailed method is used. Further analysis of yet smaller areas was reported as showing several that contained more cases than would have been expected by chance, although again one-tailed tests were used and in only one of these smaller areas were more than three cases observed. No aetiological hypotheses were suggested to explain the observed geographical distribution.

Epidemiology

A similar approach has been used in the county of Skaraborg in Sweden (Gunnarsson, 1992). Here, place of residence was analysed for 168 patients with clinical onset of disease during the period 1961–90. Standardized morbidity ratios for six contiguous municipalities within the county were significantly elevated – but only in males with onset of disease during the period 1973–84. This redefinition of the time period to delimit the cluster once the data had been inspected looks very much like the Texas sharpshooter's procedure. The author's interpretation that the cluster represents an epidemic form of motor neurone disease in men seems, on the evidence available, rather more than the data can bear.

Analysis of deaths from motor neurone disease during the period 1973–82 in the state of Wisconsin revealed three adjoining counties in the north-east of the state in which rates were significantly higher than expected (Taylor and Davis, 1989). However, the numbers on which this observation was based are very small; during the whole of the 10-year period there were only 15 cases in these three counties. Another problem with this study is that the investigators made no attempt to standardize local rates for age. The counties in which rates of motor neurone disease were highest were sparsely inhabited rural areas. The average age of their population may well have been higher than for the state as a whole because of a tendency for young people to move to cities. If so, the numbers of cases that could have been expected in these counties will have been underestimated.

18.3.4 Studies of migrants and ethnic groups

Elian and Dean (1993) have studied mortality from motor neurone disease among first-generation immigrants to England from the Indian subcontinent, the Caribbean, and East and West Africa during the period 1979–88. Unfortunately, because the population censuses of 1971 and 1981 did not collect information about ethnic group, they were obliged to estimate a population denominator from 1% samples of the population of England and Wales that made up the labour force surveys of 1985, 1986 and 1987 and from the country of birth information, without ethnic group, collected in the 1981 census. Amongst immigrants from the Indian subcontinent with Asian names, mortality from motor neurone disease was less than half of that of people born in England and Wales. Amongst immigrants with English or Irish names, which the authors judged to be an indicator of European rather than Asian ancestry, mortality was similar to that of people born in England and Wales. Immigrants from the Caribbean also experienced lower rates of mortality from motor neurone disease than the native-born population of England and Wales, though the difference did not reach statistical significance. No conclusions could be drawn about mortality from motor neurone disease in immigrants from East and West Africa because both observed and expected numbers of deaths were too low.

Although the results of this study are intriguing, they must be interpreted tentatively. The methods used to judge ethnicity and to calculate population denominators were ingenious but less than ideal. There must also be some doubt, despite the fact that Asians are known to have high rates of contact with medical practitioners, about whether motor neurone disease is always diagnosed in immigrants. Nonetheless, the study does provide prima-facie evidence of real differences in rates of motor neurone disease between ethnic groups. An observation made by Critchley and Mitchell (1990) may support this view. In their series of 235 patients with motor neurone disease seen since 1976 at a Lancashire hospital, there was not a single patient of Asian origin or descent. They made no attempt to estimate how many Asian patients might have been expected if motor neurone disease occurred at the same rate as in the rest of the Lancashire population. The 1991 census shows that 3.7% of the Lancashire population is of Asian origin (Balarajan and Soni Raleigh, 1992). No data are yet available that allow comparison of the age structure of the two ethnic groups but, if we ignore this, a very rough estimate of the number of Asian patients with motor neurone disease that could have been expected in this series is 8 or 9.

However, it is clear that motor neurone disease is not confined to White races. Mortality amongst the Japanese is similar to that of North America and most European countries (Kondo and Tsubaki, 1977). In American Blacks, mortality is about half that of Whites and is increasing at a roughly similar rate (Lilienfeld et al., 1989).

18.4 TIME TRENDS IN MOTOR NEURONE DISEASE

With the exception of Japan, where mortality from motor neurone disease fell between 1960 and 1971, and Guam, where mortality has declined rapidly since the 1950s, all studies of mortality from motor neurone disease over time have shown a rising trend. Kondo and Tsubaki (1977) updated the original study of international differences in mortality of Goldberg and Kurland (1962) and found a rise in mortality in all of the 18 countries for which data were available for two time periods. The magnitude of the increase was not clearly related to the mortality rate of the first time period (1953–58). Within the last 5 years there have been reports from England and Wales (Martyn, Barker and Osmond, 1988), the USA (Lilienfeld et al., 1989), France (Durrleman and

Epidemiology

Alperovitch, 1989), Norway (Flaten, 1989), Sweden (Gunnarsson *et al.*, 1990) and Australia and New Zealand (Dean and Elian, 1993) that mortality is continuing to increase. This rise in mortality is found in all age groups, but it is in the elderly that the increase is most marked.

Understanding the time trends in mortality from motor neurone disease is potentially very important. If the trend in mortality truly reflects a rapid increase in the incidence of the disease, it provides powerful evidence that an environmental factor is decisive in determining risk of the disease. Comparison of secular trends in disease rates with changes over time in environmental influences, including those affecting lifestyle, may lead to the formulation of hypotheses about causation. But these generalities beg the central question concerning the extent to which the rise in mortality can be explained by improved recognition, diagnosis and recording of the disease on death certificates.

Analysis of mortality data by birth cohort and period of death may give more insight into the influences that determine changes over time than simply examining age-specific death rates. Diseases in which long intervals elapse between exposure to the cause of the disease and its effect, whether indicated by onset of disease or death, tend to show changes between successive generations. Such changes are known as birth cohort effects. Diseases whose cause is more immediate are likely to affect all age groups synchronously even if different age groups are affected to different extents. Any change in mortality over time is therefore related to period of death. Changes in diagnosis, classification and treatment of disease usually influence all age groups more or less simultaneously, and tend to show up as period of death effects, rather than birth cohort effects.

Figure 18.1 shows age-specific death rates from motor neurone disease in England and Wales for men and women over three time periods. Rates are lower for women than for men in all three periods, but it is clear that mortality has increased progressively in both sexes over time. It also appears that mortality from motor neurone disease reaches a peak between the ages of 65 and 80 years and then declines. Note, though, that the peak of mortality occurs at an older age in the later time periods.

Figure 18.2 uses the same data to show how mortality has changed over time in four age groups. The pattern is similar in both sexes; rates have increased in all age groups but the increase is very much greater in the older age groups than in the younger.

The same data are used once again in Figure 18.3 to show the mortality of different birth cohorts. The mortality of the earliest cohorts – those born in the nineteenth century – declines after the age of about 70 years. In sharp contrast, all later cohorts show a continuous increase in

MALES.

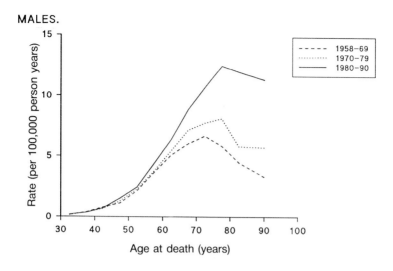

FEMALES.

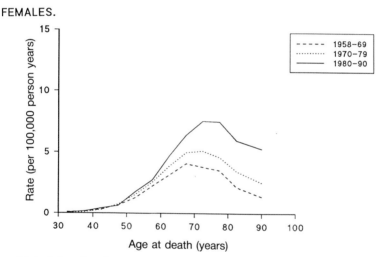

Figure 18.1 Mortality from motor neurone disease in England and Wales for men and women during the periods 1958–69, 1970–79 and 1980–90.

mortality with age. Further, all successive cohorts born after 1900 experience a progressive increase in mortality at every age. That is to say, at any age, mortality from motor neurone disease is higher for people born later.

Figure 18.3 suggests that time trends of motor neurone disease can be understood in terms of a birth cohort effect that began in the generation

405

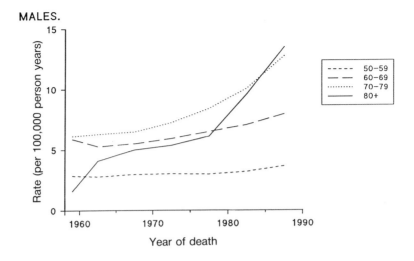

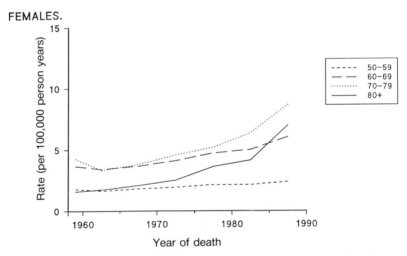

Figure 18.2 Mortality from motor neurone disease in England and Wales, 1958–1990, for men and women according to age at death.

born at the turn of the century. While this pattern is compatible with a real increase in the incidence of motor neurone disease, the analysis does not settle the question. It is possible to devise an alternative explanation by invoking a period of death effect that is age dependent. A steady improvement in diagnosis and certification of motor neurone disease over the last 30–40 years would account for the observed time

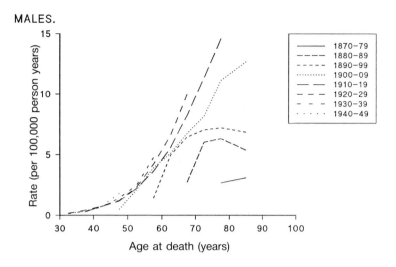

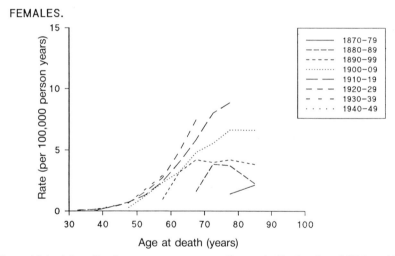

Figure 18.3 Mortality from motor neurone disease in England and Wales, 1958–90, for men and women by birth cohort.

trends if the improvement had been greater in the older than in the younger age groups.

Rather similar time trends, again on a global scale, have been reported for mortality from multiple myeloma (Cuzick, Velez and Doll, 1983). For this disease, too, it was difficult to separate the apparent increases due to changes in diagnostic capability from the true increases in myeloma incidence. The trends over time for both multiple myeloma and motor neurone disease can be resolved into either a birth cohort effect or an age-dependent period of death effect equally well. Other evidence is available that suggests that the increase in myeloma is not just a consequence of better diagnosis. The similarity of the trends in mortality from motor neurone disease in countries with very different systems of health care perhaps indicates that the increase in mortality from this disease too is not wholly the result of better recognition and certification. But we shall have to wait for repeated studies of incidence before we can be confident of this. The possibility that the rising mortality reflects, at least in part, a real increase in the frequency of occurrence of motor neurone disease cannot be excluded.

The analysis also strongly suggests that the decline in mortality in the oldest age groups, seen most clearly in Figure 18.1, is an artefact produced by the aggregation of data from a number of birth cohorts. Most of the deaths that contribute to the part of the curve in which rates are falling occurred in people from the earliest birth cohorts. Figure 18.3 shows that mortality did decline in the oldest people born in the earliest cohorts. But for people born after about the turn of the century, mortality from motor neurone disease continues to increase with age.

A rather different approach to the analysis of mortality data for motor neurone disease has recently been developed by Neilson, Robinson and Hunter (1992) using a Gompertzian model. This model assumes that mortality rises exponentially with increasing age such that:

$$R(x) = R(0) \times 10^{(ax)}$$

(where $R(x)$ is the rate at age x, $R(0)$ the rate at age 0 and a is the slope of the exponential term. They found that such a model can be made to fit the observed age- and sex-specific mortality rates closely – but only until the age of 64 years. After that age, observed mortality rates are much lower than those predicted by the model. They interpret this deviation as indicating the presence of a subpopulation of people susceptible to motor neurone disease, some of whom have died from other causes before they can develop the disease. They suggest that the increasing mortality from motor neurone disease over time can be simply explained by the decreasing mortality from other causes. The idea is that a progressively greater proportion of the susceptible subpopulation survives long enough to develop the condition. One may be forgiven for remaining sceptical about this argument. Is it reasonable to expect that just two parameters, $R(0)$ and a, will adequately describe all the factors that might influence mortality from motor neurone disease? If not, the failure of a Gompertzian model to fit the data after the age of 64 years (and more than half of all deaths from motor neurone disease occur after this age) may indicate the deficiencies of the model rather than yield useful biological insights.

18.5 RISK FACTORS FOR MOTOR NEURONE DISEASE

18.5.1 Trauma

Numerous case reports link the onset of symptoms of motor neurone disease to physical trauma. This sort of anecdotal evidence must be treated sceptically because of the obvious bias introduced by the enthusiasm of authors to document unusual cases. However, there are a number of reports of case–control studies that also suggest that mechanical trauma, bony fracture, electric shock and surgical procedures are associated with an increased risk of the disease. Differing views have been expressed about the consistency of these findings. Table 18.2 is an attempt to summarize the results of case–control studies that have investigated various categories of trauma as a possible risk factor for motor neurone disease. Readers may judge their consistency for themselves.

Many of these studies can be criticized for their small sample size, unsatisfactory selection of controls or method of ascertaining past exposure to indicators of trauma. Most weight should be given to the results of three of the larger studies – those of Chancellor et al. (1993), Deapen and Henderson (1988), and Kurtzke and Beebe (1980) – not only because of their size but because they are methodologically the most sound.

Two major difficulties must be borne in mind when interpreting evidence of a positive association between past trauma and motor neurone disease. The first concerns the extent to which the findings may be a result of a systematic difference between cases and controls in the way in which they have reported past trauma. A danger in studies that rely on recall to assess exposure is that, because of a natural interest in trying to understand why they have become ill, patients are better motivated to search their memories than controls. Most of the case–control studies summarized in Table 18.2 are vulnerable to this source of bias. However, two studies, both of which found a positive association between trauma and motor neurone disease, eliminated or minimized this problem. Kurtzke's study of US veterans used pre-existing military records rather than the subjects' own testimony to ascertain past trauma. Chancellor's study corroborated subjects' own reports of trauma by comparing them with what was recorded in medical files held by these subjects' primary care physicians. The latter study produced little

Table 18.2 Case–control studies of trauma in motor neurone disease

	Size of study	Type of trauma	Relative risk	Notes
Campbell, Williams and Barltrop, 1970	74 cases 74 controls	Bony fracture during lifetime Bony fracture in 5 years before onset of MND	1.5 3.3	Relative risk calculated by C.N. Martyn
Reed and Brody, 1975	37 cases 37 controls	Serious accidents Fracture Injury-producing unconciousness	No excess among cases	Guamanian form of MND
Felmus, Patten and Swante, 1976	25 cases 50 controls	Fractured bone Major trauma	2.9 0.6	Relative risks calculated by C.N. Martyn from the published results. No account taken of matching
Kurtzke, 1980	504 cases 504 controls (males only)	Surgical operations Injury	2.2 2.6	Ascertainment of past operation and injury free from recall bias
Pierce-Ruhland and Patten, 1981	80 cases 78 controls	Operations Injuries within 10 years of onset of motor neurone disease	No statistically significant association	
Kondo and Tsubaki, 1981	158 cases 158 controls	Mechanical injury Electrical injury Surgical operation	1.5 women 1.4 men – women 0.9 men 0.7 women 1.0 men	

Table 18.2 continued

	Size of study	Type of trauma	Relative risk	Notes
Gawel, Zaiwalla and Rose, 1983	63 cases 61 controls	Electric shock/struck by lightning Back injury Bony fracture and head injury	3.5 4.1 0.5	Relative risks calculated by C.N Martyn
Murros and Fogelholm, 1983	38 cases 146 controls	Serious injury Bony fracture Surgery	1.7 1.2 0.9	Relative risks calculated by C.N. Martyn
Angelini, Armani and Bresslin, 1983	25 cases 25 controls	Bony fractures Mechanical trauma	10 No association reported	
Roelofs-Iversen et al., 1984	105 cases 104 controls	Major surgery	Significant association – no data on magnitude of risk	
Deapen and Henderson, 1986	518 cases 518 controls	Surgery Electric shock resulting in unconsciousness Physical trauma Surgical procedure spinal surgery myelogram	No association reported 2.8 1.6 1.1 1.7 0.9	
Gresham et al., 1987	66 cases 66 controls	Bony fracture		
Granieri et al., 1988	72 cases 216 controls	Injury Operation	2.1 1.5	
Li, Alberman and Swash, 1990	560 cases 220 controls	Cumulative incidence of surgical operations	No excess among cases	

Table 18.2 *continued*

	Size of study	Type of trauma	Relative risk	Notes
Sienko *et al.*, 1990	6 cases 12 controls	Physical trauma Bony fracture Sports injury Automobile accident Electrical injury	∞ 2.5 5 3 2.2	
Provinciali and Giovagnoli, 1990	77 cases 80 controls	Skeletal trauma Surgical procedures	2.0 0.9	
Chio *et al.*, 1991	512 cases 512 controls	Mechanical injury Operation Multiple operations	1.6 No excess among cases 1.3	
Armon *et al.*, 1991b	47 cases 47 controls (males only)	Past trauma	No excess among cases	
Gunnarsson, 1992	92 cases 372 controls	Surgery within 10 years of onset of MND Surgery 11–35 years before onset of MND Bony fracture within 10 years of onset of MND Bony fracture 11–35 years before onset of MND Electric shock	0.9 0.8 1.6 0.9 1.1	Estimates of two exposure levels to electric shock combined by C.N. Martyn
Chancellor *et al.* (submitted)	103 cases 103 controls	Major surgery Bony fractures during lifetime Bony fractures within 5 years of onset of MND Non-fracture trauma	No excess among cases 1.3 15 No excess among cases	History of trauma corroborated from medical records

evidence to suggest that patients with motor neurone disease exaggerated episodes of trauma by comparison with controls. This finding suggests that it would be a mistake to write off the association with trauma as an artefact of biased recall.

The second difficulty in interpretation occurs because of the possibility that, in the presymptomatic stages of motor neurone disease, motor control has already deteriorated and that patients are predisposed to trauma as a result of their disease. Swash and Ingram (1988) have reported three patients with motor neurone disease in whom there were clear indications that some aspect of motor performance had begun to deteriorate several years before a diagnosis of motor neurone disease was made. The fact that most studies have found the association between trauma and motor neurone disease to be strongest in the years immediately before onset of symptoms does nothing to resolve the problem. While a close temporal relation between trauma and the onset of symptoms might be expected if trauma was, in fact, a causal factor, a similar relation would also be expected if the association were a result of the earliest stages of the disease.

Calculation of the attributable risk of trauma, as opposed to the relative risk, indicates that, even if the association is real and not just an effect of biased recall, it cannot account for more than a small minority of cases of motor neurone disease. Even if one takes deliberately high estimates of both the cumulative incidence of past trauma (say 20%) and its associated relative risk (say 5), the proportion of cases of motor neurone disease that could be attributed to this cause is no more than 15%.

Kurland et al. (1992) have recently carried out a comprehensive critical review of published studies in which mechanical trauma was investigated as a risk factor for classic amyotrophic lateral sclerosis. They concluded that the existing data did not suggest any association of the disease with antecedent trauma.

18.5.2 Occupational risk factors

An excess risk of motor neurone disease has been reported for truck drivers and operatives, workers using pneumatic tools, leather and textile workers and people employed in the boot and shoe industry. These are, for the most part, isolated findings that have not been confirmed in other studies.

A regular analysis of occupational mortality for England and Wales is carried out by the Office of Population Censuses and Surveys and published as a decennial supplement (Office of Population Censuses and Surveys, 1978). Mortality from motor neurone disease amongst men aged 16–64 years was highest in social class 3. A consistent excess of deaths has been found in tannery and leather workers during three separate periods: 1959–63, 1970–72 and 1975; 19 deaths occurred when 10.2 were expected. The most recent decennial supplement, based on deaths during 1979–80 and 1982–83, also reports an excess of deaths amongst male leather workers. More detailed analysis by occupational category suggests that the greater part of the excess is attributable to makers of leather goods and shoes rather than to tannery workers. Hawkes, Cavanagh and Fox (1989) have suggested that exposure to solvents used in leather industries may be relevant. Against these findings must be set the results of a follow-up study of a large cohort of workers in the boot and shoe industry; there was no excess in the observed numbers of deaths from motor neurone disease (Martyn, 1989).

Six population-based surveys have reported an increased risk for those employed in agriculture and heavy manual labour (Rosati et al., 1977; Bracco, Antuono and Amaducci, 1979; Holloway and Emery, 1982; Bharucha et al., 1983; Gunnarsson and Palm, 1984; Kalfakis et al., 1991). But as de Pedro-Cuesta and Litvan (1991) have pointed out, these investigators failed to take into account the potential confounding effects of rural environment or socioeconomic group. No confirmation of an increased risk in agricultural workers can be found in the analyses of occupational mortality carried out by the Office of Population Censuses and Surveys referred to above.

The report of the large case–control study carried out by Deapen and Henderson (1986) indicated a significantly elevated risk associated with recall of an electric shock severe enough to produce unconsciousness (see Table 18.2). The same study also showed a statistically significant increased risk of motor neurone disease associated with working in an electrically related occupation.

LEAD AND HEAVY METALS

Lead is a well-known, if now rare, cause of encephalopathy and motor neuropathy. And there are a few reports that a syndrome closely resembling motor neurone disease may result from lead poisoning. However, the evidence that exposure to lead is involved in the aetiology of sporadic motor neurone disease is conflicting. Reports of increased tissue concentrations of lead in patients with motor neurone disease are based on studies of small numbers of cases, often with poorly chosen controls, and the findings have not always been confirmed by other workers (Petkau *et al.*, 1974; House *et al.*, 1978; Conradi *et al.*, 1980, 1982). Case–control studies that have attempted to investigate past exposure to lead have always been vulnerable to recall bias and the results are inconsistent.

A matched case–control study from the Mayo Clinic examined occupational and recreational exposure to lead in 47 male patients and found a relative risk of 5.5 for a cumulative lifetime exposure of 200 h or more (Armon *et al.*, 1991b). A similarly high relative risk (5.3) for occupational exposure to lead of more than 12 months' duration was found in a recent case–control study from Scotland (Chancellor *et al.*, submitted). An earlier report of a positive association between heavy exposure to lead and risk of motor neurone disease is difficult to interpret because in the majority of exposed cases, lower motor neurone features predominated and the progression of the disease was atypically slow (Campbell, Williams and Barltrop, 1970).

Other case–control studies that investigated exposure to lead as a risk factor for motor neurone disease failed to find a statistically significant association (Deapen and Henderson, 1986; Gresham *et al.*, 1987; Granieri *et al.*, 1988; Norris and Padia, 1989; Provinciali and Giovagnoli, 1990). Nor, in a nationwide study of the geographical distribution of motor neurone disease in the USA, were mortality rates in and around counties where lead smelting took place significantly different from the US average (Bharucha *et al.*, 1983). No cohort study of workers in lead industries has shown an excess of cases of motor neurone disease.

Occupational exposure to heavy metals is very much more frequent in men than in women. If industrial exposure to lead were an important causal factor in motor neurone disease, one might reasonably expect a large excess of male cases of disease. Further, permitted levels of occupational exposure to lead have been gradually reduced over the past century. In Britain, legislation to protect workers from the toxic effects of lead-containing substances was first introduced at the beginning of the century. Levels of exposure to lead in industry are now regularly monitored and cases of lead poisoning, once a common condition, are now rare. This reduction in occupational exposure is not compatible with what is known of the time trends of motor neurone disease.

18.5.3 Past poliomyelitis

The possibility of a link between poliomyelitis and motor neurone disease was first discussed in the last century (Raymond, 1875). The idea is attractive because of the similarities in some of the clinical features of the two diseases and because both disorders have a predilection for motor neurones. There are occasional reports of cases series of motor neurone disease in which the frequency of preceding poliomyelitis seemed surprisingly high (Zilkha, 1962) but the few case–control studies that have investigated past poliomyelitis have not provided consistent evidence of a strong association (Poskanzer, Cantor and Kaplan, 1969; Pierce-Ruhland and Patten, 1981; Deapen and Henderson, 1986).

There is, however, a recent report of similarities in the geographical distribution and the trends over time of the two conditions in England and Wales (Martyn et al., 1988). Current mortality from motor neurone disease was found to correlate with past notification rates of paralytic poliomyelitis. The same report also drew attention to the parallel nature of the time trends of the two diseases. As we have seen already, mortality from motor neurone disease has increased over the last 30 years in most countries in the developed world. A similar rise in the incidence of paralytic poliomyelitis had taken place in Europe and North America half a century earlier. The authors advanced the hypothesis that the link between motor neurone disease and poliomyelitis depended upon subclinical infection. They suggested that subclinical infection of the central nervous system with poliovirus might have left an individual with reduced numbers of motor neurones and therefore both at increased risk from a second insult to the nervous system and more susceptible to age-related neuronal depletion.

Although it follows that patients with motor neurone disease would have spent their childhood and early adult life in conditions associated with increased risk of poliovirus infection, it has proved hard to test the hypothesis directly. Nearly all adults are seropositive for all strains of poliovirus and it is not possible to distinguish between those who acquired antibodies from infection with wild-type poliovirus and those who are seropositive as a result of active immunization. Population-based serological investigations carried out in the 1950s before immunization programmes had been initiated identified the major determinants of age and risk of infection as absence of domestic amenities, domestic overcrowding and a large sibship size (Backett, 1957; MacLeod et al., 1958). A case–control study that investigated these factors as indirect markers of infection with poliovirus found them to be positively associated with motor neurone disease, but the increase in risk was too small to be convincing (Martyn and Osmond, 1992). Time will eventually tell whether the hypothesis is correct; if it is, rates of motor neurone disease will begin to decline from about the year 2010, when the first cohort of people to have been immunized against poliovirus in childhood will reach the age at which the disease usually presents. The fall in incidence can be expected to occur in the youngest age groups first.

416

Table 18.3 Standardized mortality ratios for motor neurone disease by place of residence for England and Wales, 1968–78

| | *Standardized mortality ratios* | | |
	Men	*Women*	*Both sexes*
Large towns	98.9	96.3	97.7
Small towns	100.9	105.1	102.8
Rural areas	99.7	98.7	99.3

18.5.4 Urban rural differences

Although little information is available, there are no strong indications that the occurrence of motor neurone disease varies with levels of urbanization. Two case–control studies, both carried out in large geographical areas, showed no differences in risk of the disease associated with urban or rural residence either at birth or at diagnosis (Kurtzke and Beebe, 1980; Kondo and Tsubaki, 1981). Two Italian incidence surveys produced conflicting results: in one (Angelini, Armani and Bresolin, 1983), incidence of motor neurone disease was significantly higher in the rural population; in the other (Leone *et al.*, 1983), the incidence was higher in the urban area. But neither of these surveys was judged by Chancellor and Warlow (1992) to have used ideal methods for the identification of cases, and the explanation for the differences may lie in the way the surveys were carried out.

A geographical analysis of all deaths from motor neurone disease in England and Wales during the period 1968–78 using the usual place of residence as recorded on death certificates showed no significant differences between large towns (county boroughs), small towns (municipal boroughs and urban districts) and rural areas (rural districts) for mortality from motor neurone disease (C.N. Martyn, unpublished data). These results are summarized in Table 18.3.

A similar result was found in the USA when age-adjusted mortality rates were mapped at county level (Bharucha *et al.*, 1983). No relation was apparent between mortality and percentage of the population living in urban areas. There was, however, a weak but statistically significant association between mortality and percentage of the population living on rural farms.

18.5.5 Socioeconomic status

Social class and other indices of affluence or deprivation indirectly indicate risk of exposure to a whole constellation of environmental agents. Evidence that motor neurone disease was consistently more frequent in a particular socioeconomic group would be valuable in narrowing down the search for environmental risk factors. So far, however, only fragmentary data are available.

The decennial analysis of mortality by occupation carried out by the Office of Population Censuses and Surveys (1978) for deaths in England and Wales has already been mentioned. For men between the ages of 16 and 64 years, mortality from motor neurone disease was highest in social class 3. Martyn *et al.* (1990) used extracts of death certificates for the period April 1969 to December 1972 to calculate proportional mortality ratios for motor neurone disease for men at all ages. They found that mortality ratios increased progressively with higher social class, but it should be noted that the use of proportional mortality ratios may have exaggerated any social class gradient since mortality is lower generally in higher social classes. In a study of mortality in the USA (Bharucha *et al.*, 1983), death rates from motor neurone disease were highest in counties with the highest socioeconomic status as judged by median number of school years completed by the adult population. Chancellor *et al.* (1992) explored the relation between affluence and motor neurone disease in Scotland using a measure of socioeconomic deprivation based upon rates of car ownership, and unemployment and degree of overcrowding in addition to social class. Although standardized mortality ratios for motor neurone disease were highest in relatively affluent areas, they found that the association was strongest in the oldest age groups and suggested that it could be accounted for by a failure to diagnose motor neurone disease in elderly patients from deprived areas.

No definite conclusions about the relation of socioeconomic factors to risk of motor neurone disease can be drawn, but what evidence exists does not indicate that the condition is positively associated with poverty.

18.5.6 Sex differences

Mortality and incidence surveys consistently indicate that rates of motor neurone disease are higher in men than they are in women. de Pedro-Cuesta and Litvan (1991) have recently suggested that these differences may largely or wholly be a result of underdiagnosis of the condition in elderly women in the past but, as Figures 18.2 and 18.3 show, mortality from motor neurone disease is lower in women than men at all ages and in all time periods for which data are available. Nor is there any indication, within England and Wales at least, that the sex ratio is changing over time.

18.6 CONCLUSIONS

We are a long way from being able to draw even a rough map of the global distribution of motor neurone disease. There is as yet no reliable information about the incidence of the disease from any country in the southern hemisphere, and even mortality data are lacking for many developing countries. Any comment on the geography of the disease must therefore be provisional. There is, however, an impression that motor neurone disease is a 'western disease', common only in the affluent countries of the developed world. This impression is strengthened by the low rates of motor neurone disease in Asian immigrants to Britain.

It is time for the notion that motor neurone disease is homogeneous in its occurrence to be buried and forgotten. In retrospect, the rationale for the idea was always doubtful. It depended on dismissing international differences in mortality from the disease as being due to variation in diagnosis and death certification. Was it then justifiable to invert the argument and use the same inadequate data as confirmation that no differences in mortality exist? There is now, in any case, good evidence from methodologically sound surveys that the incidence of the disease varies between places.

Analysis of mortality data from England and Wales for the last 30 years suggests that mortality from motor neurone disease does not, as was previously thought, decline in the very elderly. Data from Sweden (Gunnarsson et al., 1990) and Rochester, USA (Yoshida et al., 1986) lead to the same conclusion. The apparent decline in mortality in the elderly may be a result of underdiagnosis of the condition in people born in the last century.

Studies of time trends in motor neurone disease are all based upon the retrospective analysis of data derived from death certification. The extent to which the continuing rise in mortality, seen in all countries (except Japan and Guam) for which data are available, is a result of improvements in the recognition and certification of the disease must remain a matter of individual judgment. My own view is that it would be perverse to ignore such a potentially important clue to aetiology. Mortality from motor neurone disease has doubled over the past 30 years in England and Wales. Rises of similar size have been reported from several other countries. Even if partly explained by changes in death certification, these rapid changes suggest that there must be powerful environmental determinants of motor neurone disease.

Epidemiology

No consistently strong risk factors for motor neurone disease have yet emerged. Despite numerous investigations, the evidence that trauma or exposure to heavy metals is associated with increased risk of motor neurone disease remains less than compelling. Nor are any occupational groups consistently over-represented amongst cases of motor neurone disease.

What are the priorities for epidemiological research? The view that motor neurone disease shows no interesting geographical variation in its occurrence was, until recently, hardly questioned. Now that this idea has been shown to be mistaken, one can hope that investigators will be stimulated to examine the incidence of the disease in different parts of the world. Much could be done to extend knowledge of its descriptive epidemiology. Studies in non-industrialized nations are urgently needed.

The intriguing questions about time trends in the disease raised by studies of mortality can only be completely resolved by establishing and maintaining a prospective survey of incident cases in a fairly large population over a number of years. A register of patients with motor neurone disease has been set up in Scotland (Chancellor *et al.*, 1992), which could provide a model for similar endeavours elsewhere. One useful contribution that has already emerged from this work is a practical case definition of motor neurone disease for epidemiological studies. Prospective validation of the criteria used in this definition will be possible.

Studies of environmental risk factors have not so far been very successful in generating ideas about causation. There are a number of possible explanations for this failure. It must be remembered that epidemiological investigation does not provide a powerful methodology for discovering weak associations. If each of a number of widespread environmental agents has the potential to cause the disease, the risk associated with any single one may be too small to detect except by an impracticably large study. Alternatively, a combination of exposures may be required to produce the disease; again, the associated risk for any single factor might be too small to detect. A third possibility is that an environmental agent is capable of causing disease only in individuals rendered susceptible by some genetic predisposition or antecedent insult to the nervous system. If it were feasible to identify which individuals were susceptible, investigations of environmental factors could be better targeted. Evidence that cases of motor neurone disease have a limited capacity to metabolize sulphur-containing substances is discussed in detail in Chapter 21. One implication of this work is that it may offer an opportunity for epidemiologists to define a susceptible population in which to study environmental risk factors for the disease.

ACKNOWLEDGEMENTS

The author is indebted to Andrew Chancellor and Charles Warlow for allowing him to use, in modified form, a table from their review of studies of incidence of motor neurone disease; to Lynda Wood who checked the references in this chapter; to Alistair Shiell who helped analyse mortality data; and to Clive Osmond for his comments on the manuscript.

REFERENCES

Angelini, C., Armani, M. and Bresolin, N. (1983) Incidence and risk factors of motor neuron disease in the Venice and Padua districts of Italy, 1972–1979. *Neuroepidemiology*, **2**, 236–42.

Anon. (1990) What causes motoneuron disease? (editorial). *Lancet*, **336**, 1033–5.

Armon, C., Daube, J.R., O'Brien, P.C. *et al.* (1991a) When is an apparent excess of neurologic cases epidemiologically significant? *Neurology*, **41**, 1713–18.

Armon, C., Kurland, L.T., Daube, J.R. and O'Brien, P.C. (1991b) Epidemiologic correlates of sporadic amyotrophic lateral sclerosis. *Neurology*, **41**, 1077–84.

Backett, E.M. (1957) Social patterns of antibody to poliovirus. *Lancet*, **i**, 778–83.

Balarajan, R. and Soni Raleigh, V. (1992) The ethnic populations of England and Wales: the 1991 Census. *Health Trends*, **24**, 113–16.

Bharucha, N.E., Schoenberg, B.S., Raven, R.H. *et al.* (1983) Geographic distribution of motor neuron disease and correlation with possible etiologic factors. *Neurology*, **33**, 911–15.

Bracco, L., Antuono, P. and Amaducci, L. (1979) Study of epidemiological and etiological factors of amyotrophic lateral sclerosis in the province of Florence, Italy. *Acta Neurol. Scand.*, **60**, 112–24.

Buckley, J., Warlow, C., Smith, P. *et al.* (1983) Motor neuron disease in England and Wales 1959–1979. *J. Neurol. Neurosurg. Psychiatr.*, **46**, 197–205.

Campbell, A.M.G., Williams, E.R. and Barltrop, D. (1970) Motor neurone disease and exposure to lead. *J. Neurol. Neurosurg. Psychiatry*, **33**, 877–85.

Chancellor, A.M. and Warlow, C.P. (1992) Adult onset motor neuron disease: worldwide mortality, incidence and distribution since 1950. *J. Neurol. Neurosurg. Psychiatry*, **55**, 1106–15.

Chancellor, A.M., Swingler, R.J. and Fraser, H. (1993) The utility of Scottish morbidity and mortality data for epidemiological studies of motor neurone disease. *J. Epidemiol. Community Health*, **47**, 116–20.

Chancellor, A.M., Warlow, C.P., Carstairs, V. *et al.* (1992) Affluence, age and motor neurone disease (letter). *J. Epidemiol. Community Health*, **46**, 172–3.

Chancellor, A.M., Slattery, J.M., Fraser, H. and Warlow, C.P. Risk factors for motor neuron disease: a case-control study based on patients from the Scottish Motor Neuron Disease Register. (submitted for publication).

421

Epidemiology

Chio, A., Meineri, P., Tribolo, A. and Schiffer, D. (1991) Risk factors in motor neurone disease: a case-control study. *Neuroepidemiology*, **10**, 174–84.

Chio, A., Magnani, C., Oddenino, E. *et al.* (1992) Accuracy of death certificate diagnosis of amyotrophic lateral sclerosis. *J. Epidemiol. Community Health*, **46**, 517–18.

Conradi, S., Ronnevi, L.O., Nise, G. *et al.* (1980) Abnormal distribution of lead in amyotrophic lateral sclerosis. Re-estimation of lead in the cerebrospinal fluid. *J. Neurol. Sci.*, **48**, 413–18.

Conradi, S., Ronnevi, L.O., Nise, G. *et al.* (1982) Longtime penicillamine treatment in amyotrophic lateral sclerosis with parallel determinations of lead in blood, plasma and urine. *Acta Neurol. Scand.*, **65**, 203–11.

Critchley, E.M.R. and Mitchell, J.D. (1990) What causes motoneurone disease? *Lancet*, **336**, 1380.

Cuzick, J., Velez, R. and Doll, R. (1983) International variations and temporal trends in mortality from multiple myeloma. *Int. J. Cancer*, **32**, 13–19.

Dean, G. and Elian, M. (1993) Motor neurone disease and multiple sclerosis mortality in Australia, New Zealand and South Africa compared with England and Wales. *J. Neurol. Neurosurg. Psychiatr.*, **56**, 633–7.

Deapen, D.M. and Henderson, B.E. (1986) A case-control study of amyotrophic lateral sclerosis. *Am. J. Epidemiol.*, **123**, 790–9.

Durrleman, S. and Alperovitch, A. (1989) Increasing trend of ALS in France and elsewhere: are the changes real? *Neurology*, **39**, 768–73.

Elian, M. and Dean, G. (1993) Motor neurone disease and multiple sclerosis among immigrants to England from the Indian subcontinent, the Caribbean and East and West Africa. *J. Neurol. Neurosurg. Psychiatr.*, **56**, 454–7.

Felmus, M.T., Patten, B.M. and Swante, L. (1976) Antecedent events in amyotrophic lateral sclerosis. *Neurology*, **26**, 167–72.

Flaten, T.P. (1989) Rising mortality from motoneuron disease. *Lancet*, **i**, 1018.

Forsgren, L., Almay, B.G., Holmgren, G. and Wall, S. (1983) Epidemiology of motor neuron disease in northern Sweden. *Acta Neurol. Scand.*, **68**, 20–9.

Gawel, M., Zaiwalla, Z. and Rose, F.C. (1983) Antecedent events in motor neuron disease. *J. Neurol. Neurosurg. Psychiatr.*, **46**, 1041–3.

Goldberg, I.D. and Kurland, L.T. (1962) Mortality in 33 countries from diseases of the nervous system. *World Neurology*, 444–65.

Granieri, E., Carreras, M., Tola, R. *et al.* (1988) Motor neuron disease in the province of Ferrara, Italy, 1964–1982. *Neurology*, **38**, 1604–8.

Gresham, L.S., Molgaard, C.A., Golbeck, A.L. and Smith, R. (1987) Amyotrophic lateral sclerosis and history of skeletal fracture: a case-control study. *Neurology*, **37**, 717–19.

Gunnarsson, L.-G. (1992) On the occurrence and possible causes of motor neuron disease in Sweden. *Linköping University Medical Dissertations*. **No. 364**.

Gunnarsson, L.-G. and Palm, R. (1984) Motor neuron disease and heavy manual labour: an epidemiologic survey of Varmland County, Sweden. *Neuroepidemiology*, **3**, 195–206.

Gunnarsson, L.-G., Lindberg, G., Söderfelt, B. and Axelson, D. (1990) The mortality of motor neuron disease in Sweden, 1961–1985. *Arch. Neurol.*, **47**, 42–6.

Hawkes, C.H., Cavanagh, J.B. and Fox, A.J. (1989) Motoneuron disease: a disorder secondary to solvent exposure? *Lancet*, **i**, 73–6.

Hochberg, F.H., Bryan, J.A.I. and Whelan, M.A. (1974) Clustering of amyotrophic lateral sclerosis. *Lancet*, **i**, 34.

Hoffman, P.M. and Brody, J.A. (1971) The reliability of death certificate reporting for amyotrophic lateral sclerosis. *J. Chron. Dis.*, **24**, 5–8.

Højer-Pedersen, E., Christensen, P.B. and Jensen, N.B. (1989) Incidence and prevalence of motor neuron disease in two Danish counties. *Neuroepidemiology*, **8**, 151–9.

Holloway, S.M. and Emery, A.E.H. (1982) The epidemiology of motor neurone disease in Scotland. *Muscle Nerve*, **5**, 131–3.

House, A.O., Abbot, R.J., Davidson, D.L.W. *et al.* (1978) Response to penicillamine of lead concentrations in CSF and blood of patients with motor neurone disease. *Br. Med. J.*, **2**, 1684.

Hudson, A.J., Davenport, A. and Hader, W.J. (1986) The incidence of amyotrophic lateral sclerosis in southwestern Ontario, Canada. *Neurology*, **36**, 1524–8.

Hyser, C.L., Kissell, J.T. and Mendell, J.R. (1987) Three cases of amyotrophic lateral sclerosis in a common occupational environment. *J. Neurol.*, **234**, 443–4.

Jokelainen, M. (1976) The epidemiology of amyotrophic lateral sclerosis in Finland. A study based on the death certificates of 421 patients. *J. Neurol. Sci.*, **29**, 55–63.

Kahana, E. and Zilber, N. (1984) Changes in the incidence of amyotrophic lateral sclerosis in Israel. *Arch. Neurol.*, **4**, 157–60.

Kalfakis, N., Vassilopoulos, D., Voumvorakis, C. *et al.* (1991) Amyotrophic lateral sclerosis in Southern Greece: an epidemiologic study. *Neuroepidemiology*, **10**, 170–3.

Kilnes, A.W. and Hochberg, F.H. (1977) Amyotrophic lateral sclerosis in a high selenium environment. *J. Am. Med. Assoc.*, **237**, 2843–4.

Kondo, K. (1978) Motor neuron disease, in *Advances in Neurology*, Vol. 19, *Changing Population Patterns and Clues for Etiology* (ed. B.S. Schoenberg), Raven Press, New York, pp. 509–43.

Kondo, K. and Tsubaki, T. (1977) Changing mortality patterns of motor neuron disease in Japan. *J. Neurol. Sci.*, **32**, 411–24.

Kondo, K. and Tsubaki, T. (1981) Case-control studies of motor neurone disease. Association with mechanical injuries. *Arch. Neurol.*, **38**, 220–6.

Kurland, L.T., Radhakrishnan, K., Smith, G.E. *et al.* (1992) Mechanical trauma as a risk factor in classic amyotrophic lateral sclerosis: lack of epidemiological evidence. *J. Neurol. Sci.*, **113**, 133–43.

Kurtzke, J.F. (1975a) A reassessment of the distribution of multiple sclerosis. *Acta Neurol. Scand.*, **51**, 110–36.

Kurtzke, J.F. (1975b) A reassessment of the distribution of multiple sclerosis. 2. *Acta Neurol. Scand.*, **51**, 137–57.

Epidemiology

Kurtzke, J.F. (1982) Epidemiology of amyotrophic lateral sclerosis, in *Human Motor Neuron Diseases* (ed. L. P. Rowland), Raven Press, New York, pp. 281–302.

Kurtzke, J.F. (1991) Risk factors in amyotrophic lateral sclerosis, in *Advances in Neurology*, Vol. 56, *Amyotrophic Lateral Sclerosis and other Motor Neuron Diseases* (ed. L.P. Rowland), Raven Press, New York, pp. 245–70.

Kurtzke, J.F. and Beebe, G.W. (1980) Epidemiology of amyotrophic lateral sclerosis. 1. A case–control comparison based on ALS deaths. *Neurology*, **30**, 453–62.

Leone, M., Chio, A., Mortara, P. *et al.* (1983) Motor neuron disease in the province of Turin, Italy, 1970–1980. *Acta Neurol. Scand.*, **68**, 316–27.

Li, T.-M., Alberman, E. and Swash, M. (1990) Clinical features and associations of 560 cases of motor neuron disease. *J. Neurol. Neurosurg. Psychiatry*, **53**, 1043–5.

Li, T.-M., Swash, M., Alberman, E. and Day, S.J. (1991) Diagnosis of motor neuron disease by neurologists: a study in three countries. *J. Neurol. Neurosurg. Psychiatry*, **54**, 980–3.

Lilienfeld, D.E., Ehland, J., Landrigan, P.J. *et al.* (1989) Rising mortality from motoneuron disease in the USA, 1962–84. *Lancet*, **i**, 710–12.

Macleod, R.C., Macgregor, L.G., Larminie, H.E. and Grist, N.R. (1958) Serological epidemiology of poliomyelitis in central Scotland. *Scot. Med. J.*, **3**, 76–81.

Martyn, C.N. (1989) Motoneuron disease and exposure to solvents. *Lancet*, **i**, 394.

Martyn, C.N. and Osmond, C. (1992) The environment in childhood and risk of motor neuron disease. *J. Neurol. Neurosurg. Psychiat.*, **55**, 997–1001.

Martyn, C.N. and Pippard, E.C. (1988) Usefulness of mortality data in determining the geography and time trends of dementia. *J. Epidemiol. Community Health*, **42**, 134–7.

Martyn, C.N., Barker, D.J.P. and Osmond, C. (1988) Motoneuron disease and past poliomyelitis in England and Wales. *Lancet*, **i**, 1319–22.

Melmed, C. and Krieger, C. (1982) A cluster of amyotrophic lateral sclerosis. *Arch. Neurol.*, **39**, 595–6.

Mitchell, J.D., Gibson, H.N. and Gatrell, A. (1990) Amyotrophic lateral sclerosis in Lancashire and South Cumbria, England, 1976–1986. A geographical study. *Arch .Neurol.*, **47**, 875–80.

Murros, K. and Fogelholm, R. (1983) Amyotrophic lateral sclerosis in middle-Finland: an epidemiological study. *Acta Neurol. Scand.*, **67**, 41–7.

Nielson, S., Robinson, I. and Hunter, M. (1992) Longitudinal Gompertzian analysis of ALS mortality in England and Wales, 1963–89: estimates of susceptibility in the general population. *Mechanisms of Ageing and Development*, **64**, 201–16.

Norris, F.H. and Padia, L.A. (1989) Toxic and pet exposures in amyotrophic lateral sclerosis. *Arch. Neurol.*, **46**, 945.

Office of Population Censuses and Surveys (1978) *Occupational Mortality: the Register General's Decennial Supplement for England and Wales 1970–72*. HMSO, London.

References

Olivares, L., Esteban, E.S. and Alter, M. (1972) Mexican 'resistance' to amyotrophic lateral sclerosis. *Arch. Neurol.*, **27**, 397–402.

O'Malley, F., Dean, G. and Elian, M. (1987) Multiple sclerosis and motor neurone disease: survival and how certified after death. *J. Epidemiol. Community Health*, **41**, 14–17.

de Pedro-Cuesta, J. and Litvan, J. (1990) Epidemiology of motor neurone disease, in *Neuroepidemiology. A Tribute to Bruce Schoenberg* (eds D.W. Anderson and D.G. Schoenberg), CRC Press, Boca Raton, pp. 265–96.

Petkau, A., Sawatzky, A., Hillier, C.R. *et al.* (1974) Lead content of neuromuscular tissue in amyotrophic lateral sclerosis: case report and other considerations. *Br. J. Ind. Med.*, **31**, 275–87.

Pierce-Ruhland, R. and Patten, B.M. (1981) Repeat study of antecedent events in motor neuron disease. *Ann. Clin. Res.*, **13**, 102–7.

Poskanzer, D.C., Cantor, H.M. and Kaplan, G.S. (1969) The frequency of preceding poliomyelitis in amyotrophic lateral sclerosis, in *Motor Neuron Disease* (eds F.H. Norris and L.T. Kurland), Grune & Stratton, New York, pp. 286–90.

Provinciali, L. and Giovagnoli, A.R. (1990) Antecedent events in amyotrophic lateral sclerosis: do they influence clinical onset and progression? *Neuroepidemiology*, **9**, 255–62.

Raymond, M. (1875) Paralysie essentiele de l'enfance: atrophie musculaire consecutive. *Gaz. Med. Paris Series 4*, **4**, 225–6.

Reed, D.M. and Brody, J.A. (1975) Amyotrophic lateral sclerosis and Parkinsonism–dementia on Guam, 1945–1972. I. Descriptive epidemiology. *Am. J. Epidemiol.*, **101**, 287–301.

Roelofs-Iverson, R.A., Mulder, D.W., Elveback, L.R. *et al.* (1984) ALS and heavy metals: a pilot case–control study. *Neurology*, **34**, 393–5.

Rosati, G., Pinna, L., Granieri, E. *et al.* (1977) Studies on epidemiological, clinical, and etiological aspects of ALS disease in Sardinia, Southern Italy. *Acta Neurol. Scand.*, **55**, 231–44.

Rothman, K.J. (1990) Keynote presentation. A sobering start for the cluster busters' conference. *Am. J. Epidemiol.*, **132**(Suppl. 1), S6–13.

Sanders, M. (1980) Clustering of amyotrophic lateral sclerosis. *J. Am. Med. Assoc.*, **244**, 435.

Scarpa, M., Colombo, A., Panzetti, P. and Sorgato, P. (1988) Epidemiology of amyotrophic lateral sclerosis in the province of Modena, Italy: influence of environmental exposure to lead. *Acta Neurol. Scand.*, **77**, 456–60.

Sienko, D.G., Davis, J.P., Taylor, J.A. and Brooks, B.R. (1990) Amyotrophic lateral sclerosis: a case–control study following detection of a cluster in a small Wisconsin community. *Arch. Neurol.*, **47**, 38–41.

Swash, M. and Ingram, D. (1988) Preclinical and subclinical events in motor neuron disease. *J. Neurol. Neurosurg Psychiatr.*, **51**, 165–8.

Taylor, J.A. and Davis, J.P. (1989) Evidence for clustering of amyotrophic lateral sclerosis in Wisconsin. *J. Clin. Epidemiol.*, **42**, 569–75.

World Federation of Neurology Workshop. Criteria for diagnosis of amyotrophic lateral sclerosis. World Neurology, 1991.

Epidemiology

Yoshida, S., Mulder, D.W., Kurland, L.T. *et al.* (1986) Follow-up study on amyotrophic lateral sclerosis in Rochester, Minn., 1925 through 1984. *Neuroepidemiology*, **5**, 61–70.

Zack, M.M., Levitt, L.P. and Schoenberg, B. (1977) Motor neuron disease in Lehigh county, Pennsylvania: an epidemiologic study. *J. Chron. Dis.*, **30**, 813–18.

Zilkha, K.J. (1962) Discussion on motor neurone disease. *Proc. R. Soc. Med.*, **55**, 1028–31.

19 Familial disease

DENISE A. FIGLEWICZ and GUY A. ROULEAU

19.1 INTRODUCTION

Diseases of the motor neuron constitute an important class of neurological disorders. While the etiologies of most forms of motor neuron disease remain unknown, in some instances the disease is caused by a heritable gene defect. Three classes of motor neuron diseases can be identified:

1. disorders in which only the lower motor neuron is affected – the spinal muscular atrophies;
2. disorders in which only the upper motor neuron is affected – familial spastic paraplegia; and
3. hereditary disorders in which both upper and lower motor neurons are affected – familial amyotrophic lateral sclerosis (FALS).

In this chapter, we will concern ourselves with the last two categories. See Chapter 2 for a discussion of the spinal muscular atrophies.

19.2 BACKGROUND – GENETICS, POLYMORPHISM AND LINKAGE

Since the early 1980s, the techniques of 'reverse genetics' – more precisely, genetic linkage studies followed by positional cloning strategies – have revolutionized the laboratory approaches to those genetic disorders in which a mutant protein product could not be identified. Many hereditary disorders of the nervous system fall into this category. Beginning with the assignment of the Huntington's disease gene to chromosome 4p (Gusella *et al.*, 1983), genetic linkage analysis has been successfully utilized to ascertain the chromosomal map locations of a number of neurological disorders, including neurofibromatosis type 1 (Barker *et al.*, 1987; Seizinger *et al.*, 1987), neurofibromatosis type 2 (Rouleau *et al.*, 1987), von Hippel–Lindau syndrome (Seizinger *et al.*, 1988), Friedreich's ataxia (Chamberlain *et al.*, 1988), familial amyotrophic lateral sclerosis (Siddique *et al.*, 1991), and Baltic myoclonic epilepsy (Lehesjoki *et al.*, 1991). Moreover, positional cloning strategies to isolate and characterize the diseased gene based on its chromosomal localization have resulted in the identification of the mutant gene in Duchenne muscular dystrophy (Monaco *et al.*, 1986; Koenig *et al.*, 1987), cystic fibrosis (Rommens *et al.*, 1989; Riordan *et al.*, 1989), Kennedy's disease (LaSpada *et al.*, 1991), the fragile X syndrome (Verkerk *et al.*, 1991), Kallman's syndrome (Franco *et al.*, 1991) and myotonic dystrophy (Buxton *et al.*, 1992; Harley *et al.*, 1992). Clearly, this methodology will continue to be the approach of choice for hereditary disorders in which the etiology is poorly understood.

Genetic linkage analysis is based on the concept that the more closely two DNA fragments (or loci) are located on a chromosome, the more likely it is that the two will segregate during meiosis and be passed on to the offspring together. Because crossover and exchange of homologous regions of paired chromosomes occurs during gametogenesis, the further apart the two DNA fragments, the more likely it is that the two will be separated by a crossover event and not inherited together.

The likelihood of crossover events, or genetic recombination, is the basis for one measure of distance between two DNA fragments. The 'genetic distance' is measured in centimorgans (cM). For two fixed loci spaced closely enough on a chromosome that one would expect at most one crossover in the interval, the genetic distance in cM is equivalent to the chance of recombination between the two loci. When the distance between the two loci is sufficiently large, there is the chance of multiple crossovers occurring in the interval. In addition, the occurrence of one crossover event tends to inhibit the formation of other crossovers in the immediate vicinity; this phenomenon is called interference. Mathematical functions such as the Haldane function, the Kosambi function and the Felsenstein function help to make genetic mapping more precise by correcting for these phenomena (Ott, 1985, 1991). At a sufficiently great genetic distance, there will be 50% chance of recombination between two loci on the same chromosome, resulting in random segregation as if the two loci were on separate chromosomes.

Genetic distance can give us a rough estimate of the physical distance between markers. The human genome is 3300 cM in 'genetic size' and contains approximately 3×10^9 base pairs (bp). Thus, on the average, 1 cM genetic distance is equivalent to 1×10^6 bp physical distance. However, depending on the precise location in the genome, the correlation between physical and genetic distance can vary considerably.

In a genetic linkage study, one is attempting to find a DNA marker that lies so close to a given diseased gene that its pattern of heredity is virtually identical to that of the disease phenotype when traced through a kindred segregating the disease in question. Hence, such a study depends upon the availability of polymorphic genetic markers located throughout the genome and upon DNA samples from both affected and unaffected members of kindreds.

The human genome comprises 46 chromosomes: 22 pairs of autosomes and one pair of sex chromosomes. All the genetic loci on the 22 autosomes exist in pairs, one copy on each homolog. Each member of a given pair is an allele. When an allele at a given locus can exist in two or more forms, the locus is referred to as polymorphic. Previously, the only identifiable polymorphisms showing Mendelian inheritance were those for which varying protein products were known, such as ABO blood groups, HLA markers and enzyme isoforms; or genetic variability, such as color blindness. However, in 1980, it was recognized that heritable variations in the human genome occur very frequently – on average of a single base pair difference every 500 bp (Botstein *et al.*, 1980). Clearly, the majority of these variations would fall into non-coding regions of the genome, and could serve as a rich source of polymorphic markers for linkage studies (Donis-Keller *et al.*, 1987).

One large class of polymorphic markers is based on restriction fragment length polymorphisms (RFLPs). In these markers, the polymorphism has occurred within a specific 4-, 6- or 8-bp sequence that serves as the recognition/cleavage site for one of a member of the large family of bacterial DNases called restriction enzymes. When the sequence of the recognition site (restriction site) is present, the fragment will be cleaved; in an allelic variant containing an altered sequence at the recognition site, the fragment will remain intact. Genomic DNA, digested with the restriction enzyme that recognizes the sequence in question, can be used to identify the genotype for any individual at this locus, depending on whether they have two copies of the larger (undigested) fragment, two copies of the smaller (digested) fragments or one copy of each. The laboratory methodology for genotyping an RFLP in the members of a kindred consists of restriction enzyme digestion of genomic DNA, followed by electrophoretic separation of DNA fragments (based on size), transfer of the DNA to a nylon membrane ('Southern blot') and hybridization of the membrane with a probe containing the polymorphic locus. (This procedure is described in detail in Gusella, 1986.)

In the case of RFLP-based polymorphisms, generally only two allelic variants are observed. Assuming that the two alleles are present in the human population in a 1:1 ratio (often not the case), any given individual has a 50% chance of being homozygous at this locus (two copies of the same allele) and a 50% chance of being heterozygous (one copy of each allele). The usefulness or 'informativeness' of a poly-morphic marker for linkage mapping is based on the probability that any given individual is a heterozygote, thereby allowing identification of the parental origin of each chromosome. The informativeness of a marker will increase if more than two allelic variants exist, simply because the chance of any given individual being a heterozygote at the marker locus will increase.

A second large class of polymorphic markers has been identified that satisfies the requirement of multiple allelic possibilities. These markers are all based on small, repetitive blocks of DNA and can be found throughout the genome. The number of repeat units at one of these simple sequence repeat loci can vary to provide up to 20 alleles. While these loci are obviously highly polymorphic, the variant forms are sufficiently stable to prove very useful for linkage studies. Among this class of polymorphic markers are the 'minisatellite' variable number of tandem repeats (VNTRs), in which the repetitive block of DNA contains a restriction site, or sites, making it possible to utilize the same methodology as for RFLPs (Jeffreys, Wilson and Thein, 1985; Nakamura *et al.*, 1987). There are also markers based on variation in or near Alu repeat units (Zuliani and Hobbs, 1990). Probably the most frequently used markers at the moment are the 'microsatellite' repeats based on repeating blocks of di-, tri- or tetranucleotides. In the human genome, it is estimated that dinucleotide repeat blocks occur approximately every 50–100 000 bp (Weber and May, 1989). When the number of dinucleo-tide repeats in a given block is 20 or greater, the locus is very likely to be polymorphic. These variants are also inherited in a Mendelian fashion, and dispersed throughout the genome. In addition, it has been recognized recently that microsatellite repeat blocks occur quite fre-quently in the 3' untranslated region of genes, making them an ideal resource for testing for linkage of a candidate gene. In addition to all the useful qualities described above, the methodology used to determine the genotype at a microsatellite locus is polymerase chain reaction (PCR) amplification of the polymorphic region, generally 100–300 bp, followed by resolution on a standard 6% sequencing gel. The amplified region can be labeled by a variety of means. This swift and simple technology can be applied to much smaller DNA samples than are needed for Southern blotting, making it ideal for patient studies in which the DNA supply is limited.

Once allelic information for a given marker locus has been tabulated for the members of a family segregating a disease trait, linkage or exclusion from linkage is determined statistically and expressed as a LOD score.

In the simplest analysis, two-point analysis, the segregation of alleles at one marker locus and the segregation of the alleles at the disease locus are compared. Two likelihoods are calculated. The first is the likelihood of obtaining this segregation pattern if the two loci are linked; the second is the likelihood that this pattern of alleles would have arisen as the result of random segregation. The ratio of these two probabilities tells us how much more likely the data are to have arisen under one premise (linkage) than the other (non-linkage). The $\log_{10}$ of this odds ratio is the Lod score (Lander, 1989). The Lod score is typically calculated allowing different percentages of possible recombination between the two loci.

In human genetics, a Lod score of 3.0 is accepted as the threshold for linkage. A Lod score of -2.0 or less is accepted as exclusion of the marker locus from linkage to the disease trait. Very informative families and/or very informative probes can provide exclusion data to a distance of 10 or more cM on either side of the locus tested.

Calculation of Lod scores is typically carried out using computer packages such as LIPIN or LINKAGE for data entry (Trofatter, Haines and Conneally, 1986) and storage, and LINKAGE or LIPED (Ott, 1974; Lathrop and Lalouel 1984; Lathrop et al., 1984) for the analysis.

In addition to the two-point analysis described above, more complicated analyses include multipoint analysis, in which the segregation of the disease phenotype is compared simultaneously with the segregation of several loci within the same chromosomal region (Lathrop et al., 1984, 1985). This analysis is substantially more powerful than two-point analysis, and allows more precise placement of the loci on the genetic map. Another useful analysis is the HOMOG test (Ott, 1985) for genetic heterogeneity in a group of families segregating the same disease trait, once linkage has been established. The simultaneous search strategy is another test for genetic heterogeneity in which one can ascertain the likelihood of linkage to either of a pair of marker loci (Lander and Botstein, 1986a). For more theoretical discussion of these approaches, see Lathrop et al. (1985), Lander and Botstein (1986b), Lander (1989) and Ott (1991).

19.3 FAMILIAL AMYOTROPHIC LATERAL SCLEROSIS (FALS)

19.3.1 Clinical and epidemiological characteristics

It is estimated that 5–10% of ALS cases have a familial etiology (Kurland and Mulder, 1955). While this represents only a small number of cases, we became interested in undertaking genetic linkage studies of FALS as a model of sporadic ALS because, clinically, a FALS patient (Swerts and

Familial disease

VandenBergh, 1976; Husquinet and Franck, 1980; Mulder *et al.*, 1986; Li, Alberman and Swash, 1988) is virtually indistinguishable from a patient with sporadic ALS. Epidemiologic characteristics of the two groups of patients are very similar (discussed in detail below). There is considerable agreement in the pathologic findings as well.

Together with our colleagues R.H. Brown Jr and D. McKenna-Yasek (Day Neuromuscular Laboratory, Massachusetts General Hospital, Boston, MA, USA), we undertook to identify and collect blood samples from individuals with a family history of motor neuron disease (Brown *et al.*, 1991). To date, 160 kindreds have been identified; DNA is available from over 900 individuals including 135 affecteds. Families were separated into three categories:

1. Those families in which there was unambiguous autosomal dominant mode of inheritance for the disease trait and a typical presentation of motor neuron disease (mixed upper and lower motor neuron symptoms; no sensory or cognitive impairment). Eighty per cent of FALS kindreds belong to this category.
2. Those families in which the mode of inheritance was autosomal dominant but the mean survival time after onset of the disease was unusually long (greater than 10 years).
3. Those families in which multiple affecteds were only present in a single generation. Families in this category could represent an autosomal recessive or X-linked mode of inheritance, or a non-hereditary etiology.

For the remainder of the discussion in this section, and sections 19.3.2 and 19.3.3, only affected individuals or kindreds from category 1 will be considered.

Epidemiological analyses for 268 affected individuals (survival data for 210 deceased individuals) led to the following observations:

- The mean age of onset is 50.2 ± 12 years (see Figure 19.1a):
- The ratio of male to female affecteds is 1.3:1
- Age of onset for males (48.5 ± 13 years) is earlier than for females (53.1 ± 11 years) (see Figure 19.1b). This remained true for every subcategory of patients analyzed.
- At onset, most cases are spinal (79%) as opposed to bulbar (21%). FALS rarely presents with isolated involvement of the upper motor neuron (<10% of the cases).
- The male to female ratio is higher in spinal than bulbar cases.
- Mean survival after onset of symptoms was 2.9 ± 1.9 years.
- No parameter investigated appeared to significantly alter the survival time. These parameters include sex of the affected indivi-

432

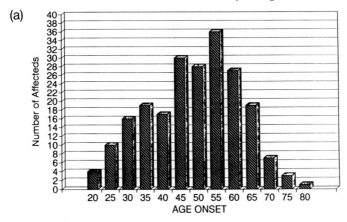

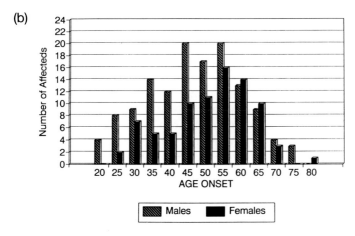

Figure 19.1 Age at onset of symptoms for familial amyotrophic lateral sclerosis (FALS) patients from kindreds displaying autosomal dominant (AD) mode of transmission. Patients are grouped in categories of five years: 20–24 years old; 25–29 years old; etc. (a) Age at onset histogram for all patients. (b) Age at onset histogram separated into male patients (striped bars) and female patients (solid bars).

dual, upper *vs.* lower motor neuron presentation and age at onset of symptoms.

Our FALS patient population strongly resembles the sporadic ALS population (Buckley *et al.*, 1983; Forsgren *et al.*, 1983; Gubbay *et al.*, 1985). We observe, in agreement with others, that the age of onset is somewhat earlier, and mean survival somewhat less, in the FALS patients. As is to be expected with an autosomal dominant trait, the male–female ratio approaches 1:1, in comparison with the sporadic patient group, in which the male–female ratio approaches 2:1. More frequent occurrence of sensory symptoms in FALS patients has been reported in the literature; however, this has not been our experience.

19.3.2 Genetic linkage studies of FALS

FALS has proved to be a particularly challenging disease for which to undertake linkage studies. The ideal resource for a linkage study of an autosomal dominant trait would be:

1. a single very large family with numerous living affected individuals in several generations; and
2. complete penetrance of the disease trait – where penetrance reflects the frequency with which the disease phenotype is expressed in an individual with the disease genotype.

In the situation of complete penetrance, unaffected siblings are as informative as affecteds.

The prevalence of ALS is estimated to be 1/20 000, making the prevalence of FALS approximately 1/200 000 individuals. In addition to this relative rarity of FALS patients, the late age of onset and short survival after onset of symptoms has made it very difficult to identify kindreds with multiple living affected individuals in the same generation, and almost impossible to obtain blood samples from affected individuals of different generations. An additional complication for FALS linkage studies is the condition of reduced penetrance. Based on information from our large family collection, we estimate the penetrance of the FALS trait to be 85%. Age-of-onset classes with the corresponding likelihood of succumbing to ALS in each decade from 20 to 70 years of age are used in the LIPED analysis to maximize the informativeness of the unaffected individuals.

Phenocopy refers to the existence of an identical phenotype (in this case, the disease trait) resulting from a non-genetic etiology. While sporadic ALS is rare enough to make the possibility of a genetic phenocopy in a FALS kindred an unlikely complication of the linkage analysis (as compared with the analysis of familial Alzheimer's, or manic depression, for example), it cannot be ruled out absolutely.

Lastly, the possibility of genetic heterogeneity for FALS could not be addressed at the outset of the study. The degree of intrafamilial variability in terms of onset age, symptoms and duration precluded any categorization of the FALS kindreds, save for the categories described above (see Espinosa et al., 1962; Horton, Eldridge and Brody, 1976; Chio *et al.*, 1987; and Appelbaum *et al.*, 1992, for additional discussion of this topic).

The reader is asked to examine Figure 19.2, which shows the chronology of motor neuron disease in a large FALS kindred. Many of the points discussed above are illustrated in this example. At the time of original contact with this family (Figure 19.2a), DNA could be obtained from only two living affected individuals – our index case, III-2, and a cousin, III-12. The onset age for individual III-2 was 59, in contrast to two siblings, III-6 and III-8, both of whom contracted FALS, and died, in their thirties.

The most likely mode of transmission of FALS in this kindred is autosomal dominant. However, there was reason to suspect a pheno-copy in individual IV-14, who had died of motor neuron disease in his thirties. Both his father (III-19) and his grandfather (II-10) remained alive, with no signs of motor neuron disease. This apparent phenocopy, or perhaps case of incomplete penetrance, provides another example of the high degree of intrafamilial variability possible with FALS. Indivi-dual II-10 did succumb to the disease in his seventies (Figure 19.2b), as did individual III-19, in his fifties (Figure 19.2c). The reader will note that, owing to the rapid progression of FALS, no more than two affected individuals in this kindred were alive at any one fixed point in time.

19.3.3 Progress with genetic studies of FALS

In order to determine if genetic linkage for the FALS trait was an achievable goal, simulated linkage analyses were performed. Based on a subgroup of well-collected families, the possibility of obtaining a Lod score of 3.0 or greater was 98%.

A genome-wide search for linkage was undertaken. In collaboration with our colleagues, T. Siddique, M. Pericak-Vance and A. Roses, linkage was established in the region 21q22.1–22.2 (Siddique *et al.*, 1991). In this collective study, 23 FALS kindreds were analyzed, using four markers spanning the region 21q21 through 21q22.1: D21S52, D21S1/S11, amyloid precursor protein (APP) and D21S58. Two-point analysis with each of these markers yielded Lod scores highly suggestive of linkage, yet no one marker gave a Lod score greater than 3.0. However, using multipoint analysis to test the FALS trait against three of these markers, a maximum Lod score of 5.03 was obtained 10 cM telomeric to the locus D21S58 (see Figure 19.3).

Once linkage was established, it was possible to test for heterogeneity of the FALS trait. A HOMOG analysis of the multipoint Lod scores for the

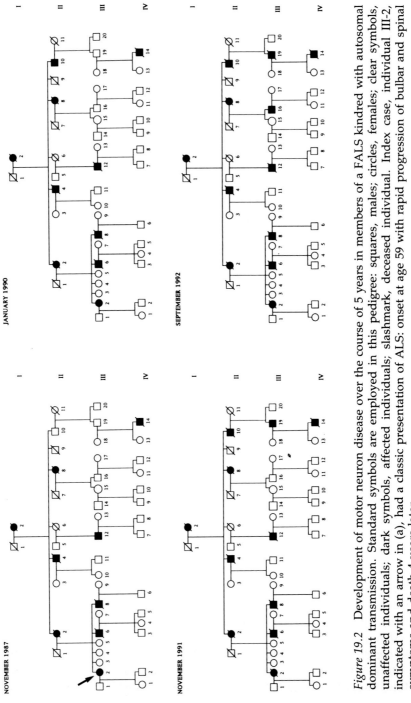

Figure 19.2 Development of motor neuron disease over the course of 5 years in members of a FALS kindred with autosomal dominant transmission. Standard symbols are employed in this pedigree: squares, males; circles, females; clear symbols, unaffected individuals; dark symbols, affected individuals; slashmark, deceased individual. Index case, individual III-2, indicated with an arrow in (a), had a classic presentation of ALS: onset at age 59 with rapid progression of bulbar and spinal symptoms and death 4 years later.

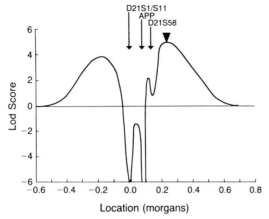

Figure 19.3 Multipoint linkage analysis of familial amyotrophic lateral sclerosis and three chromosome 21 markers (D21S1/S11; Amyloid Precursor Protein; and D21S58) spanning 21q21.1 to 21q22.3. The maximum Lod score of 5.03, obtained at a distance of 10 cM telomeric from D21S58, is indicated by the arrowhead. (Reprinted with permission from *The New England Journal of Medicine*, **324**, 1383, 1991.)

collective group of families revealed a significant probability of heterogeneity ($P < 0.0001$). Therefore, while an immediate goal is the identification and characterization of the FALS gene on chromosome 21, it is clear that at least one other FALS gene is present in the human genome.

Having established linkage, the following strategy was pursued:

1. identification of FALS kindreds that are linked to chromosome 21;
2. development of additional, and more informative, polymorphic markers in the region of linkage;
3. verification of linkage;
4. establishment of flanking markers for the FALS locus;
5. cloning of the minimal FALS region;
6. identification and testing of candidate genes within this region.

We will briefly describe our progress in each of these areas.

Based on statistically significant HOMOG analyses (M. Pericak-Vance and J. Haines, personal communication), we have been able to establish that 7 out of the 11 families analyzed in the study described above are linked to the locus on chromosome 21 with a likelihood of 84% or greater.

Plasmid, phage and cosmid clones from the region having D21S1/S11 as a centromeric boundary and D21S65 as a telomeric boundary were screened for either restriction fragment or dinucleotide repeat polymorphisms, in an attempt to saturate the region of linkage with polymorphic markers. [See the map of chromosome 21q, Figure 19.4; map information obtained from Patterson (1991) and McInnis *et al.* (1992)]. Highly informative dinucleotide repeat polymorphisms were characterized in *Sau* IIIA fragments from yeast artificial chromosomes (YACs) containing the phosphoribosylglycinamide formyltransferase (GART) (Gnirke *et al.*, 1991) and D21S65 loci (Goto *et al.*, 1992). These markers were tested in 11 FALS kindreds. In addition, a number of other highly informative dinucleotide repeat markers from the FALS region (GT02, GT12, GT11 and GT05) as well as an alumorph in the alpha interferon receptor gene (McInnis *et al.*, 1991, 1992; Warren *et al.*, 1992) were typed. Two-point analysis with each of these markers allowed us to verify linkage. The maximal (family aggregate) Lod score was obtained with the marker GT12 (D21S210): 4.14 at 10 cM. In addition, reconstruction of haplotypes in the FALS kindreds (see Figure 19.5 for an example) allowed us to identify obligate recombinant events in several of the families. The smallest FALS region was defined by the loci D21S213 on the centromeric side and D21S219 on the telomeric side. Much, if not all, of the DNA from the FALS minimal region has already been cloned into yeast accessory chromosomes (YACs) (Chumakov *et al.*, 1992; Patterson, 1992).

19.3.4 Identification of a FALS gene

There are five known transcribed sequences from human chromosome 21q22.1: the anonymous sequence at loci D21S93 (locus not shown in Figure 19.4), as well as the genes Cu/Zn superoxide dismutase 1 (SOD-1), alpha interferon receptor (INFαR), CRF2–4 (a novel member of the class II cytokine receptor family), and GART (Gardiner *et al.*, 1990; Lutfalla *et al.*, 1992; Lutfalla, 1993). The anonymous sequence at D21S93 was excluded as a candidate for the FALS gene, as it lies centromeric to the marker D21S213. The GART gene served as the telomeric boundary for the FALS region; it lies just centromeric to the marker D21S219.

These expressed sequences from the FALS region were tested for mutations in a battery of samples from 70 unrelated FALS patients. In some FALS kindreds, missense mutations were identified in SOD-1. In these families, the presence of the mutations corresponded with the occurrence of ALS (see Figure 19.6). Moreover, sequence variations in the SOD-1 gene were not seen in more than 100 control alleles (Rosen *et al.*, 1993). Screening of affected individuals from many FALS kindreds has resulted in the identification of missense mutations in all five exons of SOD-1. The lack of mutations in the SOD-1 gene in a number of FALS families confirms the genetic heterogeneity of familial ALS.

POLYMORPHIC MARKERS USED TO ESTABLISH LINKAGE AND LOCALIZE
THE FALS GENE ON CHROMOSOME 21

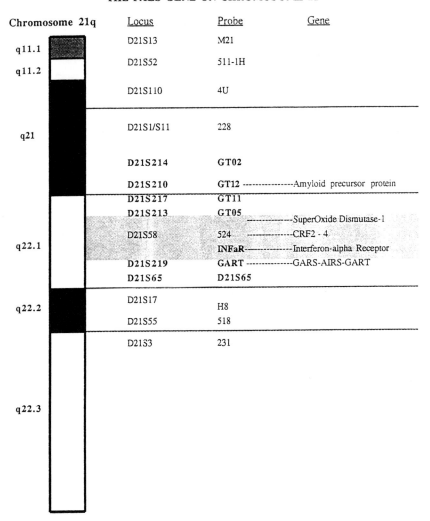

Figure 19.4 Relative position of markers on human chromosome 21q tested for linkage to familial amyotrophic lateral sclerosis (FALS). Markers in regular type represent RFLP probes which were used to establish linkage to FALS. Markers in bold type represent highly informative simple sequence repeat polymorphisms that were used to confirm linkage and narrow the FALS region. The region of chromosome 21 containing a FALS gene, indicated by stippling, has GT05 and GART as centromeric and telomeric flanking markers respectively.

Familial disease

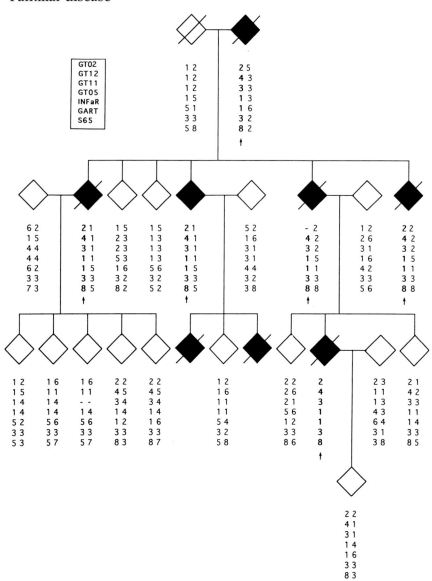

Figure 19.5 Reconstruction of haplotypes in members of an autosomal dominant FALS kindred. Allele values for seven simple sequence repeat polymorphic markers from chromosome 21q (indicated in the box in the upper left corner) are arranged under each individual in order from centromere to telomere. It is possible to reconstruct a 'FALS' haplotype; this chromosome is indicated with an arrow. In the second generation of this pedigree, all four affected members carry the FALS chromosome and two unaffected siblings do not.

440

Identification of mutations in the SOD-1 gene in some FALS families provides the first evidence for a mechanism underlying motor neuron disease. Cu/Zn SOD-1 is a cytoplasmic enzyme which is responsible for the conversion of the toxic free radical superoxide anion O_2^- to molecular oxygen and hydrogen peroxide. SOD-1 is one of three superoxide dismutase genes, each with a unique subcellular localization; a second Cu/Zn-containing SOD functions extracellularly and a Mn-containing SOD is found in mitochondria. Inefficient processing of toxic free radicals, such as the superoxide anion, has long been hypothesized as a mechanism underlying neurodegenerative processes (Calne, 1992; Fahn, 1992). We are now investigating whether SOD-1, or other members of the family of enzymes which serve to scavenge harmful free radicals, are implicated in the pathogenesis of other forms of motor neuron disease.

19.3.5 Chronic juvenile ALS

Juvenile ALS (JALS) refers to a disorder in which a bilateral pyramidal syndrome is accompanied by limb atrophy and fasciculations, with an age of onset between 2 and 25 years of age. A typical presentation is amyotrophy and fasciculation of the hands in combination with spastic paraplegia and a bulbar or pseudobulbar syndrome (BenHamida, Hentati and BenHamida, 1990). This is usually a chronic disease and most often familial, with an autosomal recessive mode of inheritance. Using both classic linkage mapping and homozygosity mapping strategies (Lander and Botstein, 1987), linkage was sought in a large Tunisian kindred in which DNA was available from 24 family members, including 10 affecteds. Linkage was established at the locus D2S72; the maximum Lod score was 6.03, with no recombination (Hentati *et al.*, 1991, 1992). This locus is being tested for linkage in other JALS kindreds. Flanking markers are currently being sought.

19.4 FAMILIAL SPASTIC PARAPLEGIA

19.4.1 Clinical and epidemiological characteristics

Spastic paraplegia of the familial type (FSP), originally described by Strumpell in 1880, is a progressive neurodegenerative disease causing spasticity chiefly in the legs (Livingstone and Robert, 1983). Age of onset varies from early childhood to over 50 years of age. In young children, early symptoms of delayed motor development are often interpreted as being cerebral palsy. In adults, initial symptoms are caused by spasticity, with difficulty walking and weakness in the feet or stiffness in the legs. As the disease progresses, patients develop scissor gait, contractures of the knees, hips and ankles with heel cord shortening – eventually confining the patient to a wheelchair. Neurologic examination in the 'pure' form of FSP shows spasticity in movements at the ankle or knees, brisk reflexes, ankle clonus and/or Babinski signs. In some families, there are other associated features such as optic atrophy, ataxia, mental retardation, tendon contractures and impaired vibration sense. Sutherland (1975) differentiated families into those with pure motor symptoms (Phanthumchinda and Somrealvongkul, 1989; Scheltens, Bruyn and Hazenburg, 1990) versus those with these other associated features (deYebenes et al., 1988; Gustavson, Modrzewska and Erikson, 1989; Sommerfelt, Kyllerman and Sanner, 1991). Inheritance in most families is autosomal dominant, though both autosomal recessive and X-linked kindreds have been reported (Wolfast, 1943; Bickerstaff, 1950; Johnston and McKusick, 1961; Fontaine et al., 1969; Behan and Maia, 1974; Holmes and Shaywitz, 1977; Harding, 1981; Cooley et al., 1990). The prevalence of the autosomal dominant variety has been estimated to be 12/100 000 (Skre, 1974). However, this figure is probably an underestimate, as many cases of FSP may be misdiagnosed.

Early reports suggest that the predominant neuropathologic lesions in FSP are a loss of myelin and axons in the lateral corticospinal tracts, particularly in the thoracic regions (Boustany et al., 1987). There may be degeneration of the fasciculus gracilis with less involvement of fasciculus cuneatus. More specific neuropathologic characteristics of FSP have not yet been described.

19.4.2 Progress with genetic studies of FSP

We have undertaken linkage studies in FSP, restricting the study to those kindreds which appear to have the 'pure' form (motor involvement without sensory, cognitive or other impairments). The involvement of motor neurons in FSP (upper motor neurons, spinal interneurons, or some combination of both) makes it an important disease to study; cloning of the gene(s) underlying this disorder will make an important contribution to our knowledge concerning the maintenance of healthy motor neurons and integrity of motor pathways.

FALS has many difficulties that make it a challenging disease for linkage studies, but FSP presents an almost ideal scenario for this approach. FSP is a crippling, but non-life-threatening, condition. Average age at onset is younger, and duration of life after onset is probably close to normal. Thus, it is possible to identify kindreds with living affecteds in three or four generations. In addition, the penetrance

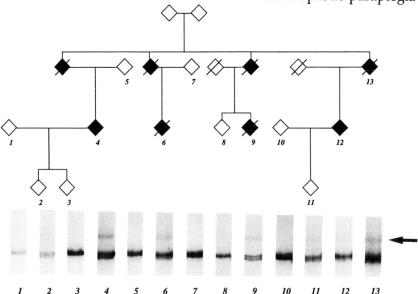

Figure 19.6 Single strand conformational analysis following PCR amplification of Exon 4 of the SOD-1 gene is shown for thirteen members of a chromosome 21-linked FALS kindred. Arrow on the right highlights an additional band which indicates the presence of a sequence variation in one copy of this exon in individuals 4, 6, 9, 11, 12 and 13. Presence of this mutation correlates exactly with the occurrence of ALS in this kindred, with the exception of individual 11, who is too young to display symptoms of ALS.

is estimated at 95%, making unaffected siblings more informative for the genetic analyses. However, the possibility of phenocopy needs to be kept in mind, as there are other syndromes that produce symptoms of spastic paraplegia: HTLV-I infection (Salazar-Grueso *et al.*, 1990), multiple sclerosis and spinal stenosis, among others. Lastly, the question of genetic heterogeneity cannot be answered at this moment. We have identified 22 kindreds segregating the pure form of FSP, and collected blood from 170 individuals in 10 of these kindreds. At least three kindreds are sufficiently informative that linkage could be established in each one on its own. One such kindred is shown in Figure 19.7; in this kindred alone, DNA samples are available from 45 individuals, including 19 affecteds.

Thus, our current strategy is two-point analysis of markers from all regions of the genome in the largest FSP kindreds. When linkage is established, all remaining FSP kindreds will be tested for linkage. *A posteriori* HOMOG analysis can then be carried out. To date, 135 polymorphic markers have been tested for linkage. One hundred of

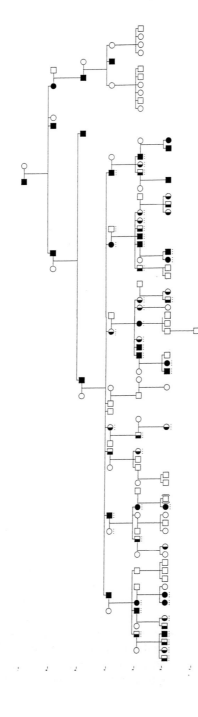

Figure 19.7 Large kindred segregating familial spastic paraplegia (FSP). Individuals indicated to be 'at risk' are those whose symptoms do not allow an absolute diagnostic of FSP. Individuals marked with stars underneath are those from whom blood/DNA samples have been obtained.

these markers demonstrated exclusion from linkage at the given locus. With these markers, we have achieved exclusion of over 40% of the genome. There have been some preliminary reports of this work (Figlewicz *et al.*, 1990; Rouleau *et al.*, 1990; Claudio *et al.*, 1992). Owing to the availability of large, cooperative, clinically well-characterized FSP kindreds, and the constantly improving quantity of highly informative polymorphic markers, we are optimistic that linkage for the pure form of FSP should be attainable within the next year or two.

19.5 CONCLUSIONS

Identification of the SOD-1 gene as the cause of ALS in some families will lead to a variety of laboratory investigations (categorization of mutations; correlation of the mutations with SOD enzyme activity, and perhaps with phenotypic variations; and establishment of *in vitro* and animal models). The aim of these studies is to understand the role of SOD-1 in the etiopathogenesis of FALS, as well as to carefully study models for clues as to the very earliest degenerative processes. In addition, protection against free radical toxicity may be an anticipated basis of clinical trials, hopefully culminating in the development of rational therapies for motor neuron disorders.

Attempts to identify genes which cause the death or malfunction of human motor neurons are continuing. Thanks to the rapid progress in both physical and genetic mapping of the human genome, and the astonishing evolution in molecular biology methodology, the approaches of genetic linkage and positional cloning to identify the diseased genes in hereditary disorders of the nervous system become ever more attractive as a means of providing insight into these inscrutable maladies. Cloning of these diseased genes, and characterization of the gene products, should contribute further to our understanding of the degenerative processes in motor neuron disease.

ACKNOWLEDGMENTS

The authors would like to thank their many collaborators in these studies, in particular:

- FALS studies: Jun Goto, Robert H. Brown Jr, Diane McKenna-Yasek, Jonathan Haines, Margaret Pericak-Vance, Teepu Siddique, Robert Horvitz, James F. Gusella, and the FALS Study Group;
- Chromosome 21: Melvin McInnis, Andrew Warren, Stylianos Antonarakis, Katheleen Gardiner, Harry Drabkin, David Kurnit, David Patterson, and the Joint YAC Screening Effort;
- FSP studies: Martin Farlow, John MacMillan, Peter Harper, George Ebers and Rosemary Boustany.

Familial disease

In addition, the authors would like to acknowledge the support of the Medical Research Council (Canada), the Muscular Dystrophy Association (USA), the Muscular Dystrophy Association (Canada) and the ALS Association of Canada.

REFERENCES

Appelbaum, J.S., Roos, R.P., Salazar-Grueso, E.F *et al.* (1992) Intrafamilial heterogeneity in hereditary motor neuron disease. *Neurology*, **42**, 1488–92.

Barker, D., Wright, E., Nguyen, K. *et al.* (1987) Gene for vonRecklinghausen neurofibromatosis is in the pericentromeric region of chromosome 17. *Science*, **236**, 1100–2.

Behan, W. and Maia, M. (1974) Strumpell's familial spastic paraplegia: genetics and neuropathology. *J. Neurol. Neurosurg. Psychiatr.*, **37**, 8–20.

BenHamida, M., Hentati, F. and BenHamida, C. (1990) Hereditary motor system diseases (chronic juvenile amyotrophic lateral sclerosis). *Brain*, **113**, 347–63.

Bickerstaff, E.R. (1950) Hereditary spastic paraplegia. *J. Neurol. Neurosurg. Psychiatr.*, **12**, 134–45.

Botstein, D., White, R.L., Skolnick, M. and Davis, R. (1980) Construction of a genetic linkage map in man using restriction fragment length polymorphisms. *Am. J. Hum. Genet.*, **32**, 314–31.

Boustany, R.-M., Fleischnick, E., Alper, C.A. *et al.* (1987) The autosomal dominant form of 'pure' familial spastic paraplegia: clinical findings and linkage analysis of a large pedigree. *Neurology*, **37**, 910–15.

Brown, R.H., Horvitz, H.R., Rouleau, G.A. *et al.* (1991) Gene linkage in familial amyotrophic lateral sclerosis: a progress report. *Adv. Neurol.*, **56**, 215–26.

Buckley, J., Warlow, C., Smith, P. *et al.* (1983) Motor neuron disease in England and Wales, 1959–1979. *J. Neurol. Neurosurg. Psychiatr.*, **46**, 197–205.

Buxton, J., Shelbourne, P., Davies, J. *et al.* (1992) Detection of an unstable fragment of DNA specific to individuals with myotonic dystrophy. *Nature*, **355**, 547–51.

Calne, D.B. (1992) The free radical hypothesis in idiopathic parkinsonism: evidence against it. *Ann. Neurol.*, **32**, 799–803.

Chamberlain, S., Shaw, J., Rowland, A. *et al.* (1988) Mapping of a mutation causing Friedreich's ataxia to human chromosome 9. *Nature*, **334**, 248–50.

Chio, A., Brignolio, F., Meineri, P. and Schiffer, D. (1987) Phenotypic and genotypic heterogeneity of dominantly inherited amyotrophic lateral sclerosis. *Acta Neurol. Scand.*, **75**, 277–82.

Chumakov, I., Heilig, R., Rigault, P. *et al.* (1992) Integrated construction of a human chromosome 21 YAC contig map. *Third International Workshop on Chromosome 21*, p. 11.

Claudio, J.O., Figlewicz, D.A., Farlow, M.R. *et al.* (1992) Genetic linkage mapping of hereditary spastic paraplegia. Proceedings of the 43rd annual meeting of the American Society of Human Genetics. *Am. J. Hum. Genet.*, **51**, A361.

References

Cooley, W.C., Melkonian, G., Moses, C. and Moeschler, J.B. (1990) Autosomal dominant familial spastic paraplegia: description of a large New England family and a study of management. *Dev. Med. Child Neurol.*, **32**, 1098–104.

deYebenes, J.G., Vazquez, A., Rabano, J. *et al.* (1988) Hereditary branchial myoclonus with spastic paraplegia and cerebellar ataxia. *Neurology*, **38**, 569–72.

Donis-Keller, H., Green, P., Helms, C. *et al.* (1987) A genetic linkage map of the human genome. *Cell*, **51**, 319–37.

Espinosa, R.E., Okihiro, M.M., Mulder, D.W. *et al.* (1962) Hereditary amyotrophic lateral sclerosis – clinical and pathologic report with comments on classification. *Neurology*, **12**, 1–7.

Fahn, S. and Cohen, G. (1992) The oxidant stress hypothesis in Parkinson's disease: evidence supporting it. *Ann. Neurol.*, **32**, 804–12.

Figlewicz, D.A., Chen, D., Farlow, M. *et al.* (1990) Linkage analysis in familial spastic paraplegia (FSP). *Am. J. Hum. Genet.*, **47S**, A179.

Fontaine, G., Dobois, B., Farriaux, J.P. and Maillard, E. (1969) Une observation familiale de maladie de Strumpell–Lorrain. *J. Neurol. Sci.*, **8**, 183–7.

Forsgren, L., Almay, B., Holmgren, G. and Wall, S. (1983) Epidemiology of motor neuron disease in northern Sweden. *Acta Neurol. Scand.*, **68**, 20–9.

Franco, B., Guioli, S., Pragliola, A. *et al.* (1991) A gene deleted in Kallmann's syndrome shares homology with neural cell adhesion and axonal pathfinding molecules. *Nature*, **353**, 529–36.

Gardiner, K., Horisberger, M., Kraus, J. *et al.* (1990) Analysis of human chromosome 21: correlation of physical and cytogenetic maps; gene and CpG island distributions. *EMBO J.*, **9**, 25–34.

Gnirke, A., Barnes, T.S., Patterson, D. *et al.* (1991) Cloning and *in vivo* expression of the human GART gene using yeast artificial chromosomes. *EMBO J.*, **10**, 1629–34.

Goto, J., Tassone, F., Demczuk, S. *et al.* (1992) Dinucleotide repeat polymorphism at the D21S65 locus. *Hum. Mol. Genet.*, **1**, 350.

Gubbay, S.S., Kahana, E., Zilber, N. *et al.* (1985) Amyotrophic lateral sclerosis. A study of its presentation and prognosis. *J. Neurol.*, **232**, 295–300.

Gusella, J.F. (1986) DNA polymorphism and human disease. *Annu. Rev. Biochem.*, **55**, 831–54.

Gusella, J.F., Wexler, N.S., Conneally, P.M. *et al.* (1983) A polymorphic DNA marker genetically linked to Huntington's disease. *Nature*, **306**, 234–8.

Gustavson, K.H., Modrzewska, K. and Erikson, A. (1989) Hereditary spastic diplegia with mental retardation in two young siblings. *Clin. Genet.*, **36**, 439–41.

Harding, A.E. (1981) Hereditary 'pure' spastic paraplegia: a clinical and genetic study of 22 families. *J. Neurol. Neurosurg. Psychiatr.*, **44**, 871–88.

Harley, H.G., Brook, J.D., Rundle, S.A. *et al.* (1992) Expansion of an unstable DNA region and phenotypic variation in myotonic dystrophy. *Nature*, **355**, 545–6.

Hentati, A., Bejaoui, K., Pericak-Vance, M.A. *et al.* (1991) Linkage of a juvenile amyotrophic lateral sclerosis gene to a chromosome 2 marker. *Satellite Symposium of the Third IBRO World Congress, Quebec City.*

Familial disease

Hentati, A., Bejaoui, K., Pericak-Vance, M.A. *et al.* (1992) The gene locus for one form of juvenile amyotrophic lateral sclerosis maps to chromosome 2. *Neurology*, **42S**, 201.

Holmes, G.L. and Shaywitz, B.A. (1977) Strumpell's pure familial spastic paraplegia: case study and review of the literature. *J. Neurol. Neurosurg. Psychiatr.*, **40**, 1003–8.

Horton, W.A., Eldridge, R. and Brody, J.A. (1976) Familial motor neuron disease: evidence for at least three different types. *Neurology*, **26**, 460–5.

Husquinet, H. and Franck, G. (1980) Hereditary amyotrophic lateral sclerosis transmitted for five generations. *Clin. Genet.*, **18**, 109–15.

Jeffreys, A.J., Wilson, V. and Thein, S.L. (1985) Hypervariable 'mini-satellite' regions in human DNA. *Nature*, **341**, 67–73.

Johnston, J.A. and McKusick, V.A. (1961) A sex-linked recessive form of spastic paraplegia. *Am. J. Hum. Genet.*, **13**, 83–93.

Koenig, M., Hoffman, E.P., Bertelson, C.J. *et al.* (1987) Complete cloning of the Duchenne muscular dystrophy cDNA and preliminary genomic organization of the DMD gene in normal and affected individuals. *Cell*, **50**, 509–17.

Kurland, L.T. and Mulder, D.W. (1955) Epidemiologic investigations of amyotrophic lateral sclerosis. 2. Familial aggregations indicative of dominant inheritance. *Neurology*, **5**, 182–268.

Lander, E. (1989) Mapping complex traits in human genetics, in *Human Genetic Disease: A Practical Approach* (ed. K. Davies) IRL Press, Oxford.

Lander, E. and Botstein, D. (1986a) Strategies for studying heterogeneous genetic traits in humans using a linkage map of restriction length polymorphisms. *Proc. Natl. Acad. Sci. USA*, **83**, 7353–7.

Lander, E. and Botstein, D. (1986b) Mapping complex genetic traits in humans: new methods using a complete RFLP linkage map. *Cold Spring Harbour Symp. Quant. Biol.*, **51**, 49–62.

Lander, E. and Botstein, D. (1987) Homozygosity mapping: a way to map human recessive traits with the DNA of inbred children. *Science*, **236**, 1567–70.

LaSpada, A.R., Wilson, E.M., Lubahn, D.B. *et al.* (1991) Androgen receptor gene mutations in X-linked spinal and bulbar muscular atrophy. *Nature*, **352**, 77–9.

Lathrop, G.M. and Lalouel, J.M. (1984) Easy calculations of lod scores and genetic risk on small computers. *Am. J. Hum. Genet.*, **36**, 460–5.

Lathrop, G.M., Lalouel, J.M., Julier, C. and Ott, J. (1984) Strategies for multilocus linkage analysis in humans. *Proc. Natl. Acad. Sci. USA*, **81**, 3443–6.

Lathrop, G.M., Lalouel, J.M., Julier, C. and Ott, J. (1985) Multilocus linkage analysis in humans: detection of linkage and estimation of recombination. *Am. J. Hum. Genet.*, **37**, 482–98.

Lehesjoki, A.E., Koskiniemi, M., Sistonen, P. *et al.* (1991) Localization of a gene for progressive myoclonus epilepsy to chromosome 21q22. *Proc. Natl. Acad. Sci. USA*, **88**, 3696–9.

Li, T., Alberman, E. and Swash, M. (1988) Comparison of sporadic and familial disease amongst 580 cases of motor neuron disease. *J. Neurol. Neurosurg. Psychiatr.*, **51**, 778–84.

References

Livingstone, I.R. and Robert, D.F. (1983) Hereditary spastic paraplegia: a clinical and genetic study of cases in the north-east of England. *J. Genet. Hum.*, **31**, 295–305.

Lutfalla, G., Gardiner, K., Proudhon, D. *et al.* (1992) The structure of the human interferon alpha/beta receptor gene. *J. Biol. Chem.*, **267**, 2802–9.

Lutfalla, G., Gardiner, K. and Uze, G. (1993) A new member of the cytokine receptor gene family maps on chromosome 21 at less than 35 kb from IFNAR. *Genomics* (in press).

McInnis, M.G., Lutfalla, G., Slaugenhaupt, S. *et al.* (1991) Linkage mapping of highly informative DNA polymorphisms within the human Interferon-alpha receptor gene on chromosome 21. *Genomics*, **11**, 573–6.

McInnis, M.G., Cox, T., Kalaitsidaki, M. *et al.* (1992) Linkage map of human chromosome 21 using SSRs and other PCR typable polymorphisms. *Third International Workshop on Chromosome 21*, p. 40.

Monaco, A., Neve, R., Colletti-Feener, C. *et al.* (1986) Isolation of candidate cDNAs for portions of the Duchenne muscular dystrophy gene. *Nature*, **323**, 646–50.

Mulder, D.W., Kurland, L.T., Offord, K.P. and Beard, C.M. (1986) Familial adult motor neuron disease: amyotrophic lateral sclerosis. *Neurology*, **36**, 511–17.

Nakamura, Y., Leppert, M., O'Connell, P. *et al.* (1987) Variable number of tandem repeats (VNTR) markers for human gene mapping. *Science*, **235**, 1616–22.

Ott, J. (1974) Estimation of the recombination fraction in human pedigrees: efficient computation of the likelihood for human linkage studies. *Am. J. Hum. Genet.*, **26**, 588–97.

Ott, J. (1985) *Analysis of Human Genetic Linkage*, Johns Hopkins University Press, Baltimore.

Ott, J. (1991) *Analysis of Human Genetic Linkage*, revised edition. Johns Hopkins University Press, Baltimore.

Patterson, D. (1991) Report of the second international workshop on human chromosome 21 mapping. *Cytogenet. Cell Genet.*, **57**, 167–74.

Patterson, D. (1992) The chromosome 21 joint YAC screening effort. *Third International Workshop on Chromosome 21*, p. 5.

Phanthumchinda, K. and Somrealvongkul, B. (1989) Familial spastic paraplegia. *J. Med. Assoc. Thai.*, **72**, 63–6.

Riordan, J.R., Rommens, J.M., Kerem, B. *et al.* (1989) Identification of the cystic fibrosis gene: cloning and characterization of complementary DNA. *Science*, **245**, 1066–73.

Rommens, J.M., Ianuzzi, M.C., Kerem, B. *et al.* (1989) Identification of the cystic fibrosis gene: chromosome walking and jumping. *Science*, **245**, 1059–65.

Rosen, D.R., Siddique, T., Patterson, D. *et al.* (1993) Mutations in Cu/Zn superoxide dismutase gene are associated with familial amyotrophic lateral sclerosis. *Nature*, **362**, 59–62.

Rouleau, G.A., Wertelecki, W., Haines, J.L. *et al.* (1987) Genetic linkage of a bilateral acoustic neurofibromatosis to a DNA marker on chromosome 22. *Nature*, **329**, 246–8.

Familial disease

Rouleau, G.A., Chen, D., Sapp, P. *et al.* (1990) Linkage analysis in familial spastic paraplegia (FSP). Proceedings of the VII International Congress on Neuromuscular Diseases, Munich, Germany. *J. Neurol. Sci.*, **985**, 185.

Salazar-Grueso, E.F., Gutierrez, B.S., Casey, J.M. *et al.* (1990) Familial spastic paraparesis syndrome associated with HTLV-I infection. *New Engl. J. Med.*, **323**, 732–6.

Scheltens, P., Bruyn, R.P. and Hazenberg, G.J. (1990) A Dutch family with autosomal dominant pure spastic paraparesis (Strumpell's disease). *Acta Neurol. Scand.*, **82**, 169–73.

Seizinger, B.R., Rouleau, G.A. Ozelius, L.J. *et al.* (1987) Genetic linkage of vonRecklinghausen neurofibromatosis to the nerve growth factor receptor gene. *Cell*, **49**, 589–94.

Seizinger, B.R., Rouleau, G.A., Ozelius, L.J. *et al.* (1988) Von Hippel–Lindau disease is genetically linked to the RAF1 oncogene on chromosome 3p. *Nature*, **332**, 268–9.

Siddique, T., Figlewicz, D.A., Pericak-Vance, M.A. *et al.* (1991) Linkage of a gene causing familial amyotrophic lateral sclerosis to chromosome 21 and evidence of genetic-locus heterogeneity. *New Engl. J. Med.*, **324**, 1381–4.

Skre, H. (1974) Hereditary spastic paraplegia in western Norway. *Clin. Genet.*, **6**, 165–83.

Sommerfelt, K., Kyllerman, M. and Sanner, G. (1991) Hereditary spastic paraplegia with epileptic myoclonus. *Acta Neurol. Scand.*, **84**, 157–60.

Sutherland, J.M. (1975) Familial spastic paraplegia, in *Handbook of Clinical Neurology*, vol. 22 (eds P.J. Vinken and G.W. Bruyn), North-Holland Publishing Co., Amsterdam, and American-Elsevier Publishing Co., New York, pp. 421–31.

Swerts, L. and Van den Bergh, R. (1976) Sclerose laterale amyotrophique familiale: Etude d'une famille atteinte sur trois generations. *J. Genet. Hum.*, **24**, 247–55.

Trofatter, J.A., Haines, J.L. and Conneally, P.M. (1986) LIPIN: An interactive data entry and management program for LIPED. *Am. J. Hum. Genet.*, **39**, 147–8.

Verkerk, A., Pieretti, M., Sutcliffe, J.S. *et al.* (1991) Identification of a gene (FMR-1) containing a CGG repeat coincident with a breakpoint cluster region exhibiting length variation in Fragile X syndrome. *Cell*, **65**, 905–14.

Warren, A.C., Kalaitsidaki, M., McInnis, M.G. and Antonarakis, S.E. (1992) New short sequence repeat (SSR) polymorphic loci on human chromosome 21. *Third International Workshop on Chromosome 21*, p. 61.

Weber, J.L. and May, P.E. (1989) Abundant class of human DNA polymorphisms which can be typed using the polymerase chain reaction. *Am. J. Hum. Genet.*, **44**, 388–96.

Wolfast, W. (1943) Eine Sippe mit recessiver geschlechtsgebundener spastischer Diplegie. *Z. menschl. Vererb.-U. Konstit.-Lehre*, **27**, 189–98.

Zuliani, G. and Hobbs, H.H. (1990) A high frequency of length polymorphisms in repeated sequences adjacent to Alu sequences. *Am. J. Hum. Genet.*, **46**, 963–9.

20 *Gene expression*

JACQUELINE DE BELLEROCHE and LISA VIRGO

20.1 INTRODUCTION

A number of distinct cellular changes occur in motor neurone disease, but despite years of study there are few clues as to the aetiology of the disease and possible causative factors. No transmissible agents, or immunological or environmental factors have yet been demonstrated consistently in the disease (Tandan and Bradley, 1985). It is therefore necessary to obtain a more detailed knowledge of the course of the disease. The approach that we have focused on is the study of gene expression in motor neurone populations in order to gain greater insight into disease initiation and progression.

Analysis of levels of specific messenger RNAs in identified cells allows a correlation to be made between morphological and functional states by means of *in situ* hybridization histochemistry. Differential changes in messenger RNA (mRNA) may be detected during the course of the disease in morphologically normal cells prior to disease progression, as well as those clearly showing morphological changes, e.g. shrunken cells and those showing loss of dendritic arborization.

20.2 PATHOLOGICAL CHANGES OCCURRING IN MOTOR NEURONE DISEASE

The course of motor neurone disease is complex. It involves a number of different sites of pathology, the degeneration of widely distributed motor neurones of the spinal cord, brainstem and cerebral cortex, and the degeneration of the corticospinal tracts. The extent of involvement of different motor neurone populations and the degree of corticospinal tract degeneration are, however, extremely variable, and considerable heterogeneity is seen. Total loss of anterior horn cells may occur in some subjects who exhibit long survival times, e.g. 10 years, whereas in other subjects minimal loss of anterior horn cells may occur, together with

451

pyramidal tract degeneration, and be associated with short survival times of less than 1 year.

20.2.1 Cortical changes in motor neurone disease

Loss of Betz cells is a consistent feature of the majority of cases of motor neurone disease, although not as extensive as the loss of anterior horn cells. Degenerating Betz cells have been observed in the absence of corticospinal tract degeneration, but whether this precedes the degeneration of the corticospinal tract and anterior horn cells has not been established. This problem has been addressed by Kiernan and Hudson (1991), who analysed cell cross-sectional area in pyramidal cells (layer V) of the precentral gyri in the foot and tongue regions, and compared this with changes in motor neurones of the hypoglossal nerve nucleus and ventral horn of the spinal cord, segment L4, in order to see whether functionally related regions showed a parallel degeneration, with one region being affected in advance of the other. The results indicated that cells in lumbar spinal cord and cerebral cortex showed independent degeneration, with no correlation between morphological changes, such as cell shrinkage in cortex, with loss of cell number in the spinal cord.

20.2.2 Neuropathology of familial forms of motor neurone disease

Approximately 5% of all cases of motor neurone disease show autosomal dominant inheritance, and a number of such cases have been analysed in order to investigate whether they show a distinctive pattern of neuropathology. One such study is that of Veltema *et al.* (1990), who examined a six-generation kindred in which affected individuals showed a mixture of lower motor neurone, bulbar and upper motor neurone signs. The morphology of these cases was similar to that shown by sporadic cases. Some variability between individuals in the same family appears to be a regular feature. The variable involvement of posterior column, Clarke's column and spinocerebellar tracts is seen both in familial cases and sporadic cases (Swash *et al.*, 1988).

20.3 DECREASES IN CELLULAR RNA IN MOTOR NEURONE DISEASE

20.3.1 Changes in RNA content in MND

A number of studies have demonstrated diminished nuclear and nucleolar volumes in motor neurones in MND, together with reduced total RNA content, determined both in tissue extracts and by micro-densitophotometry, and have concluded that there is an impaired transcription in these motor neurones (Davidson, Hartman and Johnson, 1981a,b; Mann and Yates, 1974; Murakami, 1990). In the last study, Murakami measured RNA content of nerve cells in C6 medial/lateral nuclei of anterior horn in both large neurones (>500 μm^2) and small neurones (<500 μm^2). Interestingly, RNA content of the large neurones was decreased in MND subjects in both histologically normal and abnormal large neurones, the decrease being 57% in normal cells and 42% in abnormal cells compared with RNA content in control subjects. The largest decrease seen in the small neurones was a decrease of 30% in histologically normal cells from MND cases. A study of this type therefore indicates that a decrease in RNA synthesis precedes the earliest light microscopic changes occurring in motor neurone disease.

20.3.2 Quantitation of mRNA in MND

Identification of the specific RNAs that are affected in histologically normal neurones is therefore of great interest. The first study that has been published focusing on this approach was that of Clark *et al.* (1990), who looked at the expression of four messenger RNAs both in tissue homogenates and by *in situ* hybridization. The four candidate messenger RNAs investigated were those coding for the neurofilament light chain, an abundant neuronal intermediate filament protein present in motor neurones, the amyloid precursor protein (APP_{695}), which is the form of APP predominantly expressed in neural tissue, GAP-43, a growth-associated protein, and glial fibrillary acidic protein (GFAP), an astrocyte marker. However, no change in the expression of neurofilament light-chain messenger RNA was detected by *in situ* hybridization, nor was there any change in the levels of APP, GAP-43 and GFAP messenger RNA detected in tissue extracts by Northern analysis. Thus no gross changes are detectable in glial and neuronal markers of cytoskeleton, although both neurofilament light chain and APP are known to be affected in experimental models of axotomy. The expression of GAP-43 is associated with axonal sprouting and regeneration as well as being essential during development, and hence likely to be a good marker of regenerative processes.

The lack of generalized impairment in neuronal gene expression in motor neurone disease stands in contrast to the picture obtained in Alzheimer's disease cerebral cortex, where both APP and neurofilament light chain show marked decrements below control levels (Clark *et al.*, 1989). The failure to demonstrate any changes in these neuronal messenger RNAs, despite the clear-cut loss of neurones in MND spinal cord, indicates the different specificity of the degenerating process in MND. An alternative explanation is that the remaining neurones may in fact be showing an enhanced expression of messenger RNA, but this can only be addressed further by analysis of grain counts within individual anterior horn cells.

We have selected different candidate messenger RNAs in order to focus more specifically on the changes occurring in anterior horn cells. In particular, choline acetyltransferase (ChAT) mRNA was chosen as this represents a marker of cholinergic neurones, essential for the biosynthesis of the neurotransmitter acetylcholine from acetyl CoA and choline, and therefore an abundant product of the cholinergic neurone.

20.3.3 Choline acetyltransferase messenger RNA levels as an index of neuronal function

We have characterized the distribution of ChAT messenger RNA in human spinal cord and brain using a 30mer oligonucleotide probe whose sequence was derived from the 5' region of porcine ChAT messenger RNA (Berrard et al., 1987), and a ChAT cDNA probe (Ishi et al., 1990). The oligonucleotide was 5' end-labelled with [γ-^{32}P]ATP using T4 polynucleotide kinase, and the cDNA probe was labelled by the oligolabelling method of Feinberg and Vogelstein (1983). The specificity of these probes was tested by hybridization to human spinal cord messenger RNA samples, size fractionated on Northern blots and shown to label a single RNA species of 4.2 kb in human and of similar size in the rat. ChAT messenger RNA was localized by *in situ* hybridization as described in detail by de Belleroche *et al.* (1990). High concentrations of ChAT messenger RNA were present in motor neurones throughout the spinal cord, and in the brainstem in the hypoglossal nerve nucleus and widely distributed in cerebral cortex. In the spinal cord ChAT messenger RNA is present at high concentrations in layer IX of the ventral grey matter, arranged in clusters corresponding to medial, central and lateral columns of motor neurones. In addition, other cholinergic cells are present in the spinal cord, and these show similar or moderate levels of choline acetyltransferase messenger RNA.

The three main regions outside layer IX that contain ChAT messenger RNA are layer III of the dorsal horn, the intermediate grey matter and layer X around the central canal. Lower levels of ChAT messenger RNA are detected in layers VI–VIII, and the lowest levels are found in layers I and II of the dorsal horn. This distribution of ChAT messenger RNA is similar to that reported for cells showing ChAT immunoreactivity in the rat spinal cord, determined by the use of a monoclonal antibody (Barber *et al.*, 1984), ChAT enzyme activity determined in human spinal cord

Control   MND

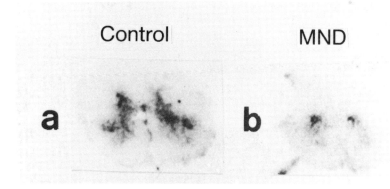

Figure 20.1 Distribution of choline acetyltransferase mRNA in lumber spinal cord of an MND patient compared to a control. The distribution of ChAT mRNA in lumbar spinal cord is shown for a control subject (a) and an MND subject (b). The age, sex and post-mortem delay (pmd) of these cases were as follows: (a) 72-year-old male, 20 h pmd; (b) 77-year-old female, 5 h pmd. Hybridization of [^{32}P]ChAT oligonucleotide probe to rat and human RNA samples (20 μg) on Northern blots showed the presence of a single labelled species whose approximate size is 4.3 kb in rat and 4.2 kb in human. [Data are taken from Virgo *et al.* (1992) with acknowledgement to *Journal of Neurological Science*, Elsevier.]

(Aquilonius, Eckernäs and Gillberg, 1981) and ChAT mRNA distribution in rat spinal cord (Ibánez, Enfors and Persson, 1991).

The distribution of ChAT mRNA in lumbar cord from a control subject is shown in Figure 20.1a. In the ventral grey matter, ChAT mRNA is localized in patches, which is consistent with the distribution of central, medial and lateral columns of motor neurones. This is particularly evident from the dark-field photomicrograph (Figure 20.2b). This signal was sensitive to treatment with RNase (Figure 20.2c). The localization of ChAT mRNA in layer III is consistent with the findings of immunohisto-chemical studies in which these cells have been further characterized and shown to be lateral neurones giving rise to an extensive innervation of the dorsal horn (Barber *et al.*, 1984).

The values obtained from densitometric analysis of the control subjects are shown in Figure 20.3. Densitometric analysis of ChAT mRNA in control samples showed no correlation with time of post-mortem delay ($r = 0.061$).

The presence of ChAT messenger RNA serves to localize cholinergic neurones, and whilst these are found in a number of areas the contribution from the anterior horn cells can be identified by *in situ* hybridization through their distinct distribution pattern. Other neur-ones present in the ventral grey matter utilizing either excitatory amino

Gene expression

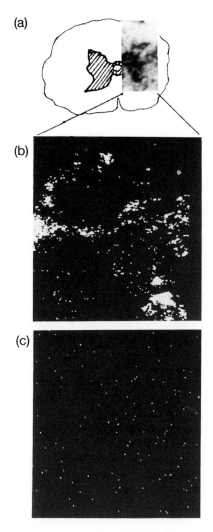

Figure 20.2 Localization of choline acetyltransferase mRNA in human spinal cord by dark-field microscopy. A dark-field view of layer IX from a control subject is shown in (b), (×40) which indicates clusters of ChAT mRNA activity corresponding to the distribution of anterior horn cells. The location of this area is shown in (a) and a corresponding dark-field RNase-treated control is shown in (c). [Data are taken from Virgo *et al*. (1992) with acknowledgement to *Journal of Neurological Science*, Elsevier.]

acids, gamma-aminobutyric acid (GABA) or glycine as neurotransmitter will not be detected, which would mask specific changes affecting only the anterior horn cells, as might be the case in the use of more

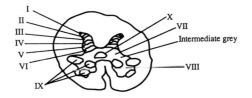

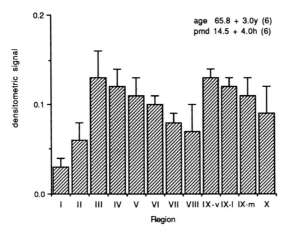

Figure 20.3 Localization of choline acetyltransferase mRNA in normal human lumbar spinal cord. The distribution of ChAT mRNA was determined in human lumbar spinal cord of six control individuals (4 M, 2 F) with no evidence of motor neurone disease aged 65.8 ± 3.0 years (mean ± SEM) at the time of death and sampled 14.5 ± 4.0 h (mean ± SEM) after death. The layers (Rexed) were defined by cytoarchitecture (above) and independently of the ChAT distribution. [Data are taken from Virgo *et al.* (1992) with acknowledgement to *Journal of Neurological Science*, Elsevier.]

generalized neuronal markers employed in the earlier study described above (Clarke *et al.*, 1990).

In situ hybridization has the additional advantage of allowing quantitative or semiquantitative analysis of messenger RNA levels, which is not possible by immunocytochemistry and localization of the protein product. For this approach it is important to match carefully control and MND cases for post-mortem delay times and age of subject. Tissue sections containing known doses of radioactivity can then be exposed in parallel and used to quantitate RNA content in areas of interest (de Belleroche *et al.*, 1990).

A marked loss of ChAT mRNA occurs in ventral grey matter of spinal cord in all cases of MND, as illustrated for an individual case in Figure

457

Gene expression

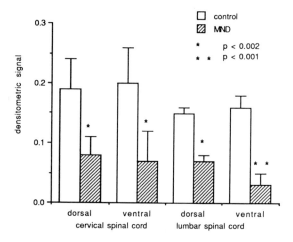

Figure 20.4 Semiquantitative analysis of choline acetyltransferase mRNA in cervical and lumbar spinal cord from controls and MND patients. Spinal cord sections were hybridized with a [^{32}P]ChAT oligonucleotide probe and analysed densitometrically to obtain the RNase-sensitive hybridization signal due to the presence of ChAT mRNA. Values are means ± SEMs. * and ** indicate that the values for the MND cases were significantly less than control values, $P < 0.002$ and $P < 0.001$ respectively (Student's t-test – unpaired samples). For studies of cervical spinal cord, the mean age and post-mortem delay (pmd) values (mean ± SEM) were 61.8 ± 3.9 years (3 M, 1 F), 24.0 ± 7.3 h pmd, for controls and 67.3 ± 5.7 years (3 F, 1 M), 13.3 ± 4.5 h pmd, for MND subjects. For studies of lumbar spinal cord, the mean age and post-mortem delay values were 63.6 ± 2.0 years (2 F, 3 M), 19.8 ± 4.4 h pmd, for controls and 63.6 ± 2.7 years (4 F, 5 M), 13.9 ± 2.1 h pmd, for MND subjects respectively. [Data are taken from Virgo *et al.* (1992) with acknowledgement to *Journal of Neurological Science*, Elsevier.]

20.1b compared with a control case. This example shows a differential loss of ChAT mRNA, which is predominantly restricted to the ventral grey matter. However, in some cases the loss of ChAT mRNA is more extensive, also affecting levels of ChAT mRNA in the dorsal grey matter and the central canal cluster cells.

Densitometric analysis of ChAT messenger RNA in dorsal and ventral grey matter from cervical and lumbar cord in control and MND cases allows quantitation of this change (Virgo *et al.*, 1992). The greatest change seen was a decrease of 77% in the ventral grey matter of lumbar spinal cord in MND cases compared with controls (Figure 20.4). In ventral grey matter of cervical spinal cord, a similar decrease of 63% was obtained.

In addition, substantial changes in other parts of the spinal cord were detected in MND subjects, especially in the dorsal grey matter, where a decrease of 58% in ChAT mRNA was seen in the cervical region, and of 51% in the lumbar region, of MND cases compared with controls. This result indicates that the pathology associated with this condition in the spinal cord is not restricted to motor neurones. In the terminal stages of the disease a much more extensive neuronal degeneration occurs, extending outside the ventral grey matter to the dorsal horn. This is also in keeping with a loss of ChAT enzyme activity seen in dorsal horn in MND (Gilberg *et al.*, 1982), and the loss of muscarinic receptors from this region (Whitehouse, Wamsley and Zarbin, 1983).

20.3.4 Specificity of mRNA changes in MND

It is important to determine the specificity of changes in mRNA levels in order to know whether this reflects cell loss or a selective effect on the expression of a single gene or a group of genes. In order to address this issue, the levels of ChAT mRNA have been compared with more widespread mRNAs such as those associated with receptor-mediated transduction, GTP-binding proteins (G-proteins). One of the most abundant G-proteins expressed in the human spinal cord is G_S alpha-subunit mRNA, which was detected by use of a cDNA probe (Itoh *et al.*, 1986). Two species of $G_{S\alpha}$ mRNA were detected in human spinal cord (Figure 20.5), and the $G_{S\alpha}$ mRNA was shown to be uniformly distributed in the grey matter of spinal cord. No widespread loss of $G_{S\alpha}$ mRNA was detected in MND subjects (Figure 20.6), which supports the specificity of the change in ChAT mRNA.

20.4 FUTURE DIRECTIONS

The results obtained in this study indicate the usefulness of assaying ChAT mRNA by *in situ* hybridization in understanding the nature of the pathophysiology of MND. This represents a specific mRNA change that occurs in anterior horn cells of all cases of MND. Changes in this mRNA also indicate the nature of more extensive degenerative processes occurring in other neurones, presumably at later stages in the course of the disease. Future work will be focused on determining whether these changes are correlated with neuronal cell loss or reflect a functional change. Current studies are in progress to use ChAT mRNA levels as a parameter to which changes in other neuronal mRNAs and receptors may be correlated in order to unravel the pathogenesis of this disease. One putative mechanism in this process is that of glutamate-mediated neurotoxicity. The *N*-methyl-D-aspartate (NMDA) glutamate receptor subtype is abundant in the ventral grey matter of spinal cord (Figure 20.7) and may mediate the selective neurotoxic effect if excess levels of

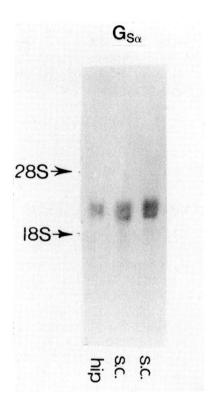

Figure 20.5 Northern blot analysis of G-protein alpha subunit ($G_{S\alpha}$ mRNA). The presence of two species of $G_{S\alpha}$ mRNA is shown in human hippocampus and spinal cord (approximate sizes of 2.8 and 3.2 kb).

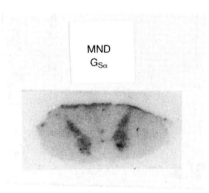

Figure 20.6 Distribution of $G_{S\alpha}$ mRNA in lumbar spinal cord from MND subjects. The distribution of $G_{S\alpha}$ mRNA is shown for a representative MND patient (66-year-old male, 4 h pmd), who shows no selective loss of mRNA from the dorsal or ventral grey matter.

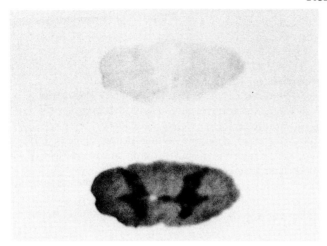

Figure 20.7 Distribution of NMDA receptors in human spinal cord. NMDA receptors were localized in frozen sections of spinal cord by incubation with [³H]MK-801 (30 nm). Non-specific binding in the presence of unlabelled ligand (TCP) is shown above to demonstrate the specificity of this signal.

glutamate or exogenous glutamate analogues are allowed to build up in the vicinity of anterior horn cells. Future experiments will investigate whether the loss of anterior horn cells is correlated with changes in NMDA receptor properties and distribution.

ACKNOWLEDGEMENTS

We are grateful to the Motor Neurone Disease Association for their financial support for this project and to the Department of Histopathology, Charing Cross Hospital, for help in obtaining post-mortem material.

REFERENCES

Aquilonius, S.M., Eckernäs, S.A. and Gillberg, P.G. (1981) Topographical localization of choline acetyltransferase within spinal cord and a comparison with other species. *Brain Res.*, **211**, 329–40.

Barber, R.P., Phelps, P.E., Houser, C.R. *et al.* (1984) The morphology and distribution of neurons containing choline acetyltransferase in the adult rat spinal cord: an immunocytochemical study. *J. Comp. Neurol.*, **229**, 329–46.

Berrard, S., Brio, A., Lottspeich, F. *et al.* (1987) cDNA cloning and complete sequence of porcine choline acetyltransferase: *in vitro* translation of the corresponding RNA yields an active protein. *Proc. Natl. Acad. Sci. USA*, **84**, 9280–94.

Gene expression

Clark, A.W., Krekoski, C.A., Parhad, I.M. *et al.* (1989) Altered expression of genes for amyloid and cytoskeletal proteins in Alzheimer cortex. *Ann. Neurol.*, **25**, 331–9.

Clark, A.W., Tran, P.M., Parhad, I.M. *et al.* (1990) Neuronal gene expression in amyotrophic lateral sclerosis. *Mol. Brain Res.*, **7**, 75–83.

Davidson, T.J., Hartman, H.A. and Johnson, P.C. (1981a) RNA content and volume of motor neurons in amyotrophic lateral sclerosis. I. The cervical swelling. *J. Neuropathol. Exp. Neurol.*, **40**, 32–6.

Davidson, J.T., Hartman, H.A. and Johnson, P.C. (1981b) RNA content and volume of motor neurons in amyotrophic lateral sclerosis. II. The lumbar intumescence and nucleus dorsalis. *J. Neuropathol. Exp. Neurol.*, **40**, 187–92.

de Belleroche, J., Bandopadhyay, R., King, A. *et al.* (1990) Regional distribution of cholecystokinin messenger RNA in rat brain during development: quantitation and correlation with cholecystokinin immunoreactivity. *Neuropeptides*, **15**, 201–12.

Feinberg, A.P. and Vogelstein, B.A. (1983) A technique for radiolabelling DNA restriction endonuclease fragments to high specific activity. *Anal. Biochem.*, **132**, 6–13.

Gillberg, P.G., Aquilonius, S.M., Eckernäs, S.A. *et al.* (1982) Choline acetyltransferase and substance P-like immunoreactivity in human spinal cord: changes in amyotrophic lateral sclerosis. *Brain Res.*, **250**, 394–7.

Ibánez, C.F., Enfors, P. and Persson, H. (1991) Developmental and regional expression of choline acetyltransferase mRNA in the rat central nervous system. *J. Neurosci. Res.*, **29**, 163–71.

Ishi, K., Oda, Y., Ichikawa, T. and Deguchi, T. (1990) Complementary DNAs for choline acetyltransferase from spinal cords of rat and mouse: nucleotide sequences, expression in mammalian cells, and *in situ* hybridization. *Mol. Brain Res.*, **7**, 151–9.

Itoh, H., Kozasa, T., Nagata, S. *et al.* (1986) Molecular cloning and sequence determination of cDNAs for alpha subunits of the guanine nucleotide binding proteins G_s, G_i and G_o from rat brain. *Proc. Natl. Acad. Sci. USA*, **83**, 3776–80.

Kiernan, J.A. and Hudson, A.J. (1991) Changes in sizes of cortical and lower motor neurons in amyotrophic lateral sclerosis. *Brain*, **114**, 843–53.

Mann, D.M.A. and Yates, P.O. (1974) Motor neurone disease, the nature of the pathogenic mechanisms. *J. Neurol. Neurosurg. Psychiatr.*, **37**, 1036–46.

Murakami, T. (1990) Motor neuron disease: quantitative morphological and micro-densitophotometric studies on neurons of anterior horn and ventral root of cervical spinal cord with special reference to the pathogenesis. *J. Neurol. Sci.*, **99**, 101–15.

Swash, M., Scholtz, C.L., Vowles, G. and Ingram, A. (1988) Selective and asymmetric vulnerability of corticospinal and spinocerebellar tracts in motor neurone disease. *J. Neurol. Neurosurg. Psychiatr.*, **51**, 785–9.

Tandan, R. and Bradley, W.G. (1985) Amyotrophic lateral sclerosis: 2, Etiopathogenesis. *Ann. Neurol.*, **18**, 419–31.

Veltema, A.N., Roos, R.A.C. and Bruyn, G.W. (1990) Autosomal dominant adult amyotrophic lateral sclerosis. A six generation Dutch family. *J. Neurol. Sci.*, **97**, 93–115.

Virgo, L., de Belleroche, J., Rossi, M. and Steiner, T.J. (1992) Characterisation of the distribution of choline acetyltransferase messenger RNA in human spinal cord and its depletion in motor neurone disease. *J. Neurol. Sci.*, **112**, 126–32.

Whitehouse, P.J., Wamsley, J.K. and Zarbin, M.A. (1983) Amyotrophic lateral sclerosis: alterations in neurotransmitter receptors. *Ann. Neurol.*, **14**, 8–16.

21 *Xenobiotic metabolism*

ROSEMARY WARING

Despite years of searching, no one single compound has been identified as the cause of motor neurone disease (MND). Although at various times solvents (Gunnarsson *et al.*, 1991), pesticides (Kurtzke, 1991) and mercury (Moriwaka, 1991) have been suggested as aetiological factors, it is clear that exposure to these agents does not automatically lead to the disease. Indeed, the relative risk for any environmental compound is fairly small. However, most cases of MND are not familial, and do not appear to involve any viral attack, so that the influence of toxins causing damage to the anterior horn cells cannot be ruled out.

Generally, when environmental agents (often referred to as xenobiotics) are ingested and absorbed, a series of enzymes are available to metabolize them. Absorption only readily takes place if compounds are lipid soluble, but excretion (which is usually via the urine) only easily occurs if the compounds are made water soluble. This process of forming polar metabolites from lipid-soluble parent compounds is usually referred to as 'detoxification'; it occurs in two phases. Firstly, the original agent, whether drug or pesticide, tends to be altered, often by oxidation using the cytochrome P450 complex, to give a more water-soluble derivative. For instance, benzene is converted to phenol. Reactions of this type usually take place in the microsomes found in the hepatic endoplasmic reticulum. Such metabolites are then often combined with endogenous water-soluble compounds to give compounds that are readily excreted in urine. For example, phenol forms conjugates with glucuronic acid or sulphate (Figure 21.1). About a dozen major pathways have been identified as detoxification reactions, and it is now generally recognized that these metabolic routes are largely genetically controlled. When they have been examined in large human populations, it is clear that there is wide variation between individuals which is reproducible. Some people, therefore, will always have relatively low capacity to detoxify certain types of compounds, while

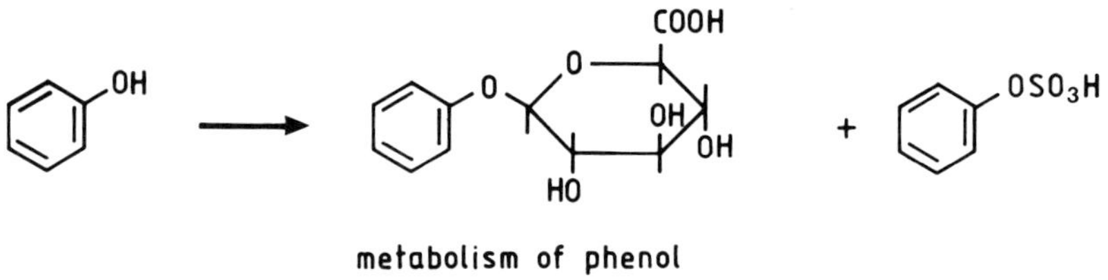

Xenobiotic metabolism

metabolism of phenol

Figure 21.1 Conjugation with glucuronic acid or sulphate.

others will metabolize them too fast to show toxicity. Analysis of the absolute capacities of these detoxification routes will provide a 'profile' for any individual, who may then have high activity for route A, but low activity for route B, etc. In the event that such an individual is challenged with a toxin requiring metabolism by route A, he will not be 'at risk' unless the exposure is sufficient to overwhelm his defences. On the other hand, toxins that would be removed by route B will be a danger; if they are neurotoxins they may lead to the symptoms of MND.

A further problem in studying the effects of environmental agents in the aetiology of MND is that acute exposure can rarely be implicated. Usually, MND patients report low chronic exposure to potential toxins or pro-toxins; this would presumably lead to slow but relentless destruction of CNS tissue, which might not lead to symptoms until either time or some other toxic event allowed further damage. If then patients with MND have responded to environmental compounds that they cannot metabolize safely, it should be possible to show that they, in general, have aberrant metabolic pathways when compared with a control population. This approach will necessarily not give a clear-cut picture, if a variety of toxins is involved in causing MND, and will be further confused if the control group contains individuals who are susceptible to MND, but by chance have not yet been exposed to the relevant agents. Nevertheless, this approach has been used in MND, and has given some interesting results. It has also proved possible to correlate known toxic compounds with common metabolic faults found in MND patients.

21.1 N-ACETYLATION IN MND

Work in the late 60s by Professor Evans established that drugs such as sulphonamides are metabolized (and made inactive pharmacologically) by N-acetylation. The enzymes involved are N-acetyltransferases, which are found in the cytosolic fraction of the cell and use acetyl CoA as the co-factor. Analysis of Caucasian populations showed that about 50% are rapid metabolizers, speedily converting drugs of this class to non-toxic

466

non-active compounds, while the other 50% are slow acetylators who had high blood levels of the parent drug, with increased therapeutic effect but also an increased risk of toxic reactions. The slow acetylator phenotype was shown by family studies to be inherited as though it were controlled by an autosomal recessive gene (Evans, 1989a,b). However, the position is complicated; current work has recently revealed that this reduced acetylation capacity is due to low levels of the A and B isoenzymes of NAT-2, the *N*-acetyltransferase involved, but it appears that the reduced enzyme levels are accompanied by lower activity (Grant *et al.*, 1991). As acetylation ability is genetic (there seems to be little environmental input on the enzyme activity), the phenotype also applies to other drugs metabolized by this pathway, such as isoniazid and, rather surprisingly, to compounds such as caffeine, where the rate-determining step of metabolism appears to be mediated by an *N*-acetyltransferase. Extremes of the *N*-acetylation phenotype range can often be determined by noting whether the individual is kept awake by coffee (slow acetylator) or finds coffee has no stimulant effect (fast acetylator).

However, studies in patients with neurological disease have shown that the phenotypic proportions seen in controls (45% fast, 55% slow acetylators) were not matched in the disease groups. Although Alzheimer's disease patients were indistinguishable from controls (46% fast, 54% slow), the values in Parkinson's disease (67% fast, 33% slow) and in MND (26% fast, 74% slow) were different, the MND result being significant ($P < 0.005$) (Heafield *et al.*, 1990a). A previous report (Zavalishin, Kovaleva and Larsky, 1986) also found that MND patients tended to be slow acetylators. Acetylation phenotype has previously been shown to be associated with increased susceptibility to disease states; slow acetylators are also more at risk from peripheral neuropathy after treatment with isoniazid (Weber and Hein, 1985). These results suggest that some cases of MND may result from chronic exposure to a neurotoxin containing an aromatic amine or sulphonamide group, both of which are detoxified by the action of the *N*-acetyltransferases. The plasticizing agent *N*-butylbenzenesulphonamide has recently been shown to induce a syndrome clinically and histologically resembling MND in rabbits (Strong *et al.*, 1990). This compound may be widely distributed in the environment, possibly as a contaminant from plastic containers and waste water effluents, so that chronic exposure to trace amounts could eventually lead to damage to the motor neurones. At least one epidemiological study has shown an increased number of cases of MND in workers in the plastics industry (Deaper and Henderson, 1986). It is not known whether neurotoxic amino acid derivatives such as β-*N*-methylamino-L-alanine (BMAA) from cycad plants, which are metabolized and detoxified by N-acetylation (Reece and Nunn, 1989), are converted by the same N-acetyltransferases. It seems unlikely that the NAT-2 genes are involved; the NAT-1 gene, which could be responsible, shows a unimodal distribution of activity but there is wide individual variation (Glowinski, Radtke and Weber, 1978). As these toxins are amino acid derivatives, they may be substrates for the enzyme systems that N-acetylate cysteine and S-substituted cysteines. Again, in a control population about 35% of individuals studied had little or no acetylation capacity for compounds of this type (Waring, 1980). These results, if applicable to the Guamian MND/ALS syndrome, would suggest that some individuals could be more resistant than others to exposure to the cycad toxins, which have been proposed as being causative agents. Recently it has been shown that levels of N-acetyl aspartate (NAA) and N-acetylaspartyl-glutamate (NAAG) are decreased in the ventral and dorsal horn and ventral column of MND patients (Tsai et al., 1991). Both compounds are involved in neurotransmission, and NAAG is co-localized in motor neurones. Reduction in NAA and NAAG could reflect some fault in N-acetylation of the appropriate precursors.

21.2 S-METHYLATION IN MND

Compounds containing aliphatic thiol groups and some sulphides are usually substrates for the aliphatic thiol methyltransferase (ATMT) enzymes. In this reaction, a methyl group is transferred from S-adenosylmethionine to 'cap' the thiol forming the $S-CH_3$ group. A number of studies (Weinshilbaum, Sladek and Klumpp, 1979; Weinshilbaum, 1992) have shown that there is wide variation within a normal population for ATMT activity. In a family study, Keith et al. (1983) concluded that ATMT in any individual was largely genetic, rather than environmentally controlled, but that inheritance appeared to be polygenic rather than following any simpler model. The enzyme is widely distributed in tissue membranes; liver microsomes and particularly the red blood cell (RBC) membranes have been used as sources in most in vitro experiments. In a study with patients with neurological diseases, it was found (Waring et al., 1989) that while Parkinson's disease patients usually had ATMT activity lower than the normal spread of values, MND patients typically had high levels. The mean ATMT activity for controls (and those with myasthenia gravis) was ~ 850 units per mg of protein, while the MND mean was 2080 units per mg of protein. There was a certain amount of overlap between the ranges, but values of up to 3200 units per mg of protein were recorded for some MND patients. This interesting result raises the question of whether the enzyme could be activated by some product of the disease process, or

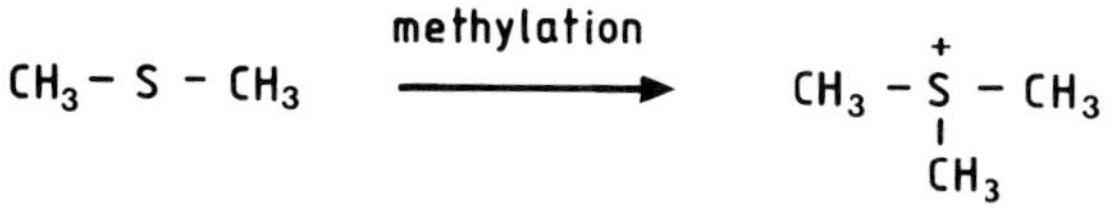

$$CH_3 - S - CH_3 \quad \xrightarrow{\textbf{methylation}} \quad CH_3 - \overset{+}{\underset{\underset{CH_3}{|}}{S}} - CH_3$$

Figure 21.2   Methylation of sulphur compounds to form thetins.

whether the ATMT found in MND patients is an isoenzyme variant. In a series of *in vitro* experiments (Peters, 1993) which measured the ATMT activity of RBC membranes from a series of individuals to both mercaptoethanol and D-penicillamine as substrates, the results suggest strongly that a different isoenzyme is present in MND. In both control and MND patients, the correlation between activities for the two substrates was good, but the gradient of the correlation line was different in each case. This result would not appear if high ATMT values in MND merely reflected some physiological enzyme activator. It seems consistent with the idea that patients with MND form a subset of the population with an isoenzyme variant that has different specificity for the two substrates tested, and probably also for any other compound that may be metabolized by this enzymic pathway. It is possible, therefore, that MND patients convert some environmental compound by this route into a neurotoxin; the rest of the population may not carry out the reaction to any great extent and so would be relatively resistant. This then raises the question of why ATMT is so widely distributed in tissues, and what is the natural substrate. This is not clear, although methylation by this enzyme system has been described as protecting against thiol toxicity (Kerremans *et al.*, 1985). Thiols (mercaptans) that have a free -SH group can alter protein configurations and often act as cell toxins. Typical examples are hydrogen sulphide (H_2S) and ethane thiol (C_2H_5SH), which both cause CNS degeneration but are converted to the less toxic thiol methyl ethers by the ATMT system (Weisiger, Pinkus and Jakoby, 1980). However, pro-toxins that have increased toxicity after methylation are less well defined. It has been suggested that two main routes could be involved. Many plants and vegetables contain sulphur compounds, often as S-substituted cysteines, disulphides or thioglycosides (Brodritz, Pollock and Wallon, 1969; Fenwick and Hanley, 1989). These are components of the typical odours and flavours of vegetables from *Brassica* and *Allium* species and may therefore make a steady contribution to dietary intake. Methylation of sulphides in the CNS (where ATMT activity is high) would form compounds called thetins, which have a positive charge on the sulphur atom (see Figure 21.2). This charge would prevent the compound from crossing the blood–brain barrier, and could lead to cell damage.

469

Xenobiotic metabolism

Anecdotal evidence suggests that some compounds of this type do in fact act as CNS toxins, causing 'knock-down' effects. As vegetables such as cabbage and onion are regularly consumed, there may be widespread but low exposure to S-methylated neurotoxins in individuals with high ATMT activity. Other sources of sulphur compounds can be found in the alicyclic tetrahydrothiophenes, which are used in the rubber industry. These have been widely used as plasticizers and may account for the slight excess of MND cases in workers in industrial rubber-moulding plants (Rowland, 1992). Another possible substrate for ATMT is metallic mercury. Inhalation of the vapour may be responsible for a few cases of MND; in personnel engaged in mining mercury the incidence of the disease is believed to be higher, while there may also be a weak link with working in the dental profession (Roelofs-Iverson *et al.*, 1984). Inorganic mercury is usually rapidly excreted, but methylation to form the mono- and dimethyl derivatives would give compounds that are much more fat soluble and also have much greater toxicity to the CNS. A similar mechanism may underlie some reported cases of MND induced by lead (Arman *et al.*, 1991), the alkyl derivatives of which are again fat-soluble CNS poisons. Whatever the natural pro-toxin, it seems probable that the existence of a high-activity isoenzyme variant of ATMT may be one of the factors leading to irreversible neuronal damage in susceptible individuals.

21.3 *S*-OXIDATION IN MND

A major enzymic fault identified in most cases of MND is a defect in oxidation of the amino acid cysteine. Although other pathways for cysteine metabolism exist, such as the formation of glutathione, protein and cysteamine, the most important catabolic reaction is the stepwise conversion of cysteine to inorganic sulphate (see Figure 21.3). The initial stage in this process, the formation of cysteine sulphinic acid, is catalysed by the enzyme cysteine oxidase, which occurs in liver and brain although at very low levels in other tissues. Analysis of a small

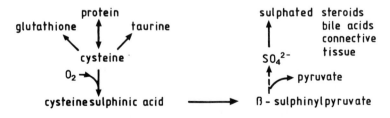

Figure 21.3 Oxidative conversion of cysteine to inorganic sulphate.

470

number (five) of post-mortem liver samples from MND patients has shown low levels of cysteine oxidase (mean ~ 23% of control values). This *in vitro* finding is reflected *in vivo*. Patients with MND have greatly reduced capacity to S-oxidize the test substrate S-carboxymethyl-L-cysteine (SCMC), which is also acted on by cysteine oxidase (Mitchell, Waring and Steventon, 1992). Analysis of plasma taken fasting at 08.00 h has shown that MND patients have high levels of cysteine, and also low levels of sulphate, the end product of the reaction sequence catalysed by cysteine oxidase (Heafield *et al.*, 1990b). Care must be taken when plasma samples are collected for assay; cysteine oxidase is diurnal, with minimum activity at night, while plasma cysteine is of course affected by intake of dietary proteins. The standard protocol for using early morning fasting samples avoids variations that might be introduced by the confounding factors of diet and time.

Family studies and twin studies using SCMC as a test substance and measuring the urinary excretion of sulphoxide metabolites have shown a strong genetic component for S-oxidation (Mitchell and Waring, 1989). Although S-oxidation capacity behaves as though it were controlled by an autosomal recessive gene, computer maximum likelihood analysis suggests that this major effect is superimposed on a background provided by two or three minor genes (Mitchell *et al.*, 1984). The proportion in a normal population who have no capacity for SCMC S-oxidation is 2%, while about 30% have reduced ability to carry out this reaction. The corresponding values in MND give 37% with absent S-oxidation and 30% with reduced levels (Steventon *et al.*, 1988). *In vivo* S-oxidation of SCMC correlates with final plasma measurements of cysteine/sulphate ratios, showing that SCMC is indeed a substrate for cysteine oxidase and, incidentally, that the oxidation of cysteine via this route is a major metabolic pathway. Both cysteine and sulphate can of course be removed by other routes, but formation of components such as proteins and glutathione or steroid and bile acid sulphates appears not to be rate limiting.

As can be seen (Table 21.1), MND patients have both high plasma levels of cysteine (mean 515 nmol per mg of protein; control 317 nmol/mg) and low levels of sulphate, with an elevated cysteine/sulphate ratio (440 compared with 114 as a control mean). The low concentrations of sulphate have 'knock-on' effects, in that the detoxification of many drugs and environmental compounds relies on formation of 'sulphate conjugates'. These non-toxic water-soluble metabolites are readily excreted; however, their formation depends on the level of available sulphate, which appears to be rate limiting (Galinsky, Slattery and Levy, 1979). As would be expected, when MND patients were challenged with a dose of paracetamol (500 mg), they produced much less of the sulphate

Xenobiotic metabolism

Table 21.1 Plasma values (0800 h) for cysteine and sulphate in MND patients and controls

	Controls (50)		MND patients (56)	
Mean age (range)	53	(26–90)	54.7	(26–88)
Plasma cysteine (μmol/ml/mg)	0.32	(0.02–1.00)	0.52*	(0.18–1.77)
Plasma sulphate (male, μmol/ml/mg)	1.92	(0.78–6.63)	1.33*	(0.23–3.29)
Plasma sulphate (female, μmol/ml/mg)	3.49	(0.53–12.3)	1.15**	(0.18–2.52)
Cysteine/sulphate ratio × 1000	114	(10–658)	440**	(110–1780)

Values are medians, with ranges in brackets.
* $P < 0.02$, ** $P < 0.0001$ (Mann–Whitney U-test).

conjugate than controls, although glucuronide formation was normal (Steventon *et al.*, 1990). Compounds that are primarily metabolized by sulphate formation may therefore be more toxic to susceptible individuals. It is intriguing that pesticides have been linked with MND and that a patient has been described who had MND-type symptoms shortly after acute exposure to high levels of a pyrethrin-based insecticide (Steventon, Williams and Waring, 1990). Pyrethrins are hydrolysed in man to compounds that normally form sulphated metabolites, and may therefore be more toxic to individuals who have less available sulphate for their removal.

The high plasma levels of cysteine may also pose problems. Cysteine is now known to be an excitotoxin that acts on the NMDA receptor, which is a subtype of the glutamate receptors. Recent work by Olney *et al.* (1990) has shown that cysteine toxicity is augmented in the presence of bicarbonate anions. While his experimental system, which involves acute exposure of neonatal rat brains to toxins, may not be a perfect model for the human CNS, it is nevertheless interesting that some of the plasma cysteine levels reported in MND patients have approached the values found to be toxic in rats. As cysteine oxidase is diurnal, and dietary proteins also impose sudden changes, the cysteine values will fluctuate *in vivo* over the course of a day. It seems possible that long-term surges in plasma cysteine may cause chronic, as opposed to acute, changes which could finally lead to MND. The metabolism of cysteine itself in the CNS has not been fully studied, so it is not possible as yet to say whether derivatives of cysteine could contribute to toxicity. However, other sulphur-containing amino acid metabolites are also excitotoxins, such as homocysteic acid (Turski, 1989) and cysteine

472

sulphinic acid (Griffiths and Dunlop, 1991). Any defects in cysteine metabolism occurring in MND could therefore lead to an imbalance in endogenous metabolic products that finally results in neuronal degradation.

21.4 GENERAL CONSIDERATIONS

Although three metabolic pathways (S-methylation, cysteine oxidation and N-acetylation) have been shown to be aberrant in MND, it is important to realize that most reactions are normal. In particular, formation of glucuronide conjugates (Steventon *et al.*, 1990), and activities of monoamine oxidase B and phenol sulphotransferase seem to be no different from controls (Steventon *et al.*, 1989a). Oxidation of the test compound debrisoquine to its 4-hydroxy metabolite (catalysed by the cytochrome P450 isoenzyme CYP II D6) has also been investigated, but the proportion of poor metabolizers with a metabolic ratio greater than 12.6 is again the same as in a control population (Steventon *et al.*, 1989b).

The realization that defects in hepatic pathways of detoxification can correlate with destruction of motor neurones may seem surprising. It is important to realize that two issues are involved. Firstly, metabolism of exogenous (environmental) compounds may lead to toxin formation, either because MND patients do not have the hepatic capacity for the appropriate detoxification pathway, or because they have aberrant activity that actually leads to synthesis of toxins from compounds which in themselves are not particularly harmful. Secondly, the hepatic enzymes appear to be very similar, if not identical, to the equivalent enzymes in brain tissue. Hence, liver enzymes, and of course enzymes from other tissues, such as the red blood cell membrane and the platelet, can be used to reflect endogenous metabolism in the brain, which is less accessible to investigation.

Results from many groups of workers suggest that MND can best be explained by multivariate analysis, where a wide range of factors exists, any or all of which may be relevant to an individual case. Environmental effects are certainly important and some toxins have been tentatively identified. The literature on the connections between MND and use of solvents suggests that these compounds are co-toxins (Gunnarsson, 1992). While they do not necessarily cause direct damage themselves, they may act synergistically with the activity of other chemicals, possibly by altering the structure of the blood–brain barrier. This could facilitate entry by contaminants that would not normally reach the tissues of the CNS. An explanation of this type may also be valid for the association of MND after viral attack; it is now known that viruses are able to soften membranes, and this would increase penetration by coexisting xeno-biotic agents, as might electric shock, which has also been linked with MND (Kurtzke, 1991; Gunnarsson, 1992). However, if the normal detoxification defences are present, environmental agents should have no effect until levels are reached which are high enough to overwhelm the body capacity. When metabolic pathways are defective, then small amounts of toxins may cause damage; if this is repeated over the years, then, since brain tissue does not regenerate, the motor neurones may finally be so depleted that the functional threshold is reached. At this point, any adverse effect, whether exogenous or endogenous, may precipitate the symptoms of MND. If this view is correct, then no single cause could be identified for all patients, and probably even in individual cases a variety of factors, both environmental and genetic, 2would contribute to the final outcome.

REFERENCES

Arman, C., Kurland, L.T., Daube, J.R. and O'Brien, P.C. (1991) Epidemiological correlates of amyotrophic lateral sclerosis. *Neurology*, **41**, 1077–84.

Brodritz, M.H., Pollock, C.L. and Wallon, P.P. (1969) Flavour components of onion oil. *J. Agric. Food Chem.*, **17**, 760–3.

Deaper, D.M. and Henderson, B.E. (1986) A case control study of amyotrophic lateral sclerosis. *Am. J. Epidemiol.*, **123**, 740–9.

Evans, D.A.P. (1989a) An improved and simplified method of detecting the acetylator phenotype. *J. Med. Genet.*, **6**, 405–7.

Evans, D.A.P. (1989b) N-acetyltransferase. *Pharmacol. Ther.*, **42**, 157–234.

Fenwick, G.R. and Hanley, A.B. (1989) Glucosinolates, alliins and cyclic disulphides: sulphur-containing secondary metabolites, in *Sulphur-Containing Drugs and Related Organic Compounds* (ed. L.A. Damani), pp. 269–315, Ellis Horwood, Chichester.

Galinksy, R.E., Slattery, J.T. and Levy, G. (1979) Effect of sodium sulphate on acetaminophen elimination by rats. *J. Pharm. Sci.*, **68**, 803–5.

Glowinski, I.B., Radtke, H.E. and Weber, W.W. (1978) Genetic variation in N-acetylation of carcinogenic arylamines by human and rabbit liver. *Mol. Pharmacol.*, **14**, 940–9.

Grant, D.M., Blum, M., Beer, M. and Meyer, V.A. (1991) Monomorphic and polymorphic human arylamine N-acetyltransferases: a comparison of liver isozymes and expressed products of two cloned genes. *Mol. Pharmacol.*, **39**, 184–91.

Griffiths, R. and Dunlop, J. (1991) Cysteine sulphinic acid as a candidate endogenous EAA ligand. *Trends Pharmacol. Sci.*, **12**, 94–5.

Gunnarsson, L.G. (1992) *On the Occurrence and Possible Causes of Motor Neurone Disease in Sweden*. Medical Dissertation No. 364, Linkoping University.

Gunnarsson, L.G., Lindberg, G., Söderfeldt, B. and Axelson, O. (1991) Amyotrophic lateral sclerosis in Sweden in relation to occupation. *Acta Neurol. Scand.*, **83**, 394–8.

Heafield, M.T.E., Waring, R.H., Sturman, S.G. et al. (1990a) N-Acetylation status in neurodegenerative disease. Med. Sci. Res., 18, 963–4.

Heafield, M.T.E., Fearn, S., Steventon, G.B. et al. (1990b) Plasma cysteine and sulphate levels in motor neurone, Parkinson's and Alzheimer's disease. Neurosci. Lett., 110, 216–20.

Keith, R.A., Van Loon, J., Wussow, L.F. and Weinshilbaum, R.M. (1983) Thiol methylation pharmacogenetics: heritability of human erythrocyte thiol methyltransferase activity. Clin. Pharmac. Ther., 34, 521–8.

Kerremans, A.L., Lipsky, J.J., Van Loon, J. et al. (1985) Cephalosporin-induced hypoprothrombinaemia: possible role for thiol methylation of 1-methyltetrazole-5-thiol and 2-methyl-1,3,4 thiadiazole-5-thiol. J. Pharmacol. Exp. Ther., 235, 382–8.

Kurtzke, J.F. (1991) Risk factors in amyotrophic lateral sclerosis. Adv. Neurol., 56, 245–70.

Mitchell, S.C. and Waring, R.H. (1989) Deficiency of the S-oxidation of S-carboxymethyl L-cysteine. Pharmacol. Therap., 43, 237–49.

Mitchell, S.C., Waring, R.H. and Steventon, G.B. (1992) Variation in the S-oxidation of cysteine derivatives, in Pharmacogenetics of Drug Metabolism (ed. W. Kalow), Pergamon Press, Oxford, pp. 367–82.

Mitchell, S.C., and Waring, R.H., Haley, C.S. et al. (1984) Genetic aspects of polymodally distributed sulphoxidation in man. Br. J. Clin. Pharmacol., 18, 507–21.

Moriwaka, F. (1991) A clinical evaluation of inorganic mercurialism and its pathogenic relationship to ALS. Rinsho Shiakeigalu, 31, 885–7.

Olney, J.W., Zorumski, C., Price, M.T. and La Bruyere, J. (1990) L-Cysteine, a bicarbonate-sensitive endogenous excitotoxin. Science, 248, 596–9.

Peters, L.M. (1993) MSc. thesis, University of Birmingham, Birmingham, UK.

Reece, D.M. and Nunn, P.B. (1989) Synthesis of ^{14}C-labelled L-α-amino-β-methylamino-propionic acid and its metabolism in the rat. Biochem. Soc. Trans., 17, 203–4.

Roelofs-Iverson, R.A., Mulde, D.W., Elveback, L.R. et al. (1984) Amyotrophic lateral sclerosis and heavy metals. Neurology, 34, 393–5.

Rowland, L.P. (1982) Diversity of MND. Adv. Neurol., 36, 1–13.

Steventon, G.B., Williams, A.C. and Waring, R.H. (1990) Pesticide toxicity and motor neurone disease. J. Neurol. Neurosurg. Psychiat., 53–7, 621–2.

Steventon, G.B., Heafield, M.T.E., Waring, R.H. et al. (1990) Metabolism of low-dose paracetamol in patients with chronic neurological disease. Xenobiotica, 20, 117–22.

Steventon, G.B., Waring, R.H., Williams, A.C. et al. (1988) Xenobiotic metabolism in motor neurone disease. Lancet, ii, 644–7.

Steventon, G.B., Sturman, S.G., Heafield, M.T.E. et al. (1989a) Platelet monoamine oxidase – B activity in Parkinson's disease. J. Neurol. Transmission, 1, 255–61.

Steventon, G.B., Heafield, M.T.E., Sturman, S.G. et al. (1989b) Degenerative neurological disease and debrisoquine-4-hydroxylation capacity. Med. Sci. Res., 17, 163–4.

Xenobiotic metabolism

Strong, M.J., Garruto, R.M., Wolff, A.V. *et al.* (1990) N-Butylbenzene sulphonamide, a novel neurotoxic plasticising agent. *Lancet*, **330**, 640.

Tsai, G., Stauch-Slusher, B., Sim, L. *et al.* (1991) Reductions in acidic amino acids and N-acetyl aspartylglutamate in amyotrophic lateral sclerosis CNS. *Brain Res.*, **556**, 151–6.

Turski, W.A. (1989) Homocysteic acids convulsant action of stereoisomers in mice. *Brain Res.*, **479**, 371–3.

Waring, R.H. (1980) Variation in human metabolism of S-carboxyymethyl cysteine. *Eur. J. Drug Metab. Pharmacokinet.*, **5** (1), 49–52.

Waring, R.H., Steventon, G.B., Sturman, S.G. *et al.* (1989) S-Methylation in motor neurone disease and Parkinson's disease. *Lancet*, **ii**, 356–7.

Weber, W.W. and Hein, D.W. (1985) N-Acetylation. *Pharmacogenet. Pharmacol. Rev.*, **37**, 25–77.

Weinshilbaum, R. (1992) Methyltransferase pharmacogenetics, in *Pharmacogenetics of Drug Metabolism* (ed. W. Kalow), Pergamon Press, Oxford, pp. 179–94.

Weinshilbaum, R.M., Sladek, S. and Klumpp, S. (1979) Human erythrocyte thiol methyltransferase: radiochemical microassay and biochemical properties. *Clin. Chim. Acta*, **97**, 58–71.

Weisiger, R.H., Pinkus, L.M. and Jakoby, W.B. (1980) Thiol S-methyltransferase: suggested role in detoxication of intestinal hydrogen sulfide. *Biochem. Pharmacol.*, **29**, 2885–7.

22 *Excitatory amino acid transmitters*

BERNARD M. PATTEN

22.1 INTRODUCTION

In the last two decades a substantial body of work has suggested that the mechanism of neuronal death in many acute and chronic neurological diseases may be related to excitatory amino acids. In particular, speculation now focuses on the role of excitotoxins, exogenous and endogenous compounds that act via excitatory amino acid (EAA) neurotransmitter receptors, as the final instruments of neuronal death. This chapter briefly reviews the background information on the biology of excitatory amino acids, including the pathways by which they are made and the mechanisms by which they act as toxins. This is followed by discussion of amino acid toxicity in general and its possible role in the pathogenesis of amyotrophic lateral sclerosis in particular. The chapter closes with some suggestions for possible therapeutic agents that might be tried in an attempt to modify this grave disease.

22.2 BACKGROUND

Vertebrate neurons contain millimolar concentrations of excitatory amino acids, usually aspartate and glutamate. These acidic amino acids play important roles in intermediary metabolism and also act as anions that contribute to the maintenance of osmotic pressure within the cell. Experiments carried out over the last three decades have provided evidence that glutamate is a neurotransmitter, and the evidence for aspartate is almost as cogent. Immunocytochemical studies localize glutamate to nerve terminals, particularly in the mossy fibers in the hippocampus. All of the enzymes necessary for glutamate synthesis are present in neurons, and the enzyme glutaminase can produce glutamate from glutamine, an abundant brain chemical. Stimulation of specific areas of the brain, such as the dentate gyrus, results in a matter of seconds in calcium-dependent release of glutamate, as one would expect

477

if it were a transmitter. Other studies have shown that pyramidal cells, particularly in the hippocampal CA_1, will depolarize in a dose-dependent manner, as one would expect from a neurotransmitter activating specific receptors. In addition, antagonists have been developed that prevent glutamate from producing a depolarization of neurons and, more recently, a high-affinity glutamate uptake has been found in astrocytes and also a temperature-dependent uptake of glutamate has been found in neuronal synaptic vesicles (Rothman and Olney, 1986).

Different excitatory amino acids have potency ratios that vary in different regions of the central nervous system, suggesting that there might be more than one type of glutamate receptor. In fact, there are at least four different glutamate receptors, three of which control ion channels and the other of which is metabolically linked. These receptor types have been named for the substances that selectively excite them. The best known of the receptors is the N-methyl-D-aspartate (NMDA) receptor, found throughout the brain, with the highest level existing in the CA_1 region of the hippocampus. High NMDA receptor concentrations are also present in many other regions of the brain, including the three outer layers of the neocortex, the basal ganglia and the dorsolateral septum, and they may actually be associated with the substantia gelatinosa, the nucleus of the solitarius tract and the medial and lateral geniculate body. These receptors have selective competitive antagonists and also non-competitive antagonists. For instance, a competitive antagonist of the NMDA receptor would be D-AP5 (D-2-amino-5-phosphonopentanoic acid); non-competitive antagonists include magnesium, ketamine, phencyclidine, MK 801 and glycine. Perhaps the second best-known receptor for excitatory amino acids is the quisqualate. These receptors seem to be more selectively bound by the agonist AMPA (amino-3-hydroxy-5-methyl-4-isoxazole propionic acid). The third best-known receptor for excitatory amino acids is the kainic acid receptor, which exists in high concentrations in layers 5 and 6 of the neocortex, in the CA_3 region of the hippocampus, the hypothalamus and the reticular nucleus of the thalamus where the NMDA receptor levels are relatively low. The fourth glutamate receptor type is the metabotropic receptor, discussion of which is beyond the scope of this chapter (Bockaert *et al.*, 1990).

22.3 FUNCTION

The function of these receptors is extremely complex. Slices in cell suspensions prepared from rat cerebellum show that activation of the NMDA receptors results in the production of nitric oxide (NO), an unstable molecule that was formerly known as the endothelium-derived relaxing factor, which crosses membranes easily to act on neighboring cells. It is highly likely that nitric oxide is the major component activating soluble guanylate cyclase, increasing cyclic GMP levels. In the cerebellum, the principal targets appear to be nerve terminal endings and astrocytes. Nitric oxide is synthesized enzymatically from guanidine nitrogen of L-arginine. Nitric oxide synthesis can be easily triggered by glutamate and is mediated almost entirely through the NMDA receptors. Non-NMDA receptors are probably also capable of inducing nitric oxide synthesis, and it is likely that the nitric oxide signaling system is not confined to the cerebellum but is widely used throughout the nervous system.

22.4   RECEPTOR ACTIVATION CURRENTS

Currents produced by kainic acid or quisqualate binding to non-NMDA receptors depend predominantly on sodium and potassium permeability. In contrast, voltage changes resulting from agonist binding to NMDA receptors depend to a great degree on calcium influx in addition to potassium and sodium ions. After agonist binding, ion fluxes at various voltages differ greatly at the two types of receptor channels. Non-NMDA channels have a linear relationship between ion influx and voltage grade. NMDA receptor channels have very little ion influx when hyperpolarized, but with depolarization undergo a marked increase in ion influx. This is because of the blocking effect of non-competitive inhibitory magnesium at the NMDA channels, which is reduced with neuronal depolarization. The depolarization caused by binding of agonist to NMDA receptors also promotes neuronal burst firing.

22.5   EXCITOTOXICITY: A BRIEF HISTORY

The history of excitotoxicity is closely linked to the history of excitatory amino acid physiology. In the late 1950s, a group of Australian scientists discovered that the acidic amino acids glutamate and aspartate have powerful excitant effects on neurons (Watkins and Evans, 1981; Albin and Greenamyre, 1992). Lucas and Newhouse in 1957 showed that systemic administration of glutamate to rats resulted in retinal degeneration. This was the first evidence that acidic amino acids might be neurotoxic. The neuroexcitant effects of the EAA were initially thought to be a non-physiologic effect, but over the course of two decades evidence has accumulated that glutamate, aspartate and closely related compounds that stimulate the excitatory receptors of the central nervous system are widely distributed throughout the brain and the spinal cord, and probably therefore play a role in the autodestruction of the nervous

Excitatory amino acid transmitters

system. Intracerebral injection of excitatory amino acids destroys neurons in the area of injection while sparing fibers of passage in the afferent terminals of distant neurons projecting to the region of injection. In addition, a robust correlation exists between the excitant and toxic properties of the excitatory amino acid analogs and correctly correlates with the neurotoxicity of the excitatory amino acids mediated through the excitatory amino acid neurotransmitter receptors. Olney (1969) summarized these investigations when he coined the term excitotoxin.

The high density of excitatory amino acids and excitatory amino acid receptors throughout the central nervous system does not cause undue neurotoxic burden within our brains because the actual concentration of excitatory amino acids within the synaptic cleft is carefully maintained at subtoxic levels by the rapid uptake and inactivation of the excitatory amino acids both by neurons and by glia (Kanner and Schuldliner, 1987; Nicholls and Attwell, 1990). Nevertheless, it is evident that a disturbance in the metabolism or physiology or receptor function or ion channel function or transmitter or secondary messenger function or any one of the number of the pathways involved in this particular aspect of neuroscience could result in a disturbance of the delicate equilibrium and cause neuronal injury by excitotoxic mechanisms.

22.6 MECHANISMS OF CELL DEATH

Several studies completed during the last decade have given insight into the pathophysiology of glutamate and aspartate's neurotoxic action. Cultures of dispersed hippocampal cells, for instance, die when exposed to glutamate in a concentration of 1 mmol for 30 min. This neuronal death can be prevented by removing sodium and chloride from the extracellular fluid and replacing them with similarly charged impermeable ions. Depolarization alone, for instance that produced by high extracellular potassium concentrations, cannot produce neurotoxicity in the absence of chloride ions. The toxic effect occurring within 1 h is quite rapid and is not dependent on extracellular calcium and pathologically consists of an initial cellular swelling followed by necrosis. Choi (1990a,b) studied dissociated mouse neurocortical neuron growth in culture. When he exposed these cells for a short period of time, in some cases 5 min, to 0.5 mmol glutamate in the presence of extracellular sodium and calcium, there initially was cellular swelling and then progressive degeneration of the neurons over the next 24 h. In the absence of calcium during glutamate exposure, there was swelling of the cells initially but they subsequently recovered. In the medium lacking sodium but containing calcium, after glutamate incubation, there was no acute swelling but several hours later there was acute neuronal degeneration. Finally, when cells were exposed to a medium without sodium or calcium, glutamate exposure did not result in either early swelling or in late neuronal loss. This leads me to conclude that there are two different but additive mechanisms that take part in producing excitatory amino acid neurotoxicity. The first is a rapid swelling caused by depolarization followed by chloride influx and water entry. If the exposure to the excitatory neurotoxin is prolonged and at a high enough concentration, this can result in acute cell death. The second mechanism, however, is delayed necrosis secondary to intra-cellular calcium accumulation, and presumably this calcium entry is the final mechanism of cell death, perhaps leading to activation of lipases and proteases and, of course, mitochondrial damage (Rothman and Olney, 1986).

22.7 EXCITATORY AMINO ACID RECEPTOR PHARMACOLOGY

NMDA receptors possess a rich pharmacology, and so do the non-NMDA receptors. The NMDA receptor has the longest list of modifying agents, including a strychnine-insensitive glycine binding site that must be occupied for receptor activation and a polyamine binding site at a separate area that enhances receptor activation. It is also known that it is possible that a block will decrease the activation of the NMDA receptor with antagonist drugs active at the glutamate NMDA site, the glycine site or the polyamine site. Phencyclidine and related drugs also act as NMDA antagonists by binding with the NMDA receptor ion channel and preventing ion passage. Naturally, the existence of drugs that can block or inhibit NMDA receptor activation emphasizes one of the most attractive features of the excitotoxic concept, namely that there might be a remedy for a disease caused by a mechanism involving these receptors. Possible treatments that might be applied to amyotrophic lateral sclerosis on the basis of this theory are discussed towards the end of this chapter.

22.8 EXCITATORY AMINO ACIDS AND NEUROLOGICAL DISEASE

It is beyond the scope of this chapter to discuss the excitotoxins and their relationship to the pathophysiology of acute neurological diseases such as hypoxia, ischemia and hypoglycemia. In all these situations the normal uptake and inactivation of excitatory amino acids is disrupted by interruption of the cellular mechanisms that release the amino acids and take them up, leading to a massive rise in the extracellular concentration of these toxic substances. When exposed to large amounts of these toxic substances under the circumstances described, neurons become more

481

depolarized, facilitating the activation of NMDA receptors, and enhancing neuronal susceptibility to the excitotoxicity. Amazingly, experimental models of focal ischemia, hypoxia and hypoglycemia show that NMDA receptor antagonists can reduce and sometimes dramatically reduce the extent of central nervous system damage (Choi, 1990a). Antagonists of the AMPA receptor are also neuroprotective against global hypoxia and ischemia (Sheardown *et al.*, 1990).

22.9 CHRONIC NEUROLOGICAL DISEASE OTHER THAN ALS

The role of excitotoxins in chronic neurological disease is probably best illustrated and has been most vigorously studied in Huntington's disease. Intrastriational injections of kainic acid produce neurochemical changes similar to those seen in Huntington's disease brains, and subsequent work has concentrated on NMDA agonists, which appear to provide a very faithful model of the pathology of Huntington's disease. While such experiments do not provide absolute proof that excitotoxicity underlies neuronal death in Huntington's chorea, the similarity of the experimental lesions to the striatal pathology of the naturally occurring disorder has made the excitotoxic model the principal testing ground of potential therapies for Huntington's disease.

Another human disease in which excitatory amino acids play a role is lathyrism. Individuals who consume substantial quantities of the chickpea (*Lathyrus sativa*), used as a food supplement during times of famine in the Indian subcontinent, will slowly develop an upper motor neuron syndrome (Spencer *et al.*, 1986; Ludolph *et al.*, 1987). It turns out that the chickling pea contains large amounts of the excitatory amino acid β-N-oxalylamino-L-alanine (BOAA). Administration of BOAA to non-human primates produces a syndrome similar to human lathyrism, but not exactly the same.

22.10 EXCITATORY AMINO ACIDS IN ALS

The history of excitatory amino acid toxicity in ALS probably goes back to 1978 when my colleagues and I reported the results of our study of free amino acids in patients with amyotrophic lateral sclerosis. We studied serum, cerebrospinal fluid and urine amino acids in 12 patients with ALS and 12 controls that had been matched for age, sex and severity of disability (Patten *et al.*, 1978). We found that ALS patients had statistically significant elevations in serum levels of tyrosine, total aromatic amino acids and total basic amino acids. ALS patients also had statistically significant elevations in the cerebrospinal fluid of total basic amino acids, lysine, essential amino acids and leucine. Perhaps the most interesting finding was that the severity of ALS correlated inversely with the acidic amino acids glutamate and aspartate and O-phosphoserine in the cerebrospinal fluid, meaning that the more severe the ALS was, the lower the levels of the amino acids glutamate and aspartate in the spinal fluid. By contrast, the activity of the ALS, that is the rate at which the disease was actually progressing, correlated directly with the serum aspartate and with acidic amino acids ($r = +0.808$, $P < 0.001$, double tail included) and this probably is a tip-off that the excitatory amino acids are playing a role in the disease. At the time we could make nothing out of the fact that the branched-chain amino acids in serum correlated with the duration of ALS ($r = +0.626$, $P < 0.05$), as did valine ($r = +0.576$, $P < 0.05$), i.e. the higher their concentration in the blood, the longer the ALS patients were living. Now we know that branched chains do stimulate the metabolism of glutamate and aspartate in the central nervous system, probably by activating glutamic dehydrogenase. So, it is possible that the more branched-chain amino acids that were present in the serum, the less effective aspartate and glutamate would be in destroying neurons, and the greater would be the duration of ALS. This particular study emphasized the need for a suitable comparison group because it showed that several ALS patients had aminoaciduria but that there was a similar incidence of aminoaciduria in the control population. The use of disabled people or people with nervous system disease as a control group is also important because it turns out that there is a non-specific effect of disease that tends to elevate the free levels of amino acids, and, therefore, having as a control group the chronically ill with nervous system illness will cancel out the non-specific abnormalities due to nervous system disease alone. Although our data showed that no amino acid was increased as much as in the aminoacidopathies, there were small but significant differences in ALS patients compared with controls, and these probably reflect some kind of defect in amino acid metabolism. The strong correlation of ALS activity with serum aspartate levels was noted at the end of our paper and it was specifically stated that aspartate, the putative excitatory neurotransmitter in spinal neurons, was the only amino acid whose average level in spinal fluid exceeded the average level in controls by more than twofold. The CSF aspartate in the ALS cases exceeded CSF aspartate in controls by 2.75. Aspartate was also the only amino acid for which the ratio of serum level to CSF level was remarkably different from controls (12 for ALS and 30 for controls). So, the evidence for excitatory function of aspartate in the gray matter was pointed out and it was postulated that excessive neuronal activity in ALS, including fibrillations and fasciculations, might be due in part to the metabolic imbalance caused by an increase in the excitatory amino acid transmitter (Patten *et al.*, 1978). The argument became more cogent when I reported that infusions of Freeamine II, a mixture of amino acids containing large amounts of aspartate and glutamate, given as a nutritional supplement to three ALS patients, were associated with a marked acceleration of ALS to death in a matter of weeks (Patten, 1980). Festoff reported an identical observation in the discussion of my paper (Patten, 1980).

Subsequently, several other papers appeared that showed alterations of glutamate and aspartate in ALS patients early in their disease (Rothstein *et al.*, 1990, 1991). Plaitakis and Caroscio (1985, 1987) took 22 patients with early-stage typical ALS and measured glutamate levels and found that glutamate was significantly elevated in the fasting plasma of patients with ALS by 100% at a *P*-value < 0.001 as compared with healthy and diseased control subjects. Moreover, oral loading with monosodium glutamate at a dose of 60 mg per kg of body weight resulted in elevations of plasma glutamate levels that were greater and of longer duration in patients with ALS than those found in control subjects, suggesting defective handling of exogenous glutamate by non-neuronal tissue in these patients. Additional studies performed in post-mortem central nervous system tissue revealed significant reduction in glutamate levels by 21–40% in several CNS regions of patients with ALS (Plaitakis, Constantakakis and Smith, 1988). Although the decrease in glutamate levels was in absolute terms the same in all central nervous system areas studied, spinal cord levels were proportionately more affected than other central nervous system areas such as the cerebellar cortex or the frontal cortex. These changes appeared to be selective, since the levels of other amino acids did not change significantly except for the content of aspartate, which was decreased significantly in spinal cord only (Plaitakis, Constantakakis and Smith, 1988). Also, levels of the *N*-acetylated form of aspartate, *N*-acetylaspartate (NAA), and the dipeptide *N*-acetylaspartyl-glutamate (NAAG) decreased significantly in the spinal cord only (Constantakakis and Plaitakis, 1988). Robinson (1988) also showed that glutamate levels or aspartate levels were both reduced in the central nervous system of patients with ALS. Perry, Hansen and Jones (1987) also showed that glutamate levels were significantly reduced in all 13 central nervous system areas studied in patients with ALS. Those changes were not found in a study of tissue from ALS patients compared with controls (Patten, Kurklander and Evans, 1980, 1982), but instead marked elevations of tissue ammonia (NH_3) were found, suggesting a defect in mitochondrial energy metabolism in ALS. So, to summarize the confusion: measurements of amino acids in the CSF of patients with ALS have been reported to show increased concentrations of lysine and leucine, no significant alteration of amino acid levels, and elevated concentrations of glutamate, glycine, alanine, threonine, isoleucine and phenylalanine. Tissue levels of glutamate and aspartate have been found to be depressed or normal in ALS. de Belleroche, Recordeti and Rose (1984) also reported that elevated CSF concentrations of glycine were clearly correlated with disease activity as determined by the severity–duration ratio in patients with ALS.

To add to the confusion, Perry, Hansen and Jones published a paper in 1990 reporting the findings of statistically increased mean glutamate concentrations in fasting plasma of patients with ALS, like those reported by Plaitakis and Caroscio (1985, 1987). Although the degree of elevation in their study was less, it was almost certainly because their patients were significantly older than normal control subjects. Regression analysis on their data seemed to indicate that the elevations in glutamate were related simply to age and not to ALS. They did find increases in concentration in ALS of leucine and lysine in the CSF, as did Patten *et al.* (1978), but found no significant increases in the concentration of glutamine or glycine in the spinal fluid of ALS patients – the same result as Patten *et al.* (1978). They also did not find a correlation between the severity of ALS and glycine levels in the spinal fluid; the same finding was reported by my group. In conclusion, the recent study of Perry, Hansen and Jones (1987) does not support the suggestion that a systemic defect in glutamate metabolism causes sporadic ALS, nor does it explain why glutamate concentrations are substantially reduced in several brain regions as well as in the spinal cord at death in ALS in some studies. They stated that they doubted that either increased concentrations of excitatory amino acids at synapses in motor neurons are potentiators of the NMDA receptor on the neurons or that increased synaptic concentrations of glycine are causing premature loss of motor neurons. They also found that it was unlikely that the sporadic form of ALS was caused by unrecognized dietary sources of BMAA or BOAA, although concentrations of those amino acids might have been detected by more sensitive analytical methods (Perry, Hansen and Jones, 1990).

How can we account for the differences between all of these studies? The patients studied by individual investigators, the control groups, the analytical methods and the methods of collecting and preparing the specimens for analysis all vary, and perhaps that accounts for the differences. Patients at a different stage of disease or who are older might actually have different levels of glutamate, and advancing disease might actually be the controlling influence on those measurements. When specimens are taken is important, and that is why in my study all blood and CSF and urine samples were taken in the mornings after an overnight fast of at least 8 h. However, the striking discrepancy between some studies, for instance the study of Rothstein *et al.* (1990) versus that of Perry, Hansen and Jones (1987), shows a tremendous difference in total glutamate and aspartate concentrations measured in the CSF. In controls, Rothstein *et al.* (1990) report glutamate concentrations of 2.9 μmol/l, which is in line with what was found by Patten *et al.* (1978), whereas the Perry group reported glutamate concentrations an order of magnitude lower at 0.2 μmol/l. These values, which represent a 15-fold difference in concentration, are not easily explained. Also, it is not easy to explain that in 1990 Perry, Hansen and Jones found normal values one-tenth the earlier revised values using seemingly identical methodology in their own same laboratory. In fact, the Perry group's current values appear to be below the sensitivity of assay for aspartate and approach the sensitivity of the assay for glutamate, and the standard deviations are large. It is possible that a more sensitive assay might have shown differences between control and ALS spinal fluid glutamate concentrations, but we simply do not know. My own feeling is that normal CSF glutamate and aspartate values make sense to the extent that the nervous system would be expected to have normal concentrations of excitatory amino acids so that neurotransmission in the normal state could not be disrupted. Although I have respect for the work of others, I tend to trust my own data more. I think that normal blood and CSF levels of glutamate and aspartate are toxic to neurons in ALS patients owing to a failure of detoxification mechanisms. If aspartate and glutamate are elevated in some ALS patients at some times (and they probably are), that can do nothing but add to the problem. Obviously, further experimentation will be needed to clarify these important issues.

Scientists owe much of their success to their ability to face facts fearlessly and disinterestedly. They recognize the danger of rejecting evidence because it proves inconvenient or accepting it because it conforms to their preconceived opinions. Darwin, for instance, found that he had to keep a special notebook in which he would write objections to his theory of evolution because he noted that in his own mind whenever he thought of an objection he quickly forgot it because his tendency was to disregard competing concepts and information. We must do the same with the theory of excitatory amino acids in ALS. Men fear thought, according to Bertrand Russell, as they fear nothing else on earth. More than ruin, more than even death because thought is subversive and revolutionary, destructive and terrible. It is merciless, especially in the light of scientific data. So, although the hypothesis that excitatory amino acids play a role in pathogenesis of ALS remains attractive and hopeful, we must constantly keep in mind that it might be wrong. The idea is still exciting because of its therapeutic implications. Indeed, two agents have been shown in double-blind prospective studies to favorably modify the course of ALS, and both agents were administered to patients based on the idea of excitatory amino acids playing a role in this disease (see below). Young (1990) has counseled us in an editorial that ALS is a tragic disease and it would be a real breakthrough if such therapy is proved effective. Nevertheless, clinical trials of preventive therapies are very expensive and labor intensive. Premature initiation of large trials without convincing preliminary data would be a mistake.

22.11 PILOT TRIALS BASED ON THE EXCITATORY TOXIC THEORY IN ALS

There have been two prospective control-blinded studies based on the excitotoxic theory of ALS. The first was a trial of branched-chain amino acids. Twenty-two patients with ALS were entered into a double-blind randomized placebo-controlled trial of a treatment with branched-chain amino acids. Eleven received daily 12 g of leucine, 8 g of L-isoleucine and 6.4 g of L-valine by mouth and the remainder received placebo. During the 1-year trial, patients in the placebo group showed a linear decline in functional status consistent with the natural history of ALS. Those treated with amino acids showed significant benefit in terms of maintenance of extremity muscle strength and continued ability to walk (Plaitakis et al., 1988). Because of the small sample size in this study, one cannot definitively conclude that treatment with branched-chain amino acids alters survival rates in ALS. The seemingly favorable results are clearly not due to differences in severity of illness and approximate duration of illness before treatment in the two groups, which were well-matched. However, the results must be viewed with caution because of the small sample size and because there is a substantial variation in the natural history of ALS. Rumor had it also that there were many protocol violations among the patients in this study. Of some concern was the fact that there were no significant differences in bulbar scores in any of the patients rated and most of the beneficial effects seemed to be on the spinal rating scales. Although this study is encouraging and may lead to a clear understanding of the pathogenesis of ALS, it is simply a preliminary trial establishing a basis for a new therapeutic approach. It should be mentioned that the theory on which this treatment was given was based on the idea that the branched-chain amino acids can induce metabolism of glutamate by correcting a partial deficiency of glutamate dehydrogenase that the authors thought they had identified in ALS. Glutamate dehydrogenase can be activated by branched-chain amino acids, particularly L-leucine and isoleucine, and those compounds are used for that purpose. The advantages of such a therapy are simply that it appears to be harmless and, if it does modify ALS, an important concept will have been established.

22.12   L-THREONINE

Patten and Klein in 1988 reported the modification of ALS by administering L-threonine. This was an open and uncontrolled study that they said showed definite benefit in terms of increased motor performance, decreased bulbar signs and decreased spasticity. L-Threonine is an essential amino acid in human nutrition and is metabolically converted to glycine in the nervous system by the operation of the enzyme threonine aldolase. Glycine is the inhibitory transmitter in the spinal cord, and it was felt that administering this would counteract some of the effects of the excitatory transmitter, as it is the actual natural inhibitory transmitter. Barbeau in 1974 had previously demonstrated that L-threonine, when administered to patients with multiple sclerosis, is safe and actually beneficial in spasticity. His doses were 2.5 g/day. Subsequently, Maher and Wurtman in 1980 demonstrated that L-threonine administration increases the concentration of glycine in the rat central nervous system. These three studies, therefore, set the scene for the administration of L-threonine in a double-blind prospective and controlled manner.

In 1989, Blin *et al.* using L-threonine reported the results with 12 patients afflicted with ALS diagnosed by strict criteria. The age range was 45–73 years and the mean was 57.9 years. They had had ALS for 10–24 months with a mean of 16.7 months. All of the patients, of course, gave informed consent in writing, and the study was fully approved by the Human Experiment Committee. Patients were given lactose placebo or L-threonine 2 g/day for 7 days; after a washout of 7 days the second session was given with the alternative agent. Thus, this was a crossover study. In this short evaluation period the objective neurological examination had demonstrated that the grip strength was very much improved in the patients taking L-threonine. The average improvement was 10.5 N with L-threonine, and those patients on placebo had actually lost strength of 15.7 N. The difference was statistically significant at $P <$ 0.05. Other improvements were observed in strength testing, and each of the patients had a self-administered scale appraising the agent they liked the best. L-Threonine was favored at a statistically significant level also. In 1991, Blin *et al.* reported their subsequent work with L-threonine, which confirmed the previous studies about the efficacy in ALS. On objective measures they found that fasciculations were reduced, cramps were reduced, motor activity was increased, strength was increased, and manual muscle testing values were improved, all at statistically significant values of less than 0.05. The investigators observed that the patients often noted a subjective improvement within 48 h of treatment, a finding that Klein and I reported in our original study (Patten and Klein, 1988). Subsequently, I discussed this with Dr Blin, and he believes that the effect of the L-threonine lasts about 3 months and then is no longer measurable. This has been my impression too. Blin did not use supplements of vitamin B_6 for his long-term treatment, and since vitamin B_6 is a co-factor in the conversion of threonine to glycine it is possible that it might actually have extended the improvement for a greater duration of time. Usually, we administer 50 mg of vitamin B_6 per day and administer the L-threonine in a dose of 500 mg four times a day by mouth between meals. Patients with bulbar palsy may notice that their speaking and swallowing improves and, strangely, the hypersalivation seems to decrease as well along with the cramps and muscle twitching. Spasticity may be modified also, as one would expect because of the known effect of L-threonine on spasticity. Further studies will have to be done to confirm these preliminary observations and also establish the role of L-threonine in the therapy of ALS, if indeed it has any role at all. At the present time, my feeling is that it is a good agent to modify some of the symptoms in the disease but that, while these symptoms are being modified, the disease continues to progress, and therefore, the benefits of L-threonine are benefits only over the short term. Incidentally, Blin *et al.* in their 1991 paper mention a study of glutamate concentrations in the serum of 18 patients compared with 16 controls and report that there was a significant elevation of glutamate. The values were 168.3 ± 52.7 μmol/l in the ALS patients compared with 57.1 ± 31.7 μmol/l in the controls, with the results statistically significant at a *P*-value of < 0.01. They were, however, unable to make any significant correlation using the Spearman rank correlation test between age of the patient, duration of the evolution of the disease and the amount of glutamate. Their patients were studied *à jeun*, that is fasting. They did not study the rate of deterioration of ALS as had been reported by Patten *et al.* in 1978.

22.13 IDEAS FOR ANTAGONIZING EXCITATORY NEUROTOXICITY

Choi (1990) has written an excellent review outlining the ranges of measures that might be used to protect neurons from excitatory damage. The organizing thesis in his review is a consideration of glutamate and aspartate neurotoxicity as a sequential three-stage process – induction, amplification and expression – each perhaps specifically amenable to therapeutic interference. Overstimulation of glutamate receptors induces intracellular accumulation of several substances, including calcium, sodium, chloride and diacylglycerol. Blockade of induction might be accomplished by antagonizing post-synaptic glutamate receptors, but could also be accomplished by reducing glutamate release from presynaptic terminals or improving glutamate clearance from synaptic clefts. Following induction, several steps may amplify the resultant rise in intracellular free calcium and promote the spread of excessive excitation to other circuit neurons. Protective strategies operating at this level might include blockade of additional calcium influx, blockade of calcium release from intracellular stores and interference with the mechanisms coupling glutamate receptor stimulation to lasting enhancements of excitatory synaptic efficacy. Following amplification, toxic levels of intracellular free calcium might trigger destructive cascades bearing direct responsibility for resultant neuronal degeneration. This, of course, is the end expression of excitotoxicity. The most important cascades to block may be those related to the activation of catabolic enzymes and the generation of free radicals. Broad consideration of possible mechanisms for antagonizing glutamate and aspartate neurotoxicity is definitely needed to develop therapies with greater efficacy and the least adverse consequences for brain function. Although a full discussion of the methods of antagonizing this particular pathogenetic mechanism in ALS is beyond the scope of this chapter, I do wish to give a few illustrations of how this might be done in a practical sense.

For instance, under induction strategies, in the presynaptic realm, it might be possible to reduce the presynaptic release of glutamate by reducing the traffic of presynaptic neuronal volleys arriving in the glutamatergic nerve terminals. One experimental drug could be tetrodotoxin, the puffer fish toxin, which inhibits action potentials generated by blocking voltage-gated sodium channels. Practical pharmaceuticals capable of reducing neuronal firing encompass an array of depressant drugs, including anesthetics, hypnotics, sedatives and anticonvulsants. We actually do not know what would happen to an ALS patient placed under general anesthesia for a long period of time. This might actually be of great benefit, and the author has certainly seen patients subjected to surgery who have improved after surgery without any relationship to what the surgical procedure was and probably in response to some beneficial effect of the anesthesia. Any drug that could reduce membrane excitability or alter circuit behavior to favor inhibition might help suppress the firing of glutamatergic neurons. Another way of interfering with presynaptic mechanisms would be to reduce glutamate synthesis, and this has been done by injection of such substances as methionine sulfoximine. Finally, in the presynaptic realm there are a number of agents that will reduce glutamate release, including adenosine A_1 agonists and adenosine A_2 antagonists. Tetanus toxin, botulinus toxin, calmodulin inhibitors, hypothermia and free radical scavengers might also be effective. One interesting agent that can block nerve terminal depolarization to transmitter release is magnesium. Elevating extracellular magnesium would be a classic method of reducing quantal transmitter release from motor nerve terminals. Magnesium also blocks the post-synaptic receptor, so it could have a double function and be beneficial in two ways. Other ions can impair the N-channels, including cadmium, manganese, nickel and cobalt. The trivalent lanthanide gadolinium^{3+} has been reported to be a relatively selective N-channel antagonist on rodent neuroblastoma glial hybrid cells. Gamma-amino butyric acid (GABA) is a well-defined presynaptic inhibitor of sensory afferent fibers projecting to the dorsal horn of the spinal cord and probably participates in presynaptic inhibition else-where in the central nervous system. Activation of presynaptic GABA receptors with the selective agonist baclofen can reduce calcium uptake and aspartate release from cultured cerebellar granular cells. In addition, the stimulation of ubiquitous post-synaptic GABA receptors can be expected to open chloride channels and reduce the circuit excitability, so baclofen would be a reasonable agent to consider.

Working down to the synaptic cleft, once glutamate release has occurred it might be possible to reduce its extracellular build-up in the synaptic cleft. This area of investigation is particularly important in ALS, as will be discussed at the end of this chapter when Rothstein's work about reuptake mechanisms in amyotrophic lateral sclerosis is reviewed. The primary process that normally limits the action of synaptically released glutamate is active cellular uptake by glia and nerve terminals. Enhancing this clearing process, which actually seems to be defective in ALS, might be accomplished by improving energy supply to the uptake pumps or by altering pump behavior or correcting the defect in the transporter protein. Of note, L-methionine sulfoximine, which inhibits glutamine synthesis by inhibiting glutamine synthetase, lowers striatal levels of glutamate. It also induces a transient fivefold increase in the V_{max} for the high-affinity glutamate uptake into striatal tissue. And lastly, working down to the post-synaptic membrane, there are a host of time-tested target sites for attenuating neurotransmitter-mediated effects in the post-synaptic region. In fact, most attempts to reduce excitotoxicity so far have been directed against the post-synaptic glutamate receptors. The target is not a stationary one and the receptor biology is very complex. Indeed, the author has attended a symposium on the subject that lasted 7 days from 8 o'clock in the morning until 8 o'clock at night each day to discuss simply these post-synaptic receptors

Excitatory amino acid transmitters

and how they might be inhibited. Abstracts for this symposium appear in *Neurochemistry International*, Vol. 16, Suppl. 1, 1990.

22.14 OTHER AGENTS

Dextromethorphan, which blocks the aspartate receptor, might be a good agent to try in some ALS patients. It is also possible that the receptors' response to transmitter could be modified using glycine, zinc, magnesium, phencyclidine (PCP), homocysteate, spermidine and other polyamines. New approaches that may be worth trying in ALS include blocking the metabotropic quisqualate receptors; inhibiting NO (nitric oxide, the second messenger) from activating the receptor; and using novel NMDA receptor antagonists such as CGP 37849 and CGP 39551, or the quinoxalinediones. One technique that is also of possible value is RADA (receptor abuse-dependent antagonism), a new strategy in drug targeting for the excitatory amino acid-induced neurotoxicity. One class of drugs that respond to the criteria of RADA are the sphingoglycolipids, both the natural ones (GM1, GD1A, GT1B) and semisynthetics (LIGA4 and LIGA20). These compounds have the unique property of preventing the protracted and exaggerated translocation of protein kinaseC (PKC), the long-acting abnormal increase of cytosol calcium levels and the neuronal death induced by abusive stimulation of excitatory amino acid receptors. The protective effect of the sphingolipids and sphingoglycolipids occurs without changing the physiologic EAA-induced signal transduction events at the ion or metabotropic receptors. Thus, natural and semisynthetic sphingolipids belong to a new class of excitatory amino acid receptor antagonists with potential therapeutic advantages over antagonists such as 2-amino-5-phosphonovalerate (APV) or 4-(3-phosphonopropyl)-2-piperazine-carboxylic acid (CPP) or the allosteric MK 801, which blocks the physiologic mechanisms of excitatory amino acid-induced signal transduction (Guidotti *et al.*, 1990).

Rapidly accumulating evidence suggests that the formation of free radicals may be clearly responsible for the brain injury associated with excitotoxins. While participation of free radicals in brain injury has been generally studied apart from consideration of excitotoxicity, there is reason to suspect that free radicals are quite important in this subject. Glutamate receptor overstimulation may cause substantial free radical formation and free radicals may be the final mediator of much of the cell destruction that occurs with the excitotoxic cascade. Perhaps administration of free radical scavenging material such as vitamin E (α-tocopherol), vitamin C or glutathione will protect the cells from damage induced by this mechanism. Other free radical scavengers include mannitol, barbiturates and chlorpromazine, and all of these drugs have been reported to have neural protective effects in certain experimental paradigms of ischemic cell injury. Free radical scavenging, therefore, may be part of the reason for the protection. Interestingly enough, methylprednisolone is also a free radical scavenger. Also of interest, allopurinol, which has been reported to reduce aspartate toxicity in mouse cerebellar cultures, is an inhibitor of xanthine oxidase, and it too might have a role in the therapy of ALS. Considering the different types and multitude of agents available, I believe a cocktail strategy is probably going to be the therapy of the future. That is an individual patient will be treated with a number of agents designed to interfere with multiple steps in the pathogenic mechanisms by which the excitotoxic amino acids damage nerve cells.

22.15 RECENT NEWS

No chapter on excitatory amino acids and amyotrophic lateral sclerosis would be complete without mentioning a recent paper by Rothstein, Martin and Kuncl (1992). They measured high-affinity sodium-dependent glutamate transport in synaptosomes from neural tissue obtained from 13 patients with ALS, 17 patients with no neurological disease and 27 patients with other neurodegenerative diseases (Alzheimer's disease in 15 patients and Huntington's disease in 12 patients). The groups were similar with respect to age and the interval between death and autopsy. Synaptosomes were prepared from the spinal cord, motor cortex, sensory cortex, visual cortex, striatum and hippocampus. They also measured sodium-dependent transport of GABA and phenylalanine in the synaptosomal preparations. In patients with ALS there was a marked decrease in the maximum velocity of transport for high-affinity glutamate uptake in synaptosomes from spinal cord. This was -59% (P-value < 0.001). Motor cortex was also affected with the value -70% and the same P-value, and somatosensory cortex was -39% with P-value < 0.05. Visual cortex, striatum and hippocampus showed no differences. The affinity of the transporter for glutamate was not altered, and no abnormalities in glutamate transport were found in synaptosomes from patients with other chronic degenerative disorders. The transport of GABA and phenylalanine was normal in patients with ALS. The authors reached the conclusion that ALS is associated with a defect in the high-affinity glutamate transporter that has disease, CNS region and chemical specificity. Defects in clearance of extracellular glutamate, because of a faulty transporter, could lead to neurotoxic levels of extracellular glutamate and thus be pathogenic in ALS. This astounding discovery is probably the most convincing evidence to date for a defect in excitatory amino acid metabolism in ALS. One should be reminded that the synaptosomal uptake for glutamate is also used by aspartate, so that the two are probably interchangeable and the defect in metabolism would affect them both.

The cause of the defect in glutamate transport is not clear, but the authors suggest numerous possible explanations. One is the loss of intrinsic glutamatergic neurons in certain regions of the brain. The reduction in high-affinity uptake in the spinal cord could reflect a loss of corticospinal fibers, which are known to be glutaminergic. However, the large reduction in uptake in the motor cortex could not be readily explained by loss of pyramidal neurons since they constitute a small minority of glutaminergic neurons in the cortex and form presynaptic terminals primarily in the spinal cord or brainstem. Another possibility is selective abnormalities in astrocytes, a possibility which I like the best. This would involve the same high-affinity glutamate transport system as present in neurons and is probably more important in taking up glutamate from the synaptic cleft than is neuronal reuptake. Thus, ALS could possibly be a primary defect in the astroglia transporter, and this defect impairs the ability to take up synaptic cleft glutamate. A third possibility is the decreased production or increased degradation of the transporter protein in either of these cell types or both. Further information will be obtained when the transporter is cloned and we know how to induce it or correct its deficiencies.

Unfortunately, Rothstein, Martin and Kuncl's results do not explain the selective loss of motor neurons. Motor neurons possess both *N*-methyl-D-aspartate and non-NMDA receptors, as anyone who has finished reading this chapter should know by now. Abnormalities in synaptic glutamate concentrations cannot explain the selective loss of motor neurons. There has to be some other missing link to explain the selective vulnerability. The proportionate subtypes of motor neuron in NMDA and non-NMDA glutamate receptors are not known. Cultured motor neurons are susceptible to toxic effects mediated selectively by non-NMDA glutamate receptors so they could be playing a special role. Whatever the mechanism for selective vulnerability, the results of the study by Rothstein, Martin and Kuncl (1992) provide important evidence for abnormal cellular metabolism of glutamate in patients with ALS, and encourage us to look further along these pathways for the ultimate solution to this dread disease.

ACKNOWLEDGMENTS

Lynn Klein RN assembled most of the early references of this chapter and read through approximately 600 references on excitatory amino acids for the author. Dale Salazar RN assembled most of the later references for the author. George Lindler generously supported this study with a gift. Pam Louis prepared this chapter for print.

REFERENCES

Albin, R.L. and Greenamyre, J.T. (1992) Alternative excitotoxic hypotheses. *Neurology*, **42**, 733–8.

Barbeau, A. (1974) A preliminary study of glycine administration in patients with spasticity. *Neurology*, **24**, 392.

Blin, O., Serratrice, G., Pouget, J. *et al.* (1989) Essai en double aveugle contre placebo a court terme de la L-Threonine dans la sclerose laterale amyotrophique. *La Press Medicale*, **18**, 1469–70.

Blin, O., Desnuelle, C., Guelton, G. *et al.* (1991) Anomalie des acides amines neurotransmetteurs dans la sclerose laterale amyotrophique: Une application therapeutique. *Rev. Neurol.*, **147**, 392–4.

Bockaert, J., Pin, J.-P., Sebben, M. *et al.* (1990) Associative stimulation of NMDA or metabotropic quisqualate receptors and depolarization are needed to trigger arachidonic acid release. *Neurochem. Int.*, **16**, 16.

Choi, D.W. (1990a) Cerebral hypoxia: some new approaches and unanswered questions. *J. Neurosci.*, **10**, 2493–501.

Choi, D.W. (1990b) Methods for antagonizing glutamate neurotoxicity. *Cerebrovasc. Brain Metab. Rev.*, **2**, 106–47.

Constantakakis, E. and Plaitakis, A. (1988) N-acetylaspartate and acetylaspartylglutamate are altered in the spinal cord in amyotrophic lateral sclerosis. *Ann. Neurol.*, **24**, 478.

de Belleroche, J., Recordate, A. and Rose, F.C. (1984) Elevated levels of amino acids in the CSF of motor neuron disease patients. *Neurochem. Pathol.*, **2**, 1–6.

Guidotti, A., Manev, H., Favaron, M. *et al.* (1990) RADA (receptor abuse dependent antagonism): a new strategy in drug targeting for the excitatory amino acid (EAA)-induced neurotoxicity. *Neurochem. Int.*, **16**, 14.

Kanner, B.I. and Schuldliner, S. (1987) Mechanism of transport and storage of neurotransmitters. *CRC Crit. Rev. Biochem.*, **22**, 1–18.

Lucas, D.R. and Newhouse, J.P. (1957) The toxic effect of sodium L-glutamate on the inner layers of the retina. *Arch. Ophthalmol.*, **58**, 193–201.

Ludolph, A.C., Hugon, J., Divivedi, M.P. *et al.* (1987) Studies on the etiology and pathogenesis of motor neuron diseases. *Lancet*, **110**, 149–65.

Maher, T.J. and Wurtman, R.J. (1980) L-Threonine administration increases glycine concentration in the rat central nervous system. *Life Sci.*, **26**, 1283–6.

Nicholls, D. and Attwell, D. (1990) The release and uptake of excitatory amino acids. *Trends Pharmacol. Sci.*, **11**, 462–8.

Olney, J.W. (1969) Brain lesion, obesity and other disturbances in mice treated with monosodium glutamate. *Science*, **164**, 719–21.

Patten, B.M. (1980) Commentary on nutritional management in amyotrophic lateral sclerosis, in *Diagnosis and Treatment of Amyotrophic Lateral Sclerosis* (ed. D.W. Mulder) Houghton Mifflin, Boston, pp. 284–6.

Excitatory amino acid transmitters

Patten, B.M. and Klein, L.M. (1988) L-Threonine and the modification of ALS. *Neurology*, **38**, 354–5.

Patten, B.M., Kurlander, H.M. and Evans, B. (1980) Amino acid content of spinal tissue from patients dying of motor neuron disease. *Trans. Am. Neurol. Assoc.*, **105**, 488–91.

Patten, B.M., Kurlander, H.M. and Evans, B. (1982) Free amino acid concentrations in spinal tissue from patients dying of motor neuron disease. *Acta Neurol. Scand.*, **66**, 594–9.

Patten, B.M., Harati, V., Acosta, L. *et al.* (1978) Free amino acid levels in amyotrophic lateral sclerosis. *Ann. Neurol.*, **3**, 305–9.

Perry, T.L., Hansen, S. and Jones, K. (1987) Brain glutamate deficiency in amyotrophic lateral sclerosis. *Neurology*, **37**, 1845–8.

Plaitakis, A. and Caroscio, J.T. (1985) Abnormal glutamate metabolism in ALS. *Ann. Neurol.*, **18**, 165.

Plaitakis, A. and Caroscio, J.T. (1987) Abnormal glutamate metabolism in amyotrophic lateral sclerosis. *Ann. Neurol.*, **22**, 575–9.

Plaitakis, A., Constantakakis, E. and Smith, J. (1988) The neuroexcitotoxic amino acids glutamate and aspartate are altered in the spinal cord and brain in amyotrophic lateral sclerosis. *Ann. Neurol.*, **24**, 446–9.

Plaitakis, A., Mandeli, J., Smith, J. *et al.* (1988) Pilot trial of branched-chain amino acids in amyotrophic lateral sclerosis. *Lancet*, 1015–8.

Robinson, N. (1988) Chemical changes in spinal cord in Friedreich's ataxia and motor neuron disease. *J. Neurol. Neurosurg. Psychiatr.*, **31**, 330–3.

Rothman, S.M. and Olney, J.W. (1986) Glutamate and the pathophysiology of hypoxic ischemic brain damage. *Ann. Neurol.*, **19**, 105–11.

Rothstein, J.D., Martin, L.J. and Kuncl, R.W. (1992) Decreased glutamate transport by the brain and spinal cord in amyotrophic lateral sclerosis. *N. Eng. J. Med.*, **326**, 1464–8.

Rothstein, J.D., Tsai, G., Kuncl, R.W. *et al.* (1990) Abnormal excitatory amino acid metabolism in amyotrophic lateral sclerosis. *Ann. Neurol.*, **28**, 18–25.

Rothstein, J.D., Kuncl, R.W., Chaudhry, V. *et al.* (1991) Excitatory amino acids in amyotrophic lateral sclerosis: an update. *Ann. Neurol.*, **30**, 224–5.

Sheardown, M.J., Nielson, E.O., Hansen, A.J. *et al.* (1990) 2,3-D-hydroxy-6-nitro-7-sulfamoyl-benzo(F)quinoxaline: a neuroprotectant for cerebral ischemia. *Science*, **247**, 571–4.

Spencer, P.S., Ludolph, A.C., Divivedi, M.P. *et al.* (1986) Lathyrism: evidence for role of the neuroexcitatory amino acid BOAA. *Lancet*, **2**, 1066–7.

Watkins, J.C. and Evans, R.H. (1981) Excitatory amino acid transmitters. *Annu. Rev. Pharmacol. Toxicol.*, **21**, 165–204.

Young, A.B. (1990) What's the excitement about excitatory amino acids in amyotrophic lateral sclerosis? *Ann. Neurol.*, **28**, 9–10.

23 Metals and free radicals

HARDEV S. PALL

The history of our knowledge of chemistry over the last two centuries shows a progression from an interest in the reactions of inorganic metal ions through the development of organic chemistry to a more recent recognition of the influence that metal ions can have on complex biochemical reactions. This evolution in chemical knowledge is mirrored by a similar bimodal interest in metal ions in human disease. Early studies measured metal ions with analytical techniques that were just becoming available and useful in metal-induced human diseases that were just being described, e.g. Wilson's disease. The recent resurgence of interest in metals and human disorders recognizes the advances in knowledge of free radical (FR) chemistry and the role of transition metals in redox reactions and recognizes the increasing knowledge of membrane metal ion channel conductances in cell signalling processes. Interactions between metal ions, for instance in their competition for transport systems or displacement of one ion from the active site of an enzyme by another metal ion, are now being given their well-deserved attention. Much of the work is now possible owing to developments in analytical techniques that not only allow measurements in biological fluids and biopsy or autopsy specimens but, with the progress in magnetic resonance spectroscopy, now make it possible to quantify metals *in vivo*. In the study of metals in human disease mechanistic considerations take us beyond asking, 'Is there an association between the disease and metal exposure?' Other pertinent questions requiring clarification include:

- Are the tissues that are damaged by the disease overloaded with the metal in question during the early stages of the disease?
- Is the biochemical form of the metal ions normal either as they enter the body or during storage, e.g. is it organic or inorganic mercury or is iron bound to ferritin rather than to haemosiderin?

497

Metals and free radicals

- Do all those exposed to the metal ions develop disease or do host susceptibility factors play a part?
- What are the effects on other metals and trace elements?
- In what subcellular compartment is the metal located and how does this differ from normal?
- What physiological processes does the metal serve or interfere with?
- What chemical processes lead to this disruption of physiological events?
- Is there a related human disease model?
- Is there a relevant animal model?
- Can the mechanisms of cell damage be studied in cell culture?
- Does metal removal improve the disease state?

According to reports dating from the 1800s the neurological and electrophysiological features of poisoning with heavy metals such as lead and mercury may be indistinguishable from those of idiopathic motor neurone disease (MND). However, with appropriate treatment the progression of metal toxicity may be prevented and, in some cases, its effects even reversed (Campbell, Williams and Barltrop, 1970), whereas no known treatment alters the progression of the idiopathic disease. Identification of metal toxicity in this setting has relied on the clinician's awareness in obtaining a history of exposure to lead or mercury. Given that the condition is invariably progressive and the outcome is fatal, it is not surprising that attempts have been made to implicate metal poisoning in the aetiology of idiopathic MND even in the absence of increased metal exposure, the hope being that metal chelation therapy will improve the prognosis if not reverse the disease. Many metals, including lead, mercury, aluminium, manganese and the group VI element selenium, are associated with MND (Ganrot, 1986; Mitchell, 1987). These elements appear to have little in common to account for their involvement in the pathophysiology of MND. However, the interactions of metal ions with one another, with reactive oxygen metabolites including FRs and with excitatory amino acid-mediated neurotransmission indicate possible mechanisms whereby poisoning with various metals could inflict cell damage by broadly similar pathological processes.

23.1 FREE RADICALS

A free radical (FR) is an atom, molecule or other chemical species that is capable of independent existence and which has one or more unpaired electrons. They are usually short-lived as a consequence of being highly reactive, an effect resulting from their intrinsic need to gain an

498

additional electron or to lose the unpaired one and hence achieve a stable electronic configuration. Considerations of the electronic configuration of molecular oxygen show that, despite its two unpaired electrons, it is relatively unreactive with organic molecules and, when it does react, it prefers to accept one electron at a time, thus producing FR intermediates (Taube, 1965).

$$O_2 + e \rightarrow O_2^{\cdot -} \tag{1}$$

$$O_2 + 2e + 2H^+ \rightarrow H_2O_2 \tag{2}$$

$$O_2 + 3e + 2H^+ \rightarrow OH^- + OH^{\cdot} \tag{3}$$

$$O_2 + 4e + 4H^+ \rightarrow 2H_2O \tag{4}$$

The oxygen-containing FRs produced by these processes include the superoxide ($O_2^{\cdot -}$) and the hydroxyl ($OH^{\cdot}$) radicals. Hydrogen peroxide is a reactive oxygen metabolite that is not a FR but which is capable of producing reactive FRs. Many biomolecules including DNA, polyunsaturated fatty acids and catecholamines are damaged by superoxide radicals (Cohen and Heikkila, 1974; Fridovich, 1983; Halliwell and Gutteridge, 1989). All these actions are inhibited, at least in part, by copper- or manganese-containing superoxide dismutase (SOD) enzymes and, in many cases, also by iron-containing native catalase, suggesting that hydrogen peroxide formation is important in mediating superoxide radical toxicity. As discussed below, the toxicity of superoxide is believed to result from production of hydroxyl FRs, possibly by a metal-catalysed Haber–Weiss reaction involving Fenton-type reactions (see Halliwell and Gutteridge, 1986) as intermediate steps.

Dismutation is the term applied to the redox reaction in which one superoxide radical reduces another to peroxide, itself becoming oxidized to oxygen in the process. This appears to be the true function of the SOD enzymes (Halliwell, 1989).

$$2 O_2^{\cdot -} + 2 H^+ \rightarrow H_2O_2 + O_2$$

The hydroxyl radical ($OH^{\cdot}$) can be produced from superoxide via hydrogen peroxide by low molecular weight/loosely bound complexes containing copper, iron and possibly manganese (Halliwell and Gutteridge, 1984). In general, protein-incorporated metal ions do not possess this capacity. Thus caeruloplasmin, ferritin, transferrin and haemoglobin have little or no capacity to produce hydroxyl free radicals (Halliwell and Gutteridge, 1989). Metal ions, notably iron and copper, are present in the human body in a form capable of catalysing these reactions (Halliwell and Gutteridge, 1985b). The mechanism of the postulated, harmful actions of copper, manganese or iron in this form is

Metals and free radicals

thought to involve a Fenton-type reaction as part of an overall metal-catalysed Haber–Weiss reaction. Possible reaction sequences are outlined below:

$$M^{n+1} + O_2^{\cdot -} \rightarrow M^n + O_2 \tag{1}$$

$$2\ O_2^{\cdot -} + 2\ H^+ \rightarrow H_2O_2 + O_2 \text{ Superoxide dismutation} \tag{2}$$

$$H_2O_2 + M^n \rightarrow M^{n+1} + OH^- + OH^{\cdot} \text{ Fenton-type reaction} \tag{3}$$

Overall:

$$\begin{array}{c} M \text{ ions} \\ O_2^{\cdot -} + H_2O_2 \rightarrow O_2 + OH^- + OH^{\cdot} \text{ Metal-catalysed Haber–Weiss} \end{array} \tag{4}$$

M = Fe or Cu or Mn.

In order to catalyse the production of hydroxyl radicals from hydrogen peroxide the transition metal ions must be present in their reduced form. Reduction of iron, manganese and copper in low molecular weight complexes may involve reactions with superoxide radicals (reaction 1 above).

Other reducing agents can also reduce metal ions, converting them to a form capable of producing hydroxyl radicals. Ascorbate is one such reducing agent present in biological fluids. The hydroxyl radicals can fragment DNA and other biomolecules such as carbohydrates or cause cross-linking of proteins resulting in loss of function of many essential enzymes. One prime target for damage is polyunsaturated lipid, which makes up an important part of cell membranes.

23.2 TRANSITION METAL IONS AND OXIDATION REACTIONS

Charge transfer (redox) reactions are involved in most metabolic pathways, including all energy-requiring processes. The need to control the sites and the timing of these charge transfers is paramount, particularly as some of the intermediates formed are unstable and consequently highly reactive and potentially damaging. Control over the sites at which certain redox reactions are allowed is exerted by accurate anatomical localization of the metal ions involved. When these are incorporated into enzymes, the intermediates are thought to be tightly bound to the protein, thereby restricting and directing their reactivity to adjacent functional groups. This fine control breaks down when the compartments, subcellular or submolecular, in which metal ions are located are disrupted. Release of metal ion complexes may result in uncontrolled damage to structures vital to cell anatomy, such as membrane lipids, or interruption of processes essential to physiological functions, such as neurotransmission, as a result of oxidative damage (Blake *et al.*, 1985). The neural manifestations of Wilson's disease and the neuro-ophthalmic complications of desferrioxamine therapy (Blake *et al.*, 1985; Pall *et al.*, 1983) might be considered examples of this form of damage. Lead and aluminium accelerate the peroxidation of membrane lipid induced by hydrogen peroxide, thereby enhancing its oxidant effect (Quinlan, 1988), and mercury at concentrations as low as 1 nM can stimulate the production of superoxide by phagocytes and can promote iron-catalysed lipid peroxidation (Halliwell and Gutteridge, 1989).

Thus:

- Transition metal ions can promote tissue damage by mechanisms involving production of oxygen-containing FRs.
- Transition metal ions in the form of metalloproteins make up a significant part of the body's defences against oxygen-containing FRs.
- Metal ions in forms capable of catalysing both uncontrolled (harmful, pro-oxidant, low molecular weight) and controlled (beneficial, antioxidant, protein-incorporated) reactions are present in the human body.
- Decompartmentalization of metal ions from antioxidant proteins not only reduces the antioxidant protection of these proteins but, by producing low molecular weight metal ion complexes, may directly increase their pro-oxidant effect.
- The oxidant/antioxidant actions of transition metal ions are altered by other metal ions such as aluminium, mercury and lead.

23.2.1 Lead

BACKGROUND

This ancient metal has been widely used in inorganic form in applications such as plumbing of water supplies, soldering, the ceramics industry, paint manufacture and protection against electromagnetic radiation and radioactive emissions, and in organic form, e.g. tetraethyl lead in petrol and lead in organometallic catalysts. Many of these uses are now outmoded, but the history of lead indicates that new applications will replace the old ones and that man's contact with this metal will not cease.

Lead encephalopathy in children and lead-induced mononeuropathies, most commonly radial neuropathy, are two of its well-recognized neurological disturbances. Van Sweiten's reports of a third type of lead-

Metals and free radicals

associated neurological disorder were highlighted nearly a century later by Aran in 1850 in a description of an MND-like syndrome. This started the interest in metals and MND. Since Wilson's (1907) description of an MND-like condition in chronic lead poisoning there have been a few reports of abnormal lead distribution and some of increased prevalence of occupational exposure to lead in MND. No report has implicated lead in the aetiology of all cases of MND, but several have suggested that in the general population of MND patients there are a number whose disease is related to lead overload and that, once identified, these patients may benefit from metal chelation therapy.

TOXICOLOGICAL ASPECTS

Much current evidence indicates that MND may arise from genetically predisposed individuals being exposed to a neurotoxin (Steventon *et al.*, 1988). In this context, it is of interest that interindividual variation in susceptibility to lead toxicity has been suggested (Conradi, Ronnevi and Vesterburg, 1978). *In vitro* studies show increased haemolysis when red cells from MND patients are exposed to lead, possibly indicating increased susceptibility to lead toxicity in this group (Ronnevi, Conradi and Nise, 1982). Lead accelerates the peroxidation of membrane lipids induced by hydrogen peroxide, thereby enhancing its oxidant effect (Quinlan, 1988). The increased red cell fragility may reflect FR-induced peroxidation of polyunsaturated fatty acids, which are required to maintain membrane fluidity and integrity. Other possible mechanisms of lead neurotoxicity include alteration in synaptic activity, changes in calcium homeostasis or altered cholinergic function. Administration of lead to mice results in impaired distribution of glutamate in the brain (Patel *et al.*, 1974). Some of the adverse effects of lead on neurotransmission are prevented by extracellular calcium ions (Cohen, 1979). The study of lead toxicity must also address the question of how lead gets into the nervous system. Several possible mechanisms exist – damage to the vascular endothelium with a breakdown in the blood–CNS barrier, retrograde axonal transport, complexes with physiological ligands such as catecholamines or negatively charged amino acids (in particular, thiol-containing ones, such as cysteine, that are known to form mercaptides with lead) or via other metals' specific receptor-mediated transport systems. Malhotra *et al.* (1984) showed that iron-deficient rats that were fed lead and manganese supplements showed marked increases in brain concentration of lead, manganese, copper and to a lesser extent iron. Zinc and calcium deficiency are also known to increase lead toxicity (Chisolm, 1980). Such complex interactions indicate that further work should perhaps focus on the effects of lead, manganese, aluminium and mercury on more physiologically relevant metals such as iron, copper, zinc, calcium and magnesium.

EPIDEMIOLOGICAL STUDIES

Some epidemiological studies of small numbers of patients show an association between lead exposure and the risk of MND (Currier and Haerer, 1968; Campbell, Williams and Barltrop, 1970; Armon et al., 1991), although other work has failed to find such a link (Kurtzke and Beebe, 1980; Kondo and Tsubaki, 1981; Gresham, Molgaard and Golbeck, 1986), and yet other studies have given inconclusive results (Scarpa et al., 1988). Currier and Haerer (1968) reported 9 of 31 patients with MND as having a history of definite or probable lead exposure, but this study had no control data for comparison. Campbell, Williams and Barltrop (1970) found 11 of 74 patients to have had severe exposure to lead with only 4 of 74 control subjects reporting similar exposure. In 74 MND patients compared with 201 matched controls Armon et al. (1991) found increased lead exposure histories and a more frequently reported contact with welding and soldering. However, in a study of 66 disease and a similar number of control patients Gresham, Molgaard and Golbeck (1986) did not find excessive lead exposure. In an Italian study in Modena, Scarpa et al. (1988) found an excess of MND in ceramics industry areas, but there was no conclusive association between the disease and lead exposure. Roelofs-Iverson et al. (1984) carried out a case–sib and case–spouse control study of 145 patients and demonstrated an increased risk of metal exposure in the patients, but their study did not examine individual metals. The balance of epidemiological evidence appears to suggest that a history of lead exposure is encountered more commonly in MND than would be expected but is still only found in a minority of patients with MND. The studies do not allow comment on whether various clinical features allow prediction of the lead-exposed patients, for instance unusually slowly progressive disease or absence of upper motor neurone or bulbar signs.

TISSUE AND FLUID MEASUREMENTS

Acute lead poisoning is relatively easy to diagnose on blood and urine tests, but more chronic effects of lead exposure are difficult to identify and may require more invasive tests such as measurement of bone lead concentrations or the mobilization of the metal's stores by the use of metal chelating agents and subsequent measurement of concentrations in body fluids. The normal concentration of lead in urine is less than 80

Metals and free radicals

μg/l; levels of 150 μg/l or more are toxic, and intermediate values have an uncertain significance (Lane, 1968). Urine lead concentrations after administration of the metal chelating agent, EDTA, have an upper limit of normal of 120 μg/l and a lower limit of the toxic range of 250 μg/l. These values are based on fairly limited data and may require revision as more information becomes available.

Conflicting results have been reported by different groups on the concentrations of lead in blood, CSF and muscle in MND (see Tandan and Bradley, 1985; Mitchell, 1987). CSF lead was reported normal by House *et al.* (1978), Manton and Cook (1979), Stobe, Stelte and Kunze (1983) and Kapaki *et al.* (1989), but Conradi *et al.* (1980) found increased levels. Erythrocyte lead has been reported to be normal (Stober, Stelte and Kunze, 1983). This contrasts with acute lead poisoning, in which erythrocyte lead is elevated. Plasma lead is increased in MND (Conradi, Ronnevi and Vesterburg, 1978). Petkau, Sawatzky and Hillier's (1974) observation of elevated muscle lead levels was not confirmed by Pierce Ruhland and Patten (1980). Spinal cord lead levels are increased in MND (Petkau, Sawatzky and Hillier, 1974; Kurlander, 1978), apparently in subgroups of both lead-exposed and unexposed patients. Kurlander and Patten (1978) showed a positive correlation of spinal cord lead concentrations with the duration of the disease, suggesting accumulation secondary to the disease process rather than a primary phenomenon. In models of inflammatory spinal cord injury (of doubtful direct relevance to MND) in experimental animals lead accumulation occurs as a secondary phenomenon, perhaps reflecting a breakdown in the blood–CNS barrier (Mandybur and Cooper, 1979). Total body lead as estimated by bone lead concentrations was no different in the MND group compared with controls (Campbell, Williams and Barltrop, 1970). Patten (1984) reported that 9 of 38 patients with MND had higher mobilized urine lead concentrations (following EDTA administration) than any of 22 control patients. The significance of this finding in relation to predicting response to chelation therapy is unclear.

CHELATION THERAPY

Many attempts have been made at chelation therapy for MND (Campbell, 1955; Currier and Haerer, 1968; Livesley and Sessons, 1968; Campbell, Williams and Barltrop, 1970; Boothby, de Jesus and Rowland, 1974; Justic and Sostarko, 1977; House *et al.*, 1978; Bousser and Malier, 1979; Conradi *et al.*, 1982). An often-quoted example of successful treatment of lead-induced MND is a case report (Campbell, 1955) of a 49-year-old woman who had a disease affecting the lower motor neurones (LMN) without any reported evidence of upper motor neurone (UMN) or bulbar involvement. There was no biochemical support for a diagnosis of lead poisoning, although there appears to have been a good response to treatment with a chelating agent. Dramatic though this patient's response to treatment was, neither a diagnosis of MND (on any criteria in use today) nor one of lead poisoning can be sustained. A subsequent study (Campbell, Williams and Barltrop, 1970) again reported that 'lead-associated MND' was predominantly a disease of the LMN and followed a more benign course than conventional MND, which also has UMN and bulbar features. This creates an uncertainty about its conclusion that lead chelation improved the outlook in the lead-associated MND. EDTA seemed to help a proportion of patients with MND-like syndromes and a clear history of occupational exposure to lead. These patients were reported to increase their urinary lead excretion, whereas the non-responders did not. The responders seemed to be mainly those with LMN problems. A more convincing patient (Simpson, Seaton and Adams 1964) had both UMN and LMN signs, had normal blood lead concentration and was anaemic. As he had a good history of lead exposure through his work as a welder he was treated with metal-chelating agents, to which he showed a good response. This patient was still alive in 1990 (J. Lewis, personal communication). Twelve patients with MND (10 with normal lead biochemistry and two with increased urinary lead excretion) failed to respond to treatment, with EDTA, penicillamine or thioctic acid (Currier and Haerer, 1968). Treatment with D-penicillamine over 6 months failed to show benefit (Conradi et al., 1982) in five patients but caused significant adverse effects, including vomiting, abnormal liver function and thrombocytopenia. A sixth patient's disease may have been slowed by the treatment, but no lasting benefit was obtained. When treatment fails to prolong survival in MND, subsequent efforts have to be directed at improving the duration of 'good-quality survival' with a minimum of symptoms. Under these circumstances the transient side-effects of medication reported by Conradi et al. (1982) assume a greater significance. Boothby, de Jesus and Rowland (1974) showed improvement in 'lead neuritis' mimicking MND when treated with chelators. Livesley and Sessons (1968) had previously suggested similar improvement. Other studies, e.g. that by House et al. (1978), failed to show any benefit. An adequately controlled, blinded trial of metal chelation therapy of sufficient numbers of patients with metal-exposed and unexposed MND has not been reported. Anecdotal and limited trial data available at present indicate a disappointing response in MND to lead chelators, with the possible exception of patients with a good history of metal exposure, other features of metal toxicity and a LMN disease of unusually slow progression.

23.2.2 Mercury

BACKGROUND

In day-to-day life in the western world contact with mercury is essentially confined to the metal in dental amalgams and in thermometers. It is also found in barometers and sphygmomanometers. Its outdated uses include its compounds in surgical dressings, mirror making, treatment of neurosyphilis, contact breakers in electrical circuits and the manufacture of felt hats. It has some newer uses, such as the purification of industrial lithium for use in the aerospace industry. Mercury mining has been a hazardous process throughout the history of its use, ranging from the mines of Idria in the fifth century BC to Minamata in Japan in the twentieth century. Mercury has also been used in gold mining. This poses major environmental problems as the safe disposal of mercury-containing waste is expensive and leads to new difficulties such as 'Brazil's mercury poisoning disaster' in the Amazon basin (Byrne, 1992).

TOXICOLOGICAL ASPECTS

Metallic mercury vaporizes at room temperature, and as this vapour can be absorbed via intact skin and also the respiratory tract (Adams, Ziegler and Lin, 1983), the toxic potential of this metal is considerable. Inorganic and non-volatile salts of mercury can be absorbed via the gastrointestinal tract. Highly toxic organic mercury compounds, including methyl mercury, can be absorbed via the respiratory mucosa and the gastrointestinal tract. Native mercury, its volatile organic compounds and its inorganic salts are all toxic to man. The chemical steps in mercury absorption or detoxification are inadequately understood. Its metabolic handling, however, involves the action of the enzyme thiol methyl transferase (TMT), which is known to be excessively active in MND (Waring *et al.*, 1989). TMT acts upon mercury to produce methyl mercury, a lipid-soluble compound with the potential to cross the blood–CNS barrier. Treatment of guinea-pigs with mercury renders their brains deficient in the important antioxidant, ascorbate (Blackstone, Hurley and Hughes, 1974). Pekkanen and Sandholm (1972) showed reduced activity of NADPH-specific glutathione reductase activity in methyl mercury toxicity. Mercury at concentrations as low as 1 nM can stimulate the production of superoxide by phagocytes and can promote iron-catalysed lipid peroxidation (Halliwell and Gutteridge, 1989). The decrease in mercury toxicity in the presence of selenium (Mano *et al.*, 1990) is further evidence favouring an interaction between thiols, the selenium-containing antioxidant, glutathione peroxidase and mercury metabolism. Polymorphisms of mercury metabolism have been suggested to explain variations in individual susceptibility with exposure to mercury (Kark, 1979).

In the rat, mercury is stored temporarily in the liver (2 weeks after intravenous injection of the nitrate) before over 80% is flushed into renal tubules (Rothstein and Hayes, 1960). Organic mercury compounds such as ethyl mercury p-toluene sulphonanilide may accumulate in hair and in nails (Kantarjian, 1961). Other than the kidney, there is no known long-term store for inorganic mercury that would provide clues to toxic exposure in the distant past. However, a provocative test using a metal-chelating agent may be able to mobilize stored mercury and allow its detection in urine.

Acute mercury poisoning causes a sore mouth with ulcerated gums, excessive salivation, tremor, irritability and sleep disorder. Gastro-intestinal upset is frequently prominent. With time, the irritability gives way to a persistent tremor, often with psychiatric disorder (hatter's shakes, mad as a hatter – from the time mercury was used in making felt hats) and then progresses to cachexia. Some patients may have a blue or dark-brown mercury line on the gum margins. Many will show a brown discoloration of the anterior capsule of the ocular lens (mercurialentis).

EPIDEMIOLOGICAL STUDIES

MND-like syndromes have been described in patients exposed to either organic or inorganic mercury (Brown, 1954; Conradi et al., 1982; Adams, Ziegler and Lin, 1983). These have included patients with progressive muscular atrophy, pyramidal degeneration and bulbar palsy. Good documentary evidence of mercury poisoning and MND is only found in a few patients (Barber, 1978). Withdrawal from the source of exposure has been reported to lead to resolution of the MND-like syndrome. Gresham, Molgaard and Golbeck (1986) found no association between mercury exposure and MND, but Roelofs-Iverson et al. (1984) reported such an association in a case–control study. Similar positive associations were reported by Felmus, Patten and Swanke (1976) and Pierce Ruhland (1981), but Norris and Padia's study (1989) failed to confirm these findings.

TISSUE AND FLUID MEASUREMENTS

Pierce Ruhland and Patten (1980) showed normal mercury concentrations in muscle tissue from 21 patients with MND. Hair and nail mercury is reported to be increased in a Japanese population with MND, including both classical ALS and cases from the Kii peninsula (see below) (Mano *et al.*, 1990). In contrast to the extensive literature on tissue lead levels, data on mercury measurement in MND are scarce, possibly reflecting the methodological difficulties in analysis rather than a lack of interest. Part of the difficulty arises from contamination of biological fluids with exogenous mercury, which is used, for instance, as a fungicide in some types of specimen bottles.

CHELATION THERAPY

No trials looking specifically at elimination of toxic mercury overload in MND have been reported to date. Variable clinical success is found with treatment with penicillamine in chronic mercury toxicity (Hoursh *et al.*, 1976). In experimental animals brain mercury was increased by treatment with penicillamine (Friedheim, Corvi and Wakker, 1976), indicating that this chelator may not be the most logical one to use in human studies. Caution needs to be exercised in using any chelating agents for diagnostic tests or as treatment – the chelating agent 2,3-dimercaptopropanol (British anti-Lewisite, BAL) can also cause an increase in brain mercury, presumably by mobilizing stores and making more circulating mercury available to the brain (Berlin and Rylander, 1964). At least in the short term, such increases in circulating metal chelates may worsen the neurological state. Friedheim, Corvi and Wakker (1976) advocated using meso-dimercaptosuccinic acid which, in their model, decreased brain mercury load. Anecdotal reports have suggested that N-acetyl-D,L-penicillamine may be more effective than D-penicillamine in treating mercury poisoning (Kark *et al.*, 1971).

Patients with MND occasionally ask about removal of mercury-containing dental fillings to reduce their exposure to the metal. At present, there is no evidence to suggest that this course of action is beneficial.

23.2.3 Aluminium

BACKGROUND

Aluminium is a ubiquitous metal that has found a number of uses in industry and in medicine. Its low density and relatively high tensile strength make it attractive for use in the aircraft industry. More mundane uses include aluminium pots and pans for use in cooking. Several antacid preparations contain aluminium. These must represent a major source of aluminium intake for a large number of patients without, so far, any clear evidence of long-term toxicity.

In the setting of chronic renal failure, aluminium toxicity is associated with the dialysis encephalopathy/dementia syndrome. The use of aluminium-free dialysis fluids has reduced the prevalence of encephalopathy. A role for this element has also been suggested in the pathogenesis of neurodegenerative disorders such as Alzheimer's disease and the ALS–parkinsonism–dementia complex of Guam (see Ganrot, 1986), and, by extension, a similar role is postulated for aluminium in the sporadic form of MND. An analogy has been drawn between MND and the chronic progressive myelopathy and motor neurone degeneration seen in the New Zealand white rabbit following the intracisternal injection of low-dose aluminium chloride (Strong and Garruto, 1991).

GUAM ALS AND ALUMINIUM

Epidemiological studies

Epidemiological considerations have suggested that the forms of MND seen commonly in the Chamorros people in Guam, the Irian Jaya of Western New Guinea and the Japanese of the Kii peninsula arise as a consequence of an environmental neurotoxin. This condition is referred to below as Guam ALS. Other neurodegenerative conditions such as a complex comprising parkinsonism and dementia also abound, and many patients with mixed disorders are seen. The prevalence of some disorders is such that in some communities these disorders are considered a part of normal ageing. Many researchers have shown a steady decline in the prevalence of MND in Guam, although it still remains higher than elsewhere by a factor of two or more (Reed et al., 1966; Garruto, Yanagihara and Gajdusek, 1985). This is not universally accepted (Lavine, 1991), and some of those involved in the early epidemiological studies have subsequently expressed concern about methodological difficulties. Since the 1960s accumulating evidence has supported the involvement of aluminium and its interactions with magnesium and calcium in the aetiology of Guam ALS (Yase, 1972, 1980; Perl et al., 1982). Soil in South Guam, where the prevalence of these disorders is at its greatest, is poor in calcium, rich in manganese and rich in iron and aluminium (see Ganrot, 1986). Aluminium and calcium co-localize in several tissues, including bone. Both can be mobilized from bone by parathyroid hormone. The deficiency of soil calcium has been postulated to result in increased aluminium absorption and deposition in bone, possibly by mechanisms involving parathormone action. It is a matter of speculation as to whether calcium deficiency, aluminium

509

excess, manganese or iron excess or even combinations of these are the initiators of the degenerative process.

Tissue and fluid studies

Spinal cord aluminium concentrations were found to be markedly increased in cases of Japanese endemic MND (Yoshimasu *et al.*, 1976, 1980). The increase was not specific for aluminium; for instance, silicon, calcium, iron, manganese and phosphorus content was also increased. About half the patients with Guam neurodegeneration are said to have increased hippocampal aluminium concentrations, particularly in cells with neurofibrillary tangles (Perl *et al.*, 1982; Garruto *et al.*, 1984). The concentrations of manganese in neural tissue from Guam ALS patients are variously reported to be normal or elevated (Yoshimasu *et al.*, 1976, 1980; Yoshida, 1977; Kurlander and Patten, 1979; Miyata *et al.*, 1980; Mizumoto *et al.*, 1980; Yasui, 1991). On current evidence, aluminium seems an unlikely candidate for the position of the sole causative environmental agent in Guam ALS.

SPORADIC MND AND ALUMINIUM

Toxicological aspects

Dietary aluminium (and manganese) supplementation in cynomolgus monkeys leads to degeneration of motor neurones in the spinal cord, suggesting a direct toxic effect (Garruto *et al.*, 1989). Aluminium is a toxic element that is stored within bone. Patients with MND are reported to have had more frequent bony fractures than control subjects, indicating that they may have a defect in bone/calcium metabolism (Kurtzke and Beebe, 1980), allowing one to postulate disordered aluminium storage. Blood aluminium is bound to transferrin and to citrate. An unconfirmed report claims elevated serum citrate concentration in MND (Saffer, Moreley and Bell, 1977), which by forming low molecular weight complexes would increase tissue availability of this metal. Plasma citrate is increased by hard physical training and by hyperparathyroidism (Julich, 1960; Toftegaard Nielsen, 1978) – both factors thought to predispose to MND (Felmus, Patten and Swanke, 1976; Bracco, Antuono and Amaducci, 1979). Aluminium accelerates the peroxidation of membrane lipids induced by hydrogen peroxide, thereby enhancing its oxidant effect (Quinlan, 1988).

Epidemiological and tissue studies

There are no clear studies of toxic aluminium exposure leading to

510

sporadic MND. Anecdotal reports suggest a role for aluminium poisoning in some patients with MND (Ganrot, 1986). Muscle aluminium levels are reported to be normal in MND (Pierce Ruhland and Patten, 1980). However, increased aluminium levels are found in the hippocampi of patients dying with MND (Piccardo *et al.*, 1988). Spinal cord aluminium has not been reported. There are no radioisotopes of aluminium that would be suitable for human studies. Gallium is another group III element that has a suitable radioisotope that can be used to study binding characteristics of proteins such as transferrin. There is some evidence that indicates disordered gallium binding (and, by extension, disordered aluminium binding) in Alzheimer's disease (Farrar *et al.*, 1990). Similar studies in a small number of MND patients have indicated normal gallium binding (unpublished data).

23.2.4 Selenium

BACKGROUND

Selenium is included in this section although it is not a metal. This group VI element has chemical similarities to sulphur and its metabolism is closely linked to sulphur's. Abnormally deficient sulphur oxidation and increased sulphur methylation have been shown in MND (Steventon *et al.*, 1988; Waring *et al.*, 1989). Biologically active selenium occurs mostly in the form of seleno-amino acids and, in particular, as selenocysteine. For instance, this amino acid forms the active site of one form of the antioxidant enzyme glutathione peroxidase (GSH-Px), which protects cells against the toxic effects of hydrogen peroxide and other peroxides. This peroxidase is believed to represent the main biological action of selenium in man. GSH-Px can reduce and hence inactivate reactive oxygen metabolites such as hydrogen peroxide, its function involving the sulphydryl-containing tripeptide, glutathione. Disordered selenium incorporation into GSH-Px would leave cells at risk of damage by peroxides and other reactive oxygen metabolites such as free radicals (FRs). GSH-Px is an inducible enzyme – under oxidant stress its concentration is increased and under these conditions the tissue content of selenium is also increased. The demonstration of altered enzyme/ selenium concentration will not, in itself, clarify whether the observed changes are primary defects or unimportant epiphenomena. Further studies measuring the products of FR-induced cell injury would be required for this. Selenium provides a bridge between the observations of disordered sulphur metabolism and the postulated metal-catalysed FR-mediated mechanism of damage in MND.

511

TOXICOLOGICAL ASPECTS

Selenium deficiency in humans has been associated with a cardiomyopathy in the Keshan area of China. Effects of selenium deficiency have also been demonstrated on skeletal muscle in lambs. Selenium excess is linked to an ataxic disorder in cattle and to a syndrome of alopecia, diarrhoea and headache in man (Kerdel-Vegas, 1966; Kilness and Hochberg, 1977).

EPIDEMIOLOGICAL AND TISSUE STUDIES

A small cluster of MND in an area of Dakota, USA, that has a high soil selenium content led to the search for a link between this element and MND (Kilness and Hochberg, 1977). In this cluster, affected subjects were said to show impaired urinary selenium excretion, but another examination failed to duplicate these results (Norris, 1978). Some of the conflicting results have been attributed to differing dietary selenium intakes (Tandan and Bradley, 1985). GSH-Px is an intracellular enzyme, and hence selenium too is located within cells. Measurements of its concentration in body fluids are therefore not very informative. Analytical problems have also hampered progress. Older methods of measuring selenium have relied on its conversion to hydrogen selenide, a gas that is not only extremely pungent but also toxic. Despite the analytical obstacles there have been reports of increased spinal cord, hepatic and blood selenium in MND. Kurlander and Patten (1979) could only find measurable concentrations of selenium in the spinal cord of one out of seven patients dying with MND. Erythrocyte selenium content has been found to be higher in MND patients than in a control population (Nagata et al., 1985). Spinal cord and hepatic selenium was said to be increased in autopsy studies on five MND patients compared with five control subjects (Mitchell et al., 1986). Selenium supplements seem to protect against mercury toxicity, possibly by increasing the availability of glutathione peroxidase or by the formation of relatively non-toxic mercury-containing selenides, analogous to the mercaptides formed with sulphur-containing molecules (Kark, 1979).

23.2.5 Manganese

BACKGROUND

This transition metal is associated with a Parkinson's disease-like syndrome with a combination of extrapyramidal and neuropsychiatric features. Outbreaks of manganese toxicity have occurred in Chilean mine workers. Manganese neurotoxicity in miners exposed to the ore (Mena *et al.*, 1967) suggests that the metal may exist in a non protein-incorporated state and may therefore catalyse the production of free radicals (FRs) (Donaldson, McGregor and La Bella, 1982) by Haber–Weiss reactions described earlier. Manganese, like copper and iron, has multiple redox states and can catalyse FR reactions (e.g. the autoxidation of dopamine), which are believed to be important in its extrapyramidal toxic effects (Halliwell and Gutteridge, 1989). Manganese superoxide dismutase (MnSOD) is a major manganese-containing antioxidant in animal cells (Weisinger and Fridovich, 1973). The overall reaction it catalyses is the same as that of the copper–zinc enzyme – but the location of MnSOD is different, it being mainly a mitochondrial protein (Halliwell and Gutteridge, 1985b). Low molecular weight manganese complexes can catalyse superoxide dismutation to produce hydrogen peroxide. MnSOD is more effective at this. An excess of manganese is likely to exert an oxidant effect by producing reactive oxygen metabolites including peroxide and the hydroxyl FR. The subcellular localization of neural manganese is largely mitochondrial or within melanosomes. Few, if any, low molecular weight manganese complexes are found in cytosol (Williams, 1982) – not an unexpected finding in view of the capability of such complexes to generate reactive oxygen metabolites, a property that would confer upon them the potential for causing damage to subcellular organelles. Manganese has an adverse effect on neurotransmission (Balnave, 1973).

TOXICOLOGICAL ASPECTS

A high manganese (and aluminium) diet fed to cynomolgus monkeys causes some degeneration of motor neurones in the spinal cord (Garruto *et al.*, 1989). The tremor caused by tremorine (1,4-dipyrrolidino-2-butyne) administered to mice may be exacerbated by co-administration of copper and manganese (Caeser and Schneiden, 1966). Manganese, when administered to experimental animals, causes an increase in brain copper levels (Chandra, Srivastava and Shukla, 1979). The concentration of manganese in neural tissue in experimental animals is increased by the administration of the parkinsonism-causing drugs reserpine and phenothiazines (Donaldson *et al.*, 1974; Weiner, Nausieda and Klawans, 1977). The neurotoxicity of phenothiazines may arise from disturbance of metal-catalysed FR reactions (Pall *et al.*, 1987a). Malhotra *et al.* (1984) showed that iron-deficient rats that were fed lead and manganese supplements showed marked increases in brain concentration of lead, manganese, copper and to a lesser extent iron. Anaemic humans have increased rates of manganese absorption, suggesting a possible interaction between the iron needed for haem synthesis and manganese. This is further supported by the finding that the main iron transport protein in plasma, transferrin, is also the main manganese transport protein (Mena, 1979). Interactions between transition metal ions seem important and disease states may result not only from the direct toxicity of an ingested metal but also from its interference with the normal activity of another metal. The interactions between iron, copper, lead and manganese may be important in the pathophysiology of manganese toxicity.

EPIDEMIOLOGICAL AND TISSUE STUDIES

In view of its abundance in the soil on Guam, manganese has been linked to Guam ALS and the parkinsonism–dementia complex prevalent there. Manganese miners in Guam have an increased incidence of Guam ALS (Yase, 1972). However, it will be apparent from the sections on aluminium that several other soil constituents are also found in abnormal concentrations, and any of these may be relevant in the pathophysiology of the disorder. A case–control study (Gresham, Molgaard and Golbeck, 1986) found no association between the development of MND and a history of prior exposure to any heavy metal including manganese, but a previous one (Roelofs-Iverson et al., 1984) had come up with precisely the opposite observation, that of a correlation with occupational heavy metal exposure.

Manganese toxicity was first implicated in causing an MND-like condition in a foundry worker (Voss, 1939). Yoshimasu et al. (1976,1980,1982) found no abnormality of spinal cord manganese in a population of Japanese patients with MND. Two groups have reported increased spinal cord manganese in MND (Miyata et al., 1983; Mitchell, 1987) and there is a suggestion that much of this may be in the ventral horns (Kurlander and Patten, 1979; Miyata et al., 1983). Some studies may have used analytical methods operating near the limits of detection; for example, Kurlander and Patten (1979) only found manganese in 3 of 19 spinal cord samples. A recent study (Kihira et al., 1990) found normal spinal cord manganese concentrations in Guam ALS but suggested altered distribution within the cord – more of the manganese being found in the anterior horns. Concentration of this metal is normal in skeletal muscle of MND patients (Pierce Ruhland and Patten, 1980). Red cell manganese concentration is reportedly lower in MND and may be lower in late disease than in the early stages (Nagata et al., 1985). No differences were found in the concentrations of manganese in other tissues. CSF manganese has not been systematically measured in MND or indeed in most other conditions. At least part of the problem lies in the much lower quantities of manganese that are present in CSF, necessitating more stringent contamination control procedures and requiring higher sensitivities from the analytical methods used. The most widely quoted and generally accepted 'normal' range of CSF manganese concentration was reported by Cotzias and Papavasiliou (1962) at 15–27 nmol/1. This study found that 93–94% of CSF manganese is non-protein bound and is ultrafiltratable. A more recent investigation (Pall *et al.*, 1987b) found a similar 'normal' range. It is far from clear whether tissue manganese concentrations are abnormal in sporadic (classical) MND and, more particularly, whether such changes are primary aetiological alterations or merely represent epiphenomena reflecting, perhaps, loss of muscle bulk and impaired diet in MND.

Preliminary studies confirm enhanced oxidant effect in MND by demonstrating ascorbate oxidation by free radical activity in the lumbar CSF of patients with MND (Pall *et al.*, 1990).

23.2.6 Iron

BACKGROUND

Iron is the most abundant metallic element in the human body. It is present chiefly in its three (III) oxidation state and is tightly incorporated into transport or storage proteins such as transferrin and ferritin respectively. Non-protein-bound iron, particularly in a reducing environment [i.e. reduced to iron (II)], such as is found in CSF and neural interstitial fluid, has the capacity to catalyse the formation of hydroxyl free radicals by Haber–Weiss-type reactions. These forms of iron are normally present in very low concentrations except in situations of iron overload or when the iron is decompartmentalized, for instance by being displaced by other metal ions or by rupture of cell or organelle membranes or by damage to the binding proteins or by disruption of the blood–brain barrier. Iron interacts in a complex way with other metal ions. Iron deficiency can increase dietary absorption of lead and hence predispose to lead toxicity (Chisolm, 1980).

A role for iron has been proposed in the pathogenesis of another human neurodegenerative disorder, Parkinson's disease (Jenner, 1989), and disordered iron metabolism is believed to be responsible for the rare condition, Hallervorden–Spatz disease. Iron is so widely present in our daily environment (in knives, needles, dust, etc.) that the methodological difficulties referred to below apply particularly to this metal.

Metals and free radicals

These are discussed in the sections above on free radicals and transition metals.

EPIDEMIOLOGICAL AND TISSUE STUDIES

Blood iron concentration is normal in patients with MND (Nagata *et al.*, 1985). Anterior horn cell tissue from seven patients with MND was found to contain higher iron concentration than that of 19 control subjects (Kurlander and Patten, 1979) but another study reported normal spinal cord and liver iron concentrations (Mitchell *et al.*, 1986). Pierce Ruhland and Patten (1980) found normal muscle iron concentration in MND. CSF iron is said to be normal in MND (Kjellin, 1967; Mitchell *et al.*, 1984). Measurement of total iron in CSF did not attract much attention between 1966 and recently. The reasons for this include the difficulties with ascertaining lack of contamination with haemoglobin iron, it being widely assumed that CSF with high iron concentrations must be contaminated with blood-derived porphyrin iron. The interest in metal-catalysed oxygen radical production has restimulated interest in CSF iron, particularly in a form capable of catalysing radical-producing reactions. The bleomycin assay described by Gutteridge, Rowley and Halliwell (1981) has been suggested to measure this catalytic form of iron. However, the concentrations measured by this method vary widely and are high in comparison with the more widely accepted 'normal' concentrations of total CSF iron.

23.2.7 Copper

BACKGROUND

Bronze-age man was aware of the usefulness of this metal, which we still have close contact with, both as the element, for instance in electrical wires or water pipes, and as its salts, as in fungicides. It is an essential trace metal, being required in maintenance of normal collagen structure (lysyl oxidase), in catecholamine neurotransmitter function (dopamine β-hydroxylase and, perhaps, a monoamine oxidase), in respiratory chain function (cytochrome oxidase) and in antioxidant activity (superoxide dismutase and caeruloplasmin). Wilson's disease and Menkes' syndrome are two well-characterized neurological problems resulting from disordered copper metabolism. Copper in proteins forms an essential part of the body's antioxidant arsenal and in a low molecular state can promote free radical or uncontrolled oxidant reactions by Haber–Weiss-type processes (see above). Impaired copper distribution has been reported in Parkinson's disease (Pall *et al.*, 1987b).

TOXICOLOGICAL ASPECTS

These are discussed in the sections above on free radicals and transition metals.

EPIDEMIOLOGICAL AND TISSUE STUDIES

Plasma caeruloplasmin concentration was said to be increased in some MND patients in one study (Mzhel'skaia *et al.*, 1989). This observation, even if duplicated by other workers, is of limited use as caeruloplasmin is an acute-phase protein and its concentration will rise, for instance, in aspiration pneumonitis. Increased copper concentration was reported in the anterior horn areas of seven patients dying with MND (Kurlander and Patten, 1979) but these results have not been supported by Yoshimasu *et al.*'s (1980) examination of Guam ALS patients. Abnormal distribution of liver copper in MND was reported by Masui, Mozai and Kakehi (1985).

An adequate examination of copper distribution in MND tissues has not been made. Previous methodological difficulties have largely been overcome so that the technology is now available for such a study. An assessment of the place of free radical reactions in the pathophysiology of MND is incomplete without investigation of the distribution and the biochemical form of tissue copper (and iron).

23.2.8 Calcium (and magnesium)

TOXICOLOGICAL ASPECTS

Calcium has a central place in the physiology of nerve and muscle function. Neural and neuromuscular processes all require influx of calcium into cells. Disorders of the concentrations of or the biochemical handling of calcium may be relevant to the pathogenesis of neurological disease. Normal homeostatic mechanisms maintain very low intracellular calcium concentrations, alterations of which can trigger neurotransmitter release, alter axonal transport and profoundly affect all aspects of high-energy phosphate metabolism. Intracellular calcium concentrations that exceed the cell's calcium buffering capacity can damage or kill the cell. Neurones have at least two types of calcium channels (Miller, 1987). One of the stimuli that results in a gated influx of calcium into neurones is activation of the N-methyl-D-aspartate (NMDA) type of the glutamate receptor. Calcium influx into cells by this receptor-operated mechanism is believed to mediate tissue injury in 'excitotoxic disorders'. Excessive excitatory neurotransmission at the NMDA receptor has been shown to be harmful, for instance in cerebral ischaemia. Blockers of this receptor site offer a hope for prevention of tissue damage, as does pharmacological manipulation of calcium either at its membrane channel or its intracellular binding. Intracellular calcium rapidly binds to calmodulin and then exerts its effects on ATPases, kinases, phosphatases, cyclases and esterases. A slower binding to parvalbumin and to calbindin allows inactivation of these calcium effects and subsequent active transport of calcium out of the cell (Williams, 1992). An area of exciting development is the effect of calcium on 'fast axon transport' (FAxT). Intracellular organelle traffic flows both away from and towards the cell body, down axoplasmic routes. This flow is calcium dependent and is altered by parathyroid hormone (PTH), and blockers of the dihydropyridine-sensitive calcium channel also affect it (Breuer, Bond and Atkinson, 1992). FAxT studies in MND show a disorder of both anterograde and retrograde organelle traffic (Breuer and Atkinson, 1988). The direct demonstration of PTH action on FAxT in human neurones (Breuer, Bond and Atkinson, 1992) suggests that these cells have PTH receptors. Thus, in conditions of altered PTH status, such as calcium deficiency, chronic renal failure or primary hyperparathyroidism, PTH receptor-mediated aberrations of metal metabolism may lead to interruption of normal neural function. This, perhaps, is a factor in the aluminium-induced dialysis encephalopathy/dementia syndrome, providing a precedent for increased aluminium toxicity in the presence of abnormal PTH metabolism. The dihydropyridine-sensitive calcium influx into isolated mammalian muscle cells can be inhibited by IgG from patients with MND (Delbono *et al.*, 1991), indicating the potential for this to be the final mediator of injury in disorders of varying aetiology ranging from the autoimmune to an exogenous neurotoxin. Using a calcium-deficient rat model Yasui, Yase and Ota (1991) showed increased aluminium absorption even in the absence of aluminium supplementation.

EPIDEMIOLOGICAL STUDIES

Yase's (1972) hypothesis of disordered calcium and magnesium metabolism leading, in the setting of increased soil and water aluminium and manganese concentrations, to development of Guam ALS has received much attention over the last two decades. Central to the hypothesis, as developed by Gajdusek and others, is the postulate that relative calcium deficiency leads to a state of hyperparathyroidism, which is known to alter the distribution and kinetics not only of calcium and magnesium but also of aluminium and lead. The last two metals have both been implicated in the aetiology of some cases of MND-like conditions. The low concentrations of calcium and magnesium and the high concentrations of aluminium and manganese in the soil and water in South Guam are frequently cited as evidence favouring Yase's (1972) hypothesis. Similar soil conditions are found in the Kii Peninsula in Japan. However, pockets of high incidence of Guam ALS are found in areas with high calcium and magnesium concentrations, e.g. in Umatic (Steele cited by Eisen and Hudson, 1987). These discrepancies point towards either a totally different aetiological factor or a complex interplay with other environmental factors, including consumption of the cycad seed. Patients with MND have been more prone to bony fractures than have control subjects, indicating a possible pre-existing defect in calcium handling (Kurtzke and Beebe, 1980).

TISSUE AND FLUID STUDIES

Six of 39 patients with MND had elevated serum calcium concentration and two had subnormal levels (Patten, 1982). The same group did not find any clinical benefit arising from the correction of the serum calcium concentrations (Mallette et al., 1977). Elevated serum citrate concentrations in MND can alter the bioavailability of calcium by making it available as a low molecular weight complex (Saffer, Moreley and Bell, 1977). Plasma citrate is increased by hard physical training and by hyperparathyroidism (Julich, 1960; Toftegaard Neilson, 1978), and these are both linked to an increased risk of MND (Felmus, Patten and Swanke, 1976; Bracco, Antuono and Amaducci, 1979). Yasui et al. (1991) demonstrated lowered brain and spinal cord magnesium, but others have found normal magnesium concentration in spinal cord (Mitchell et al., 1986). Particle induced X-ray emission analysis of neural tissue from MND patients shows increased calcium content, particularly as the hydroxyapatite (Yoshida et al., 1989). This calcium appears to co-localize with silicon (Garruto, 1986), but this may merely reflect the occurrence of aluminium in dust particles as the aluminosilicate.

23.2.9 Other metals

Zinc is an important element in the regulation of gene expression. Studies of muscle, anterior horn, spinal, CSF, hepatic and bone zinc have failed to show any abnormality (Kurlander and Patten, 1979; Pierce Ruhland and Patten, 1980; Mitchell et al., 1984, 1986). Increased CSF cobalt was reported in MND and we await results of further analyses indicated by Mitchell (1987). Chromium and the even less likely candidate elements, rubidium, caesium and antimony, are discussed by Mitchell (1987).

23.3 METHODOLOGICAL DIFFICULTIES IN TRACE METAL STUDIES

Considerable difficulties arise in the design and interpretation of trace metal investigations into disease pathogenesis. The principal areas of worry are:

1. choice of appropriate tissue;
2. choice of appropriate control subjects;
3. control of contamination during sample collection;
4. precision and accuracy of the analytical method;
5. choice of chelator for investigation or treatment.

23.3.1 Appropriate tissue

In studies in man a balance is drawn between the accessibility of tissues for investigation and the likelihood of detecting metal overload. The kidney is a site of accumulation of inorganic mercury, but the invasive nature of kidney biopsies has led to the practice of hair and nail estimations of mercury load. The distribution of metals between different tissues varies with the metal under study. For instance, lead accumulates in bone, copper in the liver and iron all through the reticuloendothelial system. The time course of metal redistribution between the blood and its ultimate site of storage also varies according to the metal, its biochemical form and the tissue levels of other metal ions. Thus acute and continuing exposure to lead may be detected by measuring whole blood lead concentration, but remote lead exposure requires examination of bone or, alternatively, a mobilization test. Mobilization tests rely on the principle of moving metal ions into body fluids from their storage site using a chelating agent and quantifying the concentration in blood or urine. The use of these tests is limited by insufficient information on the normal ranges of mobilized metal concentrations.

23.3.2 Control subjects

In addition to the familiar requirements of, for instance, age and sex matching of disease and control populations, trace metal studies require a control for occupational or environmental metal exposure. The normal range of mercury in an unexposed, healthy population is likely to be lower than that of an equally healthy group of workers dealing with elemental mercury. Clearly an investigation of possible mercury intoxication must compare the subject's mercury studies with those of a group of similarly exposed but asymptomatic people. This problem is compounded when the source of the metal under investigation is unknown. Metal biochemistry is altered by several pathological processes. The acute-phase response in a patient dying of bronchopneumonia leads to an increase in plasma copper and a decrease in plasma iron. In this context tissues obtained, for instance, from persons who died suddenly as in a road traffic accident would not be appropriate controls for a study of metals in MND.

23.3.3 Control of contamination

Measurement of trace metals in biological fluids requires care in collection, storage and analysis to avoid contamination. The levels of manganese measured in CSF are less than 1 µg/1 (<1 ng/ml or 1 part per billion). At such low concentrations the need for prevention of contamination is paramount (Zief and Mitchell, 1976). Sources of contamination include needles; syringes; collection containers; multiple steps in the collection process, e.g. connecting a manometer and three-way tap to a spinal needle during CSF collection; collection in a dust-filled, poorly ventilated room; skin flakings and dust from the collector's hands and clothes; contact of the fluid with non-acid-washed glassware, which is a frequent cause of metal ion contamination; impurities in water and reagents used in the analytical process and contaminants introduced by storage containers.

'Negative contamination' is a term sometimes used to describe losses of the ion under consideration by a variety of means including adsorption onto plastic. Such losses of ions from aqueous standard solutions should be looked for prior to starting any studies (Eicholz, Nagel and Hughes, 1965). Adsorption losses may pose real problems in trace element work, as shown by the fact that selenium losses are high when samples are stored in polyethylene tubes (Zief and Mitchell, 1976). Vaporization losses during storage may lead to an artificially increased concentration of any solute. Curtis, Rein and Yamamuro (1973) showed that storage in suitable tubes could reduce vaporization losses to less than 1%, particularly if the caps are waxed. Contamination is the main obstacle to accurate determination of tissue metal concentrations.

23.3.4 Precision and accuracy

For any analytical method to be useful it must be capable of yielding results that can be duplicated with precision quite independently of the laboratory in which the assays are carried out and also independently of the analyst. Duplicability is measured in terms of 'within-batch precision' and 'between-batch precision'. The former is a measure of the duplicability of results obtained in one assay and the latter, as its name implies, is determined from measurements carried out on one sample in several different assays.

A method may be precise without being accurate, i.e. when compared with a standard reference method or when measuring the trace metal content of a standard reference material values different from those expected are obtained even though the same values may be obtained each time the sample is assayed using the method under investigation. Recovery studies form a part of accuracy determination. Known quantities of trace metal are mixed with the material in the study and the concentration of trace metal is determined. The deviation of the amount recovered from the amount expected is determined and expressed as a percentage recovery. For an accurate method average percentage recovery approaches 100. Recovery of standard additions of metals such as lead or manganese into biological fluids such as CSF is comparatively easy and reliable but is virtually impossible for solids. However, accurate recovery of standard additions in aqueous solutions does not necessarily establish accuracy within the biological matrix of the material under examination. For this, certified standard reference materials (SRM) are required. For each tissue/fluid under examination SRMs appropriate to that biological matrix are needed. For many elements in a variety of different biological matrices such standards are available – either commercially or from the US National Bureau of Standards or the UK Bureau of Analysed Samples. It is estimated that for approximately 50% of all trace metal analyses being carried out in 1975 no SRMs were available. More have become available in the last 17 years, but for CSF studies these are still very limited, and for the measurement of lead or manganese in CSF such SRMs are not available. In the absence of SRMs a favourable comparison between two analytical methods that give good recovery data for added trace metal ions may be taken to represent accurate determinations. However, many methods that are conventionally regarded as being accurate give widely varying results; for instance, atomic absorption spectrophotometry measurements of copper in Kale Standard Reference Material differs from neutron activation analysis by greater than 10%. Inevitably, newer methods such as inductively coupled plasma emission spectroscopy and particle-induced

X-ray emission will require comparison with the older and more established methods.

23.3.5 Choice of chelator

No single chelating agent will bind and excrete all the metals discussed above. Thiol chelators such as penicillamine will bind lead, mercury and copper. Desferrioxamine will bind aluminium, iron and copper and possibly manganese. EDTA has been used as the basis of a provocation test for lead mobilization and excretion (Chisolm, 1971) but is more toxic than penicillamine. A small study of penicillamine treatment in MND (Conradi *et al.*, 1982) and wider experience of this drug in rheumatoid disease indicate a significant risk of adverse effects. Newer chelators such as *N*-acetyl penicillamine and dimercaptyl propane sulphonate may be less toxic, although it is conceivable that their toxic effects will become recognizable with more widespread use. Desferrioxamine toxicity (Blake *et al.*, 1985; Pall *et al.*, 1989) can be a severe and frightening experience for both patient and physician, and the spectrum of side-effects can vary according to the disease, highlighting the need for careful thought and risk–benefit evaluation before embarking on a course of chelation therapy. A new class of metal chelating agents, the 21-amino steroids or lazaroids, are currently being investigated for their capacity to chelate metals other than iron. These agents are lipid soluble and are therefore more likely to be effective within the nervous system. They also have a vitamin E-like function and are efficient antioxidants. Their toxicity in man is largely unknown, although studies to date have not revealed major adverse effects.

Chelating agents are only of value if the toxicity of the metal chelate is lower than that of the metal in its native state and if the chelate is more easily excreted than tissue-bound metal. British anti-Lewisite (BAL) was a chelating agent briefly used to bind mercury. There is no doubt that this agent binds mercury. However it appears to increase brain concentration of mercury, perhaps by initially mobilizing tissue stores and then presenting the lipid-soluble chelate to cross the blood–brain barrier. It is imperative to remember that metal chelation, even in tissue metal overload, is not synonymous with clinical improvement.

23.4 CURRENT STATUS OF METALS AND FREE RADICALS IN MND

Much of the trace metal research in MND over the last 20 years has examined the issue of abnormal tissue distribution of metal ions. Methodological difficulties of the sort described above combined with the small numbers of patients examined in most studies have led to conflicting results. Consistently abnormal results have not been reported for any metal in large numbers of patients with MND. Guam ALS is reported to show abnormal calcium, magnesium, aluminium and manganese concentrations in neural tissue, but much of the work in this field has come from one group of workers. In the literature a lot of effort has been put into small-scale epidemiological studies looking for excessive metal exposure in ordinary MND, and an equal amount of effort has been directed towards demonstrating abnormal tissue distribution of metal ions. The above review of this literature shows that these questions cannot be definitively answered. Basal body fluid metal content is a poor indicator of total body metal, but tissue measurements, particularly those involving relevant tissues, such as spinal cord, are highly invasive and, for practical purposes, confined to autopsy studies. There is need for non-invasive tests of total body metal load. Mobilization tests involving the use of brief-duration treatment with appropriate metal chelating agents may be more valuable than the basal measurements. These mobilization tests are not clearly defined either in the dose of chelating agents required or in the normal ranges of excretion of mobilized metal stores.

Our capacity to address the other, equally important, questions listed at the beginning of this chapter is even more limited. We are just understanding the biochemical forms of the many metals implicated. Apart from the occasional anecdotal report there is no conclusive evidence of improvement in typical MND following reduction of metal load. The interactions in living organisms between different metal ions are largely unstudied, but there are sufficient glimpses of knowledge to indicate that a metal's toxic potential may relate more to its effects on the biochemistry of another metal than its own. Polymorphisms in metal-metabolizing enzymes, e.g. in 'thiol methyl transferase', of which there is increased activity in MND and which is believed to methylate elemental mercury, may determine host susceptibility to metal toxicity. The microscopic anatomy and physiological functions of many metal ions are poorly understood, and their involvement in the pathological processes of MND have not even begun to be explored. More is understood of these processes in Guam ALS, but even in this interesting variant of MND the whole question of metal involvement is wide open. Metal-catalysed formation of free radicals (FRs) leading to oxidative tissue damage is an attractive hypothesis that has been implicated in a wide variety of medical conditions. However, little direct evidence exists of the involvement of FRs in MND. Anterior horn cell numbers in the spinal cord normally decrease with age but decline prematurely in

MND. This is accompanied by increased DNA damage and accumulation of FR reaction products as lipofuscin. In MND there is an increase in spinal cord manganese, a constituent of MnSOD. Pilot studies suggest abnormalities of MnSOD concentrations in the CSF in MND. Abnormal spinal cord selenium levels have also been reported in MND. In man, selenium is located largely in GSH-Px. MnSOD and GSH-Px act synergistically. Ascorbate is an important antioxidant that is reportedly deficient in the CSF of patients with MND. Conflicting results have been reported on the role of FR-scavenging agents in MND.

Chemical understanding of excitatory amino acid receptor stimulation leading to cation fluxes is more advanced, but to date involvement of these mechanisms in MND pathophysiology has not been shown. The occurrence of Guam ALS provides a hyperendemic focus of an MND that has given epidemiological clues to the aetiology of the sporadic, classical MND. Non-human, animal models of MND include the lead-intoxicated guinea-pig, mercury-toxic rat, aluminium-toxic rabbit, calcium-deficient rabbit and cynomolgus monkey, ascorbate-deficient guinea-pig, hereditary canine spinal muscular atrophy, 'wobbler mouse' and 'shaker calf' (Sillevis-Smitt and de Jong, 1989). None of these is satisfactory as a good model of sporadic, classical MND. The study of metal toxicity in this setting is therefore of doubtful relevance to MND. The development of cell culture techniques offers the prospect of mechanistic studies into metal-mediated neural toxicity.

There is need for a large study of tissue and fluid metal concentrations in MND to establish whether the areas of inadequate knowledge discussed above can usefully be studied in this disorder. Based on the multiple small studies already carried out, it is unlikely that gross tissue metal overload will be found in the majority of MND patients. The realistic hopes must be that (i) a subpopulation will be identified to have significant tissue metal overload, allowing a rational attempt at treatment with chelating agents, (ii) metal-catalysed free radical mechanisms in MND will allow rational treatment with appropriate antioxidants and (iii) manipulation of calcium channels, both NMDA receptor-associated ones and others, will provide hope of effective treatment. Currently, this last possibility offers the best prospect of useful treatment in MND. In common with evaluation of the results of any treatment, such attempts at treatment should form a randomized controlled trial of sufficient statistical power to come to a definite answer to the question: 'Does identification of abnormal metal metabolism and subsequent treatment with chelators, antioxidants, free radical scavengers or calcium channel modulators lead to a clinically important benefit in MND?'

23.5 CONCLUSIONS

Classical, sporadic MND does not appear to be caused by metal toxicity, and even endemic MND (Guam ALS) is not simply a manifestation of metal poisoning. It is unclear whether any patients with MND suffer through failure to identify and treat unsuspected metal poisoning. The likelihood is that the numbers of such patients must be small. In my view the main contribution of metal studies in MND to date has been to provide another piece of a large jig-saw puzzle of the aetiology of MND. Examination of the biochemical intersections and overlaps between metal ions and other recognized and putative neurotoxins offers the best prospect of identifying the molecular mechanisms of cell damage in MND. This understanding, in turn, provides our current best hope of interruption of the disease process in a way that benefits large numbers of patients.

23.6 ADDENDUM

Since completion of this manuscript an important publication reports finding 11 missense mutations within the copper zinc superoxide dismutase (CuZnSOD) gene in cases of familial motor neurone disease (FALS) (Rosen, 1993). The mutations found in the CuZnSOD gene on chromosome 21 in FALS families that show genetic linkage to this chromosome have not been found in any of more than 100 normal controls. The effects of these mutations on the functional activity of the CuZnSOD protein are unknown. Most mutations that decrease the expression of the gene product result in recessively inherited disorders whereas FALS is dominantly inherited in the majority of cases. However a decrease in the production of CuZnSOD could result from the mutations and thereby make more superoxide radicals available for interaction with transition metal ions or with nitric oxide to produce potentially cytotoxic hydroxyl free radicals. On the other hand, increased production of CuZnSOD can also promote free radical reactions in tissues deficient in selenium-containing glutathione peroxidase or catalase. Catalysing the transformation of superoxide radicals to hydrogen peroxide under these conditions can result in more Fenton-type reactions (see above) producing hydroxyl free radicals. Transcriptional regulation of CuZnSOD gene expression is dependent on the oxidant stress in the cell's environment. For instance, exposure of a cell to paraquat, a toxin that causes damage through free radical generation, results in increased SOD gene expression. In view of this it is not only important to know whether the missense mutations result in increased or decreased gene product activity in the basal state but also to determine differences in response of the mutant genes to varying degrees and types of oxidant stress. A number of FALS families do not show genetic linkage with chromosome 21. Whether the other known SOD genes, extracellular SOD (EC SOD) or manganese SOD (MnSOD) will show similar mutations in these families is not yet known. This study lends support to previous data (Pall, 1990; Miyata, 1983; Mitchell, 1986) that also indicate a role for free radical reactions in the pathophysiology of sporadic MND. These previous investigations have shown a decrease in the antioxidant form of vitamin C in the cerebrospinal fluid in MND, and an alteration in spinal cord manganese and of spinal cord selenium respectively. Preliminary data indicate decreased activity of Mn SOD in CSF from MND patients, Pall (1989). Total CSF SOD activities are normal measured using the method of Marklund (1986). In MND, more of the CSF SOD activity seems to result from CuZnSOD action rather than the other two enzymes.

REFERENCES

Adams, C.R., Ziegler, D.K. and Lin, J.T. (1983) Mercury intoxication simulating amyotrophic lateral sclerosis. *J. Am. Med. Assoc.*, **250**, 642–3.

Aran, F.A. (1850) Recherches sur une maladie non encore decrite du systeme musculaire (atrophie musculaire progressive). *Arch. Gen. Med.*, **24**, 15–35.

Armon, C., Kurland, L.T., Daube, J.R. and O'Brien, P.C. (1991) Epidemiologic correlates of sporadic amyotrophic lateral sclerosis. *Neurology*, **41**, 1077–84.

Balnave, R.J. and Page, P.W. (1973) The inhibitory effect of manganese on transmitter release at the neuromuscular junction of the toad. *Br. J. Pharmacol.*, **47**, 339–52.

Barber, T.E. (1978) Inorganic mercury intoxication reminiscent of amyotrophic lateral sclerosis. *J. Occup. Med.*, **20**, 667–9.

Berlin, M. and Rylander, R. (1964) Increased brain uptake of mercury induced by 2,3 dimercaptopropanol (BAL) in mice exposed to phenylmercuric acetate. *J. Pharmacol. Exp. Ther.*, **146**, 236–40.

Blackstone, S., Hurley, R.J. and Hughes, R.E. (1974) Some interrelationships between vitamin C (ascorbic acid) and mercury in the guinea pig. *Food Cosmet. Toxicol.*, **12**, 511–16.

Blake, D.R., Winyard, P., Lunec, J. *et al.* (1985) Cerebral and ocular toxicity induced by desferrioxamine. *Q. J. Med.*, **56**, 345–55.

Boothby, J.A., de Jesus, P.V. and Rowland, L.P. (1974) Reversible forms of motor neurone disease (lead neuritis). *Arch. Neurol.*, **31**, 18–23.

Bousser, M.G. and Malier, M. (1979) Penicillamine in amyotrophic lateral sclerosis. *Lancet*, **i**, 168.

Bracco, L., Antuono, P. and Amaducci, L. (1979) Study of epidemiological and etiological factors of amyotrophic lateral sclerosis in the province of Florence, Italy. *Acta Neurol. Scand.*, **60**, 112–24.

Breuer, A.C. and Atkinson, M.B. (1988) Fast axonal transport alterations in amyotrophic lateral sclerosis (ALS) and in parathyroid hormone (PTH)-treated axons. *Cell Motil. Cytoskeleton*, **10**, 321–30.

Breuer, A.C., Bond, M. and Atkinson, M.B. (1992) Fast axonal transport is mediated by altering trans-axolemmal calcium flux. *Cell Calcium*, **13**, 249–62.

Brown, I.A. (1954) Chronic mercurialism. A cause of the clinical syndrome of amyotrophic lateral sclerosis. *Arch. Neurol. Psychiat.*, **72**, 674–81.

Byrne, L. (1992) Brazil's mercury poisoning disaster. *Br. Med. J.*, **304**, 1397.

Caeser, P.M. and Schneiden, H. (1966) The effect of copper sulphate and manganese sulphate on the toxicity and tremor of tremorine and on the peripheral responses induced by acetylcholine, noradrenaline, dopamine and 5-hydroxytryptamine. *Biochem. Pharmacol.*, **15**, 1691–700.

Campbell, A.M.G. (1955) Calcium versenate in motor neurone disease. *Lancet*, **ii**, 376–7.

Campbell, A.M.G., Williams, E.R. and Barltrop, D. (1970) Motor neurone disease and exposure to lead. *J. Neurol. Neurosurg. Psychiat.*, **33**, 877–85.

Chandra, S.V., Srivastava, R.S. and Shukla, G.S. (1979) Regional distribution of metals and biogenic amines in the brain of monkeys exposed to manganese. *Toxicol. Lett.*, **4**, 189–92.

Chisolm Jr, J.J. (1971) Lead poisoning. *Sci. Am.*, **224(2)**, 15–23.

Chisolm Jr, J.J. (1980) Lead and other metals: a hypothesis of interaction, in *Lead Toxicity* (eds R.L. Singhai and J.A. Thomas), Urban & Schwarzenberg, Baltimore, pp. 461–82.

Cohen, G. and Heikkila, R. (1974) The generation of hydrogen peroxide, superoxide radical and hydroxyl radical by 6-hydroxydopamine, dialuric acid and related cytotoxic agents. *J. Biol. Chem.*, **249**, 2447–52.

Cohen, M.M. (1979) Biochemical aspects of lead neurotoxicity, in *Handbook of Clinical Neurology*, Vol. 36 (eds P.J. Vinken and G.W. Bruyn), North Holland Publishing, Amsterdam, pp. 65–72.

Conradi, S., Ronnevi, L.-O. and Vesterburg, O. (1978) Increased plasma levels of lead in amyotrophic lateral sclerosis compared to controls, as determined by atomic absorption spectrophotometry. *J. Neurol. Neurosurg. Psychiat.*, **41**, 389–93.

Conradi, S., Ronnevi, L.-O., Nise, G. *et al.* (1980) Abnormal distribution of lead in amyotrophic lateral sclerosis. Re-estimation of lead in the cerebrospinal fluid. *J. Neurol. Sci.*, **48**, 413–18.

Conradi, S., Ronnevi, L.-O., Nise, G. and Vesterburg, O. (1982) Long-term penicillamine-treatment in amyotrophic lateral sclerosis with parallel determination of lead in blood, plasma and urine. *Acta Neurol. Scand.*, **65**, 203–11.

Cotzias, G. and Papavasiliou, P.S. (1962) State of binding of natural manganese in human cerebrospinal fluid, blood and plasma. *Nature*, **195**, 823–4.

Currier, R.D. and Haerer, A.F. (1968) Amyotrophic lateral sclerosis. *Arch. Environ. Health*, **17**, 712–19.

Curtis, G.J., Rein, J.E. and Yamamuro, S.S. (1973) Comparative study of different methods of packaging liquid reagents. *Anal. Chem.*, **45**, 996–8.

Delbono, O., Garcia, J., Appel, S.H. and Stefani, E. (1991) IgG from amyotrophic lateral sclerosis affects tubular calcium channels of skeletal muscle. *Am. J. Physiol.*, **260**, C1347–51.

Donaldson, J., McGregor, D. and La Bella, F. (1982) Manganese neurotoxicity: a model for free radical-mediated neurodegeneration? *Can. J. Physiol. Pharmacol.*, **60**, 1398–405.

Donaldson, J., Cloutier, T., Minnich, J.L. and Barbeau, A. (1974) Trace metals and biogenic amines in rat brain. *Adv. Neurol.*, **5**, 245–52.

Eicholz, G.G., Nagel, A.E. and Hughes, R.B. (1965) Adsorption of ions in dilute aqueous solutions on glass and plastic surfaces. *Anal. Chem.*, **37**, 863–8.

Eisen, A.A. and Hudson, A.J. (1987) Amyotrophic lateral sclerosis: concepts in pathogenesis and etiology. *Can. J. Neurol. Sci.*, **14**, 649–52.

Farrar, G., Altmann, P., Welch, S. *et al.* (1990) Defective gallium transferrin binding in Alzheimer Disease and Down's syndrome. Possible mechanism for accumulation of aluminium in brain. *Lancet*, **i**, 747–50.

Felmus, M.T., Patten, B.M. and Swanke, L. (1976) Antecedent events in amyotrophic lateral sclerosis. *Neurology*, **26**, 167–72.

Fridovich, I. (1983) Superoxide radical: an endogenous toxicant. *Annu. Rev. Pharmacol. Toxicol.*, **23**, 239–59.

Friedheim, E., Corvi, C. and Wakker, C.H. (1976) Meso-dimercaptosuccinic acid: A chelating agent for the treatment of mercury and lead poisoning. *J. Pharm. Pharmacol.*, **28**, 711–12.

Ganrot, P.O. (1986) Metabolism and possible health effects of aluminium. *Environmental Health Perspectives*, **65**, 363–441.

Garruto, R.M., Yanagihara, R. and Gajdusek, D.C. (1985) Disappearance of high-incidence of amyotrophic lateral sclerosis and Parkinsonism-dementia on Guam. *Neurology*, **35**, 193–8.

Garruto, R.M., Fukatsu, R., Yanagihara, R. *et al.* (1984) Imaging of calcium and aluminium in neurofibrillary tangle-bearing neurones in Parkinsonism-Dementia of Guam. *Proc. Natl. Acad. Sci. USA*, **81**, 1875–9.

Garruto, R.M., Swyt, C., Yanagihara, R., Fiori, C.E. and Gajdusek, D.C. (1986) Intraneuronal colocalisation of silicon with calcium and aluminium in amyotrophic lateral sclerosis and parkinsonism with dementia of Guam. *N. Eng. J. Med.*, **315** (11), 711–12.

Garruto, R.M., Shankar, S.K., Yanagihara, R. *et al.* (1989) Low-calcium, high-aluminium diet-induced motor neuron pathology in cynomolgus monkeys. *Acta Neuropathol.*, **78**, 210–19.

Gresham, L.S., Molgaard, C.A. and Golbeck, A.C. (1986) Amyotrophic lateral sclerosis and occupational heavy metal exposure: a case control study. *Neuroepidemiology*, **5**, 29–38.

Gutteridge, J.M., Rowley, D.A. and Halliwell, B. (1981) Superoxide-dependent formation of hydroxyl radicals in the presence of iron salts. *Biochem. J.*, **199**, 263–5.

Halliwell, B. and Gutteridge, J.M. (1984) Oxygen toxicity, oxygen radicals, transition metals and disease. *Biochem. J.*, **219**, 1–14.

Halliwell, B. and Gutteridge, J.M. (1985a) Oxygen radicals and the nervous system. *Trends Neurosci.*, **8**, 22–6.

Metals and free radicals

Halliwell, B. and Gutteridge, J.M. (1985b) *Free Radicals in Biology and Medicine*. Clarendon Press, Oxford.

Halliwell, B. and Gutteridge, J.M. (1986) Oxygen free radicals and iron in relation to biology and medicine: some problems and concepts. *Arch. Biochem. Biophys.*, **246**, 50–14.

Halliwell, B. and Gutteridge, J.M. (1989) *Free Radicals in Biology and Medicine*, 2nd edn, Oxford, Clarendon Press.

Hoursh, J., Clarkson, T., Cherion, M. *et al.* (1976) Clearance of mercury vapour inhaled by human subjects. *Arch. Environ. Health*, **31**, 302–9.

House, A.O., Abbott, R.J., Davidson, D.L.W. *et al.* (1978) Response to penicillamine of lead concentrations in CSF and blood in patients with motor neurone disease. *Br. Med. J.*, **2**, 1684.

Jenner, P. (1989) Clues to the mechanism underlying dopamine cell death in Parkinson's disease. *J. Neurol. Neurosurg. Psychiat.*, **52** (Suppl.), 22–8.

Julich, H. (1960) The influence of physical work on the behaviour of lactic acid, pyruvic acid and citric acid in the blood. *Z. Klin. Med.*, **156**, 222–35.

Justic, A. and Sostarko, M. (1977) Improvement of spinal amyotrophy by penicillamine therapy. *Lancet*, **ii**, 1034–5.

Kantarjian, A.D. (1961) A syndrome clinically resembling amyotrophic lateral sclerosis following chronic mercurialism. *Neurology*, **1**, 639–44.

Kapaki, E., Segditsa, J., Zournas, C. *et al.* (1989) Determination of cerebrospinal fluid and serum lead levels in patients with amyotrophic lateral sclerosis and other neurological diseases. *Experientia*, **45**, 1108–10.

Kark, R. (1979) Clinical and neurochemical aspects of inorganic mercury intoxication, in *Handbook of Clinical Neurology*, Vol. 36 (eds P.J. Vinken and G.W. Bruyn), North Holland Publishing, Amsterdam, pp. 147–98.

Kark, R., Poskanzer, D., Bullock, J. *et al.* (1971) Mercury poisoning and its treatment with N-acetyl d,l-penicillamine. *New. Engl. J. Med.*, **285**, 10–16.

Kerdel-Vegas, F. (1966) The depilatory and cytotoxic action of Coco de Mono (lecythis ollaria) and its relation to chronic selenosis. *Economic Botany*, **20**, 187–95.

Kihira, T., Mukoyama, M., Ando, K. *et al.* (1990) Determination of manganese concentrations in the spinal cords from amyotrophic lateral sclerosis patients by inductively coupled plasma emission spectroscopy. *J. Neurol. Sci.*, **98**, 251–8.

Kilness, A.W. and Hochberg, F.H. (1977) Amyotrophic lateral sclerosis in a high-selenium environment. *J. Am. Med. Assoc.*, **237**, 2843–4.

Kjellin, K.G. (1967) The CSF iron in patients with neurological diseases. *Acta Neurol. Scand.*, **43**, 299–313.

Kondo, K. and Tsubaki, T. (1981) Case–control studies in motor neurone disease. *Arch. Neurol.*, **38**, 220–6.

Kurlander, H.M. and Patten, B.M. (1979) Metals in spinal cord tissue of patients dying of motor neurone disease. *Ann. Neurol.*, **6**, 21–4.

Kurtzke, J.F. and Beebe, G.W. (1980) Epidemiology of amyotrophic lateral sclerosis. 1. A case–control comparison based on ALS deaths. *Neurology*, **30**, 453–62.

References

Lane, R.E., Hunter, D., Malcolm, D. *et al.* (1968) Diagnosis of inorganic lead poisoning. *Br. Med. J.*, **iv**, 501.

Lavine, L., Steele, J.C., Wolfe, N. *et al.* (1991) Amyotrophic lateral sclerosis/ Parkinsonism dementia complex in Southern Guam: is it disappearing? *Adv. Neurol.*, **56**, 271–85.

Livesley, B. and Sessons, C.E. (1968) Chronic lead intoxication mimicking motor neurone disease. *Br. Med. J.*, **4**, 387–8.

Malhotra, K.M., Murthy, R.C., Srivastava, R.S. and Chandra, S.V. (1984) Concurrent exposure of lead and manganese to iron deficient rats: effects on lipid peroxidation and contents of some metals in the brain. *J. Appl. Toxicol.*, **4**, 22–5.

Mallette, L., Patten, B., Cook, J. *et al.* (1977) Calcium metabolism in amyotrophic lateral sclerosis. *Dis. Nerv. System*, **38**, 457–61.

Mandybur, T.I. and Cooper, G.P. (1979) Increased spinal cord lead content in amyotrophic lateral sclerosis. Possibly a secondary phenomenon. *Med. Hypotheses*, **5**, 1313–15.

Mano, Y., Takayanagi, T., Ishitani, A. and Hirota, T. (1990) Mercury in hair of patients with amyotrophic lateral sclerosis. *Rinsho Shinkeigaku*, **29**, 844–8.

Manton, W.J. and Cook, J.D. (1979) Lead content of CSF and other tissues in amyotrophic lateral sclerosis. *Neurology*, **29**, 611–12.

Marklund, S.L., Heiskala, H., Westermarck, T. *et. al.* (1986) Superoxide dismutase isoenzymes in cerebrospinal fluid and plasma from patients with neuronal ceroid lipofuscinosis. *Clin. Sci.*, **71**, 57–60.

Masui, Y., Mozai, T. and Kakehi, K. (1985) Functional and morphometric study of the liver in motor neurone disease. *J. Neurol.*, **232**, 15–19.

Mena, I. (1979) Manganese poisoning, in *Handbook of Clinical Neurology*, Vol. 36 (eds P.J. Vinken and G.W. Bruyn), North Holland Publishing, Amsterdam, pp. 217–37.

Mena, I., Marin, O., Fuenzalida, S. and Cotzias, G.C. (1967) Chronic manganese poisoning. Clinical picture and manganese turnover. *Neurology*, **17**, 128–36.

Miller, R.J. (1987) Multiple calcium channels and neuronal functions. *Science*, **235**, 46–52.

Mitchell, J.D. (1987) Heavy metals and trace elements in amyotrophic lateral sclerosis. *Neurol. Clin.*, **5**, 43–60.

Mitchell, J.D., Harris, I.A., East, B.W. *et al.* (1984) Trace elements in cerebrospinal fluid in motor neurone disease. *Br. Med. J.*, **288**, 1791–2.

Mitchell, J.D., East, B.W., Harris, I.A. *et al.* (1986) Trace element studies in amyotrophic lateral sclerosis. *Acta Pharmacol. Toxicol. Copenh.*, **59** (Suppl. 7), 454–7.

Miyata, S., Nakamura, S., Toyoshima, M. *et al.* (1980) The distribution of manganese in the spinal cord of amyotrophic lateral sclerosis. Determination of manganese by neutron activation analysis. *Clin. Neurol. (Tokyo)*, **20**, 917–23.

Miyata, S., Nakamura, S., Nagata, H. *et al.* (1983) Increased manganese level in spinal cords of amyotrophic lateral sclerosis determined by radiochemical neutron activation analysis. *J. Neurol. Sci.*, **61**, 283–93.

531

Metals and free radicals

Mizumoto, Y., Iwata, S., Sasajima, K. *et al.* (1980) Alpha particle-excited X-ray fluorescence analysis for trace metals in cervical spinal cords of amyotrophic lateral sclerosis. *Radioisotopes*, **29**, 585–7.

Mzhel'skaia, T.I., Zavalishin, I.A., Ivanova-Smolenskaia, I.A. *et al.* (1989) Ceruloplasmin activity in the blood during progressive diseases of the central nervous system. *Lab-Delo.*, **11**, 12–16.

Nagata, H., Miyata, S., Nakamura, S. *et al.* (1985) Heavy metal concentrations in blood cells in patients with amyotrophic lateral sclerosis. *J. Neurol. Sci.*, **67**, 173–8.

Norris, F.H. (1978) Amyotrophic lateral sclerosis and low selenium levels. *J. Am. Med. Assoc.*, **239**, 404.

Norris, F.H. and Padia, L.A. (1989) Toxic and pet exposures in amyotrophic lateral sclerosis. *Arch. Neurol.*, **46**, 945.

Pall, H.S. (1989) Some studies into the metal content of and metal-catalysed oxidative mechanisms in the cerebrospinal fluid in some neurological disorders. MD Thesis, Bristol University.

Pall, H.S., Williams, A.C., Blake, D.R. *et al.* (1987a) Evidence of enhanced lipid peroxidation in the cerebrospinal fluid of patients taking phenothiazines. *Lancet*, **ii**, 596–9.

Pall, H.S., Williams, A.C., Blake, D.R. *et al.* (1987b) Raised cerebrospinal fluid copper concentration in Parkinson's disease. *Lancet*, **2**, 238–41.

Pall, H.S., Blake, D.R., Good, P. *et al.* (1989) Ocular toxicity of desferrioxamine – an example of copper-promoted auto-oxidative damage? *Br. J. Ophthalmol.*, **73**, 42–7.

Pall, H.S., Williams, A.C., Chirico, S. *et al.* (1990) Concentrations of reduced and oxidised forms of ascorbic acid in serum and cerebrospinal fluid from patients with motor neurone disease. *Neurology*, **40** (Suppl. 1), 317.

Patel, A.K., Michaelson, I.A., Cremer, J.E. and Balazs, R. (1974) The metabolism of ^{14}C glucose by the brains of suckling rats intoxicated with inorganic lead. *J. Neurochem.*, **22**, 581–90.

Patten, B.M. (1982) Phosphate and parathyroid disorders associated with the syndrome of amyotrophic lateral sclerosis, in *Human Motor Neuron Diseases* (ed. L.P. Rowland), Raven Press, New York, pp. 181–200.

Patten, B.M. (1984) Mineral and metal metabolism in amyotrophic lateral sclerosis, in *Research Progress in Motor Neuron Disease* (ed. F.C. Rose), Pitman, London, pp. 217–27.

Pekkanen, T.J. and Sandholm, M. (1972) The effect of experimental methyl mercury poisoning on the activity of NADPH-specific glutathione reductase of rat brain and liver. *Acta Vet. Scand.*, **13**, 14–19.

Perl, D.P., Gajdusek, D.C., Garruto, R.M. *et al.* (1982) Intraneuronal aluminium accumulation in amyotrophic lateral sclerosis and Parkinsonism-dementia complex of Guam. *Science*, **217**, 1053–5.

Petkau, A., Sawatzky, A. and Hillier, C.R. (1974) Lead content of neuromuscular tissue in amyotrophic lateral sclerosis: case report and other considerations. *Br. J. Indust. Med.*, **31**, 275–87.

Piccardo, P., Yanagihara, R., Garruto, R.M. *et al.* (1988) Histochemical and X-ray microanalytical localisation of aluminium in amyotrophic lateral sclerosis and parkinsonism-dementia of Guam. *Acta Neuropathol. (Berlin)*, **77**, 1–4.

Pierce Ruhland, R.A. and Patten, B.M. (1980) Muscle metals in motor neurone disease. *Ann. Neurol.*, **8**, 193–5.

Quinlan, G.J. (1988) Action of lead (II) and aluminium (III) on iron-stimulated lipid peroxidation in liposomes, erythrocytes and rat liver microsomal fractions. *Biochim. Biophys. Acta*, **962**, 196–200.

Reed, D., Plato, C., Elizan, T. *et al.* (1966) The amyotrophic lateral sclerosis/Parkinsonism-dementia complex: a ten year follow-up on Guam. *Am. J. Epidemiol.*, **83**, 54–73.

Roelofs-Iverson, R.A., Mulder, D.W., Elveback, L.R. *et al.* (1984) Amyotrophic lateral sclerosis and heavy metals: a pilot case–control study. *Neurology*, **34**, 393–5.

Ronnevi, L.O., Conradi, S. and Nise, G. (1982) Further studies on the erythrocyte uptake of lead *in vitro* in amyotrophic lateral sclerosis patients and controls. *J. Neurol. Sci.*, **57**, 143–56.

Rosen, D.R., Siddique, T., Patterson, D. *et al.* (1993) Mutations in Cu Zn superoxide dismutase gene are associated with familial amyotrophic lateral sclerosis. *Nature*, **362**, 59–62.

Rothstein, A. and Hayes, A.D. (1960) The metabolism of mercury in the rat studied by isotope techniques. *J. Pharmacol. Exp. Ther.*, **130**, 166–76.

Saffer, D., Moreley, J. and Bell, P. (1977) Carbohydrate metabolism in motor neurone disease. *J. Neurol. Neurosurg. Psychiat.*, **40**, 533–7.

Scarpa, M., Colombo, A., Panzetti, P. and Sorgato, P. (1988) Epidemiology of amyotrophic lateral sclerosis in the province of Modena, Italy. Influence of environmental exposure to lead. *Acta Neurol. Scand.*, **77**, 456–60.

Sillevis-Smitt, P.A. and de Jong, J.M. (1989) Animal models of amyotrophic lateral sclerosis and the spinal muscular atrophies. *J. Neurol. Sci.*, **91**, 231–58.

Simpson, J.A., Seaton, D.A. and Adams, J.F. (1964) Response to treatment with chelating agents of anemia, chronic encephalopathy and myelopathy due to lead poisoning. *J. Neurol. Neurosurg. Psychiat.*, **27**, 536–41.

Steventon, G., Williams, A.C., Waring, R.H. *et al.* (1988) Xenobiotic metabolism in motor neurone disease. *Lancet*, **ii**, 644–7.

Stober, T., Stelte, W. and Kunze, K. (1983) Lead concentrations in blood, plasma, erythrocytes and cerebrospinal fluid in amyotrophic lateral sclerosis. *J. Neurol. Sci.*, **61**, 21–6.

Strong, M.J. and Garruto, R.M. (1991) Chronic aluminium-induced motor neuron degeneration. *Can. J. Neurol. Sci.*, **18** (Suppl. 3), 428–31.

Tandan, R. and Bradley, W.G. (1985) Amyotrophic lateral sclerosis. 2. Etiopathogenesis. *Ann. Neurol.*, **18**, 419–31.

Taube, H. (1965) Mechanisms of oxidation with oxygen. *J. Gen. Physiol.*, **49** (Suppl.), 29–52.

Toftegaard Nielsen, T. (1978) Plasma citrate during submaximal and intermittent supramaximal exercise. *Scand. J. Clin. Lab. Invest.*, **38**, 29–33.

Metals and free radicals

Voss, H. (1939) Progressive bulbar paralyse und amyotrophische lateralsklerose nach chronischer Manganvergiftung. *Arch. Gewebepath. Gewebehyg.*, **9**, 464–76.

Waring, R.H., Sturman, S.G., Williams, A.C. *et al.* (1989) S-methylation in motor neurone disease and Parkinson's disease. *Lancet*, **ii**, 356–7.

Weiner, W.J., Nausieda, P.A. and Klawans, H.L. (1977) Effect of chlorpromazine on central nervous system concentrations of manganese, iron and copper. *Life Sci.*, **20**, 1181–5.

Weisinger, R. and Fridovich, I. (1973) Mitochondrial superoxide dismutase. *J. Biol. Chem.*, **248**, 4793–6.

Williams, R. (1982) Free manganese II and iron II can act as intracellular cell controls. *FEBS Lett.*, **140**, 3–10.

Williams, R.J.P. (1992) Calcium fluxes in cells: new views on their significance. *Cell Calcium*, **13**, 273–5.

Wilson, S.A.K. (1907) The amyotrophy of chronic lead poisoning – amyotrophic lateral sclerosis of toxic origin. *Rev. Neurol. Psychiat.*, **5**, 441–55.

Yase, Y. (1972) The pathogenesis of amyotrophic lateral sclerosis. *Lancet*, **ii**, 292–6.

Yase, Y. (1980) The role of aluminium in CNS degeneration with interaction with calcium. *Neurotoxicology*, **1**, 101–9.

Yasui, M., Yase, Y. and Ota, K. (1991) Distribution of calcium in central nervous system tissues and bones of rats maintained on calcium-deficient diets. *J. Neurol. Sci.*, **105**, 206–10.

Yasui, M., Yase, Y., Ota, K. *et al.* (1991) Aluminium deposition in the CNS of patients with amyotrophic lateral sclerosis from the Kii peninsula of Japan. *Neurotoxicology*, **12**, 615–20.

Yoshida, S. (1977) X-ray microanalytic studies on amyotrophic lateral sclerosis. Part 1 (Metal distribution compared with neuropathological findings in cervical spinal cord). *Clin. Neurol.*, **17**, 299–309.

Yoshida, S., Yase, Y., Mizumoto, Y. and Iwata, S. (1989) Aluminium deposition and Ca-hydroxyapatite formation in frontal cortex tissue of amyotrophic lateral sclerosis. *Rinsho Shinkeigaku*, **29**, 421–6.

Yoshimasu, F., Uebayashi, Y., Yase, Y. *et al.* (1976) Studies on amyotrophic lateral sclerosis by neutron activation analysis. *Folia Psychiatr. Neurol. Japan*, **30**, 49–55.

Yoshimasu, F., Yasui, M., Yase, Y. *et al.* (1980) Studies on amyotrophic lateral sclerosis by neutron activation analysis. 2. Comparative study of analytical results on Guam PD, Japanese ALS and Alzheimer disease cases. *Folia Psychiatr. Neurol. Japan*, **34**, 75–82.

Yoshimasu, F., Yasui, M., Yase, Y. *et al.* (1982) Studies on amyotrophic lateral sclerosis by neutron activation analysis. 3. Systematic analysis of metals on Guamian ALS and PD cases. *Folia Psychiatr. Neurol. Japan*, **36**, 173–80.

Zief, M. and Mitchell, J. (1976) *Contamination Control in Trace Metal Analysis.* Wiley, New York.

24 *Autoimmune aspects*

STANLEY H. APPEL, R. GLENN SMITH,
JOZSEF I. ENGELHARDT and ENRICO STEFANI

24.1 INTRODUCTION

The etiology and pathogenesis of amyotrophic lateral sclerosis remain unknown despite extensive investigations from many laboratories over the last several decades. ALS has been defined from the clinical point of view as a progressive loss of motor function in upper and lower extremities as well as bulbar musculature. The pathology of ALS consists in a loss of upper and lower motor neurons, but there are few clues as to what initiates neuronal cell death. Circumstantial evidence has focused attention on processes that are known to give rise to motor neuron destruction, and these same processes have been implicated in sporadic ALS. Viruses have been implicated because poliomyelitis can attack motor neurons (Sharief, Hertges and Ciardi, 1991). Toxins have been implicated because lead can give rise to a clinical syndrome of upper and lower motor neuron compromise (Boothby, de Jesus and Rowland, 1974). Genetic disturbances such as hexosaminidase deficiency can also be demonstrated to compromise motor neurons (Johnson, 1982). In our own experience, carefully monitoring over 1000 ALS patients, fewer than 10% of our patients have a positive family history of ALS; fewer than 5% have a history of prior poliomyelitis; and it is rare to encounter evidence of toxins, viruses or genetic disturbances to explain motor neuron destruction. From our perspective, making the assumption that many different factors contribute to the etiology of sporadic ALS has not been fruitful, and it is much more likely that sporadic ALS is due to a single predominant, presently unproven, etiology.

Our own early clinical investigations described an increased incidence of autoimmune disorders in ALS patients (Appel *et al.*, 1986). The reported increased incidence of paraproteinemias also served to focus

Autoimmune aspects

attention on immune mechanisms as the most likely etiology (Shy *et al.*, 1986; Latov *et al.*, 1988; Duarte *et al.*, 1991). Autoimmunity has been implicated in the past but had been rejected primarily because most studies could not differentiate between a primary or a secondary effect of immune mechanisms, and many reports were not reproducible. Investigations of the toxicity of ALS sera on motor neuron cultures (Wolfgram and Myers, 1973) could not be confirmed (Horwich, Engel and Chauvin, 1974; Lehrich and Couture, 1978; Touzeau and Kato, 1983, 1986). A presumptive antigenic growth factor turned out to be glucose-6-phosphate isomerase (Gurney, 1984; Chaput *et al.*, 1988; Faik *et al.*, 1988), and no antibodies against this enzyme could be demonstrated in ALS sera. More recently antibodies to gangliosides have been reported in ALS patients. Careful studies from Latov's laboratory have documented several instances of motor neuron disease in patients with IgM and IgA monoclonal gammopathies in whom the monoclonal proteins were noted to react with neuronal cells by immunohistochemical techniques (Thomas *et al.*, 1990; Sadiq *et al.*, 1991). However, such cases are rare. In most ALS patients with monoclonal gammopathy, there is no direct evidence that the paraprotein specifically reacts with motor neurons. Nevertheless, the coexistence of paraproteinemia and ALS may provide circumstantial evidence that immune mechanisms contribute to both the monoclonal gammopathy and the motor neuron destruction of ALS.

In patients without monoclonal gammopathies, the role of anti-ganglioside antibodies has been unconvincing. With different techniques from 10% to 75% of ALS patients have been reported to possess anti-ganglioside antibodies (Shy *et al.*, 1987; Pestronk *et al.*, 1988, 1989). Such antibodies were also present in many other antibodies of autoimmune disorders (Endo *et al.*, 1984). Our own studies suggest that such antibodies are secondary responses and not primarily related to the pathogenesis of disease, since 14% of ALS patient were found to possess these antibodies, while 15% of control patients with other autoimmune diseases also possessed anti-ganglioside antibodies.

24.2 IMMUNE-MEDIATED MODELS OF MOTOR NEURON DESTRUCTION

To provide evidence for an immunologic origin of ALS, we have developed two immune-mediated animal models of disease; experimental autoimmune motor neuron disease (EAMND) and experimental autoimmune gray matter disease (EAGMD). EAMND is a lower motor neuron syndrome induced in guinea-pigs by five monthly injections of bovine spinal cord motor neurons prepared by differential centrifuga-

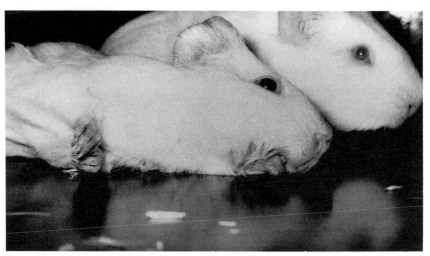

Figure 24.1 Guinea-pig with EAGMD in foreground with bulbar compromise and front paw weakness. Guinea-pig in rear without disease injected only with Freund's adjuvant (Tajti, Appel and Stefani, 1991).

tion of spinal cord ventral gray matter homogenates (Engelhardt, Appel and Killian, 1989). Following inoculation, guinea-pigs developed a slowly progressive limb weakness that was associated with EMG and morphologic evidence of denervation. Pathological examination demonstrated a depletion of motor neurons. The remaining motor neurons demonstrated a loss of Nissl substance and shrinkage of cells as well as satellitosis and neuronophagia. There was no involvement of corticospinal tracts, and no involvement of upper motor neurons. High titers of antibodies to motor neurons were demonstrated in the serum, and IgG was noted in at least one-third of the motor terminal endplates defined by α-bungarotoxin staining and in the cytoplasm of remaining spinal cord motor neurons.

EAGMD is a more acute and more rapidly progressive disorder involving lower and upper motor neurons induced by one or two inoculations of spinal cord ventral horn homogenate (Engelhardt, Appel and Killian, 1990). Over two-thirds of the inoculated animals developed disease symptoms 3 weeks after antigen injection. The symptoms appeared suddenly with 3 or 4 days of worsening followed by a period of stabilization and then further deterioration. The disease first presented with decreased tone and weakness in the hind limbs and then gradually spread to involve the front extremities. Twenty-five percent of the animals developed bulbar involvement as the initial sign (Figure 24.1). In bulbar-onset animals the disease progressed rapidly, requiring sacrifice several days after the onset of clinical signs. Denervation was also evidenced by EMG and morphologic criteria. By EMG, motor unit activity was reduced and complex repetitive discharges were noted in over half the animals. Muscle morphology demonstrated denervation with scattered atrophic fibers, some group atrophy, connective tissue proliferation and mononuclear cell infiltration. Within the CNS there were scattered perivascular inflammatory foci and a loss of spinal cord motor neurons as well as a loss of large pyramidal cells in the motor cortex (Figure 24.2). Small foci of mononuclear cells were observed in the spinal cord gray matter and in the cerebral cortex. More extensive focal inflammation was located in the spinal cord ventral white matter at sites where motor neuron axons passed to the periphery. Immuno-histochemical studies for IgG demonstrated the same intracytoplasmic staining pattern of spinal motor neurons found in EAMND (Figure 24.3). However, in addition, IgG was deposited within inflammatory foci in the CNS. In animals with long-standing disease, IgG could be detected around the external membrane of motor neurons. Intensive IgG staining was also noted at approximately 50% of the motor endplates defined by the presence of α-bungarotoxin staining.

In EAMND, serum IgG reactivity to bovine motor neurons reached a titer of 1:102 400 after the second antigen injection and was maintained continuously at this level. No detectable IgG antibodies were noted to gangliosides, cerebrosides or bovine myelin basic protein. Titers of IgM reactive with motor neurons reached a maximum level of 1:3200. In sera from animals with EAGMD, the titer of IgG reactive to bovine motor neurons was similar to that found in animals with EAMND, but EAGMD animals also developed a high titer (1:51 200) to myelin basic protein and a low titer (1:800) to cerebroside. No IgG reactivity was observed to gangliosides. No reactivity to any of these antigens was present in the sera of guinea-pigs immunized with Freund's adjuvant alone.

To provide further evidence for the role of autoimmune mechanisms, the immunosuppressant cyclophosphamide was administered prior to and after immunization with bovine ventral horn homogenate (Tajti, Appel and Stefani, 1991). Pretreatment with cyclophosphamide prevented the appearance of clinical signs of disease and decreased the loss of spinal cord motor neurons, the appearance of damaged motor neurons and the antibody titer to motor neurons (Figure 24.4). Treatment 7 days after immunization attenuated the expression of disease. Treatment immediately after signs appeared also improved the clinical and pathological findings. In all cyclophosphamide-treated animals there was less IgG within motor neurons and less inflammation. Thus cyclophosphamide altered both the clinical and pathologic

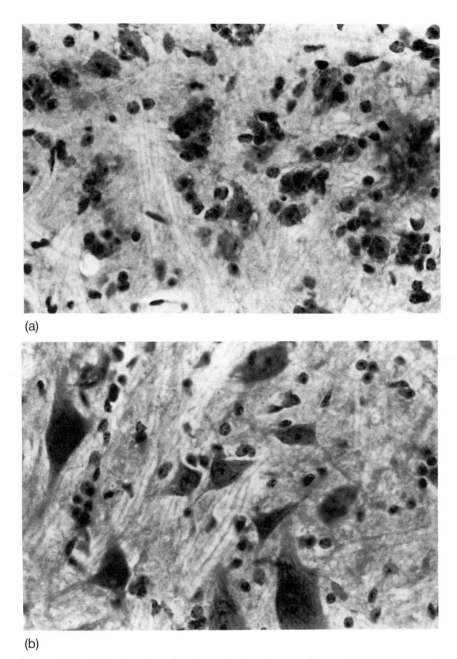

(a)

(b)

Figure 24.2 (a) Section from lumbar spinal cord ventral horn of EAGMD animal demonstrating damaged motor neurons and neuronophagia. (b) Section from lumbar spinal cord ventral horn from normal animal pretreated with cyclophosphamide and immunized with gray matter demonstrating intact motor neurons. Cresyl violet (×900) (Tajti, Appel and Stefani, 1991).

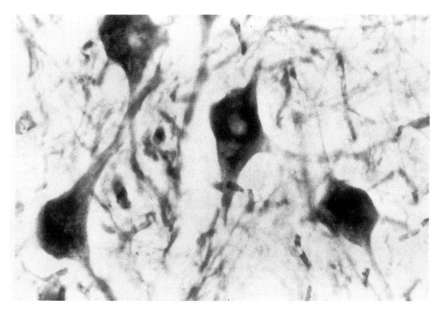

(a)

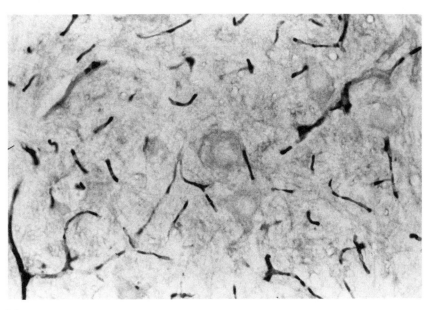

(b)

Figure 24.3   (a) Motor neurons from EAGMD guinea-pig contain IgG (×1800).
(b) Motor neurons from guinea-pig injected only with Freud's adjuvant
demonstrate no IgG staining (×900). Immunohistochemical reactions with
peroxidase-conjugated goat anti-guinea-pig IgG (Tajti, Appel and Stefani, 1991).

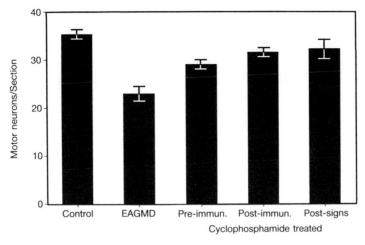

Figure 24.4 Number of intact motor neurons per lumbar cord section. Values represent mean ± SEM. Preimmune animals were injected with cyclophosphamide (5 mg or 10 mg) 2 days prior to gray matter inoculation and then three times a week. Post-immune animals were injected with cyclophosphamide 7 days after gray matter inoculation and then three times a week. Post-signs animals were injected with cyclophosphamide after the appearance of signs of EAGMD and then every other day (Tajti, Appel and Stefani, 1991).

expression of EAGMD, and such data support the role for autoimmune mechanisms in motor neuron loss in this animal model.

In both EAMND and EAGMD, distinctive changes were noted in physiological studies of the neuromuscular junction (Garcìa *et al.*, 1990). The frequency of miniature endplate potentials (mepps) was found to be increased in affected animals, especially early in the disease. Muscle fibers of these same animals had normal resting potentials, indicating the integrity of the post-synaptic membrane. Furthermore, the mepp amplitude and time constant of decay were unchanged in immunized guinea-pigs. Thus the increased mepp frequency implied a greater acetylcholine release from the axon terminal in the resting state.

24.2.1 Comparability of EAGMD and human ALS

In order to assess the comparability of the animal models in human ALS, the spinal cord and motor cortex of patients with ALS were examined with immunohistochemical techniques for the presence of IgG. In 13 of 15 spinal cords, lower motor neurons stained positively for IgG in a granular pattern characteristic of binding the rough endoplasmic reticulum (Engelhardt and Appel, 1990); and in 6 of 11 motor cortices,

Autoimmune aspects

pyramidal cells also stained positively for IgG. No such reactivity was noted in motor neurons of control human tissue, although positive IgG staining was present in astrocytes of ALS as well as control specimens. Reactive microglia and/or macrophages were detected in the territory of degenerating pyramidal tracts and ventral horns in ALS. The surface of most of these cells stained positively for IgG, and 50% stained positively for HLA-DR. Thus accumulation of IgG in motor neurons and the presence of immunologically active macrophages suggested the possible participation of immunologic factors.

The presence of inflammatory cells in the CNS of ALS patients had not been previously recognized, and this has always been an argument against conventional autoimmunity in ALS. Recent preliminary studies by Troost, Van den Oord and De Jong (1988), Lampson, Kushner and Sobel (1988), and McGeer, Itagaki and McGeer (1988), and a more extensive evaluation by Troost et al. (1989) employing monoclonal antibodies against lymphocyte antigens, had suggested that inflammatory cell infiltration in ALS CNS tissue may have been more common than previously suspected. Lampson, Kushner and Sobel (1990) demonstrated phagocytes and small numbers of T cells in degenerating white matter of four ALS spinal cords. Preliminary studies from our own laboratories demonstrated the presence of lymphocytes in the spinal cords of 10 of our 15 ALS patients using conventional histological techniques (Appel et al., 1991a). More recent studies from our own laboratory using monoclonal antibody techniques have demonstrated white and gray matter lymphocytic infiltrates in the spinal cord of 18 of 21 consecutive ALS autopsies (Engelhardt, Tajti and Appel, 1993). The lymphocytes possessed only T-cell markers, and no B-cell markers could be demonstrated. T-helper cells were found in proximity to degenerating cortical spinal tracts, while both T-helper and T-suppressor/cytotoxic cells were demonstrated in spinal cord ventral horns. Thus CD4 and CD8 lymphocytes are clearly present in ALS ventral horn as demonstrated by immunohistochemical techniques. With polymerase chain reaction technology, both V_α and V_β T-cell receptor transcripts, as well as transcripts for CD4, CD8 and the HLA class II antigens (DR, DQ, DP), have been amplified from the spinal cords and brains of ALS patients (Panzara et al., 1991). Whether these CD4 and CD8 lymphocytes are immediately related to the pathogenesis of the disease or are secondary phenomena remains to be elucidated.

Nevertheless, our animal model, especially EAGMND, resembles human ALS with respect to the loss of upper and lower motor neurons, the presence of inflammatory foci, including activated microglia within the spinal cord, and the presence of IgG within upper and lower motor neurons.

542

24.2.2 Passive transfer experiments

The presence of physiologic changes in the guinea-pig model provided a sensitive assay for the passive transfer of motor neuron dysfunction from the animal models of motor neuron disease and from human ALS patients to mice. Mice injected with serum immunoglobulin from animals with EAMND and EAGMD and patients with ALS demonstrated an uptake of IgG in spinal cord motor neurons and at the neuromuscular junction (Appel *et al.*, 1991b). The injected mice also documented an increase in mepp frequency. Individual fibers were affected to a different extent, but approximately 50% of the fibers had mepp frequencies greater than 20 mepp/s. Resting membrane potential, mepp amplitude and time constant of delay were similar in all injected animals. Thus the increased mepp frequency was not due to damage of the post-synaptic components, but reflected a presynaptic alteration with increased acetylcholine release from the nerve terminal.

The fact that immunoglobulins from immune-mediated animal models of motor neuron destruction and human ALS could passively transfer physiologic alterations of the neuromuscular junction provided important evidence for the potential primary importance of the immunoglobulins in these syndromes, just as such passive transfer experiments provided cogent evidence for the role of immunoglobulins in myasthenia gravis (Toyka *et al.*, 1975) or in the Eaton–Lambert syndrome (Lang *et al.*, 1981). The enhanced resting mepp frequency in these passive transfer experiments further defined the motor nerve terminal as a target for the immune attack. Since enhanced acetylcholine release is dependent on calcium, our data suggested the possibility that immunoglobulins from the animal model and human ALS may have induced an increase of cytoplasmic calcium to account for this increased mepp frequency. This suggestion was supported by the demonstration that Bay-K8644 can potentiate calcium currents and can increase spontaneous and evoked acetylcholine release from the neuromuscular junction (Atchinson and O'Leary, 1987; Ofirman-Uffenheimer, Rahaminoff and Shapira, 1990). It is also possible that increased cytoplasmic calcium may in turn trigger processes that lead to cell death, as has been well documented with neuronal cell death in other experimental paradigms (Dreyer *et al.*, 1990; Rich and Hollowell, 1990; Weiss *et al.*, 1990).

24.2.3 Antigenic target of ALS antibodies

The passive transfer experiments suggested the possibility that ion channels of the neuromuscular junction could represent an early target of the ALS antibodies. The immune attack of ALS would be anticipated to result in an increased entry of calcium and would differ from the Eaton–Lambert syndrome, in which an immune attack of the voltage-gated calcium channel has been reported to result in the loss of calcium channels at the neuromuscular junction and a decrease in calcium entry (Vincent, Lang and Newsom-Davis, 1989).

As a test of the hypothesis of a direct effect of ALS immunoglobulins on ion channels, the action of IgG from ALS was studied on dihydropyridine (DHP)-sensitive calcium channels in single mammalian skeletal muscle fibers (Delbono et $al.$, 1991a,b). The peak of the calcium current and the charge movement were reduced when the fibers were incubated in ALS IgG, and monitored with the Vaseline-gap voltage-clamp technique (Figure 24.5). These effects were lost when the IgGs were boiled or adsorbed with skeletal tubular membranes. The interaction of ALS IgG with the skeletal muscle L-type channel was similar to the interaction of such channels with the blocker nifedipine. ALS IgG reduced charge movement and blocked I_{Ca} in a voltage-dependent fashion. These data suggested that IgG from ALS patients reacts with the skeletal muscle DHP-sensitive calcium channel or an associated regulatory moiety.

Similar actions of blocking calcium current and reducing charge movement were observed when these same IgGs or their F_{ab} fragments were applied to highly purified L-type voltage-dependent calcium channels functionally reconstituted into an artificial lipid bilayer. In this system, the ALS IgGs only produced effects when added to the side of the bilayer corresponding to the extracellular face of the calcium channel complex. Since associated proteins do not remain with the calcium channel in the lipid bilayer, the similar actions on the skeletal muscle and in the lipid bilayer suggest a specific interaction of ALS IgG with one of the calcium channel's subunits to explain the alteration in charge movement and calcium current. To determine whether calcium channel antibodies can be identified biochemically, we have used an enzyme-linked immunosorbent assay (ELISA) technique to detect the reactivity of purified ALS immunoglobulins or antibodies with purified skeletal muscle L-type calcium channel complexes (Smith et $al.$, 1992). With this assay, 79% of sera from ALS patients have significantly higher calcium channel-binding immunoglobulins than observed for sera of other patients. Using both purified immunoglobulins and purified L-type calcium channel complexes, all ALS IgG fractions tested could be differentiated in their binding reactivity from control population IgG fractions. In ALS patients the titers of calcium channel cross-reactive antibodies correlated with the rate of ALS disease progression, rather than the stage of the disease.

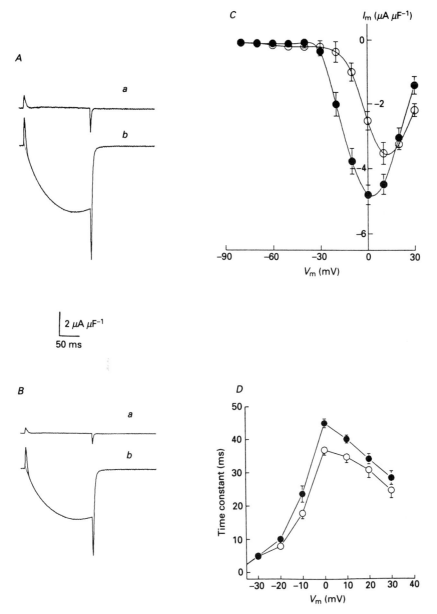

Figure 24.5 Calcium current recordings from the same fiber before (A) and after (B) 30 min of ALS IgG incubation, documenting the reduction of I_{ca} amplitude and the reduction of charge movement in the presence of ALS IgG. (C) Current–voltage relationship in control (●) and ALS IgG (○). (D) Voltage dependence of the time constant of activation in control conditions (●) and in ALS IgG (○). Values are means ± SEM (Delbono *et al.*, 1991a,b).

545

Autoimmune aspects

Thus our electrophysiological and biochemical studies suggest that the majority of ALS patients possess antibodies to the voltage-gated calcium channel. The key question is whether these antibodies are primarily involved in the pathogenesis of motor neuron destruction or are a secondary response to motor neuron destruction. Favoring a primary role is the fact that patients with familial ALS do not possess such antibodies even though in familial ALS motor neuron destruction and denervation are similar to sporadic ALS. If the antibodies were secondary, one would have anticipated that familial ALS patients would have the same elevated antibody titer as sporadic ALS patients. Also favoring a primary role is the observation that the titer of antibodies correlates with the rate of progression of disease and not the stage of disease. Patients in late stage disease with a greater loss of motor neurons and a slow course have lower titers than patients early in disease with a rapid course and less motor neuron loss. In addition, the ALS IgGs were noted to react only with the extracellular face of the calcium channel. If the antibodies were a consequence of motor neuron destruction, one would have anticipated antibodies reactive to the intracellular as well as extracellular face of the calcium channel. Thus, our data suggest that the antibodies may play a primary rather than a secondary role.

However, there are numerous stumbling blocks to implicating calcium channel antibodies in motor neuron destruction. The first is that our studies have focused on antibodies to the skeletal muscle L-type channel, and ALS is not known to influence muscle adversely. We recently carried out electrophysiological experiments on a cell line with predominantly N-type channels and no evidence of dihydropyridine receptor L-type channels (Crawford et al., 1992; Magnelli et al., 1992). In these cells, ALS IgG could also be demonstrated to block calcium currents, thereby demonstrating that the antibodies clearly react with both N-type and L-type channels, perhaps at epitopes common to both channels.

Another concern is the fact that our passive transfer experiments with ALS IgG clearly document an increased mepp frequency, and suggest increased acetylcholine release, possibly on the basis of increased intracellular calcium. Yet our acute physiological studies document a block of calcium currents that would be expected to decrease intra-cellular calcium. A resolution for this paradox is not at hand. From a theoretical point of view it is possible that the acute blocking action of ALS IgG on the voltage-dependent calcium channel may, over time, prompt the cell to up-regulate the number of channels or alter existing channels to promote an increased level of intracellular calcium. Studies are currently in progress to decide among these alternatives in an effort to resolve such discrepancies.

Another important concern is why motor neurons should show selective vulnerability if the antibodies interact with voltage-dependent calcium channels, which are present in many different tissues. Many different calcium channels are known to exist, and these differ from one another in primary structure and in tissue localization (Mori *et al.*, 1991). Motor neurons may contain unique calcium channels and thus explain the specificity of neuronal compromise. However, we suspect that a more significant role in determining selective vulnerability may be the motor neuron's relative inability to handle increased intracellular calcium. Other concerns include how upper motor neurons become compromised if IgG is responsible. How do such IgGs reach these upper motor neurons in ALS in the absence of an altered blood–brain barrier? Furthermore, what initiates the autoimmune process? What is the role of trauma? How can we explain the elevated levels of aspartate and glutamate in the CSF (Rothstein *et al.*, 1990) and the decreased levels of aspartate and glutamate within ALS spinal cord tissue (Plaitakis and Caroscio, 1987)?

Finally, the hypothesis that ALS is an autoimmune disease leads to numerous clinical questions, among the most important being the fact that standard immunotherapies used to treat most autoimmune conditions have no proven benefit in ALS (Pieper and Fields, 1957; Kellerman *et al.*, 1983; Appel *et al.*, 1988). One possible explanation for the general ineffectiveness of immunosuppression is that by the time ALS symptoms are manifest the motor neuron pool may have been significantly reduced. This may be analogous to what occurs in autoimmune type I diabetes, in which standard immunotherapies are relatively ineffective by the time clinical disease is manifest (Atkinson and MacLauren, 1990). Alternatively, once the destructive processes in ALS have been initiated, the subsequent motor neuron loss may be independent of the antibody attack that initiated the process. How calcium channel antibodies in ALS sera influence calcium channel function and calcium metabolism in neurons, and whether such interactions lead to motor neuron cell death, is currently under investigation. Nevertheless, the availability of animal models of motor neuron destruction provides an opportunity to delineate potential biologic mechanisms in motor neuron loss relevant to ALS, just as the animal models of myasthenia gravis and the myasthenic syndrome paved the way for an understanding of the relevant mechanisms responsible for neuromuscular dysfunction in these diseases in man.

Autoimmune aspects

ACKNOWLEDGMENTS

We are grateful to Mary Catherine Pond for her editorial assistance. These studies were supported by grants from the Muscular Dystrophy Association to the MDA ALS Center at Baylor College of Medicine, the M.H. 'Jack' Wagner Memorial Foundation for ALS Research and Cephalon, Inc.

REFERENCES

Appel, S.H., Stockton-Appel, V., Stewart, S.S. *et al.* (1986) Amyotrophic lateral sclerosis: associated clinical disorders and immunologic evaluations. *Arch. Neurol.*, **43**, 234–8.

Appel, S.H., Stewart, S.S., Appel, V. *et al.* (1988) A double-blind study of cyclosporine in amyotrophic lateral sclerosis. *Arch. Neurol.*, **45**, 381–6.

Appel, S.H., Engelhardt, J.I., García, J. *et al.* (1991a) Autoimmunity and ALS: a comparison of animal models of immune-mediated motor neuron destruction and human ALS, in *Advances in Neurology*, Vol. 56 (ed. L.P. Rowland), Raven Press, New York, pp. 405–12.

Appel, S.H., Engelhardt, J.I., García, J. *et al.* (1991b) Immunoglobulins from animal models of motor neuron disease and from human amyotrophic lateral sclerosis patients passively transfer physiological abnormalities to the neuromuscular junction. *Proc. Natl. Acad. Sci. USA*, **88**, 647–651.

Atchison, W.D. and O'Leary, S.M. (1987) Bay K8644 increases release of acetylcholine at the murine neuromuscular junction. *Brain Res.*, **419**, 315–19.

Atkinson, M.A. and MacLauren, N.K. (1990) What causes diabetes? *Sci. Am.*, **263**, 62–71.

Boothby, J.A., de Jesus, P.V. and Rowland, L.P. (1974) Reversible forms of motor neuron disease. *Arch. Neurol.*, **31**, 18–23.

Chaput, M., Claes, V., Portetelle, D. *et al.* (1988) The neurotrophic factor neurokinin is 90% homologous with phosphohexose isomerase. *Nature*, **332**, 454–5.

Crawford Jr, G.D., Le, W.-D., Smith, R.G. *et al.* (1992) A novel N18TG2 × mesencephalon cell hybrid expresses properties which suggest a dopaminergic cell line of substantia nigra origin. *J. Neurosci.* (in press).

Delbono, O., García, J., Appel, S.H. *et al.* (1991a) IgG from amyotrophic lateral sclerosis affects tubular calcium channels of skeletal muscle. *Am. J. Physiol.*, **260**, C1347–51.

Delbono, O., García, J., Appel, S.H. *et al.* (1991b) Calcium current and charge movement of mammalian muscle: action of amyotrophic lateral sclerosis immunoglobulins. *J. Physiol.*, **444**, 723–42.

Dreyer, E.G., Kaiser, P.I.C., Offermann, J.T. *et al.* (1990) HIV-1 coat protein neurotoxicity prevented by calcium channel antagonists. *Science*, **248**, 364–7.

Duarte, F., Binet, S., Lacomblex, L. *et al.* (1991) Quantitative analysis of monoclonal immunoglobulins in serum of patients with amyotrophic lateral sclerosis. *Neurol. Sci.*, **104**, 88–91.

Endo, T., Scott, D.D., Stewart, S.S. *et al.* (1984) Antibodies to glycosphingolipids in patients with multiple sclerosis and SLE. *J. Immunol.*, **132**, 1793–7.

Engelhardt, J.I. and Appel, S.H. (1990) IgG reactivity in the spinal cord and motor cortex in amyotrophic lateral sclerosis. *Arch. Neurol.*, **47**, 1210–16.

Engelhardt, J.I., Appel, S.H. and Killian, J.M. (1989) Experimental autoimmune motor neuron disease. *Ann. Neurol.*, **26**, 368–76.

Engelhardt, J.I., Appel, S.H. and Killian, J.M. (1990) Motor neuron destruction in guinea pigs immunized with bovine spinal cord ventral horn homogenate: experimental autoimmune gray matter disease. *J. Neuroimmunol.*, **27**, 21–31.

Engelhardt, J.I., Tajti, J. and Appel, S.H. (1993) Lymphocytic infiltrates in the spinal cord in amyotrophic lateral sclerosis. *Arch. Neurol.*

Faik, P., Walker, J.I., Redmill, A.A. *et al.* (1988) Mouse glucose-6-phosphate isomerase and neuroleukin have identical 3'sequences. *Nature*, **332**, 445–57.

García, J., Engelhardt, J.I., Appel, S.H. *et al.* (1990) Increased MEPP frequency as an early sign of experimental immune-mediated motoneuron disease. *Ann. Neurol.*, **28**, 329–34.

Gurney, M.E. (1984) Suppression of sprouting at the neuromuscular junction by immune sera. *Nature*, **307**, 538–46.

Horwich, M.S., Engel, W.K. and Chauvin, P.B. (1974) Amyotrophic lateral sclerosis sera applied to cultured human spinal cord neurons. *Arch. Neurol.*, **30**, 332–3.

Johnson, W. (1982) Hexosaminidase deficiency: a cause of recessively inherited motor neuron disease. *Adv. Neurol.*, **36**, 156–64.

Kellerman, J., Hedlund, W., Orlin, J.B. *et al.* (1983) Plasmapheresis with immunosuppression in amyotrophic lateral sclerosis. *Arch. Neurol.*, **40**, 752–3.

Lampson, L.A., Kushner, P.D. and Sobel, R.A. (1988) Strong expression of class II major histocompatibility complex (MHC) antigens in the absence of detectable T-cell infiltration in amyotrophic lateral sclerosis. *J. Neuropathol. Exp. Neurol.*, **47**, 353.

Lampson, L.A., Kushner, P.D. and Sobel, R.A. (1990) Major histocompatibility complex antigen expression in the affected tissues in amyotrophic lateral sclerosis. *Ann. Neurol.*, **28**, 365–72.

Lang, B., Newsom-Davis, J., Wray, D. *et al.* (1981) Autoimmune etiology for myasthenia (Eaton Lambert) syndrome. *Lancet*, **ii**, 224–6.

Latov, N., Hays, A.P., Donofrio, P.D. *et al.* (1988) Monoclonal IgM with unique specificity to ganglioside GM_1 and GD_{1b} and to lacto-N-tetrose associated with human motoneuron disease. *Neurology*, **38**, 763–8.

Lehrich, J.R. and Couture, J. (1978) Amyotrophic lateral sclerosis sera are not cytotoxic to neuroblastoma cells in tissue culture. *Ann. Neurol.*, **4**, 384.

McGeer, P.L., Itagaki, S. and McGeer, E.G. (1988) Expression of histocompatibility glycoprotein HLA-DR in neurological disease. *Acta Neuropathol.*, **76**, 550–7.

Autoimmune aspects

Magnelli, V., Crawford, G., Smith, R.G. *et al.* (1992) Biochemical and electrophysiological characterization of a new dopaminergic neuronal cell line. *Biophys. J.*, **61**, A248.

Mori, Y., Friedrich, T., Kim, M.-S. *et al.* (1991) Primary structure and functional expression from complementary DNA of a brain calcium channel. *Nature*, **350**, 398–402.

Ofiram-Uffenheimer, E., Rahamimoff, R. and Shapira, R. (1990) Transmitter release as the neuromuscular junction of the frog is sensitive to a dihydropyridine. *J. Physiol.*, 430–62.

Panzara, M.I., Oksenberg, J.R., Begovich, A. *et al.* (1991) Restricted T-cell receptor usage in spinal cord and brain of patients with amyotrophic lateral sclerosis. *J. Neuroimmunol.*, *Suppl. 1*, 79.

Pestronk, A., Adams, R.N., Clawson, K. *et al.* (1988) Serum antibodies to GM1 ganglioside in amyotrophic lateral sclerosis. *Neurology*, **38**, 1457–61.

Pestronk, A., Adams, R.N., Cornblath, D. *et al.* (1989) Patterns of serum antibodies to GM1 and $GD1_a$ ganglioside in ALS. *Ann. Neurol.*, **25**, 98–102.

Pieper, S.J.L. and Fields, W.S. (1957) Failure of ALS to respond to intrathecal steroid and vitamin B_{12}. *Arch. Neurol.*, **19**, 522–6.

Plaitakis, A. and Caroscio, J.T. (1987) Abnormal glutamate metabolism in amyotrophic lateral sclerosis. *Ann. Neurol.*, **22**, 575–9.

Rich, K.M. and Hollowell, J.P. (1990) Flunarizine protects neurons from death after axotomy or NGF deprivation. *Science*, **248**, 1419–21.

Rothstein, J.D., Tsai, G., Kuncl, R.W. *et al.* (1990) Abnormal excitatory amino acid metabolism in amyotrophic lateral sclerosis. *Ann. Neurol.*, **28**, 18–25.

Sadiq, S.A., van den Berg, L.-H., Thomas, F.P. *et al.* (1991) Human monoclonal antineurofilament antibody cross-reacts with a neuronal surface protein. *J. Neurosci. Res.*, **29**, 319–25.

Sharief, M.K., Hentges, R. and Ciardi, M. (1991) Intrathecal immune response in patients with post-polio syndrome. *New Engl. J. Med.*, **325**, 749–55.

Shy, M.E., Rowland, L.P., Smith, T. *et al.* (1986) Motor neuron disease and plasma cell dyscrasia. *Neurology*, **36**, 1429–36.

Shy, M.E., Evans, V.A., Lublin, F.D. *et al.* (1987) Anti-GM1 antibodies in motor neuron disease patients without plasma cell dyscrasia. *Ann. Neurol.*, **22**, 167.

Smith, R.G., Hamilton, S., Hofmann, F. *et al.* (1992) Serum antibodies to skeletal muscle-derived L-type calcium channels in patients with amyotrophic lateral sclerosis. *N. Engl. J. Med.*, **327**, 1721–8.

Tajti, J., Appel, S.H. and Stefani, E. (1991) Cyclophosphamide alters the chemical and pathological expression of experimental autoimmune gray matter disease. *J. Neuroimmunol.*, **34**, 143–51.

Thomas, F.P., Thomas, J.E., Sadiq, S.A. *et al.* (1990) Human monoclonal IgM anti-Gal (β 1–3) GalNAc autoantibodies bind to the surface of bovine spinal motoneurons. *J. Neuropathol. Exp. Neurol.*, **49**, 89–95.

Touzeau, G. and Kato, A.C. (1983) Effects of amyotrophic lateral sclerosis sera on cultured cholinergic neurons. *Neurology*, **33**, 317–22.

Touzeau, G. and Kato, A.C. (1986) ALS serum has no effect on three enzymatic activities in cultured human spinal cord neurons. *Neurology*, **36**, 573–6.

Toyka, K.V., Drachman, D.B., Prestronk, A. *et al.* (1975) Myasthenia gravis: passive transfer from man to mouse. *Science*, **190**, 397–9.

Troost, D., Van den Oord, J.J. and De Jong, J.M.B.V. (1988) Analysis of the inflammatory infiltrate in amyotrophic lateral sclerosis. *J. Neuropathol. Appl. Neurobiol.*, **14**, 255–6.

Troost, D., Van den Oord, J.J., De Jong, J.M.B.V. *et al.* (1989) Lymphocytic infiltration in the spinal cord of patients with amyotrophic lateral sclerosis. *Clin. Neuropathol.*, **8**, 289–94.

Vincent, A., Lang, B. and Newsom-Davis, J. (1989) Autoimmunity to the voltage-gated calcium channel underlies the Lambert–Eaton myasthenic syndrome, a paraneoplastic disorder. *Trends Neurosci.*, **12**, 496–502.

Weiss, J.H., Hartley, D.M., Koh, J. *et al.* (1990) The calcium channel blocker nifedipine alternates slow excitatory amino acid neurotoxicity. *Science*, **247**, 1474–7.

Wolfgram, F. and Myers, L. (1973) Amyotrophic lateral sclerosis: effect of serum on anterior horn cells in culture. *Science*, **179**, 579–80.

25 *Trophic factors*

RAE NISHI and FELIX P. ECKENSTEIN

25.1 INTRODUCTION

What are trophic factors and why are they of interest in motor neuron disease? A trophic factor can be generally defined as any molecule that supports the survival of neurons; however, such a broad definition also includes molecules that serve a nutritive function, such as glucose or pyruvate. Therefore, this chapter will confine itself to trophic factors that are polypeptides. Polypeptide trophic factors act on specific neurons by binding to the extracellular domain of a transmembrane protein, thereby inducing an intracellular signal transduction cascade that results in altered gene expression. Trophic factors are of interest in motor neuron disease because a primary cause of motor neuron degeneration may be lack of access to trophic factors. The loss of access to trophic factor may be the result of a number of causes: the muscle may be unable to synthesize or release the factor, the neuron may become unable to respond to the trophic factor or the neuron may become disconnected from the muscle during the initial process of motor neuron disease and hence become deprived of trophic factor synthesized by the muscle, all of which insures the death of the neuron.

The original concept of a neurotrophic factor was based upon the observation that many populations of neurons undergo a period of target-dependent cell death during development (reviewed in Oppenheim, 1991). This includes the spinal cord, where 60% of the neurons die in spite of the arrival of all their axons at the appropriate muscle. This developmental neuronal cell death is thought to be regulated by the limited availability of neurotrophic factors released by the target tissue. The prototypical neurotrophic factor is nerve growth factor (NGF), which supports the survival of sympathetic, sensory and cholinergic basal forebrain neurons in culture, and has been proven to regulate neuronal survival *in vivo* by the exacerbation of neuronal cell death when antibodies that block the activity of endogenous NGF are injected

553

Trophic factors

(reviewed in Thoenen and Barde, 1980; Thoenen, 1991). Adult sympathetic neurons also continue to depend upon NGF for survival and will die if axotomized unless NGF is provided exogenously.

Although target tissues were once thought to be the sole source of neurotrophic factors, it is now recognized that more ubiquitously distributed maintenance or regeneration-promoting molecules exist (see below). In fact, the survival of a particular type of neuron in culture may be promoted by more than one molecule, only one of which may be a true target-derived trophic molecule. For example sympathetic neurons in cell culture respond to four structurally distinct molecules: NGF, acidic fibroblast growth factor, basic fibroblast growth factor and growth-promoting activity (Eckenstein *et al.*, 1990). It is not known what function, if any, is subserved by these other trophic molecules *in vivo*.

If trophic molecules could be identified for motor neurons, then the local or systemic application of the trophic factor to patients with motor neuron disease might be able to slow or even halt further degeneration. Furthermore, once specific trophic molecules are identified, then specific tests could be designed to determine whether the cause of ALS is the lack of access to the appropriate trophic agent. Thus, a great deal of effort has been applied recently to identify and isolate motor neuron trophic factors.

25.2 ASSAYS FOR MOTOR NEURON TROPHIC FACTORS

Both *in vivo* and *in vitro* assays have been used for the identification of motor neuron trophic factors. *In vivo* assays include: application of putative trophic agents onto the chorioallantoic membrane of chicken embryos to test for rescue of motor neurons from normal developmental cell death (Houenou *et al.*, 1991); local application of trophic agents to axotomized nerves in adult animals to test for rescue of motor neurons from retrograde degeneration (Sendtner, Kreutzberg and Thoenen, 1990); and injection of animal models of motor neuron disease (e.g. the wobbler mouse) to test whether the onset of motor neuron degeneration can be delayed (Kozachuk *et al.*, 1987). *In vivo* assays are very expensive, require large amounts of trophic activities, and may be difficult to interpret because of the complexity of the system. They are also not suited to rapid screening of the large number of samples that are generated during purification of putative trophic factors. On the other hand, they may more accurately represent the type of degeneration encountered in motor neuron disease. Thus, *in vivo* assays may be the method of choice if a limited number of agents are to be tested for their trophic activity.

Assays for motor neuron trophic factors

In vitro assays test the ability of putative trophic factors to support survival of motor neurons in cell culture. By virtue of the fact that viable neurons from dissociated central nervous system are very difficult to obtain from adult animals, all *in vitro* testing of trophic factors must be performed on embryonic or neonatal motor neurons. Consequently, the assay may be less representative of motor neuron disease, and the age of the embryo from which the spinal cord is taken may be an important factor because motor neurons may be more sensitive to the application of muscle-derived trophic factors during normal cell death (E6–9 in chicken embryos and E14–19 in rat embryos). More importantly, the analysis of *in vitro* bioassays is complicated by the fact that ventral horn motor neurons constitute only a small proportion of the total number of neurons within the spinal cord. Thus, if motor neuron survival is to be quantified, then motor neurons must be identified in mixed cultures, or the cultures must be considerably enriched for motor neurons by sorting.

A variety of techniques to identify and sort motor neurons have been utilized. The most definitive method is to retrogradely label motor neurons by injecting a vital fluorescent dye into muscles and then sort labeled cells with a fluorescence-activated cell sorter (FACS) (Calof and Reichardt, 1984; O'Brien and Fischbach, 1986). Unfortunately, the yields of neurons obtained with such an approach are low and thus not readily suited to the screening of large numbers of samples. This method also requires a FACS, which is very expensive, takes special training to operate and is not readily available to many investigators. A technically simpler method of sorting motor neurons is to utilize density-gradient purification of large (motor) neurons from small (inter-) neurons (Berg and Fischbach, 1978; Dohrmann, Edgar and Thoenen, 1987; Arakawa, Sendtner and Thoenen, 1990). More recently, a motor neuron-specific monoclonal antibody has been used to 'pan' for motor neurons by coating the bottom of tissue culture dishes so that motor neurons selectively adhere and the other neurons are washed off (Bloch-Gallego *et al.*, 1991). The simplest motor neuron assay does not sort spinal cord cells, but quantifies trophic effects by measuring choline acetyltransferase (ChAT) activity (McManaman *et al.*, 1988). ChAT, the enzyme that synthesizes acetylcholine, is a specific marker for cholinergic neurons. ChAT levels are an accurate index of motor neuron viability if the cholinergic neurons of the preganglionic sympathetic cell column are excluded by dissection and if controls are included to demonstrate that increases in ChAT are due to general metabolic status or changes in numbers of cholinergic neurons rather than due to specific modulation of ChAT. Using the bioassays described above a number of trophic activities for motor neurons have been reported. The sections below describe these trophic factors and discuss the possibility that such an agent may be used in treating motor neuron disease.

25.3 MOTOR NEURON TROPHIC FACTORS

25.3.1 Ciliary neurotrophic factor

Of the motor neuron trophic molecules that have been identified to date, ciliary neurotrophic factor (CNTF) shows the greatest promise in treatment of motor neuron disease. CNTF was isolated and cloned from rat and rabbit sciatic nerves on the basis of its ability to support the survival in cell culture of ciliary ganglion neurons, which are para-sympathetic (Manthorpe *et al.*, 1986; Lin *et al.*, 1989; Stöckli *et al.*, 1989). Recombinant CNTF was subsequently reported to support the survival of spinal cord motor neurons *in vivo* (Oppenheim *et al.*, 1991) and *in vitro* (Arakawa, Sendtner and Thoenen, 1990). CNTF was also shown to prevent the degeneration of axotomized facial nucleus neurons when applied to the facial nerve (Sendtner, Kreutzberg and Thoenen, 1990). Most recently, CNTF prolonged the life and improved motor function of *pmn/pmn* mice, an autosomal recessive mutant that undergoes progressive caudocranial motor neuron degeneration (Sendtner *et al.*, 1992a). In spite of its trophic effect on motor neurons, CNTF is not likely to be a target-derived trophic factor because CNTF is localized in Schwann cells, and CNTF RNA is not detectable in muscle (Thoenen, 1991). In addition, CNTF is only expressed in the sciatic nerve of adult animals and not during the period of motor neuron cell death (Stöckli *et al.*, 1991). Finally, CNTF cannot be secreted by cells that are transfected with a DNA coding for CNTF (Lin *et al.*, 1989; Stöckli *et al.*, 1989; Leung *et al.*, 1992). Nonetheless, based upon its effectiveness in rescuing motor neurons from degeneration, human CNTF is currently being tested in phase I clinical trials for use in the treatment of motor neuron disease.

In light of the possible clinical use of CNTF, it would be essential to note that a variety of different biological actions have been attributed to CNTF. In addition to its ability to support neuronal survival, CNTF suppresses tyrosine hydroxylase activity while inducing choline acetyl-transferase in rat sympathetic neurons (Saadat, Sendtner and Rohrer, 1989), CNTF inhibits mitosis and induces vasoactive intestinal polypep-tide expression in embryonic chick sympathetic neurons (Ernsberger, Sendtner and Rohrer, 1989), CNTF induces the differentiation of type II astrocytes from O2A glial progenitor cells from the optic nerve (Hughes *et al.*, 1988), and CNTF induces early expression of cellular proto-oncogenes in human neuroblastoma cells (Squinto *et al.*, 1990). Long-term, chronic CNTF treatment of patients with motor neuron disease may elicit some or all of these other effects of CNTF. However, should CNTF be effective in slowing motor neuron degeneration, these potential side-effects might still be preferable to the inevitable degeneration of the motor system.

More recently, a ciliary neurotrophic factor called growth-promoting activity (GPA) was isolated from chick sciatic nerve (Eckenstein *et al.*, 1990) and its cDNA cloned from embryonic chick eyes (Leung *et al.*, 1992). Unlike CNTF, GPA is secreted by cells transfected with cDNA coding for GPA, and GPA is expressed during embryonic development. The deduced amino acid sequence of GPA is 50% identical to any of the previously cloned mammalian CNTFs. This degree of sequence identity between human CNTF and chicken GPA is considerably lower than that between human and chicken nerve growth factor and suggests that GPA may be another member of a CNTF family of trophic factors. On the other hand, GPA may simply be chicken CNTF, a molecule that has diverged considerably in structure and function. Regardless of whether or not GPA represents chicken CNTF, similarities between its sequence and that of CNTF may be of use in identifying other related molecules. In particular, the molecular weight and isoelectric point of cholinergic development factor (see below) show marked similarities to those of GPA and CNTF. Thus the true target-derived trophic factor for motor neurons may be a CNTF family member.

25.3.2 Cholinergic development factor

The first motor neuron trophic factor to be purified from muscle was cholinergic development factor (CDF; McManaman *et al.*, 1988). Its name was derived from the bioassay that was used to identify, characterize and purify this molecule. Embryonic day 14 rat spinal cord neurons were plated in culture and various fractions were tested for their ability to enhance ChAT activity 2 days after plating. CDF seems to be present in relatively high concentration in rat muscle because it is purified to apparent homogeneity after only a 5500-fold enrichment in specific activity over the crude extract. The biochemical properties of CDF are similar to those of CNTF (Manthorpe *et al.*, 1986; McManaman *et al.*, 1988; Stöckli *et al.*, 1989) – the molecular weight of CDF is approximately 20.5 kDa, whereas that of CNTF is 21.5 kDa (chick) or 22.5 kDa (rat); the isoelectric point (pI) of CDF is 4.8, whereas the pI of CNTF is 5.0 (chick) or 5.6 (rat); the amino acid compositions of CDF and rat CNTF are also similar. It is impossible to determine directly whether CDF is CNTF or a related molecule because CDF has not been cloned, nor has any amino acid sequence been made publicly available. Although initially it was not clear whether CDF promoted the survival of cholinergic (motor) neurons or whether CDF simply enhanced the ChAT activity of cholinergic neurons that were not killed by lack of muscle extract, more recent studies have shown that embryonic chick motor neurons are rescued from cell death by application of CDF to the chorioallantoic membrane (Oppenheim *et al.*, 1988). Should CDF prove to be different from CNTF, then CDF would be another possible pharmacological agent in treating motor neuron disease.

25.3.3 Fibroblast growth factor (FGF)

Recently FGFs have been identified as having neurotrophic effects on a number of neuronal populations, including motor neurons (see Thoenen, 1991). FGFs are peptide growth factors that were isolated in a number of different systems on the basis of their abilities to stimulate cell division; hence they have received a great deal of attention in the field of cancer biology and growth control. The FGF family of growth factors has seven members, each of which shares about 50% amino acid identity with the other members. The two most abundant and best-studied members are acidic FGF (aFGF) and basic FGF (bFGF). Basic FGF, and to a lesser extent aFGF, has been shown to support motor neuron survival *in vitro* (McManaman *et al.*, 1989; Arakawa, Sendtner and Thoenen, 1990). The effect of bFGF is additive with CNTF at saturating concentrations (Arakawa, Sendtner and Thoenen, 1990), suggesting that the two trophic factors are acting through two independent mechanisms or on two different populations of spinal cord neurons. Interestingly, the application of bFGF to chicken embryos *in ovo* does not rescue motor neurons from cell death, whereas CNTF does (Oppenheim *et al.*, 1991). Thus bFGF may already be sufficiently supplied to the motor neurons *in vivo*, or FGF may not play an essential role in regulating developmental cell death. In light of this observation, it should be noted that bFGF and aFGF are distributed specifically and in non-overlapping domains of the central nervous system – virtually all of the bFGF is found in astrocytes (Woodward *et al.*, 1992), whereas the aFGF is localized in specific neuronal populations including bulbar and spinal cord motor neurons (Elde *et al.*, 1991; Stock *et al.*, 1992). The precise function of the aFGF in neurons is not yet understood, but the combined effects of aFGF with other trophic factors may be essential for full trophic support of motor neurons.

25.3.4 Nerve growth factor and other members of the neurotrophin family

Although nerve growth factor (NGF) does not support survival or promote regeneration of spinal cord motor neurons, other members of the NGF-related trophic factors or neurotrophin family may do so. As described in the introduction to this chapter, NGF is the prototypical target-derived trophic factor for sympathetic and sensory neurons. In 1982 a trophic molecule called brain-derived neurotrophic factor (BDNF) was purified (Barde, Edgar and Thoenen, 1982). After BDNF was cloned it was found to have significant homology to NGF (Leibrock et al., 1989). Regions of homology between NGF and BDNF were, in turn, used to clone other related molecules by polymerase chain reaction. Currently, three molecules in addition to NGF and BDNF have been identified: neurotrophin (NT)-3 (Ernfors et al., 1990; Hohn et al., 1990; Jones and Reichardt, 1990; Maisonpierre et al., 1990; Rosenthal et al., 1990), NT-4 (Hallböök, Ibáñez and Persson, 1991) and NT-5 (Berkemeier et al., 1991). All of these molecules share approximately 50% amino acid identity with NGF. NGF, BDNF and the neurotrophins have now been grouped together as the neurotrophin family of trophic factors.

Embryonic motor neurons in the spinal cord express a neurotrophin-binding molecule known as P75, which was originally called the low-affinity NGF receptor (Eckenstein, 1988). The expression of P75 is not detectable in adult spinal cord, but it reappears when the motor neurons are axotomized (Koliatsos, Crawford and Price, 1991). All neurons that respond to neurotrophins express P75, and P75 binds all neurotrophins equally well. Specificity of neurotrophin binding and signal transduction is conferred by another membrane glycoprotein, trk (reviewed in Chao, 1992). To date, three different trk proteins that share amino acid homology with one another have been identified. NGF binds specifically to trk-A (Kaplan et al., 1991) whereas BDNF binds more specifically to trk-B (Squinto et al., 1991). The expression of P75 in motor neurons after injury suggests that a neurotrophin may be a trophic factor for motor neurons. Since motor neurons do not respond to NGF (Yan et al., 1988), they may respond to BDNF, NT-3, NT-4 or NT-5. The expression of specific trks in axotomized motor neurons or in post-mortem tissue of patients with motor neuron disease has not been investigated. Specific trk expression would indicate which of the neurotrophins is the likeliest ligand for motor neurons. Neurotrophin action on motor neurons remains a largely unexplored area.

Recent reports have suggested that brain-derived neurotrophic factor (BDNF) may be the neurotrophin that interacts with the p75 receptor expressed on embryonic and axotomized motor neurons. BDNF has been shown to prevent the death of motor neurons in newborn rats after axotomy (Yan *et al.*, 1992; Sendtner *et al.*, 1992b); and to rescue avian motor neurons from developmental cell death (Oppenheim *et al.*, 1992).

23.3.5 Neuroleukin

Neuroleukin initially received attention as a potential trophic factor whose inactivation by an autoimmune response was a possible cause for some cases of ALS (Gurney, 1984; Gurney *et al.*, 1986). The basis for this claim was as follows. Rabbit antisera against an antigen in medium conditioned by a denervated rat hemidiaphragm were isolated. Some were able to suppress botulinum toxin-induced terminal sprouting in the mouse gluteus muscle. The antisera that suppressed sprouting recognized a 56-kDa protein from rat hemidiaphragm that was not recognized by non-blocking antisera. The same sprouting assay was also used to test sera from 19 sporadic ALS patients with both upper and lower motor neuron signs. Sprouting was significantly suppressed by 8/19 ALS sera, and the three most effective ALS sera also recognized a 56-kDa protein from hemidiaphragm (Gurney, 1984). Monoclonal antibodies against this 56-kDa protein were subsequently prepared and used to identify the molecule in order to biochemically purify the antigen from mouse salivary glands (Gurney *et al.*, 1986). The antigen was sequenced and the sequence information used to clone a cDNA. The 56-kDa molecule was shown to support the survival of spinal and sensory neurons in cell culture and also acted as a potent lymphokine (Gurney *et al.*, 1986), hence its naming as 'neuroleukin'.

Unfortunately, neuroleukin is no longer thought to be relevant to ALS for several reasons. First, recombinant neuroleukin is not recognized by the three ALS sera that blocked sprouting in mouse muscle (Gurney *et al.*, 1986); thus it is not the same 56-kDa protein that was originally described. Secondly, if autoimmune antibodies against neuroleukin are a cause of ALS, then the complete lack of sensory degeneration and immune dysfunction in ALS is not consistent with the abilities of neuroleukin to support sensory neuron survival and to act as a lymphokine. Finally, it has been reported that the amino acid sequence of neuroleukin is identical to that of mouse glucose-6-phosphate isomerase, a ubiquitous enzyme that is a part of the glycolytic metabolic pathway (Faik *et al.*, 1988). Indeed, the rabbit polyclonal and the mouse monoclonal antibodies against neuroleukin that were described above cross-react with highly purified glucose-6-phosphate isomerase from rabbit heart (Sigma, Type XI) (Gurney, reply to Faik *et al.*, *Nature*, **332**, 456). It seems unlikely that an intracellular enzyme would also be a secreted neurotrophic factor. As a result, interest in neuroleukin as a motor neuron trophic factor has receded.

25.3.6 Neuropeptides

Neuropeptides that are localized to terminal boutons surrounding spinal cord and bulbar motor neurons have been reported to have neurotrophic effects. These include thyrotrophin-releasing hormone (TRH), cholecystokinin, vasoactive intestinal polypeptide, vasopressin and somatostatin (Schmidt-Ackert, Askanas and Engel, 1984; Iwasaki *et al.*, 1991; Weill, 1991). Peptides have several advantages over larger proteins as a pharmacological agent. Peptides are more stable, readily diffusible and more inexpensive to produce because they can be synthesized. However, because most of these peptides also function as neurotransmitters, it is possible that their effectiveness in supporting survival may be by depolarization of motor neurons. The ionic fluxes associated with chronic depolarization are known to support neuronal survival in cell culture. For example, increasing the potassium concentration of the medium increases neuronal survival in cell culture (Lasher and Zagon, 1972; Bennett and White, 1979; Chalazonitis and Fischbach, 1980). However, the physiological status of chronically depolarized neurons is suboptimal and is further enhanced by addition of trophic factor (Nishi and Berg, 1981). If the peptide must act at synapses within the CNS, then the peptide must cross the blood–brain barrier or it must be administered intrathecally. In either case, possibly unacceptable side-effects may result from the overall changes in neuronal activity.

Clinical investigations using TRH for treating motor neuron disease have been reported since 1983 (reviewed in Brooks, 1989). Whether TRH has any long-term beneficial effect on patients with motor neuron disease has been controversial because many conflicting results have been published. The effectiveness of TRH appears to depend upon whether the patient is male or female and whether the patient exhibits bulbar or non-bulbar signs. In addition receptors for TRH appear to decrease with the progression of motor neuron disease, TRH administration becomes less effective as the disease progresses. Thus the use of TRH may have some short-term beneficial effect by increasing muscular strength, probably by enhancing motor neuron activity; however, TRH is unlikely to improve the long-term prognosis of patients with motor neuron disease.

25.4 FUTURE DIRECTIONS

The isolation and cloning of a target-derived trophic factor for motor neurons remains a priority with respect to motor neuron disease. A true target-derived trophic factor may be considerably more potent than the molecules described above in promoting the repair and survival of

Trophic factors

motor neurons. More importantly, the information obtained by cloning the muscle-derived trophic factor can be used to test whether the cause of motor neuron disease is a lack of availability of trophic factor. For example, when the nucleic acid sequence of the mRNA coding for the factor is obtained, then the extremely sensitive polymerase chain reaction technique could be used to assay for the presence of trophic factor RNA in small biopsies of muscles from patients with motor neuron disease. In addition, antibodies against the factor could be used to develop highly sensitive two-site immunoassays to quantify trophic factor protein levels in muscle and in sera. The availability of recombinant trophic factor would allow one to test sera from patients with motor neuron disease for autoantibodies that may inactivate endogenous trophic factor. Finally, one avenue that remains largely unexplored is to determine whether there is a trophic reason for the relatively high resistance of oculomotor and sacral motor nuclei to the degenerative process that occurs in motor neuron disease.

25.5 SUMMARY

Significant progress in the identification and characterization of neuro-trophic factors has been made over the last decade. Trophic factors are essential for the survival of many neuronal cell types and have proven to be potent agents in stimulating axonal regeneration and neuronal cell repair. Several candidate trophic factors have been identified for motor neurons. One trophic factor, CNTF, is undergoing testing for the treatment of motor neuron disease; however, a true target-derived trophic factor for motor neurons has yet to be cloned. If the degenerative process has not permanently impaired the capacity of the neurons of patients with motor neuron disease to respond to trophic factors, then the administration of motor neuron trophic factors may hold some promise for slowing or even halting the progressive neuronal degeneration associated with motor neuron disease.

REFERENCES

Arakawa, Y., Sendtner, M. and Thoenen, H. (1990) Survival effect of ciliary neurotrophic factor (CNTF) on chick embryonic motoneurons in culture: comparison with other neurotrophic factors and cytokines. *J. Neurosci.*, **10**, 3507–15.

Barde, Y.-A., Edgar, D. and Thoenen, H. (1982) Purification of a new neurotrophic factor from mammalian brain. *EMBO J.*, **1**, 549–53.

Bennett, M.R. and White, W. (1979) The survival and development of cholinergic neurons in potassium-enriched media. *Brain Res.*, **173**, 549–53.

References

Berg, D.K. and Fischbach, G.D. (1978) Enrichment of spinal cord cell cultures with motoneurons. *J. Cell Biol.*, **77**, 83–98.

Berkemeier, L.R., Winslow, J.W., Kaplan, D.R. *et al.* (1991) Neurotrophin-5: a novel neurotrophic factor that activates trk and trkB. *Neuron*, **7**, 857–66.

Bloch-Gallego, E., Huchet, M., El M'Hamdi, H. *et al.* (1991) Survival *in vitro* of motoneurons identified or purified by novel antibody-based methods is selectively enhanced by muscle-derived factors. *Development*, **111**, 221–32.

Brooks, B.R. (1989) A summary of the current position of TRH in ALS therapy. *Ann. N.Y. Acad. Sci.*, **553**, 431–61.

Calof, A.L. and Reichardt, L.F. (1984) Motoneurons purified by cell sorting respond to two distinct activities in myotube-conditioned medium. *Dev. Biol.*, **106**, 194–210.

Chalazonitis, A. and Fischbach, G.D. (1980) Elevated potassium induced morphological differentiation of dorsal root ganglionic neurons in dissociated cell culture. *Dev. Biol.*, **78**, 173–83.

Chao, M.V. (1992) Growth factor signaling: where is the specificity? *Cell*, **68**, 995–7.

Dohrmann, U., Edgar, D. and Thoenen, H. (1987) Distinct neurotrophic factors from skeletal muscle and the central nervous system interact synergistically to support the survival of cultured embryonic spinal motor neurons. *Dev. Biol.*, **124**, 145–52.

Eckenstein, F. (1988) Transient expression of NGF-receptor-like immunoreactivity in postnatal rat brain and spinal cord. *Brain Res.*, **446**, 149–54.

Eckenstein, F.P., Esch, F., Holbert, T. *et al.* (1990) Purification and characterization of a trophic factor for embryonic peripheral neurons: comparison with fibroblast growth factors. *Neuron*, **4**, 623–31.

Elde, R., Cao, Y., Cintra, A. *et al.* (1991) Prominent expression of acidic fibroblast growth factor in motor and sensory neurons. *Neuron*, **7**, 349–64.

Ernfors, P., Ibanez, C.F., Ebendal, T. *et al.* (1990) Molecular cloning and neurotrophic activities of a protein with structural similarities to nerve growth factor: developmental and topographical expression in the brain. *Proc. Natl. Acad. Sci. USA*, **87**, 5454–8.

Ernsberger, U., Sendtner, M. and Rohrer, H. (1989) Proliferation and differentiation of embryonic chick sympathetic neurons: effects of ciliary neurotrophic factor. *Neuron*, **2**, 1275–84.

Faik, P., Walker, J.I.H., Redmill, A.A.M. and Morgan, M.J. (1988) Mouse glucose-6-phosphate isomerase and neuroleukin have identical 3' sequences. *Nature*, **332**, 455–7.

Gurney, M.E. (1984) Suppression of sprouting at the neuromuscular junction by immune sera. *Nature*, **307**, 546–8.

Gurney, M.E., Heinrich, S.P., Lee, M.R. and Yin, H. (1986) Molecular cloning and expression of neuroleukin, a neurotrophic factor for spinal and sensory neurons. *Science*, **234**, 566–73.

Hallböök, F., Ibáñez, C.F. and Persson, H. (1991) Evolutionary studies of the nerve growth factor family reveal a novel member abundantly expressed in *Xenopus* ovary. *Neuron*, **6**, 845–8.

Trophic factors

Hohn, A., Leibrock, J., Bailey, K. and Barde, Y.-A. (1990) Identification and characterization of a novel member of the nerve growth factor/brain-derived neurotrophic factor family. *Nature*, **344**, 339–41.

Houenou, L.J., McManaman, J.L., Prevette, D. and Oppenheim, R.W. (1991) Regulation of putative muscle-derived neurotrophic factors by muscle activity and innervation: *in vivo* and *in vitro* studies. *J. Neurosci.*, **11**, 2829–37.

Hughes, S.M., Lillien, L.E., Raff, M.C. *et al.* (1988) Ciliary neurotrophic factor induces type-2 astrocyte differentiation in culture. *Nature*, **335**, 70–3.

Iwasaki, Y., Kinoshita, M., Ikeda, K. *et al.* (1991) Trophic effect of angiotensin II, vasopressin and other peptides on the cultured ventral spinal cord of rat embryo. *J. Neurol. Sci.*, **103**, 151–5.

Jones, K.R. and Reichardt, L.F. (1990) Molecular cloning of a human gene that is a member of the nerve growth factor family. *Proc. Natl. Acad. Sci. USA*, **87**, 8060–4.

Kaplan, D.R., Hempstead, B.L., Martin-Zanca, D. *et al.* (1991) The trk proto-oncogene product: a signal transducing receptor for nerve growth factor. *Science*, **252**, 558–60.

Koliatsos, V.E., Crawford, T.O. and Price, D.L. (1991) Axotomy induces nerve growth factor receptor immunoreactivity in spinal motor neurons. *Brain Res.*, **549**, 297–304.

Kozachuk, W.E., Mitsumoto, H., Salanga, V.D. *et al.* (1987) Thyrotropin-releasing hormone (TRH) in murine motor neuron disease (the wobbler mouse). *J. Neurol. Sci.*, **78**, 253–60.

Lasher, J. and Zagon, R. (1972) The effect of potassium on neuronal differentiation in cultures of dissociated newborn rat cerebellum. *Brain Res.*, **41**, 482–8.

Leibrock, J., Lottspeich, F., Hohn, A. *et al.* (1989) Molecular cloning and expression of brain-derived neurotrophic factor. *Nature*, **341**, 149–52.

Leung, D.W., Parent, A.S., Cachianes, G. *et al.* (1992) Cloning, expression during development, and evidence for release of a trophic factor for ciliar ganglion neurons. *Neuron*, **8**, 1045–53.

Lin, L.-F.H., Mismer, D., Lile, J.D. *et al.* (1989) Purification, cloning, and expression of ciliary neurotrophic factor (CNTF). *Science*, **246**, 1023–5.

Maisonpierre, P.C., Belluscio, L., Squinto, S. *et al.* (1990) Neurotrophin-3: a neurotrophic factor related to NGF and BDNF. *Science*, **247**, 1446–51.

Manthorpe, M., Skaper, S.D., Williams, L.R. and Varon, S. (1986) Purification of adult rat sciatic nerve ciliary neuronotrophic factor. *Brain Res.*, **367**, 282–6.

McManaman, J.L., Crawford, F.G., Stewart, S.S. and Appel, S.H. (1988) Purification of a skeletal muscle polypeptide which stimulates choline acetyltransferase activity in cultured spinal cord neurons. *J. Biol. Chem.*, **263**, 5890–7.

McManaman, J., Crawford, F., Clark, R. *et al.* (1989) Multiple neurotrophic factors from skeletal muscle: demonstration of effects of basic fibroblast growth factor and comparisons with the 22-kilodalton choline acetyltransferase development factor. *J. Neurochem.*, **53**, 1763–71.

Nishi, R. and Berg, D.K. (1981) Two components from eye tissue that differentially stimulate the growth and development of ciliary ganglion neurons in cell culture. *J. Neurosci.*, **1**, 505–13.

O'Brien, R.J. and Fischbach, G.D. (1986) Isolation of embryonic chick motoneurons and their survival *in vitro. J. Neurosci.*, **6**, 3265–74.

Oppenheim, R. (1991) Cell death during development of the nervous system. *Ann. Rev. Neurosci.*, **14**, 453–501.

Oppenheim, R.W., Haverkamp, L.J., Prevette, D. *et al.* (1988) Reduction of naturally-occurring motoneuron death *in vivo* by a target-derived neurotrophic factor. *Science*, **240**, 919–22.

Oppenheim, R.W., Prevette, D., Qin-Wei, Y. *et al.* (1991) Control of embryonic motoneuron survival *in vivo* by ciliary neurotrophic factor. *Science*, **251**, 1616–18.

Oppenheim, R.W. *et al.* (1992) *Nature*, **360**, 755–7.

Rosenthal, A., Goeddel, D.V., Nguyen, T. *et al.* (1990) Primary structure and biological activity of a novel human neurotrophic factor. *Neuron*, **4**, 767–73.

Saadat, S., Sendtner, M. and Rohrer, H. (1989) Ciliary neurotrophic factor induces cholinergic differentiation of rat sympathetic neurons in culture. *J. Cell Biol.*, **108**, 1807–16.

Schmidt-Ackert, K.M., Askanas, V. and Engel, W.K. (1984) Thyrotropin releasing hormone enhances choline acetyltransferase and creatine kinase in cultured spinal ventral horn neurons. *J. Neurochem.*, **43**, 586–9.

Sendtner, M., Kreutzberg, G.W. and Thoenen, H. (1990) Ciliary neurotrophic factor prevents the degeneration of motoneurones after axotomy. *Nature*, **345**, 440–1.

Sendtner, M., Schmalbruch, H., Stöcklie, K.A. *et al.* (1992a) Ciliary neurotrophic factor prevents degeneration of motor neurons in mouse mutant progressive motor neuronopathy. *Nature*, **358**, 502–4.

Sendtner, M. *et al.* (1992b) *Nature*, **360**, 757–9.

Squinto, S.P., Aldrich, T.H., Lindsay, R.M. *et al.* (1990) Identification of functional receptors for ciliary neurotrophic factor on neuronal cell lines and primary neurons. *Neuron*, **5**, 757–66.

Squinto, S.P., Stitt, T.N., Aldrich, T.H. *et al.* (1991) trkB encodes a functional receptor for brain-derived neurotrophic factor and neurotrophin-3 but not nerve growth factor. *Cell*, **65**, 885–94.

Stock, A., Kuzis, K., Woodward, W.R. *et al.* Localization of acidic fibroblast growth factor in specific subcortical neuronal populations: overlap with populations expressing the low affinity nerve growth factor receptor. *J. Neurosci.*, **12**, 4688–700.

Stöckli, K.A., Lottspeich, F., Sendtner, M. *et al.* (1989) Molecular cloning, expression and regional distribution of rat ciliary neurotrophic factor. *Nature*, **342**, 920–3.

Stöckli, K.A., Lillien, L.E., Näher-Noé, M. *et al.* (1991) Regional distribution, developmental changes and cellular localization of CNTF-mRNA and protein in the rat brain. *J. Cell Biol.*, **115**, 447–59.

Thoenen, H. (1991) The changing scene of neurotrophic factors. *Trends Neurosci.*, **14**, 165–70.

Trophic factors

Thoenen, H. and Barde, Y.-A. (1980) Physiology of nerve growth factor. *Physiol. Rev.*, **60**, 1284–335.

Weill, C.L. (1991) Somatostatin (SRIF) prevents natural motoneuron cell death in embryonic chick spinal cord. *Dev. Neurosci.*, **13**, 377–81.

Woodward, W., Nishi, R., Meshul, C.K. *et al.* (1992) Nuclear and cytoplasmic localization of basic fibroblast growth factor in astrocytes and CA2 hippocampal neurons. *J. Neurosci.*, **12**, 142–52.

Yan, Q., Snider, W.D., Pinzone, J.J. and Johnson, E.M. (1988) Retrograde transport of nerve growth factor (NGF) in motoneurons of developing rats: assessment of potential neurotrophic effects. *Neuron*, **1**, 335–43.

Yan, Q. *et al.* (1992) *Nature*, **360**, 753–5.

26 Chemical toxins

PETER B. NUNN

This chapter is dedicated to the memory of Mr Reginald S. Kay, a sufferer from motor neurone disease, who was a generous benefactor to the author's laboratory.

26.1 INTRODUCTION

While there is an anecdotal belief that toxic compounds may be implicated in the aetiology of sporadic motor neurone disease and in other disorders in which neuronal death is a prominent feature (see for example Tandan and Bradley, 1985), there is little firm evidence to support this contention. However, the more considered view that, under some circumstances, food-borne toxic compounds may cause neurodegeneration in man, in domestic or experimental animals or in laboratory test systems is readily substantiated. This chapter attempts to bring together data concerning some neurotoxic compounds that occur in plants, considers the evidence for their involvement in specific disease states and reviews the mechanisms by which they may act. Because of their origins it is convenient to consider these compounds in the context of their botanical vectors. A recent general review of some of the principles discussed here is available (Meldrum and Garthwaite, 1990).

26.2 *LATHYRUS SATIVUS*

This leguminous plant (common names chickling pea; grass pea) has been known since historical times to cause in man the chronic neurological disease neurolathyrism (Sarma and Padmanaban, 1969; Ludolph *et al.*, 1987). This is regrettable because *L. sativus* is rich in protein and other nutrients. As a nitrogen-fixing legume it thrives on poor soils without the need for nitrogen fertilizers. It is resistant to both

567

Chemical toxins

drought and flooding and it can be grown in harsh environments that will not support other crop plants. *L. sativus* is a robust, reliable and dependable food for many thousands of people; it can be regarded as the nutritional equivalent of the Volkswagen Beetle to the Third World.

Neurolathyrism is characterized by a spastic paraparesis and appears to be non-progressive in that the condition of afflicted subjects changes little once consumption of the seed ceases. Today neurolathyrism is endemic in Ethiopia, India, Bangladesh, Nepal and China. The active principle is generally believed to be the non-protein amino acid, β-*N*-oxalyl-L-α,β-diaminopropionic acid (β-ODAP; synonym, β-oxalyl-amino-L-alanine, BOAA) (Nunn, 1989), which was first isolated by Rao, Adiga and Sarma (1963). This compound was quickly found to be a neuroexcitant in cat spinal motor neurones and Betz cells (Watkins, Curtis and Biscoe, 1966). Subsequently the compound was shown to cause a similar neuropathology (Olney, Misra and Rhee, 1976) to that which characterized the group of acidic amino acids that Olney termed 'excitotoxins' (Olney, Ho and Rhee, 1971). The principle underlying the 'excitotoxic theory of neuronal death' (see Olney, 1978) is that excitatory amino acids overactivate neuronal receptors, allowing entry of sodium, which depolarizes the cell membrane; the energy supplies of the cell are depleted in a vain attempt (by the membrane-bound Na^+/K^+-ATPase) to re-establish ionic homeostasis, but osmotic vacuolation occurs within the neurone due to the influx of Na^+, Cl^- and water, which leads to subsequent physical damage to the cell. This simplistic mechanism is now known to be rather more elaborate; vacuolation need not necessarily give rise to neurodegeneration provided the situation is reversed rapidly; neurodegeneration appears to be Ca^{2+}-dependent (Choi, 1985, 1987) which, to add to the cellular damage caused by the osmotic effects, would activate Ca^{2+}-dependent proteases and lipases (see Eberhard and Holz, 1988) and also increase the expression of immediate-early genes in neurones (Sheng and Greenberg, 1990).

The subdivision of receptors for excitatory amino acids (Watkins and Evans, 1981) stimulated analysis of the specific subgroup of glutamate receptors that were activated by β-ODAP. Judged by the effects of a group of antagonists the compound was active against non-NMDA receptors, i.e those glutamate receptors that are not activated by the model compound *N*-methyl-D-aspartate (Pearson and Nunn, 1981; MacDonald and Morris, 1984). Binding studies revealed that β-ODAP binds to α-amino-3-hydroxy-5-methyl-4-isoxazolepropionate (AMPA) receptors (see Monaghan, Bridges and Cotman, 1989) at low concentrations and to kainate receptors and AMPA receptors at higher concentrations (Bridges *et al.*, 1988; Ross, Roy and Spencer, 1989). Activation of non-NMDA receptors would cause neurones to depolarize allowing the influx of Na^+, but Ca^{2+} does not enter cells through the ion channels that are regulated by these receptors. However, Ca^{2+} influx would result from the activation of voltage-sensitive calcium channels, and these two mechanisms probably account for the excitotoxic pathology shown by Olney, Misra and Rhee (1976) in the mouse pup.

The question must be asked as to whether these mechanisms are responsible for the signs and symptoms seen in sufferers from neurolathyrism. Perhaps neuroexcitation may account for the muscle cramps that are commonly experienced. However, evidence from clinical studies suggests that clonus (due to upper motor neurone dysfunction) is a prominent early feature of neurolathyrism. This evidence suggests that upper motor neurones are specifically damaged in this disorder, demonstrating a specificity that is difficult to reconcile with the known neuropharmacological properties of the cell types that carry kainate and AMPA receptors (see for example Schwob *et al.*, 1980). On this basis it might be expected that, once β-ODAP entered the central nervous system and reached a suitable concentration, it would activate all cell types that carried non-NMDA receptors, but the human clinical condition appears to contradict that simplistic impression. It is possible that β-ODAP might cause excitotoxicity by a presynaptic mechanism in that, at least in guinea-pig hippocampal mossy fibre synaptosomes, the compound causes the release of glutamate (Gannon and Terrian, 1989). However, β-ODAP (200 μM) released only the cytosolic pool of glutamate and not the vesicular pool and, therefore, it is difficult to assess the extent to which this effect might stimulate post-synaptic excitotoxicity *in vivo*. No attempt was made in these experiments to antagonize the effect of β-ODAP. However, at least some kainate receptors are thought to be located presynaptically and it is conceivable, in view of the pharmacological specificity of β-ODAP, that the effect was mediated by these receptors. A further effect of β-ODAP that is mediated presynaptically is that of inhibition of glutamate uptake by synaptosomes (Lakshmanan and Padmanaban, 1974), which would result in glutamate being retained in the synaptic cleft after release from presynaptic stores.

Attempts to model neurolathyrism in experimental animals have had only limited success and direct administration into the cerebrospinal fluid has been used as a means of achieving acute responses. When β-ODAP is administered direct into the cerebrospinal fluid in macaques, a flaccid paralysis occurs with extensive neuropathology (Mani *et al.*, 1971); in the rat the compound also causes extensive neuropathological damage (Chase *et al.*, 1985), but a spastic extensor paralysis is generated. In the carefully designed experiments of Spencer *et al.* (1986), in which macaques were fed on diets containing *L. sativus* or purified β-ODAP for several months, the animals developed to a stage that the authors believed was equivalent to an early stage of neurolathyrism in man (Hugon *et al.*, 1988). However, on returning these animals to normal food the signs and symptoms were lost. There was no neuropathology except for a mild chromatolysis in some neurones (P.S. Spencer, personal communication). Such a reversible effect seems unlikely to be perpetrated against neurones, and more recent work has suggested non-excitotoxic mechanisms by which such a reversible effect might come about.

β-ODAP appears to interact with facets of the monoamine system in the central nervous system. In rat brain slices the compound inhibits the adrenaline-stimulated hydrolysis of phosphoinositides. The inhibition is concentration dependent with an IC_{50} of 300 μM and is insensitive to excitatory amino acid antagonists. These results resemble those obtained with quisqualate and the authors (Ormandy and Jope, 1990) proposed that the two compounds might act at a unique common site for which β-ODAP was the more selective agonist. Further evidence of a non-excitotoxic mechanism involving monamines is that the amino acid inhibits the uptake of noradrenaline into cortical synaptosomes (Lindstrom *et al.*, 1990). It is not clear whether there is a relationship between these two effects.

An additional non-excitotoxic mechanism mediated by β-ODAP is that of glial toxicity. The early experiments of Olney in which a wide range of acidic amino acids were administered to the mouse pup revealed that L-α-aminoadipate (the higher homologue of L-glutamate) was not neurotoxic in that system but instead was a glial toxin (Olney, Ho and Rhee, 1971). No satisfactory explanation for the dramatic differences in the activities of these two compounds is available. Relatively high concentrations (2 mM) of β-ODAP were also toxic to cultured astrocytes (Bridges *et al.*, 1991), using as an indicator of cell death the release of the cytosolic enzyme lactate dehydrogenase into the incubation medium (Koh and Choi, 1987). Under the same conditions 47% of astrocytes survived after 48 h treatment with β-ODAP; only 19% survived the same concentration of L-α-aminoadipate. Thus by comparison with L-α-aminoadipate β-ODAP is an effective gliotoxin, but it is difficult to evaluate the importance of this effect at such a relatively high concentration. Neither AMPA nor kainate was gliotoxic under these conditions which, since the cells carry non-MNDA receptors, suggests that the cytotoxicity was not mediated by these receptor subtypes. It is not clear at present whether the effects seen here with β-ODAP are mediated by similar mechanisms to those seen when astrocytes are treated with quisqualate (1 mM). Here the gliotoxic response was seen to be a transient phenomenon dependent upon the number of days that the cells had spent *in vitro* (Haas and Erdo, 1991); unfortunately, no antagonist studies were reported. It is evident that β-ODAP can also cause metabolic changes in cultured astrocytes that are probably independent of effects on metabotrophic glutamate receptors at which β-ODAP is a weak agonist (R.J. Bridges, personal communication). Thus, β-ODAP causes the induction of glutamine synthetase in these cells by a mechanism that requires the compound to enter the cells (as judged by the inhibitory effect of the transport inhibitor dihydrokainate) and to increase the activity of glutamine synthetase by a process that is affected at the translational level (Millar, Nunn and Bridges, in Press). This effect has an EC_{50} of approximately 55 μM, which is below the level of cytotoxicity in the cultured astrocyte preparation and, as the effect appears to require intracellular β-ODAP, could be important even at low extracellular concentrations of the amino acid provided that a sufficiently high intracellular concentration could be maintained.

26.3 CYCAS CIRCINALIS

Culinary use of the seed of the false sago palm (*Cycas circinalis*) from Guam has been known since towards the end of the eighteenth century (Steel and Guzman, 1987). The island has also been known since 1945 for the high incidence there of a chronic neurological disease termed amyotrophic lateral sclerosis (motor neurone disease)–parkinsonism–dementia (ALS–PD). The relationship between the consumption of *C. circinalis* seed and ALS–PD was proposed by Kurland and Mulder (1954) and explored by Whiting (1963), whose comprehensive review of the subject summarizes a model investigation. *Cycas* species are known to contain a glycoside, cycasin, in which the carbohydrate residue is glucose, but a number of other sugars form glycosides with the same aglycone, methylazoxymethanol (MAM). Unwashed cycad seed is known to be both an emetic and to cause diarrhoea, and the native Chamorros of Guam have evolved the cultural habit of washing the seed extensively before use. Cycasin was investigated as a tumorigenic agent (Laqueur, 1965); hydrolysis of the β-glycosidic bond by gastrointestinal bacteria to yield MAM was required in rats before hepatic tumour generation. No neurotoxicity was known until it was shown that MAM causes changes in the cerebellar development of newborn mice (Jones, Yang and Michelson, 1972). Recent evidence suggests that cycasin is taken up by mouse cortical tissue and that this process competes for transport with 2-deoxyglucose, which is itself an indicator of glucose transport into neural tissue. Further, cycasin causes selective neuronal degeneration in mouse cortical explants that is antagonized by D-2-

amino-7-phosphonoheptanoate (D-AP7), a competitive antagonist towards NMDA receptors, which implies that the mechanism is mediated by these receptors (Kisby *et al.*, 1992).

During a purposeful search for acidic amino acids in *C. circinalis* seed Vega and Bell (1967) discovered α-amino-β-methylaminopropionic acid (MeDAP; synonym; β-methylamino-L-alanine). This compound was neurotoxic to chicks, rats and mice, which gave rise to speculation that MeDAP was indeed the neurotoxic principle involved in Guam ALS–PD. Although the acute toxicity of the compound was beyond doubt, chronic treatment of rats for 78 days showed no obvious neurological deficits (Polsky, Nunn and Bell, 1972). Subsequently, oral ingestion of the compound over several weeks by macaques gave rise to a neurological dysfunction with pronounced changes in conduction velocity from motor cortex to the periphery and with neuropathological features particularly associated with upper motor neurones (Spencer *et al.*, 1987). These effects were clearly different from those seen in acute experiments in the rat, which were shown to be associated with neuropathological features in the cerebellum (Seawright *et al.*, 1990). The thorough washing procedure adopted by the native people of Guam might be expected to remove soluble material such as MeDAP and MAM. Duncan *et al.* (1990) showed that the concentration of MeDAP varied from 0.74 to 15.2 mg per 100 g of dry flour and concluded that the compound could not be responsible for Guam ALS–PD. However this explanation is itself not beyond criticism in that it is difficult to extrapolate from the content of a potential toxin in a food source to its effects, especially long term, in man. Cycad flour tends to be produced by small-scale units on Guam, and the concentration of residual toxins would be expected to vary widely. It is of interest in this context that [^{14}C]MeDAP is accumulated by mouse cortical explants and the Na$^+$-dependent accumulation of the compound was observed in synaptosomes prepared from Swiss mice (Kisby *et al.*, 1992).

Although the role, if any, that MeDAP might play in Guamanian ALS–PD is in doubt [see Garutto and Yase (1986) for a consideration of other aetiological factors], considerable efforts have been made to establish the mechanism by which its toxicity is expressed. Only the natural L-isomer is toxic to experimental animals (Vega, Bell and Nunn, 1968) and organotypic cultures of fetal mouse spinal cord (Nunn *et al.*, 1987). The vacuolation seen in cultured fetal mouse spinal cord dorsal root ganglia is similar to, but kinetically different from, that seen when excitotoxic amino acids are applied to the same preparation (Nunn *et al.*, 1987). The compound is also less effective than, for example, NMDA in that it produces a response in the mM, rather than μM, concentration range. The effectiveness of MeDAP in producing typical excitotoxic damage is surprising in that MeDAP is a basic rather than an acidic amino acid. This behaviour suggests that a metabolite or an indirect action of MeDAP might be responsible for the observed neuronotoxicity of the compound. Antagonist studies revealed that MeDAP was active at NMDA receptors, judged by the antagonism by MK 801 and D-AP7 (Ross, Seelig and Spencer, 1987). However, in fetal mouse mixed cortical cell cultures the neurotoxicity of the compound was more complex in that cells containing NADPH diaphorase (now known to be nitric oxide synthase; see Bredt and Snyder, 1992) were especially sensitive to the lower concentrations of MeDAP and were protected by kynurenate, which is a general antagonist at non-MNDA receptors. A striking discovery was that the neurotoxic effects of MeDAP were dependent upon the presence of bicarbonate in the medium (Weiss and Choi, 1988). Increasing the bicarbonate concentration within the physiological range up to 24 mM greatly increased the neuronotoxicity of MeDAP. The effect of bicarbonate was also clearly seen in outside-out membrane patches from murine cortical neurones, where an increased frequency of opening of NMDA-regulated ion channels was apparent in the presence of 12 mM sodium bicarbonate (Weiss, Christine and Choi, 1989).

The explanation for the neurotoxicity of MeDAP in the presence of bicarbonate probably lies in the formation of carbamates. The amino group of MeDAP reacts with bicarbonate or carbon dioxide to yield an α-carbamate, but the reaction does not go to completion, and about 10% of the free amino acid reacts (Nunn and O'Brien, 1989). The formation of the α-carbamate causes an apparent inversion of configuration at the α-carbon atom and the product appears to be a structural analogue of NMDA. The β-methylcarbamate is also formed in a reaction of MeDAP with bicarbonate, and at equilibrium the concentration is approximately one-third that of the α-carbamate (Myers and Nelson, 1990). A mixture of MeDAP and 25 mM bicarbonate in equilibrium with carbon dioxide would yield at equilibrium approximately 10% α-carbamate, 3% β-methylcarbamate and 87% of the free amino acid. Carbamate formation also appears to be a factor in the toxicity of cysteine (Olney *et al.*, 1990; Nunn, Davies and O'Brien, 1991).

MeDAP is also an exceptionally good chelator of copper and zinc, and with zinc forms a 2:1 complex in the *cis* configuration (Nunn *et al.*, 1989). It is difficult to evaluate the effect that metal chelation might have in terms of neurotoxicity, but both zinc and copper have complex functions within the central nervous system. One effect that would be expected to assume importance depends upon the desensitization of NMDA receptors by zinc (Peters, Koh and Choi, 1987). Removal of this zinc by avid chelating agents would increase the sensitivity of NMDA receptors, thus making neurones more susceptible to the effects of neuroexcitants.

Chemical toxins

Apart from the effects of MeDAP upon ionotrophic glutamate receptors, it is now clear that the compound also activates metabo-trophic receptors, which are linked to inositol phospholipid hydrolysis. MeDAP enhanced inositol phospholipid hydrolysis in hippocampal slices from 9-day-old rats. The effect at 1 mM was greater than that of glutamate itself, but less than that of 1-amino-1,3-cyclopentane-*trans*-dicarboxylate (*trans*-ACPD). This agonist specifies the receptor subtype; see Monaghan, Bridges and Cotman (1989). Antagonist studies showed that the effect was not mediated by NMDA receptors. As with the excitatory amino acids [^{3}H]inositol phosphate formation was much greater in slices from immature animals than in adult tissue (Copani, Canonico and Nicoletti, 1990; Copani *et al.*, 1991). It is not clear from these studies whether the effect of MeDAP at metabotrophic receptors is dependent upon the presence of bicarbonate.

Using primary cultures of striatal neurones with MK 801 and 6-cyano-7-nitroquinoxaline-2,3-dione (CNQX) to antagonize the effects of NMDA and non-NMDA receptors, respectively, revealed that MeDAP was a full agonist at metabotrophic receptors, but was less potent than *trans*-ACPD. However, this result was obtained in the presence of only 3 mM bicarbonate, which is submaximal in terms of the effect of MeDAP on NMDA receptors, so that the calculated EC_{50} of 0.95 mM might have been lower had the bicarbonate concentration been higher (Manzoni, Prezeau and Bockaert, 1991).

26.4 *NITZSCHIA PUNGENS*

Domoic acid was first isolated from *Chondria armata* as a result of an investigation into the ascaric properties of this seaweed. The compound is also an excellent insecticide (see Takamoto, 1978), and proved to be a powerful neuroexcitant at rat spinal interneurones and frog motor neurones (Biscoe *et al.*, 1975). Domoic acid appears to act solely at kainate receptors (see for example Young and Fagg, 1990).

In Canada in 1987 there occurred an acute illness with gastrointestinal and neurological symptoms that included vomiting, diarrhoea, head-ache and loss of short-term memory in people who had consumed cultivated mussels (Perl *et al.*, 1990). Mussels from a specific region of Prince Edward Island, Vancouver, were incriminated, and it was rapidly discovered that the molluscs contained domoic acid as a result of their becoming infested with the phytoplankton *Nitzschia pungens* (Wright *et al.*, 1989). The compound has since been identified in phytoplankton in the Gulf of Mexico (Dickey *et al.*, 1992).

The toxic response in the patients was to some extent complicated by the age range of the afflicted subjects. However, the most frequently

574

experienced signs and symptoms were confusion and disorientation, seizures and myoclonus. Positron emission tomography revealed low values of glucose utilization in the hippocampus and amygdala of the two most severely affected patients, and this deficit correlated well with their memory scores. Thus excitotoxic damage to the neurones in these areas of the brain seemed likely in view of the known effects of kainic acid in experimental animals (Schwob *et al.*, 1980). All patients were unsteady and showed generalized weakness, and there were varied symptoms, including fasciculations, in some patients; some experienced spastic hemiparesis. Nine of 10 patients showed evidence of acute denervation on electromyography. The authors concluded that domoic acid caused a non-progressive neuropathy involving anterior horn cells or a diffuse axonopathy predominantly affecting motor neurones. Neuropathology of one patient who succumbed to the intoxication revealed the expected losses of neurones in the hippocampus, but no lesions were found in the motor nuclei of the brainstem or thoracic spinal cord. Thus, despite the presence in the spinal cord of excitatory amino acid receptors that are sensitive to domoic acid, no evidence was found that the excitotoxin caused the death of these neurones.

These observations generated an explosion of research activity, of which the following account is representative of a large number of publications. Bilateral injection of domoic acid into the rat hippocampus produced degeneration of neurones in the CA1 and CA3 pyramidal cells and in the dentate gyrus. Animals thus treated performed poorly in a test of spatial awareness, which suggested that the experiment was modelling the anterograde amnesia seen in subjects who had been intoxicated with domoic acid (Sutherland, Hoesing and Whishaw, 1990).

More detailed studies (Stewart *et al.*, 1990) in rats showed that domoic acid caused seizure activity and subsequent neuropathological damage to the cerebral cortex, hippocampus, amygdala and thalamus; the basal forebrain and basal ganglia showed regions of intermediate damage, while the midbrain, hindbrain and spinal cord were largely spared. The pathopharmacology of the substance in the chick embryo retina preparation was also investigated in this study. Retinal neurones underwent acute degeneration, and oedematous swelling characteristic of the effects of excitatory amino acids in this preparation occurred. The threshold concentration required to achieve this effect was lower (3 μM) than that of kainate (25 μM), quisqualate (15 μM) or NMDA (80 μM). The pattern of damage resembled that of kainate, and the effect was antagonized by CNQX but not by MK 801, which protects against NMDA receptor agonists in this test system. The neurophysiological response to domoic acid in cultured hippocampal neurones produced an effect that was identical to that produced by kainate, but was distinguishable from that given by NMDA. CNQX again antagonized the response, which was insensitive to D-2-amino-5-phosphonoheptanoate (D-AP5), a competitive antagonist at NMDA receptors.

Hippocampal damage caused by domoic acid following its systemic injection into mice was examined in considerable detail by Strain and Tasker (1991). These studies revealed that the toxin damaged the CA1 region of the hippocampus most extensively. Whether this effect is significant may depend upon the data of Novelli et al. (1992), who showed that, in primary cultures of cerebellar granule cells, domoic acid was more active in the presence of other excitotoxic amino acids, i.e. glutamate and aspartate, than when given alone. Both studies used extracts of infected muscles, instead of purified domoic acid, and these preparations contained glutamate, aspartate and presumably other compounds. Unfortunately, the use of such extracts, though expedient, does not mimic the conditions of oral consumption. Moreover, extracts of muscles contaminated with *Nitszchia pungens* are known to contain other isomeric forms of domoic acid in addition to the compound itself, and the pathopharmacological activities of these compounds are unknown (Wright et al., 1990).

Although the majority of this work interprets the effects of domoic acid primarily in terms of its action on post-synaptic receptors, there is some evidence that the compound can also act presynaptically. In a preparation of guinea-pig hippocampal mossy fibre synaptosomes domoic acid potentiated the K^+-stimulated release of glutamate in a concentration-dependent manner up to 300 μM. This effect was also found with kainate and appeared to be receptor mediated as it was antagonized with CNQX (Terrain et al., 1991). It is clear that the response of this preparation to domoic acid is quite different to that of the *Lathyrus* excitotoxin α-ODAP (see section 26.1.1).

This episode reveals the potential dangers of excitatory amino acids in food chains and brings to mind the well-established case of neurolathyrism (described in section 26.1.1). There the lack of a suitable animal model is a hindrance to a thorough analysis of the subject. However, although the acute effects of domoic acid cause behavioural and pathological changes that might be predicted from a laboratory model, the lack of excitotoxic damage to neurones that are known to carry receptors for domoic acid is surprising. Presumably, complex mechanisms prevent the toxin reaching these cells in sufficient concentration to set in train the characteristic excitotoxic damage. Unfortunately, this work appears to shed little light on the long-term effects that such a toxin might have on neuronal survival, which is necessary for an understanding of the effects of chronic toxicity on the aetiology of chronic neurological disease.

26.5 *MANIHOT ESCULENTA*

This plant (common name cassava) was originally cultivated in the lowland tropics of South America and was introduced first into west Africa in the sixteenth century and subsequently into East Africa and Asia. Its thick starchy roots are a staple source of carbohydrate across central Africa and, as is true of *L. sativus* (section 26.1.1), the crop is cultivated because of its ability to thrive in poor soils. Interesting accounts of the history and current use of this plant are available (Cock, 1982; Cooke and Cock, 1989). Cassava contains a cyanogenic glycoside, linamarin (see Davis, 1991); this compound is not unique to this species, but assumes special importance here because processing disrupts the root tissue, liberating an endogenous β-glucosidase that hydrolyses linamarin to yield, ultimately, hydrogen cyanide via acetone cyanohydrin. Cultural experience dictates that the root is prepared thoroughly (e.g. by soaking, roasting or fermenting), which effectively removes the toxic components. This practice recalls that on Guam, where *C. circinalis* seed is also soaked for several days to remove the toxic glycoside cycasin and the free amino acid MeDAP (section 26.1.2).

Consumption of improperly prepared cassava starch leads to a number of disorders associated with the high cyanide content, and fatalities have occurred as a result of cyanide poisoning. An important account of the relationship between the consumption of cassava and cyanide intoxication in Nigeria is available (Osuntokan, 1981). The main route for the detoxication of cyanide is its reaction with inorganic sulphate in a reaction that is catalysed by thiosulphate:cyanide sulphurtransferase, yielding thiocyanate:

$$\text{Thiosulphate} + \text{cyanide} \rightleftharpoons \text{sulphite} + \text{thiocyanate}$$

High circulating concentrations of thiocyanate produced by this reaction may lead to a goitrous condition due to the competition of thiocyanate with iodide for transport into thyroid tissue. Such a mechanism probably explains the cretinism in regions where high concentrations of cyanogenic glycosides are consumed without adequate preparation (Davis, 1991). The extent to which ingested cyanide can be removed by this reaction depends upon the availability of inorganic sulphate, which itself is derived from the dietary sulphur amino acids, cystine and methionine (Sabry *et al.*, 1965; Griffiths, 1987). Since cassava contains low levels of these compounds (FAO, 1970), the trapping of cyanide into thiocyanate may be suboptimal compared with diets that are rich in sulphur-containing amino acids.

People who consume cassava containing high concentrations of laminarin (or its hydrolysis products) may develop a spastic paraparesis

Chemical toxins

(Cliff *et al.*, 1985) called mantakassa in Mozambique (Ministry of Health, 1984) or konzo in Zaire (Tylleskar *et al.*, 1992). This disorder has been characterized as an upper motor neurone dysfunction (Tylleskar *et al.*, 1991, 1992). Those at risk excrete very large amounts of thiocyanate, although urinary sulphate, which is low by European standards, is not significantly different from control samples (Cliff *et al.*, 1985; Tylleskar *et al.*, 1992).

The main biochemical function of cyanide is its inhibition of cytochrome oxidase and, as this reaction is the terminal reaction of the electron transport chain, the result is a cataclysmic cessation of oxidative cellular energy metabolism. Although the evidence is convincing, the targeting of the central nervous system (and more especially a specific part judged from the clinical manifestation of the disease) remains problematic. The reaction of cyanide with inorganic sulphate would reduce the availability of the latter, which is used mainly as a substrate for ATP-sulphurylase in the following reaction:

$$\text{Sulphate} + \text{ATP} \rightleftharpoons \text{adenosine 5'-phosphosulphate (APS)}$$

The product once formed can react with a second molecule of ATP in a reaction that is catalysed by adenosine 5'-phosphosulphate kinase:

$$\text{Adenosine 5'-phosphosulphate} + \text{ATP} \rightleftharpoons$$
$$\text{adenosine 3'-phosphate 5'-phosphosulphate (PAPS)}$$

PAPS can then act as the sulphuryl group donor, for example for the synthesis of sulphated peptide aminoglycans, sulphated steroids and cerebroside sulphates. However, there appears to be no specific requirement for these components in the central nervous system consistent with the upper motor neurone dysfunction, although cerebroside sulphates are components of myelin (see Cumar *et al.*, 1968). Alternatively, the drain on dietary sulphate and lack of sulphur amino acids might reduce the availability of cysteine for glutathione synthesis, but there is no evidence that might suggest that such an effect need be brain specific, though there is evidence that neural tissue depleted of glutathione is more sensitive to the effects of excitotoxic agents.

An attractive, though speculative, possibility is that some at least of the glycoside linamarin might escape hydrolysis in the gastrointestinal tract (Davis, 1991), become absorbed, circulate in the blood and accumulate in the central nervous system by means of the glucose transporter. Work with the glycoside cycasin (from *C. circinalis*, see section 26.1.2) suggests that this compound is accumulated into cultured neural tissue and that the aglycone, MAM, is released there, presumably by β-glucosidase activity (Kisby *et al.*, 1992). Were this mechanism available to linamarin it would explain the specificity of delivery of the

578

glycoside, and hence cyanide, to the central nervous system. The targeting of upper motor neurones would still require explanation.

26.6 *INDIGOFERA* SPECIES

Indigophera species (*I. spicata, I. dominii and I. linnaei*) are leguminous plants that are associated with the poisoning of horses in Australia (Birdsville disease) and America (reviewed by Morton, 1989). There is prominent central nervous system involvement in animals that have browsed these legumes, and two toxic components produced by these plants have been identified: 3-nitropropionic acid, which was isolated from *I. endecaphylla* (Cooke, 1955); and indospicine, isolated from *I. spicata* (Hegarty and Pound, 1968). It seems likely that nitropropionic acid causes neurotoxicity, whereas the toxicity of indospicine is directed mainly at the liver (Hegarty *et al.*, 1988).

Probably because of its central involvement, but also because of its interesting biochemistry, 3-nitropropionic acid has been the subject of thorough investigation. However, it has become apparent that the compound is widely distributed not only in leguminous plants (especially *Astragalus*), but also in some fungi, e.g. *Aspergillus* and *Penicillium* species. *Aspergillus oryzae* may contaminate a variety of foods (e.g. cheeses) by synthesizing 3-nitropropionic acid (Penel and Kosik-owski, 1990), and sugar cane infected with *Arthrinium* (see He, Zhand and Zhang, 1990) gives rise to central nervous system toxicity in children.

The biochemical mechanism that has attracted most research interest is that by which 3-nitropropionic acid acts as a suicide inhibitor of succinate dehydrogenase (Alston, Mela and Bright, 1977; Coles, Edmondson and Singer, 1979). Thus, the type of lesion that would be anticipated is that associated with inhibition of the Krebs cycle, which would point to a generalized toxicity of oxidative cell types. However, rats intoxicated with 3-nitropropionic acid (subcutaneous 30 mg/kg) develop signs of a generalized central nervous dysfunction. A light and electron microscopic study revealed a specific pattern of neuropathy in the caudate putamen, hippocampus and thalamus (Hamilton and Gould, 1987a,b) that resembles at its most extreme the excitotoxic lesions caused by excitatory amino acids (Olney, Ho and Rhee, 1971).

The mechanism by which 3-nitropropionic acid exerts its effects has been the subject of a recent electrophysiological study. 3-Nitropropionic acid (1 mM) produces in the pyramidal layer of the CA1 region of the hippocampus a long-lasting depolarization (presumably due to the inhibition of ATP synthesis) followed by a hyperpolarization that is due to the activation of ATP-dependent K^+ channels. Despite the histological

Chemical toxins

appearance the effects of 3-nitropropionic acid were not attenuated by antagonists of the excitatory amino acid receptors (Riepe *et al.*, 1992).

26.7 CONCLUSION

The foregoing account of neurotoxic compounds that have the potential to cause pathological damage to the central nervous system does not specifically answer the question of whether environmental compounds, including those in foods, are a factor in the aetiology of sporadic motor neurone disease. However, the case has been made for the existence of specific disease states, which may be geographically localized, in which a disorder of motor neurones (and in some cases other neuronal types) can be related to the presence of specific neurotoxins in foodstuffs. This work has led to an understanding of some basic mechanisms involved in the mode of action of these toxins, which enables predictive judgements to be made in the search for further environmental compounds and assessment of the risks of known neurotoxic agents. Whether exogenous compounds contribute to the aetiology of motor neurone disease remains an open question, but the sheer variety of noxious compounds contained in common foods (see D'Mello, Duffus and Duffus, 1991) suggests that vigilance is necessary. Moreover, dysfunction of the liver, the primary organ concerned with the homoeostatic regulation of circulating plasma amino acids, could lead to loss of regulatory control of the free concentrations of potentially excitotoxic amino acids, such as glutamate, aspartate (Plaitakis and Caroscio, 1987) and cysteine (Heafield *et al.*, 1989). Further, the inability of subjects suffering from motor neurone disease and other neurodegenerative conditions to metabolize food-borne compounds is strongly suggested from experiments with model compounds (see Chapter 21).

ACKNOWLEDGEMENTS

I am grateful to the Motor Neurone Disease Association for a grant that supported my work on α-amino-β-methylaminopropionic acid and to Professor E.A. Bell for his helpful criticism of the manuscript.

REFERENCES

Alston, T.A., Mela, L. and Bright, H.J. (1977) 3-Nitropropionate, the toxic substance of *Indigofera*, is a suicide inhibitor of succinate dehydrogenase. *Proc. Natl. Acad. Sci. USA*, **74**, 3767–71.
Biscoe, T.J., Evans, R.H., Headley, P.M. *et al.* (1975) Domoic and quisqualic acids

580

are potent amino acid excitants of frog and rat spinal neurones. *Nature*, **255**, 166–7.

Bredt, D.S. and Snyder, S.H. (1992) Nitric oxide, a novel neuronal messenger. *Neuron*, **8**, 3–11.

Bridges, R.J., Kadri, M.M., Monaghan, D.T. *et al.* (1988) Inhibition of ^{3}H-AMPA binding by the excitotoxin β-N-oxalyl-L-α,β-diaminopropionic acid. *Eur. J. Pharmacol.*, **145**, 357–9.

Bridges, R.J., Hatalski, C., Shim, S.N. and Nunn, P.B. (1991) Gliotoxic properties of the *Lathyrus* excitotoxin β-N-oxalyl-L-α,β-diaminopropionic acid (β-L-ODAP). *Brain Res.*, **561**, 262–8.

Chase, R.A., Pearson, S., Nunn, P.B. and Lantos, P.L. (1985) Comparative toxicities of α- and β-N-oxalyl-L-diaminopropionic acids to rat spinal cord. *Neurosci. Lett.*, **55**, 89–94.

Choi, D.W. (1985) Glutamate neurotoxicity in cortical cell culture is calcium dependent. *Neurosci. Lett.*, **58**, 293–7.

Choi, D.W. (1987) Ionic dependence of glutamate neurotoxicity. *J. Neurosci.*, **7**, 369–79.

Cliff, J., Lundqvist, P., Martensson, J. *et al.* (1985) Association of high cyanide and low sulphur intake in cassava-induced spastic paraparesis. *Lancet*, **ii**, 1211–13.

Cock, J.H. (1982) Cassava: a basic energy source in the tropics. *Science*, **218**, 755–62.

Coles, C.J., Edmondson, D.E. and Singer, T.P. (1979) Inactivation of succinate dehydrogenase by 3-nitropropionate. *J. Biol. Chem.*, **254**, 5161–7.

Cooke, A.R. (1955) The toxic constituent of *Indigofera endecaphylla*. *Arch. Biochem. Biophys.*, **55**, 114–20.

Cooke, R. and Cock, J. (1989) Cassava crops up again. *New Sci.*, No. 1669, 63–8.

Copani, A., Canonico, P.L. and Nicoletti, F. (1990) β-N-Methylamino-L-alanine (L-BMAA) is a potent agonist of 'metabotropic' glutamate receptors. *Eur. J. Pharmacol.*, **181**, 327–8.

Copani, A., Canonico, P.L., Catania, M.V. *et al.* (1991) Interaction between β-N-methylamino-L-alanine and excitatory amino acid receptors in brain neuronal cultures. *Brain Res.*, **558**, 79–86.

Cumar, F.A., Barra, H.S., Maccioni, H.J. and Caputto, R. (1968) Sulfation of glycosphingolipids and related carbohydrates by brain preparations from young rats. *J. Biol. Chem.*, **243**, 3807–16.

Davis, R.H. (1991) Cyanogens, in *Toxic Substances in Crop Plants* (eds J.P.F. D'Mello, C.M. Duffus and J.H. Duffus), The Royal Society of Chemistry, London, pp. 202–25.

Dickey, R.W., Fryxell, G.A., Granade, H.R. and Roelke, R. (1992) Detection of the marine toxins okadaic acid and domoic acid in shellfish and phytoplankton in the Gulf of Mexico. *Toxicon*, **30**, 355–9.

D'Mello, J.P.F., Duffus, C.M. and Duffus, J.H. (eds) (1991) *Toxic Substances in Crop Plants*, The Royal Society of Chemistry, London.

Duncan, M.W., Steele, J.C., Kopin, I.J. and Sanford, P.M. (1990) 2-Amino-3-(methylamino)-propanoic acid (BMAA) in cycad flour: an unlikely cause of

Chemical toxins

amyotrophic lateral sclerosis and parkinsonism–dementia of Guam. *Neurology*, **40**, 767–72.

Eberhard, D.A. and Holz, R.W. (1988) Intracellular Ca^{2+} activates phospholipase C. *Trends Neurosci.*, **11**, 517–20.

FAO (1970) *Amino-Acid Content of Foods and Biological Data on Proteins*. Food and Agricultural Organisation of the United Nations, Rome.

Gannon, R.L. and Terrian, D.M. (1989) BOAA selectively enhances L-glutamate release from guinea pig hippocampal mossy fiber synaptosomes. *Neurosci. Lett.*, **107**, 289–94.

Griffiths, O.W. (1987) Mammalian sulfur amino acid metabolism: an overview, in *Methods in Enzymology*, Vol. 143 (eds W.B. Jakoby and O.W. Griffiths), Academic Press, New York, pp. 366–76.

Gurruto, R.M. and Yase, Y. (1986) Neurodegenerative disorders of the western Pacific: the search for mechanisms of pathogenesis. *Trends Neurosci.*, **9**, 368–74.

Haas, J. and Erdo, S.L. (1991) Quisqualate-induced excitotoxic death of glial cells: transient vulnerability of cultured astrocytes. *Glia*, **4**, 111–14.

Hamilton, B.F. and Gould, D.H. (1987a) Nature and distribution of brain lesions in rats intoxicated with 3-nitropropionic acid: a type of hypoxic (energy deficient) brain damage. *Acta Neuropathol.*, **72**, 286–97.

Hamilton, B.F. and Gould, D.H. (1987b) Correlation of morphologic brain lesions with physiologic alterations and blood–brain barrier impairment in 3-nitropropionic acid toxicity in rats. *Acta Neuropathol.*, **74**, 67–74.

He, F., Zhang, S. and Zhang, C. (1990) Mycotoxin induced encephalopathy and dystonia in children, in *Basic Science in Toxicology* (ed. G.N. Volans), Taylor & Francis, London, pp. 596–604.

Heafield, M.T., Fearn, S., Steventon, G.B. *et al.* (1990) Plasma cysteine and sulphate levels in patients with motor neurone, Parkinson's and Alzheimer's disease. *Neurosci. Lett.*, **110**, 216–20.

Hegarty, M.P. and Pound, A.W. (1968) Indospicine, a new hepatotoxic amino acid from *Indigofera spicata*. *Nature*, **217**, 354–5.

Hegarty, M.P., Kelly, W.R., McEwan, D. *et al.* (1988) Hepatotoxicity to dogs of horse meat contaminated with indospicine. *Aust. Vet. J.*, **65**, 337–40.

Hugon, J., Ludolph, A., Roy, D.N. *et al.* (1988) Studies on the etiology and pathogenesis of motor neurone diseases. II. Clinical and electrophysiologic features of pyramidal dysfunction in macaques fed *Lathyrus sativus* and IDPN. *Neurology*, **38**, 435–42.

Jones, M., Yang, M.G. and Michelsen, O. (1972) Effects of methylazoxymethanol glucoside and methylazoxymethanol acetate on the cerebellum of the postnatal Swiss albino mouse. *Fed. Proc.*, **31**, 1508–11.

Kisby, G.E., Ross, S.M., Spencer, P.S. *et al.* (1992) Cycas and BMAA: candidate neurotoxins for western Pacific amyotrophic lateral sclerosis/parkinsonism–dementia complex. *Neurodegeneration*, **1**, 73–82.

Koh, J. and Choi, D.W. (1987) Quantitative determination of glutamate mediated cortical neuronal injury in cell culture by lactate dehydrogenase efflux assay. *J. Neurosci. Methods*, **20**, 83–90.

582

References

Kurland, L.T. and Mulder, D.W. (1954) Epidemiological investigations of amyotrophic lateral sclerosis. 1. Preliminary report on geographic distribution, with special reference to the Mariana Islands, including clinical and pathological observations. *Neurology*, **4**, 355 78; **5**, 438–48.

Lakshmanan, J. and Padmanaban, G. (1974) Effect of β-N-oxalyl-L-α,β-diaminopropionic acid on glutamate uptake by synaptosomes. *Nature*, **249**, 469–71.

Laqueur, G.L. (1965) The induction of intestinal neoplasms in rats with the glycoside cycasin and its aglycone. *Virshows Arch. Path. Anat.*, **340**, 151–63.

Lindstrom, H., Luthman, J., Mouton, P. *et al.* (1990) Plant-derived neurotoxic amino acids (β-N-oxalylamino-L-alanine and β-N-methylamino-L-alanine): effects on central monoamine neurons. *J. Neurochem.*, **55**, 941–9.

Ludolph, A.C., Hugon, J., Dwivedi, M.P. *et al.* (1987) Studies on the aetiology and pathogenesis of motor neuron diseases. 1. Lathyrism: clinical findings in established cases. *Brain*, **110**, 149–65.

MacDonald, J.F. and Morris, M.E. (1984) *Lathyrus* excitotoxin: Mechanism of neuronal excitation by L-2-oxalylamino-3-amino- and L-3-oxalylamino-2-aminopropionic acid. *Exp. Brain Res.*, **57**, 158–66.

Mani, K.S., Sriramachari, S., Rao, S.L.N. and Sarma, P.S. (1971) Experimental neurolathyrism in monkeys. *Ind. J. Med. Res.*, **59**, 880–5.

Manzoni, J.J., Prezeau, L. and Bockaert, J. (1991) β-N-methylamino-L-alanine is a low-affinity agonist of metabotrophic glutamate receptors. *NeuroReport*, **2**, 609–11.

Meldrum, B. and Garthwaite, J. (1990) Excitatory amino acid neurotoxicity and neurodegenerative disease. *Trends Pharmacol. Sci.*, **11**, 379–87.

Miller, S., Nunn, P.B. and Bridges, R.J. Induction of astrocyte glutamine synthetase by the *Lathyrus* toxin β-N-oxalyl-L-α,β-diaminopropionic acid (β-L-ODAP). *Glia* (in press).

Ministry of Health, Mozambique (1984) Mantakassa: an epidemic of spastic paraparesis associated with chronic intoxication in a cassava staple area of Mozambique. 1. Epidemiology and clinical findings in patients. 2. Nutritional factors and hydrocyanic acid content of cassava products. *Bull. World Health Organization*, **62**, 477–84 and 485–92.

Monaghan, D.T., Bridges, R.J. and Cotman, C.W. (1989) The excitatory amino acid receptors: their classes, pharmacology and distinct properties in the function of the central nervous system. *Annu. Rev. Pharmacol. Toxicol.*, **29**, 365–402.

Morton, J.F. (1989) Creeping indigo (*Indiofera spicata* Forsk.) (Fabaceae) – a hazard to herbivores in Florida. *Econ. Bot.*, **43**, 314–27.

Myers, T.G. and Nelson, S.D. (1990) Neuroactive carbamate adducts of β-N-methylamino-L-alanine and ethylenediamine. *J. Biol. Chem.*, **265**, 10193–5.

Novelli, A., Kispert, J., Fernandez-Sanchez, M.T. *et al.* (1992) Domoic acid-containing toxic mussels produce neurotoxicity in neuronal cultures through a synergism between excitatory amino acids. *Brain Res.*, **577**, 41–8.

Nunn, P.B. (1989) *Lathyrus sativus* toxins: identification and possible mech-

Chemical toxins

anisms, in *The Grass Pea: Threat and Promise* (ed. P.S. Spencer), Third World Medical Research Foundation, New York, pp. 89–96.

Nunn, P.B. and O'Brien, P. (1989) The interaction of L-β-methylaminoalanine with bicarbonate: an 1H n.m.r. study. *FEBS Lett.*, **251**, 31–5.

Nunn, P.B., Davies, A.J. and O'Brien, P. (1991) Carbamate formation and the neurotoxicity of L-α-amino acids. *Science*, **251**, 1619–20.

Nunn, P.B., Seelig, M., Zagoren, J.C. and Spencer, P.S. (1987) Stereospecific acute neuronotoxicity of 'uncommon' plant amino acids linked to human motor-system diseases. *Brain Res.*, **410**, 375–9.

Nunn, P.B., O'Brien, P., Pettit, L.D. and Pyburn, S.I. (1989) Complexes of zinc, copper and nickel with the non-protein amino acid α-amino-β-methylaminopropionic acid: a naturally occurring neurotoxin. *J. Inorg. Biochem.*, **37**, 175–83.

Olney, J.W. (1978) Neurotoxicity of excitatory amino acids, in *Kainic Acid as a Tool in Neurobiology* (eds E.G. McGeer, J.W. Olney and P.L. McGeer), Raven Press, New York, pp. 95–121.

Olney, J.W., Ho, O.L. and Rhee, V. (1971) Cytotoxic effects of acidic and sulphur containing amino acids in the infant mouse central nervous system. *Exp. Brain Res.*, **14**, 61–76.

Olney, J.W., Misra, C.H. and Rhee, V. (1976) Brain and retinal damage from lathyrus excitotoxin β-N-oxalyl-L-α,β-diaminopropionic acid. *Nature*, **264**, 659–61.

Olney, J.W., Zorumski, C., Price, M.T. and Labruyere, J. (1990) L-Cysteine, a bicarbonate-sensitive endogenous excitotoxin. *Science*, **248**, 596–9.

Ormandy, G.C. and Jope, R.S. (1990) Inhibition of phosphoinositide hydrolysis by the novel neurotoxin β-N-oxalyl-L-α,β-diaminopropionic acid (L-BOAA). *Brain Res.*, **510**, 53–7.

Osuntokun, B.O. (1981) Cassava diet, chronic cyanide intoxication and neuropathy in Nigerian Africans. *Wld. Rev. Nutr. Diet.*, **36**, 141–73.

Pearson, S. and Nunn, P.B. (1981) The neurolathyrogen, β-N-oxalyl-L-α,β-diaminopropionic acid, is a potent agonist at 'glutamate preferring' receptors in frog spinal cord. *Brain Res.*, **206**, 178–82.

Penel, A.J. and Kosikowski, F.V. (1990) β-nitropropionic acid production by *Aspergillus oryzae* in selected high protein and carbohydrate-rich foods. *J. Food Prot.*, **53**, 321–3.

Perl, T.M., Bedard, L., Kosatsky, T. *et al.* (1990) An outbreak of toxic encephalopathy caused by eating mussels contaminated with domoic acid. *New Engl. J. Med.*, **322**, 1775–80.

Peters, S.J., Koh, J. and Choi, D.W. (1987) Zinc selectively blocks the action of N-methyl-D-aspartate on cortical neurones. *Science*, **236**, 589–93.

Plaitakis, A. and Caroscio, J.T. (1987) Abnormal glutamate metabolism in amyotrophic lateral sclerosis. *Ann. Neurol.*, **22**, 575–9.

Polsky, F.I., Nunn, P.B. and Bell, E.A. (1972) Distribution and toxicity of α-amino-β-methylaminopropionic acid. *Fed. Proc.*, **31**, 1473–5.

Rao, S.L.N., Adiga, P.R. and Sarma, P.S. (1964) Isolation and characterization of

584

β-N-oxalyl-L-α,β-diaminopropionic acid: a neurotoxin from the seeds of *Lathyrus sativus*. *Biochemistry*, **3**, 432–6.

Riepe, M., Hori, N., Ludolph, A.C. *et al.* (1992) Inhibition of energy metabolism by 3-nitropropionic acid activates ATP-sensitive potassium channels. *Brain Res.*, **586**, 61–6.

Ross, S.M., Seelig, M. and Spencer, P.S. (1987) Specific antagonism of excitotoxic action of 'uncommon' amino acids assayed in organotypic mouse cortical cultures. *Brain Res.*, **425**, 120–7.

Ross, S.M., Roy, D.N. and Spencer, P.S. (1989) β-N-oxalylamino-L-alanine action on glutamate receptors. *J. Neurochem.*, **53**, 710–15.

Sabry, Z.I., Shadarevian, S.B., Cowan, J.W. and Cambell, J.A. (1965) Relationship of dietary intake of sulphur amino-acids to urinary excretion of inorganic sulphur in man. *Nature*, **206**, 931–3.

Sarma, P.S. and Padmanaban, G. (1969) Lathyrogens, in *Toxic Constituents of Plant Foodstuffs* (ed. E. Leiner), Academic Press, New York, pp. 265–91.

Schwob, J.E., Fuller, T., Price, J.L. and Olney, J.W. (1980) Widespread patterns of neuronal damage following systemic or intracerebral injections of kainic acid: a histological study. *Neuroscience*, **5**, 991–1014.

Seawright, A.A., Brown, A.W., Nolan, C.C. and Cavanagh, J.B. (1990) Selective degeneration of cerebellar cortical neurones caused by the cycad neurotoxin, L-β-methylaminoalanine (L-BMAA), in rats. *Neuropathol. Appl. Neurobiol.*, **16**, 153–69.

Sheng, M. and Greenberg, M.E. (1990) The regulation and function of c-fos and other immediate early genes in the nervous system. *Neuron*, **4**, 477–85.

Spencer, P.S., Roy, D.N., Ludolph, A.C. *et al.* (1986) Lathyrism: evidence for the role of the neuroexcitatory amino acid BOAA. *Lancet*, **ii**, 1066–7.

Spencer, P.S., Nunn, P.B., Hugon, J. *et al.* (1987) Linkage of Guam amyotrophic lateral sclerosis–parkinsonism–dementia to a plant excitant neurotoxin. *Science*, **237**, 17–522.

Steel, J.C. and Guzman, T. (1987) Observations about amyotrophic lateral sclerosis and the parkinsonism-dementia complex of Guam with regard to epidemiology and etiology. *Can. J. Neurol. Sci.*, **14** (Suppl.), 358–62.

Stewart, G.R., Zorumski, C.F., Price, M.T. and Olney, J.W. (1990) Domoic acid: A dementia-inducing excitotoxic food poison with kainic acid receptor specificity. *Exp. Neurol.*, **110**, 127–38.

Strain, S.M. and Tasker, R.A.R. (1991) Hippocampal damage produced by systemic injections of domoic acid in mice. *Neuroscience*, **44**, 343–52.

Sutherland, R.J., Hoesing, J.M. and Whishaw, I.Q. (1990) Domoic acid, an environmental toxin, produces hippocampal damage and severe memory impairment. *Neurosci. Lett.*, **120**, 221–3.

Takemoto, T. (1978) Isolation and structural identification of naturally occurring excitatory amino acids, in *Kainic Acid as a Tool in Neurobiology* (eds M.G. McGeer, J.W. Olney and P.L. McGeer), Raven Press, New York, pp. 1–15.

Tandan, R. and Bradley, W.G. (1985) Amyotrophic lateral sclerosis. 2. Etiopathogeneis. *Ann. Neurol.*, **18**, 419–31.

Teitelbaum, J.S., Zatorre, R.J., Carpenter, S. *et al.* (1990) Neurologic sequelae of domoic acid intoxication due to the ingestion of contaminated mussels. *New Engl. J. Med.*, **322**, 1781–7.

Terrian, D.M., Conner-Kerr, T.A., Privette, T.H. and Gannon, R.L. (1991) Domoic acid enhances the K⁺-evoked release of endogenous glutamate from guinea pig hippocampal mossy fiber synaptosomes. *Brain Res.*, **551**, 303–7.

Tylleskar, T., Banea, M., Bikangi, N. *et al.* (1991) Epidemiological evidence from Zaire for a dietary aetiology of konzo, an upper motor neurone disease. *Bull. World Health Org.*, **69**, 581–9.

Tylleskar, T., Banea, M., Bikangi, N. *et al.* (1992) Cassava cyanogens and konzo, an upper motor neuron disease found in Africa. *Lancet*, **339**, 208–11.

Vega, A. and Bell, E.A. (1967) α-Amino-β-methylaminopropionic acid, a new amino acid from seeds of *Cycas circinalis*. *Phytochemistry*, **6**, 759–62.

Vega, A., Bell, E.A. and Nunn, P.B. (1968) The preparation of L- and D-α-amino-β-methylaminopropionic acids and the identification of the compound isolated from *Cycas circinalis* as the L-isomer. *Phytochemistry*, **7**, 1885–7.

Watkins, J.C. and Evans, R.H. (1981) Excitatory amino acid transmitters. *Annu. Rev. Pharmacol. Toxicol.*, **21**, 165–204.

Watkins, J.C., Curtis, D.R. and Biscoe, T.J. (1966) Central effects of β-N-oxalyl-α,β-diaminopropionic acid and other *Lathyrus* factors. *Nature*, **211**, 637.

Weiss, J.H. and Choi, D.W. (1988) β-N-methylamino-L-alanine neurotoxicity: requirement for bicarbonate as a cofactor. *Science*, **241**, 973–5.

Weiss, J.H., Christine, C.W. and Choi, D.W. (1989) Bicarbonate dependence of glutamate receptor activation by β-N-methylamino-L-alanine: channel recording and study with related compounds. *Neuron*, **3**, 321–6.

Whiting, M.G. (1963) Toxicity of Cycads. *Econ. Bot.*, **17**, 271–302.

Wright, J.L.C., Boyd, R.K., De Freitas, A.S.W. *et al.* (1989) Identification of domoic acid, a neuroexcitatory amino acid, in toxic mussels from eastern Prince Edward Island. *Can. J. Chem.*, **67**, 481–90.

Wright, J.L.C., Falk, M., McInnis, A.G. and Walter, J.A. (1990) Identification of isodomoic acid D and two new geometrical isomers of domoic acid in toxic mussels. *Can. J. Chem.*, **68**, 22–5.

Young, A.B. and Fagg, G.E. (1990) Excitatory amino acids in the brain: membrane binding and receptor and receptor autoradiographic approaches. *Trends Neurosci.*, **11**, 26–133.

27   Viruses and motor neuron disease: the viral hypothesis lives

DOROTHY C. KELLEY-GERAGHTY and
BURK JUBELT

Since the viruses that have been directly associated with motor neuron disease (MND) have been recently reviewed (Dalakas and Pezeshkpour, 1988; Jubelt, 1991; Salazar-Grueso and Roos, 1992), we thought that we would diverge from reviewing strictly the viral data and review instead additional data on MND as support for the viral hypothesis. We will try to show how the epidemiological evidence, virus infections in MND, latent virus infection in other diseases and finally the immunological findings all support a viral hypothesis.

Viruses are the most common cause of disease, including chronic disease, and viral infections occur frequently without overt symptoms (Fields and Knipe, 1985). There certainly are viruses that have caused MND in man (Sever and Gibbs, 1988; Harter, 1982; Jubelt 1991), and there are certainly cases of MND in which no virus has been identified (Viola et al., 1979; Miller et al., 1980; Kohne et al., 1981; Bartfeld et al., 1989; Kohne, 1990).

27.1   VIRAL HYPOTHESIS OF MND

Viruses can selectively infect different host cell populations. Specific viruses infect specific cells resulting in specific CNS syndromes (Johnson, 1988). Syndromes caused by viruses include diffuse encephalitis (togaviruses infecting cortical neurons), focal encephalitis (herpesvirus infecting temporal lobe neurons; rabies infecting limbic system neurons), demyelinating disease (papovaviruses and coronaviruses infecting oligodendroglia), meningitis (mumps, echo and coxsackieviruses infecting meningeal and ependymal cells) and acute poliomyelitis (poliovirus infecting anterior horn cells). In addition, viruses can cause chronic disease with continuous infection (SSPE, PML, etc.) or chronic disease without ongoing infection (post-polio syndrome, mumps hydrocephalus, multiple sclerosis). Therefore, it is theoretically possible that specific viruses could chronically infect motor neurons or cause their chronic degeneration.

27.2 EPIDEMIOLOGY

The viral hypothesis has been historically supported by evidence from epidemiological studies that link MND with viral outbreaks by identifying clusters of MND where antecedent clusters of virus infections have occurred. In general, clustering occurs when the incidence of MND is greater than 1:100 000. The ability to identify an agent by epidemiology alone requires direct association or large numbers. Neither of these possibilities has been the case with MND. Sometimes the numbers have been very small (Sienko et al., 1990), and sometimes the link to a virus is suggested but unproven, especially when there is a large time lapse (Currier and Conwill, 1988; Frecker et al., 1990; Hudson and Rice, 1990). In other instances the clusters have not even been that (see Pamphlett (1990) for explanation). Most of the reports are of a few cases, and an environmental insult other than virus has not been eliminated. However, the epidemiological data of MND reported for England and Wales show a close geographical relation with the incidence of poliomyelitis reported 40 years ago (Martyn, Barker and Osmond, 1988; Martyn, 1991). Do the putative rises in incidence reported in France (Durrleman and Alperovitch, 1989), Sweden (Gunnarsson et al., 1990) and the USA (Kurtzke, 1991) also correlate with the worldwide poliomyelitis epidemic 40 years ago? The study of Hudson and Rice (1990) has implicated a previous influenza infection with MND incidence. Epidemiological studies of ALS have tried to determine risk factors in general (Kurtzke, 1991) or specific sectors of the population at risk, as in Harris County (Annegers et al., 1991). These studies have correlated risk with exercise and labor, neither of which contradicts a viral cause. In fact there is a definite relationship between increased physical activity/exercise and increased duration and/or severity of viral illness including poliomyelitis (Russell, 1949; Roberts, 1986; Ilback, Fohlman and Friman, 1989; Jubelt and Lipton, 1989; Montague et al., 1989; Rudoff, 1989; Tvede et al., 1989; Esterling et al., 1990; Vacek and Smith, 1990).

27.3 VIRUSES IN MND

Direct evidence for a role of viruses in causing MND exists, since there are reported cases of MND in which a virus has been identified. For recent reviews of these cases see Jubelt (1991), Irkec et al. (1989), Mora

Table 27.1 Viruses and other agents associated with motor neuron disease

Agent	Clinical disease[a]
Picornaviruses	
Poliovirus	Acute poliomyelitis
	PPMA
	ALS
	Acute LMN
	Chronic LMN
Coxsackie	(agammaglobulinemics)
Echovirus	Acute poliomyelitis
	Acute poliomyelitis
Enterovirus 70, 71	Acute poliomyelitis
Flaviviruses	
Russian spring–summer encephalitis	Chronic cervical LMN
Schu virus	ALS
Paramyxovirus	
Mumps virus	ALS
Retroviruses	
HIV	ALS
	Chronic UMN (myelopathy)
	Chronic LMN
HTLV-I	Chronic UMN (myelopathy)
Adenovirus 26	ALS
Herpesviruses	
Varicella-zoster	ALS (in immunodeficient patient)
Herpes simplex	Chronic LMN
Other agents	
Creuzfeldt–Jakob disease agent	ALS
	Chronic UMN
	Chronic LMN
	Atypical MND
Vilyuisk encephalitis	ALS
Encephalitis lethargica	ALS
SMON agent	ALS
Recurrent meningitis	ALS

[a] See Jubelt (1991), Harter (1982) and Salazar-Grueso and Roos (1992) for details.

et al. (1988), Evans *et al.* (1989), Hayward *et al.* (1989) and Salazar-Grueso *et al.* (1990a). Table 27.1 shows the viruses that have been associated with MND. The viruses that have been isolated from MND patients are positive and negative stranded, RNA and DNA, double and single stranded, enveloped and non-enveloped. However, the viral theory remains controversial because there are certainly cases of MND in which no virus has been identified. If so many different viruses have caused neurological manifestations even though their main target tissue is non-neuronal, clearly the isolation of the CNS by the blood–brain barrier is fragile, or many viruses enter the CNS at the neuromuscular junction. For simplicity and brevity, we will examine only those viruses with a high probability of being factors in MND.

27.3.1 Retroviruses

Even though association of MND with these infections is not as common as other neurologic manifestations, human immunodeficiency virus (HIV) and human T-cell leukemia virus (HTLV) types I and II have been associated with some cases of MND. As the incidence of HIV infection rises, there will be a large component of neurological diseases that are HIV associated (Sever and Gibbs, 1988). Statistically this rise may make MND look like another manifestation of HIV. In fact, it may be that retroviruses are associated causes in human MND, as in the mouse model. On the other hand, like oncoviruses and oncogenes in cancer, they might cause this effect by selective integration in the genome at a critical locus or by subtle mutations in a normal cellular protein picked up and transmitted by the retrovirus. To date the number of retrovirus-associated cases of MND is very low. As with any virus, this paucity may be associated with difficulties in identifying virus by culturing [see Brooks *et al.* (1979) for more details]. It is possible that the application of *in situ* hybridization techniques to archived tissue may cause the actual occurrence of retroviruses in MND to increase. Unfortunately, integrated retroviruses have been found in human tissue samples from patients with and without neurological disease (Fine, 1988; Gajdusek, 1988; Koprowski and DeFreitas, 1988; Greenberg *et al.*, 1989; Bohannon, Donehower and Ford, 1991), which could complicate the interpretation of *in situ* results. Since retroviruses (HTLV-I and -II) are a causative agent of lymphoma, it is important to note that an association of lymphoma with MND has been reported (Younger *et al.*, 1991). This association of lymphoma with MND also suggests that retroviruses might cause MND.

Retroviruses have been found in neurons, but it is unclear whether any replication is taking place (Sharpe *et al.*, 1990). Since HIV has not been shown to replicate without cell division, it is not known whether it can replicate in adult neurons (Kunsch and Wigdahl, 1990); however, this seems to be the same situation as occurs in non-dividing macrophages, which putatively serve as a reservoir of infectious particles *in vivo* (Gendelman and Meltzer, 1989). Furthermore, the viruses isolated from neural tissue have a tissue tropism distinct from those isolated in peripheral blood, and will infect macrophages but not T cells (Anand, 1988; Watkins *et al.*, 1990). In retroviral MND, the neurons are probably killed indirectly, not by the virus (Jolicoeur, 1990; Kunsch and Wigdahl, 1990; Sharpe *et al.*, 1990; Berger *et al.*, 1991; Jolicoeur *et al.*, 1991). The association of a retrovirus with MND still needs to be clarified. For a viral hypothesis, though, they are good candidates since they can infect neurons, they have a long latency and they can alter cellular function indirectly by integration events or by possible receptor-mediated dysfunction. Neither HIV nor HTLV seems capable of solely infecting neurons, so are probably not themselves the agents. Possibly another retrovirus will be identified.

27.3.2 Spongiform encephalopathy agents

Spongiform encephalopathies in mice and man can be caused by different agents. In humans the known spongiform encephalopathies are Creutzfeldt–Jakob disease (CJD), Kuru and Gerstmann–Straussler syndrome (GSS). The identification of the spongiform encephalopathy agent associated with CJD disease is itself controversial (Brunori, Silvestrini and Pocchiari, 1988; Murdoch *et al.*, 1990). However, the implication of its involvement in MND is less so, since lower motor neuron symptoms and signs occur in about 10% of the transmissible cases of CJD. The CJD agent – we will refer to it as a prion (Prusiner, Stahl and De Armond, 1988) – causes both the transmissible and inherited disease. Recently evidence has arisen that even the inherited form is transmissible (Baker *et al.*, 1990). More importantly for our discussion of the viral theory of MND, it now appears that a genetic mutation confers susceptibility to the agent (Westaway *et al.*, 1987; Wu *et al.*, 1987; Simpson, 1988; Doh-ura *et al.*, 1989). Even though the agent is probably not nucleic acid containing, this mutation could be viewed as a susceptibility mutation for a conventional viral disease, e.g. a receptor. The proposed model involves a mutant protein (prion) interacting with a cellular protein with a one amino acid substitution that allows it to form a beta-sheet in conjunction with the mutant. So the cellular protein is like a receptor for the mutant. The result is a shift of the soluble barrel-shaped cellular proteins in a cascading event into an insoluble sheet-like structure. The biggest problem with prions as causative agents in MND is that the characteristic pathology of prion disease is absent in MND, although we find no references in the literature to studies specifically trying to identify prion protein in MND autopsy samples. On the positive side of the argument, prions do not cause lymphocytic

591

infiltration and they certainly have a long latency period from infection to disease, both of which are characteristics of MND. Since MND does occur in 10% of CJD patients, which is more frequent than is seen in retrovirus diseases, a linkage of prions and MND is definitely possible. Furthermore, as Calne and Eisen (1989) point out, there are similar cytoskeletal changes in MND and Alzheimer's with accumulation of neurofilaments, and there is also shared amyloid plaque pathology between CJD and Alzheimer's. Are they all related at some crucial level involving protein degradation? Could a different prion particle cause different neurological manifestations? There are differences in a slow and fast disease caused by prions in mice (Westaway *et al.*, 1987). Is it also occurring in man? It may be that an unconventional 'viral' agent (the spongiform encephalopathy agent) or a close relative is involved in MND (Wills, 1986).

27.3.3 Poliovirus and other enteroviruses

What probably is more interesting, though, is the continual association of enteroviruses and picornaviruses with neurological disease in general and with MND specifically. They are the major agents of viral infections in man (Melnick, 1985). The attempt to link enteroviruses with MND has a long history based on the shared symptoms of MND and poliomyelitis, the shared cells infected and the cases of ALS with antecedent poliomyelitis (Roos *et al.*, 1980). Furthermore, males have a higher incidence of MND and also more frequently have enteroviral infections (Moore and Morens, 1984; Kurtzke, 1991). Is it coincidental that the incidence of both in males is 1.5–2.0 times greater than in females?

The problems of directly relating enteroviral infection to MND are many. Until recently the lytic nature of enterovirus and the rapid replication have been hard to reconcile with slow, possibly latent infections. Furthermore, the presence of poliovirus in CNS tissue or CSF in cases of MND has been clearly demonstrated in only a few instances (Brahic *et al.*, 1985). Enterovirus-specific antibodies or an ongoing immune response to an enterovirus have not been consistently demonstrated (Salazar-Grueso *et al.*, 1989; Sharief, Hentges and Giardi, 1991). These results by themselves are not promising of a causal connection. However, molecular biology has made strides, especially with polymerase chain reaction, and very low levels of virus are now detectable (Kennedy, 1990). In general, as with retroviruses, testing archived samples may be helpful in elucidating an agent. In support of the viral hypothesis in general and of enteroviral involvement in MND specifically are the recently accumulated data on persistent enteroviral infections in diseases.

Is the immune response in MND due to virus?

Although enteroviruses have been shown to persist in lymphoid tissue, only recently has a persistent enteroviral infection of neurons been shown to occur. Colbere-Garapin *et al.* (1990) have demonstrated a poliovirus infection that has been passaged for years in tissue culture. These viruses were characterized *in vitro* and found to have mutated (Pelletier *et al.*, 1991). Our own data using a non-virulent strain of type 2 poliovirus has shown that the virus persists, causing late paralysis in a high percentage of immunosuppressed mice (Jubelt and Meagher, 1984; Jubelt *et al.*, 1989). These viruses have also mutated (Rohzon, Wilson and Jubelt, 1984). In a Theiler virus model, neutralization escape mutants have a different disease phenotype than the parent (Roos *et al.*, 1989). It may be that a latent or persistent CNS infection requires some mutation in the enteroviral genome.

Latent enteroviral infections of presumably immunocompetent humans have been identified in at least four diseases (Kandolf *et al.*, 1987; Yousef *et al.*, 1988; Rosenberg *et al.*, 1989; Gow *et al.*, 1991). In some cases of post-viral fatigue syndrome, enteroviral RNA has been shown to still be present after 20 years (Archard *et al.*, 1988; Gow *et al.*, 1991; Hotchin *et al.*, 1989). In other instances, serum antibody has been found which is specific for enterovirus coat proteins (Muir, Singh and Banatvala, 1990; Tracy *et al.*, 1990). Furthermore, there is a strong linkage of enteroviruses with myocarditis and cardiomyopathies (Kandolf *et al.*, 1987; Tracy *et al.*, 1990; Archard *et al.*, 1991), diabetes type 1 (Muir, Singh and Banatvala, 1989; Muir *et al.*, 1989; Foulis *et al.*, 1990), pancreatitis (Vuorinen *et al.*, 1989; Foulis *et al.*, 1990) and dermatomyositis (Plotz *et al.*, 1989; Rosenberg *et al.*, 1989). In one agammaglobulinemic child, enterovirus was shown by *in situ* hybridization to have persisted in the CNS even though virus was not culturable (Rotbart, Kinsella and Wasserman, 1990). In many respects, these data support the idea that persistent or latent enteroviruses may be responsible for chronic disease in tissues where they would normally cause a typical lytic viral disease and immune response. In light of the data from Colbere-Garapin and our laboratory, it is possible that the latent or persistent viruses are mutants spontaneously arising during a lytic infection. All of these examples of persistent infection with a disease of late onset are supportive of the possible involvement of enteroviruses in MND.

27.4 IS THE IMMUNE RESPONSE IN MND DUE TO VIRUS?

In a study on viral antibodies in ALS patients, Irkec (1989) found higher antibody levels to herpes simplex virus (HSV) and poliovirus in patients with ALS than in controls. However, 80% of the population at large has HSV antibody, and in one study HSV sequences were found by *in situ* detection in brains from both controls and Alzheimer's disease patients (Jamieson *et al.*, 1991). HSV has also been found in the brains from patients with Alzheimer's and Parkinson's diseases (Deatly *et al.*, 1990). One might expect a similar problem with poliovirus antibodies in a population that has been vaccinated. It may be that a statistically significant difference could be found in general for these antigens in MND, but so far this has not proven to be the case (Deatly *et al.*, 1990).

In two animal models of picornavirus-induced disease, diabetes induced by a coxsackievirus (Blay *et al.*, 1989) and demyelinating disease caused by a defective Theiler virus (Roos *et al.*, 1989), the disease is initiated by the virus but is definitely mediated by the immune system. In both of these cases the T cells of the animals respond to the infection by destroying the cells initially infected. In the animal diabetes model, the virus is no longer present at any detectable level. This appears also to be the case in enterovirus-induced pancreatitis and diabetes in humans (Yoon, 1991). In virally induced diabetes, an anti-idiotype antibody to the virally induced antibody prevented ADCC from occurring and killing persistently infected cells (Vlaspolder *et al.*, 1990). On the other hand, in myocarditis, a second enteroviral infection brought on the disease (Beck *et al.*, 1990) in persistently infected animals. The involvement of cytotoxic T cells is not clearly evident in MND, although there is a fairly large body of conflicting data. In these enterovirus late diseases, there is a definite increase in the $CD4^+/CD8^+$ T-cell ratio as compared with controls (Tracy *et al.*, 1990; Barger and Craighead, 1991). This ratio has also been seen in MND (Provinciali *et al.*, 1988). Immune infiltrates have also been identified in a high percentage of MND autopsy samples and include increased macrophages, no B cells, cytotoxic T cells and increased expression of MHC I and II antigens (Troost, Van den Oord and Vianney de Jong, 1990). In healthy males, Beck and Tracy (1990) have found T cells of the $CD4^+$ variety that respond to many enteroviruses, even though antibodies to some of these viruses are not detected. Furthermore, viruses can induce an autoimmune T-cell response by up-regulating MHC antigens on a cell surface where they normally are not expressed (Schwartz and Datta, 1989).

Other immune responses have also been characterized in MND, including complement activation (Lampson, Kushner and Sobel, 1990) and autoantibodies (Srinivasan *et al.*, 1990). There is a large body of evidence that IgM antibodies occur with high frequency in MND (Pestronk *et al.*, 1988; Drachman and Kuncl, 1989; Pestronk *et al.*, 1989; Salazar-Grueso *et al.*, 1990b; Santoro *et al.*, 1990; Sadiq *et al.*, 1990; Shy *et al.*, 1990; Pestronk and Li, 1991). Since enterovirus has been shown to mediate a T-cell-mediated autoimmune disease in mice, the presence in MND of antibody against host tissue that does not react with enterovirus could be indicative of an autoimmune disease induced by enterovirus. The mechanisms by which a virus can cause an antibody response that is specific to the host can be molecular mimicry (the viral antigen looks like a cellular antigen) (Fujinami and Oldstone, 1985), epitope uncovering (the virus causes a conformational change in a cellular protein causing a new epitope to be exposed) (Mishiro *et al.*, 1990) or new antigen presentation (the virus causes a normally sequestered protein to be presented outside the cell) (Schwartz and Datta, 1989; Craighead, Huber and Sriram, 1990; Yoon, 1991).

These mechanisms can be postulated to occur for any virus. Can poliovirus, which has a long associated history with MND, cause the production of anti-ganglioside antibodies observed in MND? Poliovirus replication requires the production of large amounts of new membrane to which viral replication is linked (Koch and Koch, 1985), and since the membranes of neurons contain GM1 it is possible that the specific rise in anti-ganglioside antibodies in the MND process is due to the presence of the virus. It is unclear how poliovirus can persistently infect a cell, be released and not be lytic (Colbere-Garapin *et al.*, 1989). Possibly the mechanism for release is the reverse of infection and involves fusion of the new membranes associated with virus to the cellular membrane and consequent exocytosis. Whatever the mechanism, even in a normal poliovirus infection there is some virus released prior to the lytic release (Koch and Koch, 1985). If these particles are enclosed in host membrane, and are consequently phagocytosed, they could induce a response to the cell of origin (i.e. the motor neuron). The immune response in this scenario is purely speculative. Chaudhry and Pestronk (1992) found a reactivity of serum anti-gangliosides in rats that were immunized with human CNS material different from that which is evident in LMN disease patients with anti-ganglioside antibodies. They concluded that the anti-gangliosides seen in MND could not therefore arise as a result of CNS destruction. We are not sure that this is clearly demonstrated by their experiments but believe it is still possible.

27.5 CONCLUSION

Taken together, the data about persistent viruses and the cellular and humoral immune responses in MND do not preclude viral agents as initiators of MND. In looking at viral causes of disease, it is well to keep in mind what Mims (1989) has said: 'We must maintain a healthy skepticism as we await the reproducibility and specificity that is needed.' In arguing the case for a viral hypothesis of MND, we are well aware that not all the available data truly support this theory. However, though the certain evidence for a viral etiology of all MND is not

Viruses and motor neuron disease

presently available, the sum of all the evidence does lean heavily toward a possible viral etiology for some MND. It may be that MND in the future will, like diabetes in the recent past, be dissociated into a common phenotype with a number of different etiologies. Neurons are unlike other cells in the body, and the CNS has derived its unique manner of development. Possibly our dissection of its diseases and functions will have to be equally unique. The complex interaction between viruses and the immune system in general is made more complex by the containment yet leakiness of the CNS. We know that viruses can persist, we know that viruses cause many chronic CNS diseases, we know that viruses initiate an autoimmune response, but we do not know how this comes together for MND. Clearly we have a large jigsaw puzzle with many small pieces; with perseverance we may be able to assemble the data during this decade of the brain.

REFERENCES

Anand, R. (1988) Natural variants of human immunodeficiency virus from patients with neurological disorders do not kill T4+ cells. *Ann. Neurol.*, **23** (Suppl.), S66–70.

Annegers, J.F., Appel, S., Lee, J.R. and Perkins, P. (1991) Incidence and prevalence of amyotrophic lateral sclerosis in Harris County, Texas, 1985–1988. *Arch. Neurol.*, **48**, 589–93.

Archard, L.C., Bowles, N.E., Behan, P.O. *et al.* (1988) Postviral fatigue syndrome: persistence of enterovirus RNA in muscle and elevated creatine kinase. *J.R. Soc. Med.*, **81**, 326–9.

Archard, L.C., Bowles, N.E., Cunningham, L. *et al.* (1991) Molecular probes for detection of persisting enterovirus infection of human heart and their prognostic value. *Eur. Heart J.*, **12** (Suppl. D), 56–9.

Baker, H.F., Duchen, L.W., Jacobs, J.M. and Ridley, R.M. (1990) Spongiform encephalopathy transmitted experimentally from Creutzfelt-Jakob and familial Gerstmann–Straussler–Scheinker diseases. *Brain*, **113**, 1891–909.

Barger, M.T. and Craighead, J.E. (1991) Immunomodulation of encephalomyocarditis virus-induced disease in A/J mice. *J. Virol.*, **65**, 2676–81.

Bartfeld, H., Dham, C., Donnenfeld, H. *et al.* (1989) Enteroviral-related antigen in circulating immune complexes of amyotrophic lateral sclerosis patients. *Intervirology*, **30**, 202–12.

Beck, M.A. and Tracy, S.M. (1990) Evidence for a group-specific enteroviral antigen(s) recognized by human T cells. *J. Clin. Microbiol.*, **28**, 1822–7.

Beck, M.A., Chapman, N.M., McManus, B.M., Mullican, J.C. and Tracy, S. (1990) Secondary enterovirus infection in the murine model of myocarditis. Pathologic and immunologic aspects. *Am. J. Pathol.*, **136**, 669–81.

Berger, J.R., Raffanti, S., Svenningsson, A. *et al.* (1991) The role of HTLV in HIV-1 neurologic disease. *Neurology*, **41**, 197–202.

Blay, R., Simpson, K., Leslie, K. and Huber, S. (1989) Coxsackievirus-induced disease. CD4+ cells initiate both myocarditis and pancreatitis in DBA/2 mice. *Am. J. Pathol.*, **135**, 899–907.

Bohannon, R.C., Donehower, L.A. and Ford, R.J. (1991) Isolation of a type D retrovirus from B-cell lymphomas of a patient with AIDS. *J. Virol.*, **65**, 5663–72.

Brahic, M., Smith, R.A., Gibbs Jr, G.J. *et al.* (1985) Detection of picornavirus sequences in nervous tissue of amyotrophic lateral sclerosis and control patients. *Ann. Neurol.*, **18**, 337–43.

Brooks, B.R., Jubelt, B., Swarz, J.F and Johnson, R.T. (1979) Slow viral infections. *Annu. Rev. Neurosci.*, **2**, 309–40.

Brunori, M., Silvestrini, M.C. and Pocchiari, M. (1988) The scrapie agent and the prion hypothesis. *Trends Biochem. Sci.*, **13**, 309–13.

Calne, D.B. and Eisen, A. (1989) The relationship between Alzheimer's disease, Parkinson's disease and motor neuron disease. *Can. J. Neurol. Sci.*, **16**, 547–50.

Chaudhry, V. and Pestronk, A. (1992) Different patterns of glycolipid antibody reactivity: lower motor neuron syndromes vs. immunization. *J. Neuroimmunol.*, **36**, 127–34.

Colbere-Garapin, F., Christodoulou, C., Crainic, R. and Pelletier, I. (1989) Persistent poliovirus infection of human neuroblastoma cells. *Proc. Natl. Acad. Sci. USA*, **86**, 7590.

Craighead, J.E., Huber, S.A. and Sriram, S. (1990) Animal models of picornavirus-induced autoimmune disease: their possible relevance to human disease. *Lab. Invest.*, **63**, 432–46.

Currier, R.D. and Conwill, D.E. (1988) Is ALS caused by influenza and physical exercise – results of a twin study. *Ann. Neurol.*, **24**, 148.

Dalakas, M.C. and Pezeshkpour, G.H. (1988) Neuromuscular diseases associated with human immunodeficiency virus infection. *Ann. Neurol.*, **23** (Suppl.), S38–48.

Deatly, A.M., Haase, A.T., Fewster, P.H. *et al.* (1990) Human herpes virus infections and Alzheimer's disease. *Neuropathol. Appl. Neurobiol.*, **16**, 213–23.

Doh-ura, K., Tateishi, J., Sasaki, H. *et al.* (1989) Pro–leu change at position 102 of prion protein is the most common but not the sole mutation related to Gerstmann–Straussler syndrome. *Biochem. Biophys. Res. Commun.*, **163**, 974–9.

Drachman, D.B. and Kuncl, R.W. (1989) Amyotrophic lateral sclerosis: an unconventional autoimmune disease? *Ann. Neurol.*, **26**, 269–74.

Durrleman, S. and Alperovitch, A. (1989) Increasing trend of ALS in France and elsewhere: are the changes real? *Neurology*, **39**, 768–73.

Esterling, B.A., Antoni, M.H., Kumar, M. and Schneiderman, N. (1990) Emotional repression, stress disclosure responses, and Epstein–Barr viral capsid antigen titers. *Psychosom. Med.*, **52**, 397–410.

Evans, B.K., Gore, I., Harrell, L.E. *et al.* (1989) HTLV-I-associated myelopathy and polymyositis in a US native. *Neurology*, **39**, 1572–5.

Fields, B.N. and Knipe, D.M. (1985) *Virology* (ed. B.N. Fields), Raven Press, New York, pp. 1–6.

Viruses and motor neuron disease

Fine, R.M. (1988) HTLV-V: a new human retrovirus associated with cutaneous T-cell lymphoma (mycosis fungoides). *Int. J. Dermatol.*, **27**, 473–4.

Foulis, A.K., Farquharson, M.A., Cameron, S.O. *et al.* (1990) A search for the presence of the enteroviral capsid protein VP1 in pancreases of patients with type 1 (insulin-dependent) diabetes and pancreases and hearts of infants who died of coxsackieviral myocarditis. *Diabetologia*, **33**, 290–8.

Frecker, M.F., Fraser, F.C., Andermann, E. and Pryse-Phillips, W.E. (1990) Association between Alzheimer disease and amyotrophic lateral sclerosis? See comments. *Can. J. Neurol. Sci.*, **17**, 12–14.

Fujinami, R.S. and Oldstone, M.B.A. (1985) Amino acid homology between the encephalitogenic site of myelin basic protein and virus: mechanism for autoimmunity. *Science*, **230**, 1043–8.

Gajdusek, D.C. (1988) Retrovirus encephalomyelitides. *Ann. Neurol.*, **23** (Suppl.), S207.

Gendelman, H.E. and Meltzer, M.S. (1989) Mononuclear phagocytes and the human immunodeficiency virus. *Curr. Opin. Immunol.*, **2**, 414–19.

Gow, J.W., Behan, W.M., Clements, G.B. *et al.* (1991) Enteroviral RNA sequences detected by polymerase chain reaction in muscle of patients with postviral fatigue syndrome. See comments. *Br. Med. J.*, **302**, 692–6.

Greenberg, S.J., Ehrlich, G.D., Abbott, M.A. *et al.* (1989) Detection of sequences homologous to human retroviral DNA in multiple sclerosis by gene amplification. *Proc. Natl. Acad. Sci. USA*, **86**, 2878–82.

Gunnarsson, L.G., Lindberg, G., Soderfelt, B. and Axelson, O. (1990) The mortality of motor neuron disease in Sweden. *Arch. Neurol.*, **47**, 42–6.

Harter, D.H. (1982) *Human Motor Neuron Diseases* (ed. L.P. Rowland), Raven Press, New York, pp. 339–42.

Hayward, J.C., Gillespie, S.M., Kaplan, K.M. *et al.* (1989) Outbreak of poliomyelitis-like paralysis associated with enterovirus 71. *Pediatr. Infect. Dis. J.*, **8**, 611–16.

Hotchin, N.A., Read, R., Smith, D.G. and Crawford, D.H. (1989) Active Epstein-Barr virus infection in post-viral fatigue syndrome. *J. Infect.*, **18**, 143–50.

Hudson, A.J. and Rice, G.P. (1990) Similarities of guamanian ALS/PD to postencephalitic parkinsonism/ALS: possible viral cause. *Can. J. Neurol. Sci.*, **17**, 427–33.

Ilback, N.G., Fohlman, J. and Friman, G. (1989) Exercise in coxsackie B3 myocarditis: effects on heart lymphocyte subpopulations and the inflammatory reaction. *Am. Heart. J.*, **117**, 1298–302.

Irkec, C. (1989) The role of viral antibodies in the pathogenesis of degenerative and demyelinating diseases. *Mikrobiyol. Bul.*, **23**, 40–50.

Irkec, C., Ustacelebi, S., Ozalp, K. *et al.* (1989) The viral etiology of amyotrophic lateral sclerosis. *Mikrobiyol. Bul.*, **23**, 102–9.

Jamieson, G.A., Maitland, N.J., Wilcock, G.K. *et al.* (1991) Latent herpes simplex virus type 1 in normal and Alzheimer's disease brains. *J. Med. Virol.*, **33**, 224–7.

Johnson, R.T. (1988) Virus in the nervous system. *Ann. Neurol.*, **23** (Suppl.), S210.

Jolicoeur, P. (1990) *Amyotrophic Lateral Sclerosis: Concepts in Pathogenesis and Etiology* (ed. A.J. Hudson), University of Toronto Press, Toronto, pp. 53–82.

Jolicoeur, P., Rassart, E., DesGroseillers, L. *et al.* (1991) Retrovirus-induced motor neuron disease of mice: molecular basis of neurotropism and paralysis. *Adv. Neurol.*, **56**, 481–93.

Jubelt, B. (1991) Viruses and motor neuron diseases. *Adv. Neurol.*, **56**, 463–72.

Jubelt, B. and Lipton, H.L. (1989) *Viral Disease. Handbook of Clinical Neurology*, Vol. 12, 12th edn (eds. R.R. McKendall, P.J. Vinken, G.W. Bruyn and H.L. Klawsan), Elsevier, Amsterdam, pp. 307–47.

Jubelt, B. and Meagher, J.B. (1984) Poliovirus infection of cyclophosphamide-treated mice results in persistence and late paralysis. II. Virologic studies. *Neurology*, **34**, 494–9.

Jubelt, B., Wilson, A.K., Ropka, S.L. *et al.* (1989) Clearance of a persistent human enterovirus infection of the mouse central nervous system by the antiviral agent disoxaril. *J. Infect. Dis.*, **159**, 866–71.

Kandolf, R., Ameis, D., Kirschner, P. *et al.* (1987) In situ detection of enteroviral genomes in myocardial cells by nucleic acid hybridization: an approach to the diagnosis of viral heart disease. *Proc. Natl. Acad. Sci. USA*, **84**, 6272–6.

Kennedy, P.G.E. (1990) On the possible role of viruses in the aetiology of motor neurone disease: a review. *J.R. Soc. Med.*, **83**, 784–7.

Koch, F. and Koch, G. (1985) *The Molecular Biology of Poliovirus*, Springer, Vienna.

Kohne, D.E. (1990) The use of DNA probes to detect and identify micro-organisms. *Adv. Exp. Med. Biol.*, **263**, 11–35.

Kohne, D.E., Gibbs, C.J., White, L. *et al.* (1981) Virus detection by nucleic acid hybridization: examination of normal and ALS tissues for the presence of poliovirus. *J. Gen. Virol.*, **56**, 223–33.

Koprowski, H. and DeFreitas, E. (1988) HTLV-I and chronic nervous diseases: present status and a look into the future. *Ann. Neurol.*, **23** (Suppl.), S166–70.

Kunsch, C. and Wigdahl, B. (1990) Analysis of nonproductive human immunodeficiency virus type 1 infection of human fetal dorsal root ganglia glial cells. *Intervirology*, **31**, 147–58.

Kurtzke, J.F. (1991) Risk factors in amyotrophic lateral sclerosis. *Adv. Neurol.*, **56**, 245–70.

Lampson, L.A., Kushner, P.D. and Sobel, R.A. (1990) Major histocompatibility complex antigen expression in the affected tissues in amyotrophic lateral sclerosis. *Ann. Neurol.*, **28**, 365–72.

Martyn, C.N. (1991) Childhood infection and adult disease. *Ciba Found. Symp.*, **156**, 93–102.

Martyn, C.N., Barker, D.J. and Osmond, C. (1988) Motoneuron disease and past poliomyelitis in England and Wales. *Lancet*, **i**, 1319–22.

Viruses and motor neuron disease

Melnick, J.L. (1985) *Virology* (ed. B.N. Fields) Raven Press, New York, pp. 739–94.

Miller, J.R., Ramareddy, M., Guntaka, V. and Myers, J.C. (1980) Amyotrophic lateral sclerosis: search for poliovirus by nucleic acid hybridization. *Neurology*, **30**, 884–6.

Mims, C.A. (1989) Important diseases with a possible viral aetiology. *Adv. Exp. Med. Biol.*, **257**, 135–45.

Mishiro, S., Hoshi, Y., Takeda, K. *et al.* (1990) Non-A, non-B hepatitis specific antibodies directed at host-derived epitope: implication for an autoimmune process. Published erratum appears in *Lancet*, 1990, Jan 26; **337** (8735), 252; see comments. *Lancet*, **336**, 1400–3.

Montague, T.J., Marrie, T.J., Klassen, G.A. *et al.* (1989) Cardiac function at rest and with exercise in the chronic fatigue syndrome. *Chest*, **95**, 779–84.

Moore, M. and Morens, D.M. (1984) *Textbook of Human Virology* (ed. R.B. Belshe) PSG-Wright, Littleton, pp. 407–83.

Mora, C.A., Garruto, R.M., Brown, P. *et al.* (1988) Seroprevalence of antibodies to HTLV-I in patients with chronic neurological disorders other than tropical spastic paraparesis. *Ann. Neurol.*, **23** (Suppl.), S192–5.

Muir, P., Singh, N.B. and Banatvala, J.E. (1990) Enterovirus-specific serum IgA antibody responses in patients with acute infections, chronic cardiac disease, and recently diagnosed insulin-dependent diabetes mellitus. *J. Med. Virol.*, **32**, 236–42.

Muir, P., Nicholson, F., Tilzey, A.J. *et al.* (1989) Chronic relapsing pericarditis and dilated cardiomyopathy: serological evidence of persistent enterovirus infection. *Lancet*, **i**, 804–7.

Murdoch, G.H., Sklaviadis, T., Manuelidis, E.E. and Manuelidis, L. (1990) Potential retroviral RNAs in Creutzfeldt–Jakob disease. *J. Virol.*, **64**, 1477–86.

Pamphlett, R. (1990) 'Clusters' of patients with motor neurone disease. *Med. J. Aust.*, **153**, 742–3.

Pelletier, I., Couderc, T., Borzakian, S. *et al.* (1991) Characterization of persistent poliovirus mutants selected in human neuroblastoma cells. *Virology*, **180**, 729–37.

Pestronk, A. and Li, F. (1991) Motor neuropathies and motor neuron disorders: association with antiglycolipid antibodies. *Adv. Neurol.*, **56**, 427–32.

Pestronk, A., Adams, R.N., Clawson, L. *et al.* (1988) Serum antibodies to GM1 ganglioside in amyotrophic lateral sclerosis. *Neurology*, **38**, 1457–61.

Pestronk, A., Adams, R.N., Cornblath, D. *et al.* (1989) Patterns of serum IgM antibodies to GM1 and GD1a gangliosides in amyotrophic lateral sclerosis. *Ann. Neurol.*, **25**, 98–102.

Plotz, P.H., Dalakas, M., Leff, R.L. *et al.* (1989) Current concepts in the idiopathic inflammatory myopathies: polymyositis, dermatomyositis, and related disorders. *Ann. Intern. Med.*, **111**, 143–57.

Provinciali, L., Laurenzi, M.A., Vesprini, L. *et al.* (1988) Immunity assessment in the early stages of amyotrophic lateral sclerosis: a study of virus antibodies and lymphocyte subsets. *Acta. Neurol. Scand.*, **78**, 449–54.

600

Prusiner, S.B., Stahl, N. and DeArmond, S.J. (1988) Novel mechanisms of degeneration of the central nervous system – prion structure and biology. *Ciba Found. Symp.*, **135**, 239–60.

Roberts, J.A. (1986) Viral illnesses and sports performance. *Sports Med.*, **3**, 298–303.

Rohzon, E.J., Wilson, A.K. and Jubelt, B. (1984) Characterization of genetic changes occurring in attenuated poliovirus 2 during persistent infection in mouse central nervous system. *J. Virol.*, **50**, 137–44.

Roos, R.P., Viola, M.V., Wollmann, R. *et al.* (1980) Amyotrophic lateral sclerosis with antecedent poliomyelitis. *Arch. Neurol.*, **37**, 312–13.

Roos, R.P., Stein, S., Routbort, M. *et al.* (1989) Theiler's murine encephalomyelitis virus neutralization escape mutants have a change in disease phenotype. *J. Virol.*, **63**, 4469–73.

Rosenberg, N.L., Rotbart, H.A., Abzug, M.J. *et al.* (1989) Evidence for a novel picornavirus in human dermatomyositis. *Ann. Neurol.*, **26**, 204–9.

Rotbart, H.A., Kinsella, J.P. and Wasserman, R.L. (1990) Persistent enterovirus infection in culture-negative meningoencephalitis: demonstration by enzymatic RNA amplification. *J. Infect. Dis.*, **161**, 787–91.

Rudoff, J. (1989) Physical activity after viral illness (letter). *Chest*, **96**, 703.

Russell, W.R. (1949) Paralytic poliomyelitis – the early symptoms and the effect of physical activity on the course of the disease. *Br. Med. J.*, **1**, 465–71.

Sadiq, S.A., Thomas, F.P., Kilidireas, K. *et al.* (1990) The spectrum of neurologic disease associated with anti-GM1 antibodies. *Neurology*, **40**, 1067–72.

Salazar-Grueso, E.F. and Roos, R.P. (1992) *Handbook of Amyotrophic Lateral Sclerosis* (ed. R.A. Smith) Marcel Dekker, New York, pp. 453–77.

Salazar-Grueso, E.F., Grimaldi, L. M., Roos, R.P. *et al.* (1989) Isoelectric focusing studies of serum and cerebrospinal fluid in patients with antecedent poliomyelitis. See comments. *Ann. Neurol.*, **26**, 709–13.

Salazar-Grueso, E.F., Holzer, T.J., Gutierrez, R.A. *et al.* (1990a) Familial spastic paraparesis syndrome associated with HTLV-I infection. *N. Engl. J. Med.*, **323**, 732–7.

Salazar-Grueso, E.F., Routbort, M.J., Martin, J. *et al.* (1990b) Polyclonal IgM anti-GM1 ganglioside antibody in patients with motor neuron disease and variants. *Ann. Neurol.*, **27**, 558–63.

Santoro, M., Thomas, F.P., Fink, M.E. *et al.* (1990) IgM deposits at nodes of Ranvier in a patient with amyotrophic lateral sclerosis, anti-GM1 antibodies, and multifocal motor conduction block. *Ann. Neurol.*, **28**, 373–7.

Schwartz, R.S. and Datta, S.K. (1989) In *Fundamental Immunology*, 2nd edn (ed. W.E. Paul) Raven Press, New York, pp. 819–66.

Sever, J.L. and Gibbs, C.J. (eds) (1988) Retroviruses in the nervous system. Proceedings of a symposium sponsored by the National Institutes of Health, Bethesda, Maryland, May 4–6, 1987. *Ann. Neurol.*, **23** (**Suppl.**), S1–217.

Sharief, M.K., Hentges, R. and Ciardi, M. (1991) Intrathecal immune response in patients with the post-polio syndrome. *N. Engl. J. Med.*, **325**, 749–55.

Sharpe, A.H., Hunter, J.J., Chassler, P. and Jaenisch, R. (1990) Role of abortive retroviral infection of neurons in spongiform CNS degeneration. *Nature*, **346**, 181–3.

Shy, M.E., Heiman-Patterson, T., Parry, G.J. *et al.* (1990) Lower motor neuron disease in a patient with autoantibodies against Gal(beta 1–3)GalNAc in gangliosides GM1 and GD1b: improvement following immunotherapy. *Neurology*, **40**, 842–4.

Sienko, D.G., Davis, J.P., Taylor, J.A. and Brooks, B.R. (1990) Amyotrophic lateral sclerosis. A case–control study following detection of a cluster in a small Wisconsin community. *Arch. Neurol.*, **47**, 38–41.

Simpson, N.E. (1988) The map of chromosome 20. *J. Med. Genet.*, **25**, 794–804.

Srinivasan, J., Hays, A.P., Thomas, F.P. *et al.* (1990) Autoantigens in human neuroblastoma cells. *J. Neuroimmunol.*, **26**, 43–50.

Tracy, S., Chapman, N.M., McManus, B.M. *et al.* (1990) A molecular and serologic evaluation of enteroviral involvement in human myocarditis. *J. Mol. Cell. Cardiol.*, **22**, 403–14.

Troost, D., Van den Oord, J.J. and Vianney de Jong, J.M. (1990) Immunohisto-chemical characterization of the inflammatory infiltrate in amyotrophic lateral sclerosis. *Neuropathol. Appl. Neurobiol.*, **16**, 401–10.

Tvede, N., Heilmann, C., Halkjaer-Kristensen, J. and Pedersen, B.K. (1989) Mechanisms of B-lymphocyte suppression induced by acute physical exercise. *J. Clin. Lab. Immunol.*, **30**, 169–73.

Vacek, J.L. and Smith, G.S. (1990) The effects of exercise during viremia on the signal-averaged electrocardiogram. *Am. Heart. J.*, **119**, 702–5.

Viola, M.V., Myers, J.C., Gann, K.L. *et al.* (1979) Failure to detect poliovirus genetic information in amyotrophic lateral sclerosis. *Ann. Neurol.*, **5**, 402–3.

Vlaspolder, F., Oosterlaken, T.A., Harmsen, M. *et al.* (1990) Blocking by anti-idiotypic antibodies of monoclonal antibody mediated protection in mice against encephalomyocarditis virus induced diabetes and lethal disease. *Arch. Virol.*, **110**, 277–85.

Vuorinen, T., Kallajoki, M., Hyypia, T. and Vainionpaa, R. (1989) Coxsackievirus B3-induced acute pancreatitis: analysis of histopathological and viral parameters in a mouse model. *Br. J. Exp. Pathol.*, **70**, 395–403.

Watkins, B.A., Dorn, H.H., Kelly, W.B. *et al.* (1990) Specific tropism of HIV-1 for microglial cells in primary human brain cultures. *Science*, **249**, 549–53.

Westaway, D., Goodman, P.A., Mirenda, C.A. *et al.* (1987) Distinct prion proteins in short and long scrapie incubation period mice. *Cell*, **51**, 651–62.

Wills, P.R. (1986) Scrapie, ribosomal proteins and biological information. *J. Theor. Biol.*, **122**, 157–78.

Wu, Y., Brown, W.T., Robakis, N.K. *et al.* (1987) A PvuII RFLP detected in the human prion protein (PrP) gene. *Nucleic Acids Res.*, **15**, 3191.

Yoon, J.W. (1991) Role of viruses in the pathogenesis of IDDM. *Ann. Med.*, **23**, 437–45.

Younger, D.S., Rowland, L.P., Latov, N. *et al.* (1991) Lymphoma, motor neuron diseases, and amyotrophic lateral sclerosis. *Ann. Neurol.*, **29**, 78–86.

Yousef, G.E., Bell, E.J., Mann, G.D. *et al.* (1988) Chronic enterovirus infection in patients with postviral fatigue syndrome. *Lancet*, **i**, 146–50.

28 Neuropeptides: occurrence in motor nerves and relevance to motor neurone disease

JULIA M. POLAK and SALLY J. GIBSON

28.1 INTRODUCTION

Neuropeptides are small biologically active amino acid molecules and represent a large family of neurochemicals that are produced by neurones and regulate many important functions in the nervous system (Polak and Van Noorden, 1986; Polak, 1989). The discovery of small peptide molecules, the endogenous enkephalins, as ligands for opiate receptors in the central nervous system was the inital impetus for the intensive neuropeptide research over the past 15 years. Since this time more than 40 pharmacologically active peptides have been localized to the mammalian brain and spinal cord, and studies on their distribution, receptors, physiological actions and behavioural effects have radically altered our perception of nervous system function (Emson, 1979; Hokfelt et al., 1980; Salt and Hill, 1983; Gibson and Polak, 1986; Holzer, 1988). Immunocytochemical studies have localized peptides to all classes of neurones in the nervous system, not only to those involved with sensory and autonomic actions, but also to motor nerves, where a number of peptides are known to have profound effects on the functional status. This chapter will concentrate on the occurrence of peptides in motor nerves and their potential significance in disorders of motor function. The presence of many peptides in functionally specialized regions of the nervous system and the mounting evidence that they may act as neurotransmitters or neuromodulators, as well as exerting long-term neurotrophic effects (Laufer and Changeux, 1987; Strand et al., 1991), has encouraged speculation that they may be involved in the pathogenesis of nervous diseases. Localization studies of classical neuro transmitters and neuropeptides have contributed much to our under-standing of how certain regions of the central nervous system function in health and disease. This in turn has led to the realization that some neurological disorders are caused by imbalances of these substances. Loss of dopaminergic neurones in Parkinson's disease, cholinergic cortical

Neuropeptides

neurones in Alzheimer's disease and selective loss of striatal neurones, which contain the peptides somatostatin and neuropeptide Y, in Huntington's chorea, are amongst the most well-documented examples.

In motor neurone disease (MND) the precise cause of neuronal degeneration is unresolved. One possibility is that change in biosynthesis and expression of a specific neurochemical or growth factor will promote neuronal degeneration. Motor neurone function is influenced via a number of sources. The cell body receives synaptic input from other neurones in the central nervous system and its efferent axon receives signals from the target muscle it innervates. Trophic interactions between neurones and target tissues are important for neuronal maintenance and performance (Lewis, 1977). Motor neurones also contribute anterograde trophic influences to target tissues (see Chapter 25). Defective production of peptides with nerve–muscle trophic actions in the motor neurone and delivery to motor nerve terminals in the neuromuscular junction may thus induce defects in muscle function and subsequently deficits in muscle trophic factors needed to maintain homeostasis. Thus, reduced production of peptides in motor neurones may result in muscle wasting and eventually motor neurone death. In order to determine the potential importance of any peptide in the aetiology of MND it must first be established which peptides are associated with and/or are produced by motor neurones and whether specific alteration in their expression in motor nerves is evident in examples of dysfunction and diseases of the motor system.

Many peptides are present in the spinal cord, most of which are listed in Table 28.1. Interest was originally focused on neuropeptides in the spinal cord, because of their abundance in the dorsal horn, with high densities of peptide-containing fibres in laminae I and II, the region in which afferent fibres from small-sized (nociceptive) primary sensory neurones terminate. Roles for a number of peptides as sensory neurotransmitters and/or modulators were proposed and subsequently established. All peptides identified to date in the spinal cord are found in fibres (some also in neuronal cell bodies) in the adult mammalian dorsal horn, with the exception of thyrotrophin-releasing hormone. In autonomic nuclei of thoracolumbar and lumbosacral spinal cord segments peptide-containing fibres (less frequently cell bodies) are also prevalent. By comparison the ventral spinal cord is not so well endowed, but peptides are present and occur in substantial amounts (for reviews, see Hunt, 1983; Gibson and Polak, 1986; Ruda, Bennett and Dubner, 1986). Peptides that appear to be of major importance in relation to motor neurones in the adult mammalian spinal cord include substance P and TRH (present in fibres) and calcitonin gene-related peptide (CGRP), endothelin, cholecystokinin (CCK) and pro-

604

Table 28.1 Immunocytochemical localization of peptides in the ventral spinal cord grey matter of normal adult rat

Peptide	Lamina			
	VII	*VIII*	*IX*	*X*
ACTH	−	−	−	+
BN	+	−	+	+
CGRP	+ (+)	+ (+)	+ (+++)	++
CCK	+ (+)	+ (+)	++ (++)	+++ (+)
DYN	+	+	+	++
ET[a]	+ (+)	++ (+)	++ (+++)	+++
ENK	+	++	+++	+++
FMRF	+	+	+	+
GAL	++ (+)	+ (+)	+	++ (+)
MCH	−	−	+	+
NnB	−	−	+	+
NnN	−	−	+	+
NnU	−	−	−	−
NT	−	−	+	+
NPY/CPON	+	+	++	++
NP	++	+	+	++
OXY	+	+	+	++
PANC[b]	++ (+)	++ (+)	++ (++)	++
PHI	−	−	+	+
SOM	++	+	++	++
SP	++	++	+++	+++
TRH	+	++	+++	++
VP	−	−	−	+
VIP	−	−	+	+

Relative abundance of peptide immunoreactivities in the spinal cord. The distribution of fibres is shown with distribution of cell bodies in parentheses. Key: −, immunoreactive fibres not seen. Number of fibres and cell bodies: +++, dense; ++ moderate; + sparse. The distribution in a mid-lumbar segment is described: [a] human spinal cord; [b] porcine spinal cord. [From Hunt (1983), Palkovits (1984), Gibson and Polak (1986); see also Giaid *et al.* (1989) for endothelin, Ballesta *et al.* (1987) for neuromedin U, Kar, Gibson and Polak (1990) for pancreastatin and Schiffman *et al.* (1991) for CCK.]

Abbreviations: ACTH, adrenocorticotrophin; BN, bombesin/growth hormone-releasing peptide; CGRP, calcitonin gene-related peptide; CCK, cholecystokinin; FRMF, FRMF-amide-like peptide; GAL, galanin; MCH, melanin concentrating hormone; NnB, neuromedin B; NnN, neuromedin U; NT, neurotensin; NPY/CPON, neuropeptide Y/CPON; NPY, neurophysin; OXY, oxytocin; PANC, pancreastatin; PHI, peptide histidine isoleucine; SOM, somatostatin; SP, substance P; TRH, thyrotrophin-releasing hormone; VP, vasopressin; VIP, vasoactive intestinal polypeptide.

opiomelanocortin (POMC)-related peptides (β-endorphin and α-melanocortin). [For further details of discovery, amino acid sequences, localization and actions not directly related to motor nerves see Cortes *et al.* (1990), Strand *et al.* (1991) and Rubanyi (1992).]

Of the peptides present in the ventral horn and/or nerve terminals in the neuromuscular junction (Table 28.1 and section 28.3.3), particular significance must be imparted to the peptides CGRP and endothelin, which have recently been identified in adult human motor neurones. The distributions and actions of these peptides in relation to motor nerves are discussed in this chapter, and some general aspects are summarized below.

CGRP is a 37 amino acid peptide, produced by alternative processing of the primary transcript of the calcitonin gene (Amara *et al.*, 1982; Rosenfeld *et al.*, 1983). CGRP immunoreactivity has been localized to various areas of the central and peripheral nervous system, and it is particularly abundant in sensory neurones, where it coexists with the pain neurotransmitter, substance P (Gibson *et al.*, 1984). A number of actions have been ascribed to CGRP (Goodman and Iversen, 1986; Holzer, 1988). Behavioural and electrophysiological studies have shown that CGRP plays a part in the processing of painful stimuli, and that it potentiates a number of substance P-induced effects, including hyperalgesia, scratch/biting behaviour in rats and the facilitation of the flexor withdrawal response (Woolf and Wiesenfeld-Hallin, 1986). Although relatively inactive on its own, CGRP potentiates oedema induced by other mediators of increased microvascular permeability, including substance P (Brain and Williams, 1985). A trophic role for CGRP in the sensory nervous system has been recently proposed (Denis-Donini, 1989). CGRP is also a potent vasodilator, capable of inducing a protracted increase in microvascular flow following extravascular injection (Brain *et al.*, 1989).

Endothelin is a recently discovered 21 amino acid peptide, originally isolated from the supernatant of porcine endothelial cell cultures (Yanagisawa *et al.*, 1988). At least three separate isoforms have been described, encoded by different genes (Rubanyi, 1992). Endothelin has been localized to a variety of cell types, including endothelial, epithelial and some endocrine cells (Gibson, Springall and Polak, 1992). Receptors for endothelin are present in the peripheral and central nervous system and in man the peptide and its messenger RNA (mRNA) are widespread in brain neurones of the hypothalamus, cortex, hippocampus, cerebellum and brainstem, including the raphe nuclei, as well as in the spinal cord (Giaid *et al.*, 1989; Giaid *et al.*, 1991; Lee *et al.*, 1990) (see also sections 28.3.2 and 28.5.2). Localization of endothelin to glial cells has also been reported. A variety of actions have been attributed to endothelin, including bronchoconstriction, and it is one of the most potent pressor agents recognized to date (Yanagisawa *et al.*, 1988). Trophic properties for endothelin have been shown in several cell types, fibroblasts and smooth muscle cells, and include calcium mobilization and oncogene expression (Komuro *et al.*, 1988). In the central nervous system, endothelin modulates the release of other peptides (vasopressin, substance P) from the hypothalamus and possibly of substance P in the spinal cord (Yoshizawa *et al.*, 1989; Calvo *et al.*, 1990). Endothelin administered intra-aortically does not cross the blood–brain barrier, whereas intracerebroventricular injection induces behavioural changes associated with cerebellar function, suggesting that this peptide is released via a neuronal source (Moser and Pelton, 1991). Finally endothelin has an effect on neuronal excitability in the spinal cord and elicits a ventral root depolarization in newborn rats [Yoshizawa *et al.* (1989) and section 28.3.2].

28.2 TECHNIQUES

To establish the role of neuropeptides and other neurally borne substances in normal function and disease, useful information can be obtained from a knowledge of peptide storage/translation, synthesis and site of action. Since it is also of importance to determine changes that occur at the cellular level in diseases such as MND (i.e. motor neuronal soma, dendritic and axonal processes, neuromuscular junction) microscopical methods are ideally suited to provide precise knowledge of the cellular localization of stored peptide (immunocytochemistry), synthetic machinery (*in situ* hybridization) and receptor sites (*in vitro* autoradiography). By means of computerized image analysis, all of these techniques can be rendered quantitative.

28.2.1 Immunocytochemistry

The principal method for investigating cellular localization is immunocytochemistry, at either the light or electron microscopic level, using specific antibodies (Varndell and Polak, 1984; Gibson and Polak, 1986; Polak and Van Noorden, 1986). Such techniques are highly sensitive and because of novel enhancing methods peptides stored even in low concentrations within neurones can be accurately and reliably analysed (McBride *et al.*, 1990). Several techniques are available for immunocytochemical detection of peptide storage sites, the most popular at the light level being those giving permanent preparations, mainly the unlabelled antibody enzyme (peroxidase antiperoxidase) and avidin–biotin complex methods using various chromogens to visualize the antigen–antibody complex (Hsu, Raine and Fanger, 1981; Sternberger, 1979). Radioactive ligands (e.g. [^{3}H]biotin–avidin complex) have also been

been successfully used (Dietl *et al.*, 1989; Hunt, Allanson and Mantyh, 1986), because of ease of quantification from densitometric analyses of autoradiograms; however, resolution is poor. Immunofluorescence remains popular for the study of neural networks in animals, but in the human central nervous system tissue autofluorescence and lipofucsin accumulation often hamper visualization. At the electron microscopic level, gold-labelled antibodies provide the most accurate subcellular localization of peptides (Varndell and Polak, 1984; Merighi *et al.*, 1989). Computerized morphometric techniques are now widely employed for quantitative immunocytochemical data (Springall *et al.*, 1982; Zoli *et al.*, 1986; Arvidsson *et al.*, 1990a; Zhang and Vacca-Gallaway, 1992). Information regarding translated/stored peptide can also be obtained by radioimmunoassay of extracts of whole tissue or microdissected, anatomically defined, regions of tissue, which permits peptide content to be analysed and also allows a biochemical characterization of peptides present by various chromatographic procedures (Bloom and Long, 1982). Recently, a high degree of sophistication has been achieved from the combination of biochemical data and quantitative immunocyto-chemistry to provide relative concentrations of different subsets of neuro-chemically defined varicosities (substance P, TRH and 5-hydroxytryp-tamine) in the spinal cord (Arvidsson *et al.*, 1990a).

28.2.2 *In situ* hybridization

Using molecular biological techniques it is possible to determine whether a cell has the synthetic machinery to produce a peptide, and this provides a new dimension to the study of gene expression in the nervous system (see Chapter 16). The methods involve the detection by hybridization with labelled 'probes' of specific mRNAs encoding the peptide [see Polak and McGee (1990) for review]. Studies can be performed either at the whole-tissue level on extracts by Northern blotting, the nucleic acids being separated by gel electrophoresis followed by transfer to a membrane for hybridization to detect the mRNA of interest, or on tissue sections by hybridization of the mRNA species *in situ*. *In situ* hybridization is the only method available to the morphologist that allows cellular localization of DNA and RNA sequences in a heterogeneous cell population. The general principle relies upon the fact that for each strand of DNA- or RNA-containing (complementary) probe there is a predetermined strand of sequences in the tissue, and the probe will bind specifically to form stable hybrids in the tissue. This precise nature of complementary base pairing thus permits detection of both high- and low-abundance copy numbers of gene sequences. Several different types of probes are in current use,

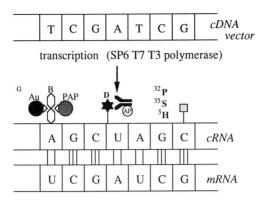

Figure 28.1 Diagrammatic representation of the method of *in situ* hybridization with riboprobes. cDNA sequences are subcloned adjacent to a promoter within a plasmid vector, linearized and transcribed to produce a sequence complementary to the messenger RNA (mRNA) (cRNA or antisense probes). The RNA probe is detected by a nucleotide labelled radioisotopically or non-radioactively. Alternate control sections are hybridized with a non-complementary ('sense') RNA probe as a method control. The labelled cRNA that has hybridized is visualized by use of an appropriate technique to allow localization of the tissue mRNA. Labels include radioisotopes (^{3}H, ^{35}S, ^{32}P), detected by autoradiography; biotin (B), detected by gold (Au)- or peroxidase (PAP)-labelled streptavidin or antibody to biotin; and digoxigenin (D), detected by alkaline-phosphatase-labelled antibody.

including double-stranded cDNAs, cRNAs (riboprobes) and synthetic oligonucleotides (Gibson and Polak, 1990). The probes can be labelled isotopically (^{3}H, ^{32}P, ^{35}S) and localized by autoradiography or non-isotopically with substances subsequently localized by immunocytochemistry (e.g. biotin, digoxigenin) (Figure 28.1). Isotopic labelling has been used extensively for studies in the central nervous system, and quantification can be achieved from either directly apposing the labelled slide to X-ray film to produce an autoradiogram for densitometric analysis of gross anatomical structures or from dipping the slides directly into liquid photographic emulsion, which allows the density of silver grains to be counted at the cellular level as well as the number of cells expressing the mRNA to be evaluated (Davenport and Nunez, 1990; Popper and Micevych, 1990).

28.2.3 Receptor localization

The use of isolated membranes from tissue homogenates is the classical method for investigations of binding site kinetics and determination of the amount of radiolabelled ligand binding. However, for the precise

Neuropeptides

localization of binding sites (and hence site of action) within any tissue, *in vitro* receptor autoradiography, first introduced by Young and Kuhar (1979), is the method of choice. *In vitro* autoradiography combines binding site localization with histochemical analysis and can be quantified [see Palacios and Dietl (1989) for review] (Figure 28.2). Radioligands are used to identify peptide binding sites in tissue sections, and these are visualized either (a) at the microscopic level in emulsion-coated slides or coverslips, which allows comparisons to be made with tissue histology or immunocytochemistry and other techniques such as *in situ* hybridization, or (b) at the gross level in autoradiographs generated by the apposition of tissue sections to photographic film, which can be quantified by image analysis and the optical density of the autoradiographs compared with those of standards containing known concentrations of radioactive material (Davenport, Hill and Hughes, 1989).

Immunocytochemistry using divalent ligands (Lackie *et al.*, 1984) and anti-idiotypic antibodies (Gaulton and Greene, 1986) and *in situ* hybridization employing probes for the mRNA coding for a particular receptor have also been employed to localize binding sites for peptide products on their target cells, but as yet these methods have not been widely exploited in the CNS.

28.3 NORMAL DISTRIBUTION OF MOTOR NERVES

28.3.1 Neuropeptide fibres in the ventral spinal cord of vertebrates and man

In the ventral spinal cord (laminae VII–IX), the relative abundance of peptide-immunoreactive fibres is low compared with the dorsal horn and central canal region and is reflected in lower concentrations of peptides as determined by radioimmunoassay (Figure 28.3). It is not within the scope of this chapter to describe the localization of each peptide in the ventral spinal cord; a summary of some and their distributions is shown in Table 28.1 [see also reviews by Hunt (1983), Palkovits (1984), Gibson and Polak (1986) and Katagiri *et al.* (1988), and, for man, Schoenen *et al.* (1985a) and Gibson *et al.* (1988a)]. Receptors for a number of these peptides have been identified and characterized in the ventral horn of man and other mammals (Charlton and Helke, 1985; Manaker *et al.*, 1985, 1988; Dietl *et al.*, 1989; Kar, Chabot and Quirion, 1991). In the majority of mammalian species fibres immunoreactive for substance P, enkephalin, CCK, somatostatin, neuropeptide Y (NPY) and its C-flanking peptide (CPON) and pancreastatin (pig) are most prevalent and present in all laminae of the ventral horn. In particular, fibres immunoreactive for these peptides are present in close apposition

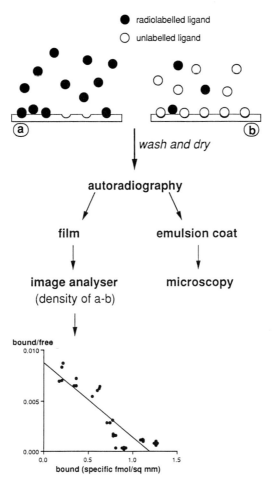

Figure 28.2 Schematic illustration of receptor localization using the method of *in vitro* autoradiography. Tissue sections are incubated with radiolabelled ligand without (a) or with (b) an excess of the unlabelled ligand. This allows for detection of non-specific binding of the ligand (competitive displacement). Following autoradiography, optical densities of anatomically defined areas on the films may be quantified using image analysis and, when compared with co-exposed standards, kinetic data can be determined and the specific binding derived (e.g. by Scatchard plot; see diagram).

to motor neurones of laminae VIII and IX (Figures 28.3 and 28.4B and C). Immunocytochemical analyses of human spinal cord are less well documented, but it appears that in man peptide-containing fibres (namely substance P, enkephalin, somatostatin and TRH) have a more

611

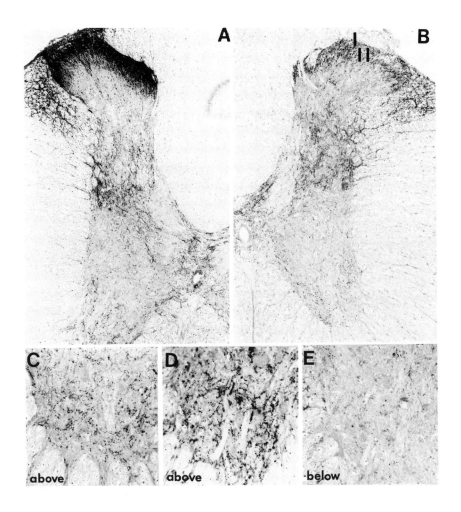

Figure 28.3 Substance P-immunoreactive fibres in the thoracic spinal cord of the rat. (A and B) Half-transverse sections showing the dorsal and ventral horns. Substance P is reduced dramatically from laminae I and II (I,II) and from the region ventral to the central canal in the adult spinal cord following neonatal administration of the sensory neurotoxin capsaicin (B) compared with the control (A). There is no change in the distribution of fibres in the ventral horn, confirming an intrinsic origin for substance P-immunoreactive fibres. (C–E) Substance P-immunoreactive fibres in the ventral horn of the rat spinal cord rostral (C), immediately rostral (D) and (E) caudal to spinal cord transection at the mid-thoracic level. Note build-up of immunoreactivity above (D) and almost complete loss (E) below the lesion, demonstrating that substance P-immunoreactive fibres in the ventral horn are of supraspinal origin.

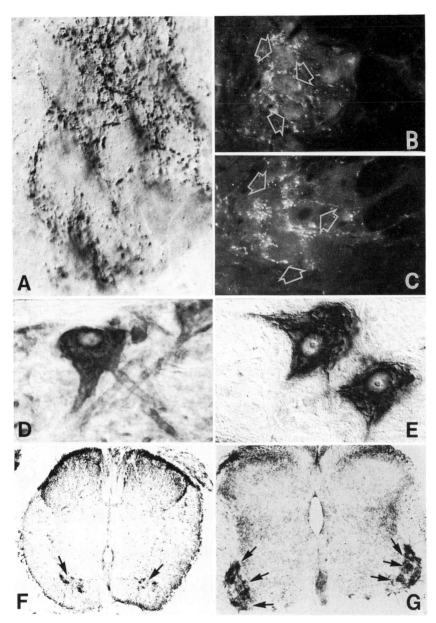

Figure 28.4 (A) Substance P-immunoreactive fibres concentrated around the cremaster motor neurones in the L2 ventral spinal cord segment of rat. (B) NPY- and (C) ENK-immunoreactive fibres concentrated around motor neurones (some arrowed) of the pudendal motor nuclei (Onuf's nuclei) in the L6 ventral spinal cord segment. (D) A galanin-immunoreactive motor neurone in rat lumbar spinal cord showing strong accumulation of immunoproduct following colchicine treatment. (E) CGRP-immunoreactive motor neurones in the rat sacral spinal cord. (F and G) Developing rat lumbosacral spinal cord at (F) E21 and (G) E16 immunostained for CGRP and galanin respectively – note strong immunoreactivity in the motor nuclei (arrows point to motor neurones).

intimate association with the motoneuronal soma and processes than in other species (see Figure 28.11I–L). High densities of peptide-immunoreactive fibres are also localized to specific groups of motor neurones. In rat, the cremaster motor nucleus of segments L1–L2 is densely innervated by substance P and CCK fibres (Kar, Gibson and Polak, 1990) and the pudendal motor nucleus (Onuf's nucleus) (segments L6–S1 rat, S2–S3 man, S1–S3 cat) by fibres immunoreactive for enkephalin, somatostatin and NPY/CPON (Gibson *et al.*, 1988a; Katagiri *et al.*, 1986) (Figure 28.4A–C).

In developing spinal cord, galanin-, NPY/CPON-, somatostatin- and substance P-immunoreactive fibres are among the first to appear between embryonic days 15 and 17 (rat) and the sixth to tenth fetal week (man) (Marti *et al.*, 1987; Suburo *et al.*, 1992), and most of these are associated with motor neurones expressing immunoreactivity for the same peptides (section 28.3.2) (Figure 28.4F and G). Most other peptides, as well as the catecholamine-synthesizing enzyme tyrosine hydroxylase and 5-HT, appear perinatally (Table 28.2). The density of fibres, in particular those immunoreactive for enkephalin, NPY/CPON, somatostatin, substance P and TRH, increases until birth in man and the second post-natal week in rat. Subsequently, their distributions are similar to that of the adult.

The origin of peptide-immunoreactive fibres in the ventral horn is from (a) primary afferent collaterals, (b) intrinsic spinal neurones and/or (c) supraspinal descending afferents. Origins for some but not all peptides in the ventral horn have been established. Vasopressin and oxytocin fibres originate in the paraventricular hypothalamic nuclei (Millan *et al.*, 1984). In the brainstem raphe, 5-hydroxytryptamine (5-HT) neurones have been shown to co-localize substance P, enkephalin and TRH (Johansson *et al.*, 1981; Mantyh and Hunt, 1984). Experiments employing 5-HT neurotoxins (5,6- or 5,7-dihydroxytryptamine) and spinal cord transections have shown by immunocytochemistry and radioimmunoassay that, like 5-HT, most substance P- and TRH-immunoreactive fibres in the ventral horn originate from the raphe (Johansson *et al.*, 1981; Gilbert *et al.*, 1982; Arvidsson *et al.*, 1990a; and Ruda, 1988, for reviews), and at least a proportion of CCK and enkephalin immunoreactivity derives from bulbospinal pathways (Figure 28.3C–E). The source of CGRP-immunoreactive fibres in the ventral spinal cord from the raphe nuclei has also been recently suggested (Arvidsson *et al.*, 1991).

Electrophysiological actions have been shown for some peptides present in nerve terminals synapsing on motor neurones. TRH, substance P, neurotensin and bombesin induce depolarization of ventral roots and motor neurones *in vivo* and *in vitro* (Nicoll, 1978; Ono and

Table 28.2 Temporal appearance of peptide-immunoreactive fibres and cells in the ventral spinal cord of man and rat

Peptide	Ventral grey matter	
	C	Γ
CGRP	E15	E21
	(6W)	(6W)
GAL	E15	E21
	(6W)	(6W)
SOM	E15	E15
	(8W)	(10W)
SP	*	E18
	(*)	(6W)
NPY/CPON	E17	E15
	(6–11W)	(8W)
ENK	*	E21
	(*)	(10W)
TRH	*	E21
	(*)	(*)
VIP	*	P1
	(*)	(20W)

Appearance in rat is shown with appearance in human fetal spinal cord in parentheses.
From Marti *et al.* (1985) and Suburo *et al.* (1992).
Abbreviations: C, cell bodies; F, fibres; E, embryonic day; W, gestational week. *, not seen; CGRP, calcitonin gene-related peptide; GAL, galanin; SOM, somatostatin; SP, substance P; NPY/CPON, neuropeptide Y and its C-flanking peptide; ENK, enkephalin; TRH, thyrotrophin-releasing hormone; VIP, vasoactive intestinal polypeptide.

Fukuda, 1982; Nistri, Fisher and Gurnell, 1990; and review by Strand *et al.*, 1991). Substance P also potentiates the excitatory effects of 5-HT. However, the action of neurotensin and bombesin is thought to be indirect, mediated via interneurones, as depolarization is blocked by tetrodotoxin (Nicoll, 1978). Endothelin induces a dose-dependent ventral root depolarization *in vivo* that is attenuated by nicardipine (dihydropyridine-sensitive Ca^{2+} channel blocker) or the substance P analogue spantide (Yoshizawa *et al.*, 1989), and while no direct effects on motor neurone excitability are reported for somatostatin, intrathecal administration decreases spontaneous motor activity [see Strand *et al.* (1991) for review]. Alterations in the production and release of peptides with transmitter-like effects that may also provide trophic interactions (section 28.3.2) from nerves terminating on motor neurones therefore have important implications for motor nerve function in the diseased state.

Neuropeptides

28.3.2 Neuropeptide-containing motor neurones in vertebrates and man

Particularly exciting has been the revelation that motor neurones contain neuropeptides. CGRP was the first peptide discovered in adult motor neurones (Gibson et al., 1984). Cholecystokinin (CCK) (Abelson and Micevych, 1991; Cortes et al., 1991; Schiffman et al., 1991), galanin (Ch'ng et al., 1985; Moore, 1989), endothelin (Shinmi et al., 1989), pancreastatin (Kar et al., 1989) and in dystrophic mice POMC-related peptides (Haynes and Smith, 1985; Haynes, Smith and Li, 1985) have been subsequently identified (Figures 28.4D and E and 28.5).

CGRP immunoreactivity and mRNA have been localized to brainstem and spinal motor neurones (Gibson et al., 1988a,b; Rethelyi, Metz and Lund, 1989; Haas, Streit and Krentzberg, 1990; Piehl et al., 1991; Rethelyi et al., 1990) and binding site densities are high in the spinal cord (Tschopp et al., 1985) (Figures 28.5A and B). Reports vary with respect to the relative abundance of CGRP immunoreactivity and mRNA in rat spinal motor neurones, and there appears to be a differential distribution in some motor nuclei (Gibson et al., 1988a,b; Matteoli et al., 1990; Popper and Micevych, 1990; Arvidsson et al., 1991; Piehl et al., 1991; Hietanen-Peltola, 1992), but in adult rat and in motor neurone-enriched cell cultures of chick spinal cord, CGRP immunoreactivity is present in the majority of motor neurones and has therefore been proposed to be a good marker (Gibson et al., 1988a,b; Juurlink, Munoz and Devon, 1990). Ultrastructurally, CGRP immunoreactivity localizes to Golgi complex membranes in multivesicular bodies and vesicles adjacent to the Golgi complex (Striet et al., 1989; Hietanen-Peltola, 1992). CGRP-immunoreactive motor neurones also contain acetylcholinesterase (AChe) and/or ChAT immunoreactivity (Takami et al., 1985a; Hietanen, Pelto-Huikko and Rechardt, 1990) and a subpopulation express protein kinase C β-subtype immunoreactivity (a cell-surface signal transduction enzyme for cell function and proliferation). Coexistence of CGRP and CCK mRNAs has recently been shown in numerous motor neurones of rat, but in guinea-pigs few motor neurones express message for CCK (Cortes et al., 1990). In normal adult mammalian spinal cord the remaining peptides are not so abundant; a few motor neurones show galanin (rat) or endothelin (pig) immunoreactivities, whereas POMC-related peptides occur only in adult dystrophic mice (Ch'ng et al., 1985; Haynes and Smith, 1985; Moore, 1989; Shinmi et al., 1989).

In adult human spinal cord, CGRP and endothelin immunoreactivities and their mRNAs localize to motor neurones (Gibson et al., 1988a,b; Giaid et al., 1989) (Figures 28.5, 28.11G and 28.13A,C and E). Although most motor neurones express CGRP transcripts, in contrast to other

616

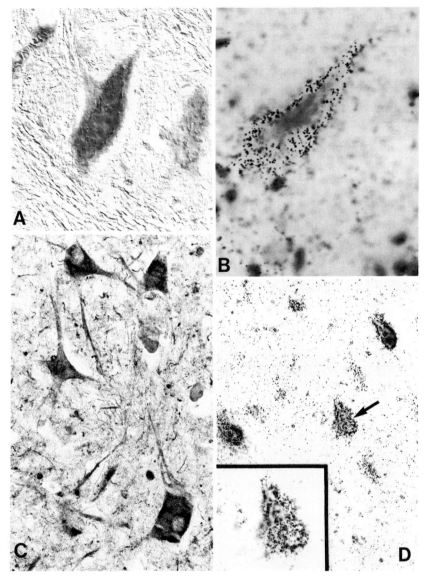

Figure 28.5 (A) CGRP-immunoreactive motor neurone in normal human spinal cord – note granular appearance of immunostaining. (B) Autoradiograph of a motor neurone from normal human spinal cord following *in situ* hybridization with ^{35}S-labelled CGRP cRNA. (C) Endothelin-immunoreactive motor neurones in normal human sacral spinal cord. Many motor neurones in the lateral motor columns are endothelin immunoreactive. (D) Autoradiograph of normal adult human lumbar motor neurones following *in situ* hybridization with a [32]S-labelled endothelin-1 cRNA probe. High-power photomicrograph of one motor neurone (arrowed) is shown in the inset; note high density of silver grains, depicting mRNA sites overlying the motor neurone cytoplasm.

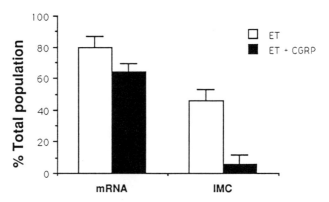

Figure 28.6 Histogram depicting the abundance of motor neurones expressing endothelin immunoreactivity and mRNA and CGRP immunoreactivity and mRNA in the lumbar ventral spinal cord of normal adult tissue. Average cell counts from three cases ± standard error of means (SEM).

animals, relatively small numbers are CGRP-immunoreactive (Gibson *et al.*, 1988a,b; Harmann, Chung and Briner, 1988; Giaid *et al.*, 1989; Kato, Hirano and Manaka, 1991). Many endothelin-producing motor neurones are present even though there are low densities of binding sites for endothelin in the spinal cord (Hoyer, Waeber and Palacios, 1989; Jones *et al.*, 1989), suggesting the synthesized peptide exerts an action on receptors located in distant structures in the nervous system.

In a study of neurologically normal spinal cords ($n = 10$, 4–7 h post mortem), the distribution of endothelin peptide and message was investigated using an antiserum to human/porcine endothelin and a ^{32}P-labelled cRNA probe specific for endothelin-1 respectively. The distribution of immunoreactivity and mRNA was similar, although motor neurones labelled with the cRNA probe were more abundant. Densest labelling was found in lamina XI (motor nuclei) (Giaid *et al.*, 1989). Endothelin and CGRP immunoreactivities or their mRNAs were often co-localized, and a semiquantitative analysis of the numbers of motor neurones that expressed endothelin alone or in combination with CGRP showed that few motor neurones were CGRP reactive, but 10 times as many were endothelin immunoreactive. Nearly all motor neurones contained CGRP mRNA, and 75–80% of these were also labelled with the endothelin-1 cRNA probe (Giaid *et al.*, 1989) (Figure 28.6).

During development, some peptides not visible in the adult are transiently present and/or found in greater proportions in vertebrate motor neurones. In chick, somatostatin-, vasoactive intestinal peptide (VIP)- and CGRP-immunoreactive motor neurones occur in the embryonic period, and some somatostatin-containing motor neurones co-localize with VIP or CGRP. Few somatostatin or VIP motor neurones are seen in post-hatch chicks, whereas CGRP persists with minor loss of immunoreactivity (Villar *et al.*, 1988). In rat motor neurones somato-statin, CPON, galanin and CGRP appear around embryonic day 15, peaking between day 17 and birth (Table 28.2) (Figure 28.4F and G). No somatostatin or CPON and only 1–2 galanin cells persist in the adult (Marti *et al.*, 1987). CGRP-containing motor neurones remain in considerable numbers, but expression of immunoreactivity and mRNA is down-regulated in adults compared with embryonic and neonatal stages (Marti *et al.*, 1987; Matteoli *et al.*, 1990). A similar pattern occurs in human fetal motor neurones. Somatostatin, CPON, galanin and CGRP immunoreactivity appears between 6 and 11 weeks of gestation, peaking at around 10–14 weeks and then declining to birth, with only small numbers of CGRP-immunoreactive motor neurones present in the juvenile and adult (Marti *et al.*, 1987; Suburo *et al.*, 1992) (Table 28.2 and Figure 28.7). Transient expression of neuro-peptide-containing motor neurones may be attributable to loss of these cells during the period of natural cell death; alternatively, neurochemical expression could vary during development prior to acquisition of the adult phenotype, and thus the neuropeptides may be of importance in neuronal differentia-tion. However, down-regulation of CGRP occurs after the time of cell death in the rat and, therefore, is perhaps related to maintenance and maturation of neuromuscular function (Matteoli *et al.*, 1990). A further hypothesis is that the remaining CGRP-producing motor neurones represent a specific subset of motor neurones (Matteoli *et al.*, 1990; Piehl *et al.*, 1991). Recent studies suggest that motor neuronal CGRP may be re-expressed in MND (Kato, Hirano and Manaka, 1991; and section 28.5.2), so investigations of possible re-expression of other embryonic neuropeptide phenotypes in motor neurones of MND patients are currently in progress in our laboratory.

It has been hypothesized that MND and other degenerative diseases involving motor neurones result in an impairment of trophic inter-actions between muscle and motor neurones (Appel, 1981). Trophic actions have been attributed to a number of neuropeptides present in motor neurones and/or fibres synapsing on them. CGRP is now recog-nized as an anterograde trophic factor released by motor neurones (New and Mudge, 1986; Laufer and Changeux, 1987; Fontaine, Klarsfeld and Changeux, 1986). Developmentally, CGRP appears in motor neurones and motor endplates when the neuromuscular junction is forming and contributes to maintenance of high densities of acetylcholine (ACh) receptors when myotubes develop (Moss *et al.*, 1991, section 28.3.3; Roa and Changeaux, 1991), as well as effecting neuronal sprouting of motor

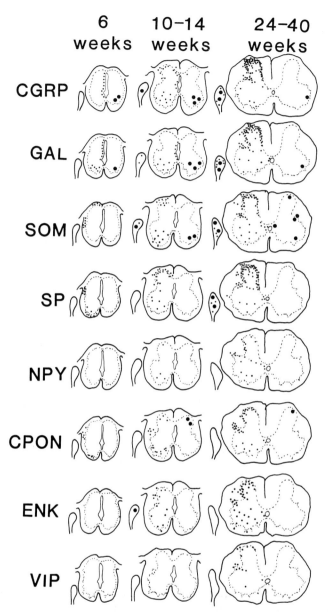

Figure 28.7 Diagrammatic representation of the distribution of peptide-immunoreactive structures in man during early (6–14 weeks) fetal life and in late fetal and early neonatal life (24–40 weeks). Immunoreactive fibres (small dots, left-hand side of spinal cord) and cell bodies (large dots, right-hand side of spinal cord) are shown. The distribution of peptide immunoreactivity in the dorsal root ganglia is depicted on the left-hand side of the corresponding spinal cord.

nerves after injury (Tsjimoto and Kuno, 1988; White and Zimmerman, 1988). Functional roles for most other peptides present in motor neurones remain to be fully substantiated, but motor neurotrophic actions *in vitro* and *in vivo* have been reported for some. CCK has significant effects on promotion of neurite formation in cultures of embryonic rat ventral spinal cord explants (Iwasaki *et al.*, 1989); by contrast, CGRP has no effect. Substance P, bombesin and TRH, which are present in fibres in close proximity to motor neurones, have similar neurite-promoting effects in the same preparations (Iwasaki *et al.*, 1991), and this action is presumably mediated via receptors located on the motor neuronal membrane. In accord with these observations, receptors for substance P and TRH are reduced in MND (Manaker *et al.*, 1985; Dietl *et al.*, 1989) and immunoreactivity is reduced in other conditions that influence motor neurone homeostasis (Post *et al.*, 1987). TRH also enhances production of choline acetyltransferase and creatine kinase in cultured rat embryonic ventral horn neurones (Schmidt-Achert, Askanas and Engel, 1984). TRH administration in man ameliorates motor neurone function in MND and improves neurological recovery after spinal injury (Faden *et al.*, 1981; Engel, Siddique and Nicoloff, 1983; Stober *et al.*, 1985; Freedman *et al.*, 1986; and see review by Strand *et al.*, 1991). A similar therapeutic use has been postulated for substance P (Schoenen, 1990). Somatostatin enhances neurite outgrowth in regenerating gastropod neurones (Bullock, 1987; Grimm-Jorgensen, 1987). The importance of this peptide in neuronal differentiation is underlined by the fact that when it is administered exogenously natural motor neuronal cell death is inhibited *in vivo* in chick embryos, possibly via activation of intraneuronal calcium, and thus acts it as an antagonist of cell death in development and perhaps also in neurodegenerative diseases of motor systems (Weill, 1991).

Although endothelin is expressed in the majority of motor neurones, no direct motor neurotrophic actions have yet been demonstrated for this recently discovered neuropeptide. However, endothelin has mitogenic actions on a number of cell types (Komuro *et al.*, 1988; Simonson *et al.*, 1989; Takuwa *et al.*, 1989) and modulates neurite outgrowth in chick embryonic sensory neurones in culture (Hsu, Savage and Jeng, 1992). POMC-related peptides (including β-endorphin and α-melanocortin) have a wide spectrum of neurotrophic actions [Strand *et al.*, 1989; see Strand *et al.* (1991) for review]. Effects include enhancement of peripheral nerve regeneration, promotion of neurite outgrowth from damaged nerve trunks, acceleration of neuromuscular development and amelioration of pathological loss of evoked muscle action potentials (section 28.3.3) as well as influencing the patterns of regenerating motor neurones and their function (Saint-Come, Acker and Strand, 1985; Saint-

Neuropeptides

Come and Strand, 1988; Strand *et al.*, 1981). However, direct trophic actions on motor neurones *in vitro* have not yet been established (Iwasaki *et al.*, 1990).

28.3.3 Neuropeptides in motor nerves of the neuromuscular junction

In normal adult mammalian neuromuscular junction CGRP- and POMC-related peptide-immunoreactive (β-endorphin, α-melanocortin) and in amphibians substance P-immunoreactive (Matteoli, Haimann and De Camilli, 1991) nerve terminals have been demonstrated. CGRP-immunoreactive nerves (namely motor endplates) are present in a number of mammalian species (Rodrigo *et al.*, 1985a,b; Takami *et al.*, 1985a; Terenghi *et al.*, 1986; Kruger *et al.*, 1989; Popper and Micevych, 1989; Matteoli *et al.*, 1990), including man (Mora *et al.*, 1989), in both striated muscles of the upper gastrointestinal tract and somatic skeletal muscles (Figure 28.8A). The presence of receptors for CGRP (Jennings and Mudge, 1989; Popper and Micevych, 1989; Roa and Changeux, 1991) and its release from striated muscle (Hiromasa *et al.*, 1990) have been established. In certain muscles CGRP coexists with ACh (Takami *et al.*, 1985a; Matteoli *et al.*, 1988) and enhances release of ACh (Jinnai *et al.*, 1989). At the subcellular level, in contrast to ACh (present in small clear vesicles), CGRP is stored in large dense-core vesicles (Matteoli *et al.*, 1988).

CGRP immunoreactivity is highly expressed in somatic muscle motor nerve terminals in embryonic and neonatal animals (Fontaine, Klarsfeld and Changeux, 1986; Matteoli *et al.*, 1990; New and Mudge, 1986), but decreases with age and in adult rat occurs only in muscle spindles of intrafusal fibres, in accord with the down-regulation of CGRP synthesis in motor neurones (Matteoli *et al.*, 1990; and section 28.3.2).

There is a spectrum of actions for CGRP *in vivo* and *in vitro* in skeletal muscle including (a) enhancement of neuromuscular transmission and the excitation–contraction mechanism, (b) inhibition of glycogen bio-synthesis, (c) increased rate of insertion of nicotinic ACh receptors and mRNA levels coding for its subunit in the muscle plasmalemma, (d) stimulation of adenylate cyclase activity and phosphoinositide turnover via activation of adenylate cyclase and elevation of cyclic AMP and (e) increased rate of densitization of ACh receptors (see Roa and Changeux, 1991). These actions, together with the demonstration that CGRP is synthesized and transported from motor neurones and appears in motor neurones and nerve terminals during the period of synapto-genesis in the neuromuscular junction, support a role for CGRP as an anterograde nerve/muscle trophic factor that is important for muscle

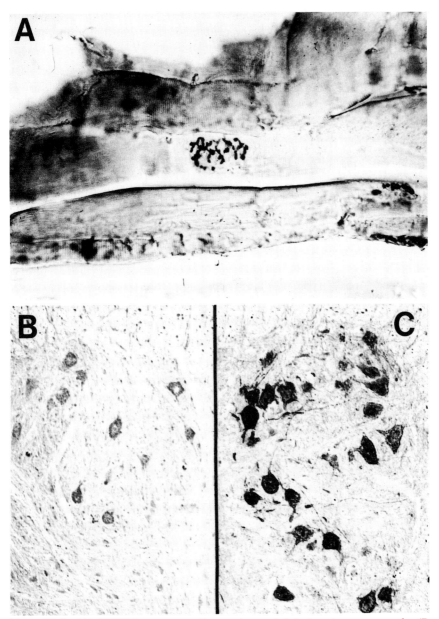

Figure 28.8 (A) CGRP-immunoreactive motor endplate in rat psoas muscle. (B and C) Rat L4 ventral spinal cord segments showing the distribution of CGRP-immunoreactive motor neurones in normal (B) and colchicine-treated (C) animals. Note intensely immunoreactive motor neurones and processes after colchicine administration.

623

Neuropeptides

fibre development in the biogenesis and maturation of the neuromuscular junction. A role for CGRP in maintenance of the adult neuromuscular junction is suggested by the following facts:

1. CGRP immunoreactivity is re-expressed in motor endplates (Matteoli, 1991) (although receptor binding is slightly decreased – Roa and Changeux, 1991) following denervation; and
2. treatment of dysgenic myotubes with CGRP restores normal ultrastructural features (Garcia *et al.*, 1990).

β-Endorphin- (β-END) and α-melanotrophin- (α-MT) immunoreactive nerve terminals and opioid receptors (β-END) are present in a small population of somatic skeletal neuromuscular junctions of normal adult rodents (Haynes, Smyth and Zakarian, 1982; Haynes and Smith, 1985; Hughes and Smith, 1990). There are greater numbers of immunoreactive motor terminals in embryonic rodents, and β-END release can be evoked from immature nerve–muscle preparations in response to nerve stimulation (Haynes, Smith and Li, 1985). As with CGRP, the number of immunoreactive endplates declines after birth to the low levels attained in the adult. In adult denervated mouse muscles there are considerable increases in β-END- and α-MT-immunoreactive motor terminals as well as in mice with motor neurone disease (wobbler mice) and muscular dystrophy (Hughes and Smith, 1988, 1989). In the latter myopathy, there are also significantly greater numbers of muscle fibres expressing binding sites for β-END (Hughes and Smith, 1990). POMC-related peptides possess many trophic actions [see Strand *et al.* (1991) for review and section 28.4.2], including increased endplate branching and promotion of nerve growth after nerve section and amelioration of muscle atrophy after denervation. Enhancement of neuromuscular synaptogenesis mediated by POMC-related peptides is of particular significance and supports a role for these peptides in regulation and maintenance of the neuromuscular junction and an involvement with pathological conditions of motor neurones.

Although this chapter is devoted to peptides that are present in motor nerves, it would give an incomplete picture of nerve–muscle relationships if mention of the polypeptide N-CAM (neural-cell adhesion molecule) was omitted. N-CAM was originally identified as a cell-surface antigen that mediates adhesive interactions between cells in the nervous system during neurogenesis (Cunningham, 1991) and is thought to play a part in axonal guidance in myogenesis and regeneration of nerves (including motor terminals) and muscles (Edelman, 1987; Rutishauser and Jessell, 1988). The mechanisms involved in neural degeneration/regeneration in muscles include fundamental cell–cell interactions. One of the earliest appearing (primary) molecules involved in these events is N-CAM, a member of the immunoglobulin superfamily (Cunningham *et al.*, 1987). Developing muscle (myoblasts) express N-CAM, but after innervation is completed N-CAM is down-regulated (Daniloff *et al.*, 1986; Rutishauser and Jessell, 1988; Cunningham, 1991). However, if the sciatic nerve is cut or crushed in experimental animals, N-CAM and its mRNA increase in the muscle and distal stumps of the transected nerves (Daniloff *et al.*, 1986; Tacke and Martini, 1990; Mallonga and Ontell, 1991), returning to the normally low levels found in the adult after reinnervation of the denervated muscle. In man also, myofibre N-CAM is present in denervated and myopathic muscles, as well as in non-diagnostic biopsies from MND patients, but is not present in normal or abnormal muscle showing no sign of denervation/reinnervation (Cashman *et al.*, 1987). Furthermore, axonal motor nerve terminal sprouting is inhibited in paralysed mouse muscles by an antibody to N-CAM (Booth, Kemplay and Brown, 1990). In wobbler mice increased N-CAM levels also occur in the muscle, where there is intense axonal sprouting, but activity is reduced in the majority of neuromuscular contacts, which has been suggested as a specific defect of the motor neurone (Melki *et al.*, 1991).

28.4 EXPERIMENTAL ANIMAL STUDIES

A summary of neuropeptide changes associated with motor nerves in experimental animals is shown in Table 28.3.

28.4.1 Motor nerve manipulations

PERIPHERAL NERVE TRANSECTION

Peripheral nerve axotomy has profound effects on motor nerves and motor function. Motor neurones become chromolytic and protein synthesis changes in response to regeneration of severed axons. In brainstem and spinal cord motor neurones, CGRP immunoreactivity increases up to twofold and is evident by 15 h after axotomy, when staining occurs throughout the cell body, dendritic extensions and some myelinated fibres (presumably representing degenerating axons). Levels return to normal from between 2 and 6 weeks later (Moore, 1989; Streit *et al.*, 1989; Villar *et al.*, 1989; Arvidsson *et al.*, 1990b; Piehl, 1991). A strong induction of CGRP mRNA expression is also evident by 16 h, peaking at 48 h post-operatively (Haas, Streit and Krentzberg, 1990). In contrast to CGRP immunoreactivity, which normalizes, Piehl *et al.* (1991) showed that mRNA levels remained elevated even after 2 weeks, indicative of increased synthesis/release of CGRP from motor nerves as a

Neuropeptides

Table 28.3 Summary of neuropeptide changes in experimental animals

Animal study	Observations
Peripheral axotomy	↑ CGRP-IR, CGRP mRNA motor neurones
	↑ GAL-IR motor neurones
	↑ α-MT-IR motor neurones
	↑ β-END, α-MT motor endplates
Colchicine	↑ CGRP-IR, CGRP mRNA motor neurones
	↑ GAL-IR motor neurones
Castration	↑ CGRP-IR, CGRP mRNA motor neurones
Spantide	↓ CGRP-IR motor neurones
Wobbler mice	↓ CGRP-IR motor neurones
	↑ TRH-, SP-, ENK-, NPY-, GAL, CCK-IR ventral horn fibres
	↑ β-END, α-MT-IR motor endplates
Ataxic mice	↑ TRH-IR in lumbar cord
Shambling mice	↑ TRH-, SP-IR in motor neurones
Arthritic rats	↓ CGRP-IR motor neurones
Leprae mice	↓ CGRP-IR motor neurones
Dystrophic mice	↑ β-END-, α-MT-IR motor neurones and endplates
Botulinum A toxin	↑ TRH mRNA raphe neurones

Abbreviations: CCK, cholecystokinin; CGRP, calcitonin gene-related peptide; β-END, β-endorphin; GAL, galanin; α-MT, α-melanotrophin; NPY, neuropeptide Y; SP, substance P; TRH, thyrotrophin-releasing hormone; IR, immunoreactivity; ↑ increase, ↓ decrease.

response to axon injury. Ventral root section induced similar changes. Phenotypic re-expression of α-MT and galanin in spinal motor neurones has also been suggested (Hughes and Smith, 1987; Polak *et al.*, 1991) following sciatic nerve section. In the severed nerve trunks and neuromas small increases, followed by reduced levels, of CGRP-immunoreactive nerves are found 1 week post-operatively; by contrast, galanin fibres remain increased. The majority of these fibres are of sensory origin, so whether there are alterations of peptide expression in motor axons as a consequence of alterations in transport due to increased synthesis in the motor neurone is not clear (White, Leah and Zimmerman, 1989; Fried, Brodin and Theodorsson, 1990; Villar *et al.*, 1989). Twenty-four hours after nerve ligation accumulation of CCK immunoreactivity is present in large axonal swellings proximal to the ligature, which also contain CGRP, supporting the recent observations that CCK is also a peptide produced by and transported from motor neurones (Abelson and Micevych, 1991; Cortes *et al.*, 1991; Schiffman *et al.*, 1991).

In denervated mouse muscles, 24 h after unilateral sciatic nerve section, when most axons have degenerated, numbers of endplates immunoreactive for β-END and α-MT increase to 50% and 25%, respectively, of total endplates. The increase is also apparent in the contralateral limb muscle. The mechanism for the contralateral effect may be transneuronal via the spinal cord or by an uptake of circulating peptides produced from the pituitary in response to injury.

COLCHICINE

Use of this antimitotic drug blocks axonal transport, and in spinal and brainstem motor neurones increases in CGRP immunoreactivity and mRNA and in galanin immunoreactivity have been reported, demonstrating that there is also an effect on peptide synthesis (Gibson et al., 1984; Ch'ng et al., 1985; Rethelyi et al., 1991; Hietanen-Peltola, 1992) (Figure 28.4D and 28.8B and C).

CASTRATION

Castration has a similar effect on CGRP-producing motor neurones to that of peripheral nerve section and colchicine administration. The mechanism for the change in castration, however, is likely to be more complicated. In male rats, motor neurones located in the spinal nucleus of the bulbocavernosus (SNB) in lower lumbar segments innervate the bulbocavernosus, levator ani and anal sphincter muscles (Schroder, 1980). These neurones accumulate testosterone and are androgen sensitive, which implies that they bear androgen receptor sites that play a key role in gene transcription (Breedlove and Arnold, 1980; Evans, 1988), which is up-regulated after nerve injury (Kinderman and Jones, 1991). CGRP expression in SNB motor neurones is sensitive to circulating levels of testosterone. Following castration, numbers of SNB motor neurones expressing CGRP immunoreactivity and mRNA are significantly increased; this effect is reversed by testosterone replacement in the castrates, and penile reflexes are also restored (Popper and Micevych, 1990). It appears that testosterone directly influences CGRP gene transcription and expression in SNB motor neurones. Alternatively, the increase may reflect increased release of a neurotrophic factor or factors from the denervated target muscles (Popper, Ulibarri and Micevych, 1992). Increased numbers of CGRP SNB motor neurones are also found after muscle (bulbocavernosus, levator ani) inactivation with local anaesthetic (Popper and Micevych, 1990). It seems probable that CGRP may be one of these neurotrophic factors, consistent with the actions of CGRP in regulation of muscle function (Laufer and Changeux, 1987) and sprout formation during muscle regeneration and disuse

Neuropeptides

(Tsujimoto and Kuno, 1988; White and Zimmerman, 1988). If so, increased synthesis in accord with elevated levels of CGRP mRNA in SNB motor neurones is in accord with the raised levels seen in motor neurones after peripheral nerve section (Arvidsson *et al.*, 1989; Moore, 1989; Streit *et al.*, 1989).

SPANTIDE

Spantide, a substance P analogue, developed as a antinociceptive agent, also affects motor behaviour (Akerman, Rosell and Folkers, 1982). Intrathecal injection has a neurotoxic action in rat (but not mouse) motor neurones, resulting in loss of CGRP and motor ridigity (Freedman *et al.*, 1986; Post *et al.*, 1987). Interestingly, these effects are counteracted by TRH administration, supporting the use of TRH as a preventative against neuronal damage (Freedman *et al.*, 1989; see review by Strand *et al.*, 1991).

28.4.2 Models of motor nerve dysfunction

Animal models involving motor nerve abnormalities, either genetically inherited or experimentally induced, are discussed fully in Chapter 29. Neuropeptides have been studied in some animals with motor nerve dysfunction and these are summarized below.

WOBBLER MICE

Wobbler mice are considered to be models of human MND and infantile spinal muscular atrophy (Duchen, Falconer and Strich, 1966; Puchen, Strich and Falconer, 1968). They exhibit recessively inherited degeneration of motor neurones and other ventral horn neurones, which is most apparent in the cervical spinal cord. Vacca-Galloway and co-workers have made extensive studies of neuropeptide and 5-HT changes in the spinal cord and brainstem of wobbler mice (Tang, Cheung and Vacca-Galloway, 1990; Vacca-Galloway *et al.*, 1987; Yung *et al.*, 1990; Zhang and Vacca-Galloway, 1992). Initial studies found that substance P-, TRH- and 5-HT-immunoreactive fibres were increased in the ventral horn of wobbler mice in well-advanced stages of the disease compared with controls. These findings are consistent with interneuronal sprouting of neurochemically defined subsets of neuronal processes that is most likely linked to degeneration of motor neurones (Vacca-Galloway *et al.*, 1987). Increased concentrations of TRH have also been found in spinal cords of ataxic mice (Mitsuma *et al.*, 1990) as well as of substance P in shambling mutant mice (Mitsuma *et al.*, 1988), which may further indicate that neuronal sprouting occurs in some examples of motor dysfunction. More recent qualitative and quantitative immunochemical studies (for determination of fibre density using computerized morphometry and point counting on a grid) in wobbler mice mutants have confirmed and extended earlier observations (Zang and Vacca-Galloway, 1992). In the later stages of the disease fibres immunoreactive for substance P, CCK, NPY, galanin and 5-HT were significantly increased in the lateral ventral horn of cervical segments. In addition, there was an increase of enkephalin-immunoreactive fibres, in agreement with previous observations by radioimmunoassay (Tang, Cheung and Vacca-Galloway, 1990; Yung et al., 1990). By contrast, CGRP-immunoreactive fibres and cell bodies were decreased. Alterations in immunoreactivity for CCK, CGRP and enkephalins were evident in early stages of the disease, when motor neuronal degeneration is barely detectable, whereas changes in substance P, NPY and galanin were more exaggerated in later stages when compared with pair-matched phenotypic controls. In the brainstems of wobbler mice substance P-immunoreactive fibres were also increased in sensory cranial nuclei, whereas CGRP was reduced in sensory (fibres) and motor (fibres and motor neurones) cranial nuclei. The fact that no change was noted in corticospinal tracts that degenerate in MND suggests that the wobbler does not exactly mimic the pathology of MND in man. In addition, alterations of neuropeptides were found in the dorsal horn (increased CCK, enkephalins; reduced CGRP) and lamina X (increased substance P; reduced CGRP) sensory regions of the spinal cord and in the autonomic nuclei (increased substance P, unchanged CGRP). An involvement of these areas is not characteristic of MND and suggests that in wobbler mice the disease process is not only restricted to motor neurones. The cause of the increase of fibres is unknown, but Vacca-Galloway et al. (1987) suggested that the progressive loss of AChe, which hydrolyses substance P, from degenerating cholinergic motor neurones, (Chubb, Hodgson and White, 1980), could explain the increase of substance P. However, this does not hold for the remaining neuropeptides, and the authors speculate that the peptide-containing fibres increase as a result of motor neurone degeneration in an attempt to protect from and ameliorate the disease process (Zhang and Vacca-Galloway, 1992). However, in MND in which degeneration is more severe, decreases of fibres immunoreactive for substance P, enkephalin, TRH and NPY have been noted (section 28.5.1 and Table 28.3); thus, in early stages of MND, when degeneration is not pronounced, sprouting of peptide nerve fibres may take place prior to their loss in the final stage. Since CGRP influences regeneration (Streit et al., 1989) and neuronal sprouting (White and Zimmerman, 1988; McNeill et al., 1990), it may exert a more direct effect on the disease process. The loss of CGRP from cervical motor neurones and motor cranial nuclei, and hence loss of trophic support to the neuromuscular junctions (Fontaine, Klarsfeld and Changeux, 1986; New and Mudge, 1986; Laufer and Changeux, 1987), correlates with atrophy of facial and triceps muscles respectively that are characteristically associated with the mutant wobbler mice.

Degeneration and regeneration of motor neurones, unlike in human MND, is a feature of wobbler mutants (Mitsumoto and Bradley, 1982). Further evidence that neuropeptides participate in the repairing effect has been demonstrated by the increased abundance of POMC-related peptides (β-END and α-MT) in motor endplates of wobbler mice compared with controls (Hughes and Smith, 1989). These peptides are not normally expressed in adult motor nerves but are present during development [see Hughes and Smith (1989) for further references]. Both β-END and α-MT promote synaptogenesis and motor function and are neurotrophic (Strand et al., 1991). Phenotypic re-expression of POMC-related peptides in wobbler mice suggests they are of importance in the reinnervation of the neuromuscular junction in this disease.

ARTHRITIC RATS AND LEPROMATOUS MICE

Adjuvant-induced arthritis has been used as an animal model for the study of chronic pain (De Castro Costa et al., 1981; Colpaert et al., 1982), but decreased locomotor activity also accompanies this condition (Dardick, Basbaum and Levine, 1986). A significant loss of CGRP-immunoreactive motor neurones from the lumbar (L4) spinal cord is evident 28 days after induction of arthritis, although numbers of motor neurones are unchanged (Kar et al., 1991) (Figure 28.9A and B). Furthermore, in animals with unilateral sciatic nerve section, prior to induction of arthritis a few CGRP-immunoreactive motor neurones are present in the contralateral ventral horn, but ipsilateral to the axotomy numbers of CGRP motor neurones are significantly greater than in the contralateral side (but not equal to that of normal litter mate controls; Figure 28.10). Loss of CGRP from motor neurones of arthritic rats is consistent with their reduced muscular activity and also with loss of target (muscle)-derived trophic factors (Oppenheim, Haverkamp and Prevette, 1988), which may depend on CGRP for their production or vice versa. The presence of considerable numbers of CGRP-immunoreactive motor neurones in the ipsilateral ventral horn of arthritic rats with sciatic nerve section suggests that the leg on the lesioned side may be used in preference to the intact, 'painful' limb (contralateral side). Alternatively, the ipsilateral increase (relative to the intact side) could be a conse-

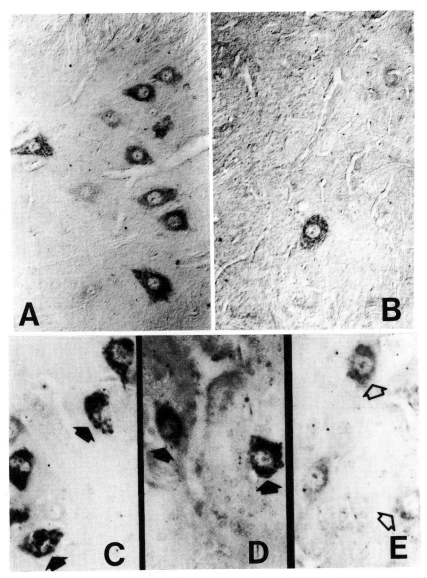

Figure 28.9 CGRP-immunoreactive motor neurones in the rat (A and B) and mouse (C–E) ventral horn of L4 spinal cord segments. (A) Control rat. (B) Adjuvant-induced arthritic rat. There is a marked loss of CGRP-immunoreactive motor neurones in the diseased state. (C) Control mouse. (D and E) Mice 6 and 12 months, respectively, after injection of *Myobacterium leprae* into the footpad. Note reduction of immunoreactivity with time post injection; by 12 months immunoreactive product is absent from the motor neurones (open arrows), although the motor neurones are still present.

631

Neuropeptides

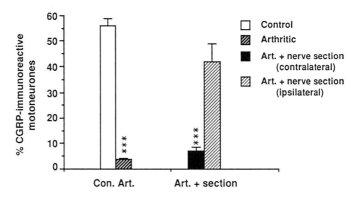

Figure 28.10 Histogram to show the percentage of CGRP-immunoreactive motor neurones in the L4 segment of control, adjuvant-induced arthritic and arthritic rats with unilateral sciatic nerve section. Columns and bars represent means ± standard error of means (SEM); *** $P < 0.001$.

quence of severance of motor nerve axons and induce increased expression of CGRP in a population of motor neurones that does not display the CGRP phenotype in adult motor neurones.

Loss of CGRP-immunoreactive motor neurones has also been noted in lepromatous mice (Karanth *et al.*, 1991). Although this condition is primarily associated with sensory deficits, there is muscle weakness and in the later stages of leprosy in man there is significant muscle atrophy (Goodwin and Watson, 1968). In mice injected with *Myobacterium leprae*, a progressive loss of CGRP-immunoreactive motor neurones, from a few present at 6 months to total disappearance at 12 months post infection, was reported (Figure 28.9C–E). Thus, as in the arthritic condition, the importance of CGRP in motor neurones and the integrity of normal muscle function is underlined.

DYSTROPHIC MICE

The majority of neuropeptide studies in dystrophic mice relate to POMC-related peptides. These animals are characterized by abnormalities of motor neurones, delayed development of neuromuscular junctions and acceleration of degeneration and regeneration of motor nerves (Crowe and Baskin, 1982). Atypical of adult rodents, POMC-related peptides (α-MT and to a lesser extent β-END) are found in motor nerve terminals and motor neurones of dystrophic mice, but do occur during development (Haynes, Smyth and Zakarian, 1982; Haynes and Smith, 1985). In dystrophic mice, digitorum muscles have elevated numbers of immunoreactive motor nerve terminals as well as increased numbers of opioid receptors (β-END and naloxone) (Hughes and Smith,

Table 28.4 Distribution of peptide-immunoreactive fibres in MND spinal cord compared with normal controls

Peptide	Dorsal horn	Autonomic nuclei	Ventral horn
CCK	N[a]	N[a]	N[a]
CGRP	N[b-e]	N[b,c]	N[b,c]
CPON	N[b]	N[b]	N[b]
ENK	N[a-c]	N[a-c]	↓ N[a-c]
GAL	N[b,c]	N[b,c]	N[b,c]
NPY	N[c]	N[c]	N[c]
PHI	N[c]	N[c]	N[c]
SOM	N[b,c]	N[b,c]	↓ N[b,c]
SP	↓ N[a-c,f]	N[a-c]	↓ N[a-c,f]
TRH	n.p	N[b,g]	↓ N[b,g]
VIP	N[b,c]	N[b,c]	N[b,c]

From: [a] Schoenen *et al.* (1985b); [b] Gibson *et al.* (1988a); [c] Katagiri *et al.* (1988); [d] Kato *et al.* (1991a); [e] Kato *et al.* (1991b); [f] Patten and Croft (1984); [g] Jackson *et al.* (1986).
Abbreviations: CCK, cholecystokinin; CGRP, calcitonin gene-related peptide; CPON, C-flanking peptide of neuropeptide Y; ENK, enkephalin; GAL, galanin; NPY, neuropeptide Y; PHI, peptide histidine isoleucine; SOM, somatostatin; SP, substance P; TRH, thyrotrophin-releasing hormone; VIP, vasoactive intestinal polypeptide. N, normal distribution of immunoreactive fibres, ↓ decrease of immunoreactive fibres; n.p., not present.

1990). Two days after section of the sciatic nerve (when the majority of nerves degenerate) there is a marked increase in β-END (less significantly α-MT, as this is already highly expressed) in the denervated and contralateral muscles in comparison with unoperated dystrophic mice (Hughes and Smith, 1988). These data suggest that a phenotypic re-expression of POMC-like peptides may occur as a general response to perturbation of motor nerves, in addition to their participation in acceleration of nerve growth/regeneration (section 28.4.2) (Strand *et al.*, 1981; Edwards *et al.*, 1986).

28.5.1 Distribution of peptide-containing fibres in MND spinal cord

Several immunocytochemical studies have investigated the localization of peptide-containing nerves in the spinal cords of MND patients. The peptides studied and the reported changes are summarized in Table 28.4. The results of these investigations are briefly described below.

As it is widely agreed that MND is characterized by progressive degeneration of the corticospinal tracts and lower motor neurones, it is the motor system that is exclusively affected in this neurological disease

Neuropeptides

(Chapter 15). Thus, it was to be expected that the distribution of peptide-containing nerves in the dorsal horn (region associated with sensory processing) or autonomic nuclei would not show drastic change in MND (Figure 28.11A–F). There is only one report that evidences changed peptide immunoreactivity, substance P, in the dorsal horn and nucleus proprius (Patten and Croft, 1984). Although a few clinicopathological studies suggest that there is some sensory pathway involvement in MND (Dyck et al., 1975; Jamal et al., 1985) and substance P is largely confined to sensory nerves (and is therefore a good marker), more recent immunocytochemical studies have not reported a similar trend (Schoenen et al., 1985b; Gibson et al., 1988a; Katagiri et al., 1988).

In the ventral horn of diseased spinal cords, a loss of fibres immunoreactive for enkephalin, somatostatin and TRH has been established (Schoenen et al., 1985b; Gibson et al., 1988a; Patten and Croft, 1984) (Figure 28.11I–L). Reduction of substance P fibres was clearly demonstrated by Schoenen et al. (1985b), who by mapping exactly the distribution of substance P-containing fibres in the ventral cord found the loss of immunoreactivity was restricted to the large motor neurone columns (lamina IX) in four patients with sporadic MND (interestingly, however, these changes were not visible in a case of familial MND). Loss of substance P from the ventral horn is consistent with our own studies (Gibson et al., 1988a) and with Patten and Croft (1984). Radioimmunoassay, however, by two independent groups failed to find any significant change in substance P concentrations in the ventral cord of MND patients (Otsuka et al., 1978; Gillberg et al., 1982). The apparent contradiction between these reports remains unexplained. But since motor neurones degenerate, the immunoreactive fibres normally associated with them are also lost and the overall concentration of peptide-immunoreactive fibres should be less than that in control tissues. In support of this speculation, TRH measured per mg of protein gave similar values in control and MND cases; measurement per wet weight of tissue showed a decrease of TRH concentrations in MND (Mitsuma, Nagimori and Adachi, 1984; Jackson et al., 1986). Although in the study by Jackson et al. (1986) TRH-immunoreactive fibres were apparently unaltered in the ventral spinal cord of MND patients, later work (Gibson et al., 1988a) noted a loss of small TRH-positive fibres, which are found normally in close proximity to motor neuronal cell bodies and processes. It is interesting that enkephalin-, somatostatin-, substance P- and TRH-immunoreactive fibres were decreased in MND patients (Table 28.4), and it may be of some significance to consider changes that take place in the cells that give rise to these fibres in the ventral spinal cord to establish whether they may contribute to motor

634

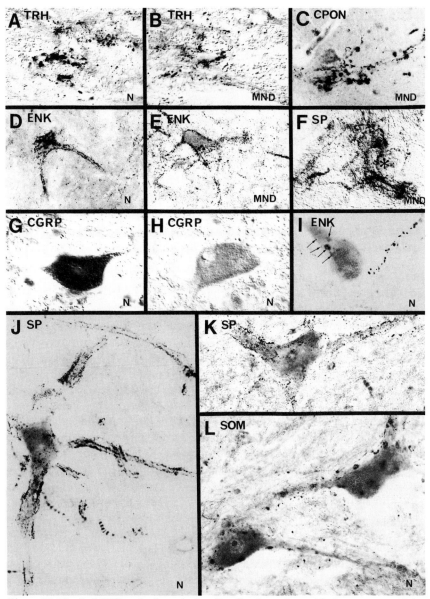

Figure 28.11 In MND spinal cord, the distribution of peptide immunoreactivity in the intermediolateral cell columns is similar to that of normal controls. (A and B) TRH-immunoreactive fibres in the thoracic intermediolateral cell columns. (C) CPON-immunoreactive fibres in the thoracic intermediolateral cell column. (D and E) ENK-immunoreactive fibres in the thoracic intermediolateral cell column outlining non-immunoreactive preganglionic neurones. (F) Substance P (SP)-immunoreactive fibres in the sacral intermediolateral cell column. Asterisks, non-immunoreactive preganglionic neurone. (G–L) Ventral horn of normal human spinal cord. (G) CGRP-immunoreactive motor neurone in lamina IX in the lumbar spinal cord. (H) A motor neurone from same patient as (G), which is not immunoreactive. (I) ENK-, (J and K) substance P and (L) somatostatin (SOM)-immunoreactive fibres in close apposition to motor neurones in lamina IX of the lumbar spinal cord. N, normal; MND, motor neurone disease.

neuronal degeneration. Many of these fibres originate from the raphe nuclei of the brainstem, and there is a notable degree of coexistence between enkephalin, substance P and TRH (Hunt, 1983; Ruda, Bennett and Dubner, 1986). It is possible that a neurochemically coded cell type in the raphe nucleus is also selectively vulnerable in MND. Interestingly, *in situ* hybridization has shown that TRH mRNA expression increases in raphe neurones of rats treated with botulinum toxin A (Vandenbergh, Octave and Lechan, 1991), indicating that neurochemical changes do occur in these neurones as a consequence of muscle denervation and that TRH may exert a trophic influence on spinal motor neurones.

Several reports have analysed the distribution of peptide-containing fibres in a small nucleus located in sacral segments, known as Onuf's nucleus (see above; Schoenen *et al.*, 1985b; Gibson *et al.*, 1988a; Katagiri *et al.*, 1988). This nucleus is of particular interest in MND, as even in the most advanced stages of the disease the neurones are preserved (Mannen *et al.*, 1977; Iwata and Hirano, 1979; Sung, 1982; Oyanagi, Makifuchi and Ikuta, 1983; Konno *et al.*, 1986). Onuf's nucleus is characterized by the rich supply of nerve fibres immunoreactive for enkephalin, somatostatin and CPON that innervate it in man. Consistent with the selective sparing of this nucleus in MND, no change in the density of immunostaining has been found in the diseased spinal cords (Schoenen *et al.*, 1985b; Gibson *et al.*, 1988a; Katagiri *et al.*, 1988) (Figure 28.12).

Neurones of Onuf's nucleus are thought to innervate perineal striated muscle, and therefore should be classically regarded as somatic motor neurones (Mannen *et al.*, 1977). But there has long been speculation as to whether these neurones are somatic, autonomic or of mixed types of neurones (Onuf, 1900; Laruelle, 1937; Pons-Tortella, Roca-de-Vinales and Rodriguez-Arias, 1951; Rexed, 1954; Nakano, 1969; Mannen *et al.*, 1977). Several lines of evidence support the view that Onuf's nucleus may be autonomic.

1. Vesicorectal function relies upon the integrity of Onuf's nucleus and the parasympathetic autonomic nucleus (Yamamoto *et al.*, 1977; Sung, 1979).
2. Neurones of Onuf's nucleus share a common selective vulnerability together with autonomic neurones in neurological conditions such as Shy-Drager syndrome and Fabry's disease (Konno *et al.*, 1986; Mannen *et al.*, 1977; Sung *et al.*, 1979; Sung 1982, but see also Oyanagi *et al.*, 1983).
3. Some parasympathetic neurones are thought to be located in the ventral horn (Jacobsohn, 1908; Jacobsohn-Lask, 1931; Laurelle, 1937).

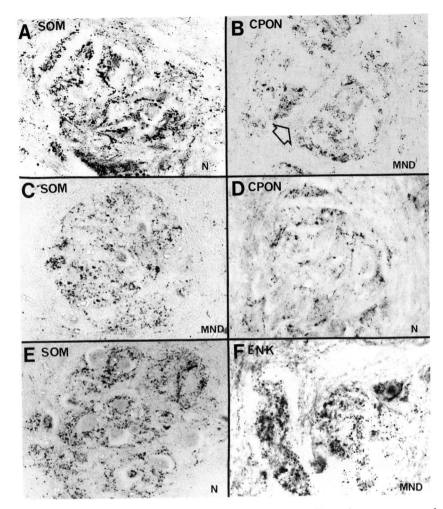

Figure 28.12 Peptide-immunoreactive fibres surrounding the neurones of Onuf's nucleus in the S2 segment of diseased (MND) and normal (N) spinal cord. (A, C and E) Somatostatin-immunoreactive fibres. (A and C) Cryostat sections. (E) Wax section. (B and D) Fibres immunoreactive for NPY/CPON. Note the distinct dendritic bundle (open arrow), which is characteristic of Onuf's nucleus. (F) ENK-immunoreactive fibres.

4. A cellular bridge connects Onuf's nucleus with the parasympathetic nucleus (Konno *et al.*, 1986).
5. The neurones of Onuf's nucleus are smaller than somatic motor neurones (Shroder, 1981).

Neuropeptides

However, most convincing evidence for at least a partly autonomic nature derives from the immunocytochemical studies demonstrating that the rich peptidergic (namely enkephalin, somatostatin and CPON) innervation of Onuf's nucleus is common to the autonomic nuclei, neither of which is affected in MND. Whether this innervation reflects only the autonomic nature of Onuf's neurones (Anand and Bloom, 1984) or directly influences preservation of the neurones by providing a protective action remains to be established.

28.5.2 Distribution of neuropeptide-containing motor neurones in MND

Since to date relatively few neuropeptides have been identified in motor neurones of adult man, studies that address the possibility of changes of expression of peptide-containing motor neurones in MND are not extensive. However, as expected, most reports have centred on the distribution and change in localization of CGRP.

Our early studies (Gibson et al., 1988a) analysed by immunocyto-chemistry the presence of CGRP-immunoreactive motor neurones in spinal cords of 52 neurologically normal subjects and 36 patients with MND. Where possible, samples were matched for age and post-mortem times (age range 14–84 years; post-mortem times 12–220 h normal, 53–79 h MND). Similar segmental levels (cervical, thoracic, lumbar and sacral) were also studied, but most samples had varying fixation times, some samples having been optimally fixed for immunocytochemistry (i.e. 8–12 h in fixative), whilst other were obtained after formalin fixation for between 1 and 9 years. As perhaps expected, we found that there was a severe loss of motor neurones from the MND spinal cords and that there was an overall reduction in numbers of CGRP-immunoreactive motor neurones when compared with controls (Figure 28.11G and H). More recent preliminary studies of spinal cords obtained within 3–4 h post mortem, in which antigenicity was more optimally preserved, showed that in two of the six spinal cords from MND patients there were also reduced numbers of CGRP-containing motor neurones. In the remainder, however, some motor neurones were strongly labelled with CGRP antiserum. It would seem therefore that the relationship between CGRP expression in motor neurones of MND spinal cords is not always clear cut. Indeed, the later and more extensive studies of Kato et al. (1991a,b) on tissues also obtained relatively soon after death (2–12 h post-mortem delay) have shown in a detailed analysis of spinal cords from patients with familial ($n = 3$) and sporadic ($n = 7$) MND that CGRP immuno-reactivity in the ventral spinal cord shows an increase over and above

638

that which is found normally in controls. CGRP immunoreactivity was identified in a half to a third of motor neurones in MND spinal cords. Most of these neurones displayed central chromatolysis, but the presence of CGRP in motor neurones from a patient with vincristine neuropathy, in which chromolytic neurones are also found, was not evident, suggesting that CGRP expression is not a general feature of chromolytic cells and may have a special role in MND (Kato et al., 1991a). In the same study, immunostaining of serial sections with antibodies to neurofilaments and ubiquitin revealed that the presence of CGRP in motor neurones that were neurofilament and ubiquitin positive was a common occurrence. Some motor neurones contained hyaline inclusions that were intensely ubiquitin positive, and here also weak labelling with the CGRP antiserum was present in the cores, with more intense staining of the haloes and surrounding areas of the inclusions. Furthermore, studies by the same group (Kato et al., 1991a,b) have also revealed that CGRP immunoreactivity occurs in spheroids, neurofilament-rich abnormal swellings of spinal neurites that are often an early pathological feature (Chou et al., 1970; Hirano and Inoue, 1980; Kato et al., 1989) in MND spinal cords. Approximately half of the spheroids showed CGRP immunoreactivity, having a range of distribution patterns (rod, rings and irregular profiles and some homogeneously stained). Immunostaining of globules (small axonal swellings) showed also some CGRP immunoreactivity in both MND patients and controls.

The relationship between presence of CGRP and MND motor neurones that show ubiquitin deposition is unclear. Ubiquitin has not yet been identified in normal spinal motor neurones (Kato et al., 1988; Leigh, Anderton and Dodson, 1988; Lowe et al., 1988; Murayama et al., 1989; Chapter 16). Ubiquitin is thought to have a major role in regulation of the ATP-dependent non-lysosomal proteolytic system; thus subsequent to ubiquitination of proteins degeneration of the protein ensues (Hershko, 1983; Ciechanover, Finley and Varshowsky, 1984; Chapter 16). Thus, the presence of CGRP and ubiquitin in motor neurones of MND may be related to degeneration of motor neurones in this disease.

Kato et al. (1991a,b) postulate that their findings of CGRP accumulation in motor neurones and neuritic swellings of MND spinal cords may be caused by defects in axonal transport, which causes an entrapment of CGRP, which may in turn induce a loss of CGRP supply to the neuromuscular junction. Other factors many explain their observations. In support of these studies, however, although we have been unable to detect a clear increase in CGRP immunoreactivity in MND motor neurones, we have in a pilot study of spinal cords (3–4 h post mortem) shown that in two cases the message is reduced when compared with normal controls. In situ hybridization employing a ^{32}P radioactively labelled cRNA probe for α-CGRP [see Gibson *et al.* (1988b) for details of probe] revealed fewer CGRP transcripts in MND motor neurones (Figure 28.13A and B). Thus if there is reduced synthesis of the peptide, reduced axonal transport could also be expected.

CGRP has a well-described action as a motor neurone-derived anterograde muscle trophic factor that is released from the neuromuscular junction (Fontaine *et al.*, 1986) and a number of motor actions have been described for this peptide, including contraction of striated muscle (Takami *et al.*, 1985b), increasing the level of cAMP in muscle and myocytes (Takami *et al.*, 1985b; Laufer and Changeux, 1987; Jennings and Mudge, 1989) and regulation of acetylcholine receptor channel properties at the neuromuscular junction (Laufer and Changeux, 1987; New and Mudge, 1986; Ohhashi and Jacobowitz, 1988). The ability of motor neurones to synthesize and transport this peptide to the motor endplates may thus have a direct trophic effect on muscle fibre function and in turn on the integrity of the motor neurone. As MND may be caused by an impairment of trophic mechanisms between muscle and neurones, CGRP is likely to be of importance to motor neurone survival.

Endothelin, therefore, remains as the only other major peptide found in motor neurones of human adults (Giaid *et al.*, 1989). The fact that endothelin immunoreactivity and mRNA for the peptide occur in considerable numbers of motor neurones suggests that its biosynthesis may be linked to normal functioning of motor nerves. To date, however, this peptide has not yet been fully investigated in MND spinal cords. Our preliminary investigations on spinal cords (3–4 h post mortem) using immunocytochemistry and *in situ* hybridization with a ^{32}P-labelled endothelin-1 cRNA indicate a generalized loss of motor neurones expressing endothelin immunoreactivity and its mRNA in two patients with MND compared with controls (Figure 28.13C–F). These studies need to be extended but are encouraging. However, the possible role of endothelin in the motor neurone has not yet been identified, and no action on skeletal muscle activity has so far been demonstrated (Wilkund *et al.*, 1989). Thus, whether endothelin, like CGRP, will prove to be a nerve muscle trophic factor remains conjectural. Demonstration of the presence of receptors for endothelin and release from the neuromuscular junction would further underline the importance of this peptide in the motor neurone and axonal projections.

28.5.3 Neuropeptide receptor studies in MND

Receptor localization of neuropeptides in MND spinal cord adds support to the reports using immunocytochemical and radioimmuno-assay techniques (Mitsuma, Nagimori and Adachi, 1984; Patten and

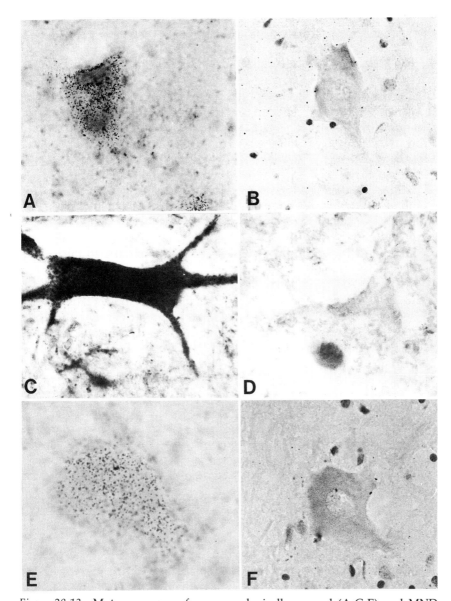

Figure 28.13 Motor neurones from neurologically normal (A,C,E) and MND (B,D,F) lumbar spinal cords. (A,B) Autoradiographs hybridized with ^{32}P-labelled CGRP cRNA probes. In the normal spinal cord most motor neurones express CGRP transcripts (A) but in MND only background levels of labelling are seen in the vicinity of the motor neurones (B). (C) Strongly endothelin-immunoreactive motor neurone in normal spinal cord, in the diseased state (D) most motor neurones are non-immunoreactive. (E and F) Autoradiographs hybridized with ^{32}P-labelled endothelin cRNA. Most motor neurones express endothelin transcripts in control tissues (E), but in MND the density of silver grains over motor neuronal soma is low (F).

Neuropeptides

Croft, 1984; Schoenen *et al.*, 1985b; Jackson *et al.*, 1986; Gibson *et al.*, 1988a) of losses of TRH and substance P from the ventral spinal cord. By means of quantitative *in vitro* autoradiography and analysis of auto-radiograms with densitometry, concentrations of TRH receptors have been reported to be reduced by up to 50% in lamina IX (region containing motor neurones) (Manaker *et al.*, 1985, 1988), and this is attributable to reduced numbers of receptors and not to changes in the binding affinity of the radioligand. Receptors for substance P were also studied in MND by *in vitro* autoradiography, and in addition adjacent sections were examined for substance P immunoreactivity employing radioimmunohistochemistry [Dietl *et al.*, 1989; see Hunt, Allanson and Mantyh (1986) for the immunocytochemical method]. Substance P binding was decreased in MND patients, notably in the ventral spinal cord (lamina IX). By contrast, immunoreactivity for the peptide did not show marked changes.

Whether TRH and substance P receptors are localized post-synaptically to motor neurones or presynaptically to the nerve fibres that innervate them is not clear, since loss of both motor neurones and fibres containing TRH and substance P occurs in MND. Physiological studies suggest a post-synaptic localization (Nicoll, 1977, 1978; Ono and Fukuda, 1982), but further studies are necessary to determine whether distant brain structures, e.g. raphe nucleus, which contains cells that send TRH and substance P projections to motor neurones (Hunt, 1983; Ruda, Bennett and Dubner, 1986 for reviews), are also altered, thus supporting a presynaptic location. These studies, however, confirm a role for TRH and substance P in the function of motor neurones, and also implicate them in the pathological processes involved in MND, since other receptors for neurotransmitters remain intact in the ventral spinal cord even when associated with severe motor neurone loss (e.g. β-adrenergic receptors, noradrenaline binding) (Manaker *et al.*, 1988).

28.6 CONCLUSIONS

The study of neuropeptides has considerably expanded current know-ledge of the neurobiology of motor nerves. Motor neurone function is regulated by peptide-containing nerve fibres synapsing upon the cell body, and which themselves also produce bioactive peptides. Changes in biosynthesis and expression of peptides present in motor nerves (and nerves in close contact with motor neuronal cell bodies) occur in experimental animals with abnormal motor function and in MND, consistent with motor neurotrophic effects provided by the peptides, and further highlights their importance in the preservation and maintenance of motor nerve integrity. Of particular significance is the demonstration that CGRP and the newly described peptide, endothelin, are synthesized and stored in adult human motor neurones and in MND their expression is altered. CGRP has well-established trophic actions on the neuromuscular junction, but the role of endothelin in human spinal motor neurones is not yet fully characterized. Future studies to establish the significance of endothelin to motor nerves and its interactions with CGRP and other peptides present in motor neurones or derived from synapsing nerve terminals on the motor neuronal cell body present an exciting future direction for research in MND.

ACKNOWLEDGEMENTS

Studies conducted in our laboratory were supported by the Motor Neurone Disease Association, the Colt Foundation, the Grand Charity of Freemasons, BUPA Medical Foundation and the Arthritis and Rheumatism Council.

REFERENCES

Abelson, L. and Micevych, P.E. (1991) Distribution of preprocholecystokinin messenger RNA in motoneurons of the rat brainstem and spinal cord. *Mol. Brain Res.*, **10**, 327–35.

Akerman, B., Rosell, S. and Folkers, K. (1982) Intrathecal [D-Pro2, D-Try7,9]-SP elicits hypoalgesia and motor blockade in the rat and antagonizes noxious responses induced by substance P. *Acta Physiol. Scand.*, **114**, 631–3.

Amara, S.G., Jonas, V., Rosenfeld, M.G. *et al.* (1982) Alternative RNA processing in calcitonin gene expression generates mRNAs encoding different polypeptide products. *Nature*, **298**, 240–4.

Anand, P. and Bloom, S.R. (1984) Neuropeptides are selective markers of spinal cord autonomic pathways. *Trends Neurosci.*, **7**, 267–8.

Appel, S.H. (1981) A unifying hypothesis for the cause of amyotrophic lateral sclerosis, Parkinsonism and Alzheimer disease. *Ann. Neurol.*, **10**, 499–505.

Arvidsson, N., Cullheim, S., Ulfhake, B. *et al.* (1989) Altered levels of calcitonin gene-related peptide (CGRP)-like immunoreactivity of cat lumbar moto-neurones after chronic spinal cord transection. *Brain Res.*, **48**, 9387–91.

Arvidsson, N., Ulfhake, B., Cullheuin, B. *et al.* (1991) Calcitonin gene-related peptide in monkey spinal cord and medulla oblongata. *Brain Res.*, **558**, 330–4.

Arvidsson, U., Cullheim, S., Ulfhake, B. *et al.* (1990a) 5-Hydroxytryptamine, substance P and thyrotrophin-releasing hormone in the adult cat spinal cord segment L7: immunohistochemical and chemical studies. *Synapse*, **6**, 237–70.

Arvidsson, U., Johnson, H., Piehl, F. *et al.* (1990b) Peripheral nerve section induces increased levels of calcitonin gene-related peptide (CGRP)-like immunoreactivity in axotomized motoneurones. *Exp. Brain Res.*, **79**, 212–16.

Ballesta, J., Carlei, F., Bishop, A.E. *et al.* (1987) Occurrence, projections and developmental pattern of neuromedin U-immunoreactive nerves in the gastrointestinal tract and brain of rat. *Neuroscience*, **25**, 797–816.

Bloom, S.R. and Long, R.G. (1982) *Radioimmunoassay of Gut Regulatory Peptides*. W.B. Saunders, London.

Booth, C.M., Kemplay, S.K. and Brown, M.C. (1990) An antibody to neural cell adhesion molecule impairs motor nerve terminal sprouting in a mouse muscle locally paralysed with botulinum toxin. *Neuroscience*, **35**, 85–91.

Brain, S.D. and Williams, T.J. (1985) Inflammatory oedema induced by synergism between calcitonin gene-related peptide and mediators of increased vascular permeability. *Br. J. Pharmacol.*, **86**, 855–60.

Brain, S.D., Williams, T.J., Tipins, J.R. *et al.* (1989) Calcitonin gene-related peptide is a potent vasodilator. *Nature*, **813**, 54–64.

Breedlove, S.M. and Arnold, A.P. (1980) Hormone accumulation in a sexually dimorphic motor nucleus of the rat spinal cord. *Science*, **210**, 564–6.

Bullock, A.G.M. (1987) Somatostatin enhances neurite outgrowth in *Helisoma*. *Brain Res.*, **412**, 6–17.

Calvo, J.J., Gonzalez, R., Carvalhos *et al.* (1990) Release of substance P from rat hypothalamus and pituitary by endothelin. *Endocrinology*, **126**, 2288–95.

Cashman, N.R., Covault, J., Wollman, R.L. *et al.* (1987) Neural cell adhesion molecule in normal, denervated and myopathic human muscle. *Ann. Neurol.*, **21**, 481–9.

Ch'ng, J.L.C., Christofides, N.D., Anand, P. *et al.* (1985) Distribution of galanin immunoreactivity in the central nervous system and the responses of galanin-containing neuronal pathways to injury. *Neuroscience*, **2**, 343–54.

Charlton, C. and Helke, C.J. (1985) Autoradiographic localization and characterisation of spinal cord substance P binding sites: high densities in sensory, autonomic, phrenic and Onuf's motor nuclei. *J. Neurosci.*, **5**, 1653–61.

Chou, S.M., Martin, J.D., Gutrecht, J.A. *et al.* (1970) Axonal balloons in subacute motor neuron disease. *J. Neuropathol. Exp. Neurol.*, **29**, 141–2.

Chubb, I.W., Hodgson, A.J. and White, G.H. (1980) Acetylcholinesterase hydrolyses substance P. *Neuroscience*, **5**, 2065–72.

Ciechanover, A., Finley, D. and Varshowsky, A. (1984) Ubiquitin dependence of selective protein degradation demonstrated in the mammalian cell cycle mutant. *Cell*, **34**, 57–66.

Colpaert, F.C., Meert, T., De Witte, P. *et al.* (1982) Further evidence validating adjuvant arthritis as an experimental model of chronic pain in the rat. *Life Sci.*, **31**, 67–75.

Cortes, R., Arvidsson, U., Schalling, M. *et al.* (1990) In situ hybridization studies on mRNAs for cholecystokinin, calcitonin gene-related peptide and choline acetyltransferase in the lower brain stem, spinal cord and dorsal root ganglia of rat and guinea pig with special reference to motoneurones. *J. Chem. Neuroanat.*, **3**, 467–85.

Cortes, R., Aman, K., Arvidsson, U. *et al.* (1991) Immunohistochemical study of cholecystokinin peptide in rat spinal motoneurones. *Synapse*, **9**, 103–10.

Crowe, L.M. and Baskin, R.J. (1982) Quantitative ultrastructural differences in the development of normal and dystrophic muscle. *Exp. Neurol.*, **78**, 303–15.

Cunningham, B.A. (1991) Cell adhesion molecules and the regulation of development. *Am. J. Obst. Gynae.*, **164**, 939–48.

Cunningham, B.A., Hemperley, J.J., Murray, B.A. *et al.* (1987) Neural cell adhesion molecule: structure, immunoglobulin-like domains, cell surface modulation and alternative RNA splicing. *Science*, **236**, 799–806.

Daniloff, J.K., Levi, G., Grumet, M. *et al.* (1986) Altered expression of neuronal cell adhesion molecules induced by nerve injury and repair. *J. Cell Biol.*, **103**, 929–45.

Dardick, S.J., Basbaum, A.I. and Levine, J.D. (1986) The contribution of pain disability in experimentally induced arthritis. *Arthr. Rheumat.*, **29**, 1017–22.

Davenport, A.P. and Nunez, D.J. (1990) Quantification of radioactive mRNA in situ hybridization signals, in *In situ Hybridization: Principles and Practice* (eds J.M. Polak and J.D. McGee), Oxford University Press, Oxford, pp. 95–113.

Davenport, A.P., Hill, R.G. and Hughes J. (1989) Quantitative analysis of autoradiograms, in *Regulatory Peptides* (ed. J.M. Polak), Birkhauser, Basle, pp. 137–53.

De Castro Costa, M., De Sutter, P., Gybels, J. *et al.* (1981) Adjuvant-induced arthritis in rats: a possible animal model of chronic pain. *Pain*, **10**, 173–85.

Denis-Donini, S. (1989) Expression of dopaminergic phenotypes in the mouse olfactory bulb induced by the calcitonin gene-related peptide. *Nature*, **339**, 701–3.

Dietl, M.M., Sanchez, M., Probst, A. *et al.* (1989) Substance P receptors in the human spinal cord: decrease in amyotrophic lateral sclerosis. *Brain Res.*, **483**, 39–49.

Duchen, L.W., Falconer, D.S. and Strich, J.S. (1966) Hereditary progressive neurogenic muscular atrophy in the mouse. *J. Physiol.*, **183**, 53–5.

Duchen, L.W., Strich, S.J. and Falconer, D.S. (1968) A hereditary motoneuron disease with progressive denervation of muscle in the mouse, the mutant 'Wobbler'. *J. Neurol. Neurosurg. Psychiat.*, **31**, 535–42.

Dyck, P.J., Stevens, J.C., Mulder, D.W. *et al.* (1975) Frequency of nerve fiber degeneration of peripheral motor and sensory neurones in amyotrophic lateral sclerosis. Morphometry of deep and superficial perineal nerves. *Neurology*, **25**, 781–5.

Edelman, G.M. (1987) CAMs and Igs: cell adhesion and the evolutionary origins of immunity. *Immunol. Rev.*, **100**, 11–16.

Edwards, P.M., Kinters, R.R.F., Boer, G.I. *et al.* (1986) Recovery from peripheral nerve transection is accelerated by local application of a-MSH by means of microporous polypropylene tubes. *J. Neurol. Sci.*, **74**, 171–6.

Emson, P.C. (1979) Peptides as neurotransmitter candidates in the mammalian CNS. *Prog. Neurobiol.*, **13**, 16–116.

Engel, W.K., Siddique, T. and Nicoloff, J.T. (1983) Effect on weakness and spasticity in amyotrophic lateral sclerosis of thyrotrophin-releasing hormone. *Lancet*, 273–5.

Evans, E.M. (1988) The steroid and thyroid hormone receptor superfamily. *Science*, **240**, 889–95.

Faden, A.I., Jacobs, T.P. and Holaday, J.W. *et al.* (1981) Thyrotrophin-releasing hormone improves neurologic recovery after spinal trauma in cats. *New Engl. J. Med.*, **305**, 1063–6.

Fontaine, B., Klarsfeld, A. and Changeux, J.-P. (1986) Calcitonin gene-related peptide and muscle activity regulate acetylcholine receptor subunit mRNA levels by distinct intracellular pathways. *J. Cell Biol.*, **105**, 1337–42.

Freedman, J., Hokfelt, T., Jonsson, G. *et al.* (1986) Thyrotrophin-releasing hormone TRH counteracts neuronal damage induced by a substance P antagonist. *Exp. Brain Res.*, **62**, 175–8.

Freedman, J., Hokfelt, T., Post, C. *et al.* (1989) Immunohistochemical and behavioral analysis of spinal lesions induced by a substance P antagonist and protected by thyrotrophin releasing hormone. *Exp. Brain Res.*, **74**, 279–92.

Fried, K., Brodin, E. and Theodorsson, E. (1990) Substance P, CGRP and NPY-immunoreactive nerve fibres in rat sciatic nerve-end neuromas. *Neurosci. Lett.*, **24**, 43–7.

Garcia, L., Pincon-Raymond, M., Raney, T. *et al.* (1990) Induction of normal ultrastructure by CGRP treatment in dysgenic myotubes. *FEBS Letts.*, **263**, 147–52.

Gaulton, G.N. and Greene, M.I. (1986) Idiotypic mimicking of biological receptors. *Annu. Rev. Immunol.*, **4**, 253–80.

Giaid, A., Gibson, S.J. and Ibrahim, N.B.N. *et al.* (1989) Endothelin 1, an endothelium-derived peptide is expressed in neurones of the human spinal cord and dorsal root ganglia. *Proc. Natl. Acad. Sci. USA*, **86**, 7634–8.

Giaid, A., Gibson, S.J., Herrero, M.T. *et al.* (1991) Topographical localisation of endothelin mRNA and peptide immunoreactivity in neurones of the human brain. *Histochemistry*, **95**, 303–14.

Gibson, S.J. and Polak, J.M. (1986) Neurochemistry of the spinal cord, in *Immunocytochemistry: Modern Methods and Applications* (eds J.M. Polak and S. Van Noorden), John Wright, Bristol, pp. 360–90.

Gibson, S.J. and Polak, J.M. (1990) Principles and applications of complementary RNA probes, in *In situ Hybridization: Principles and Practice* (eds J.M. Polak and J.O.D. McGee), Oxford University Press, Oxford, pp. 81–95.

Gibson, S.J., Springall, D.R. and Polak, J.M. (1992) Endothelin, a ubiquitous peptide: morphological demonstration of immunoreactive and synthetic sites and receptors in the respiratory tract and central nervous system, in *Endothelin* (ed. G.M. Rubanyi), Oxford University Press, New York, pp. 179–208.

Gibson, S.J., Polak, J.M., Bloom, S.R. *et al.* (1984) Calcitonin gene-related peptide (CGRP) immunoreactivity in the spinal cord of man and of eight other species. *J. Neurosci.*, **4**, 3101–11.

Gibson, S.J., Polak, J.M., Katagiri, T. *et al.* (1988a) A comparison of the distributions of eight peptides in spinal cord from normal controls and cases of motor neuron disease with special reference to Onuf's nucleus. *Brain Res.*, **474**, 255–78.

Gibson, S.J., Polak, J.M., Giaid, A. *et al.* (1988b) Calcitonin gene-related peptide messenger RNA is expressed in sensory neurones of the dorsal root ganglia and also in spinal motoneurones in man and rat. *Neurosci. Lett.*, **91**, 283–8.

Gilbert, R.F.T., Emson, P.C., Hunt, S.P. *et al.* (1982) The effects of monoamine neurotoxins on peptides in the rat spinal cord. *Neuroscience*, **7**, 69–87.

Gillberg, P.-G., Aquilonius, S.M., Eckernas, S. *et al.* (1982) Choline acetyltransferase and substance P-like immunoreactivity in the human spinal cord: changes in amyotrophic lateral sclerosis. *Brain Res.*, **250**, 394–7.

Goodman, E.C. and Iversen, L.L. (1986) Calcitonin gene-related peptide: novel neuropeptide. *Life Sci.*, **38**, 2169–78.

Goodwin, C.S. and Watson, J.M. (1968) Neuritis and paralysis in leprosy. *Physiotherapy*, **54**, 327–32.

Grimm-Jorgensen, Y. (1987) Somatostatin and calcitonin promote neurite regeneration in vitro in cultured gastropod neurons. *Brain Res.*, **403**, 121–6.

Haas, C.A., Streit, W.J. and Krentzberg, M. (1990) Rat facial motoneurones express increased levels of calcitonin gene-related peptide mRNA in response to axotomy. *J. Neurosci. Res.*, **27**, 270–5.

Harmann, P.A., Chung, K. and Briner, B.P. (1988) Calcitonin gene-related peptide in the human spinal cord. A light and electron microscopic analysis. *J. Comp. Neurol.*, **269**, 371–80.

Haynes, L.W. and Smith, M.E. (1985) Presence of immunoreactive α-melanotropin and β-endorphin in spinal motoneurones of the dystrophic mouse. *Neurosci. Lett.*, **58**, 13–18.

Haynes, L.W., Smith, M.E. and Li, C.H. (1985) *CRC Handbook of Comparative Aspects of Opioid and Related Neuropeptide Mechanisms* (ed. G.B. Stefano), Oxford University Press, Oxford and New York, pp. 65–79.

Haynes, L.W., Smyth, D.G. and Zakarian (1982) *Brain Res.*, **232**, 115–28.

Hershko, A. (1983) Ubiquitin: roles in protein modification and breakdown. *Cell*, **34**, 11–12.

Hietanen, M., Pelto-Huikko, M. and Rechardt, L. (1990) Immunocytochemical study of the relations of acetylcholinesterase, enkephalin-, substance P-, choline acetyltransferase- and calcitonin gene-related peptide-immunoreactive structures in the ventral horn of rat spinal cord. *Histochemistry*, **93**, 473–7.

Hietanen-Peltola, M. (1992) Colocalization of protein kinase C β-subtype and calcitonin gene-related peptide in rat spinal cord. *Histochemistry*, **97**, 19–23.

Hirano, A. and Inoue, K. (1980) Early pathological changes of amyotrophic lateral sclerosis. Electron microscopic study of chromatolysis, spheroids and Bunina bodies. *Neurol. Med.*, **13**, 148–60.

Hiromasa, S., Yamamoto, H., Iio, S. *et al.* (1990) Release of calcitonin gene-related peptide-like immunoreactive substance from neuromuscular junction by nerve excitation and its action on striated muscle. *J. Neurochem.*, **54**, 1000–3.

Hokfelt, T., Johansson, O., Lungdahl, A. *et al.* (1980) Peptidergic neurons. *Nature*, **284**, 515–18.

Holzer, P. (1988) Local effector functions of capsaicin-sensitive sensory nerve endings: involvement of tachykinins, calcitonin gene-related peptide and other neuropeptides. *Neuroscience*, **24**, 739–68.

Hoyer, D., Waeber, C. and Palacios, J.M. (1989) [125I] endothelin-1 binding sites: autoradiographic studies in the brain and periphery of various species including humans. *J. Cardiovasc. Pharmacol.*, **13**, S162–5.

Hsu, L., Savage, P. and Jeng, A.Y. (1992) Dual effects of endothelin-1 on neurite outgrowth induced by 12–O-tetradecanoyl-phorbol-13-acetate. *Neurosci. Lett.*, **136**, 219–22.

Hsu, S.M., Raine, L. and Fanger, H. (1981) Use of avidin-biotin-peroxidase complex (ABC) in immunoperoxidase techniques: a comparison between ABC and unlabelled antibody (PAP) procedures. *J. Histochem. Cytochem.*, **29**, 577–80.

Hughes, S. and Smith, M.E. (1987) β-endorphin and α-melanotropin immunoreactivity in degenerating and contralateral motoneurones of the rat. *J. Physiol.*, **388**, 52P.

Hughes, S. and Smith, M.E. (1988) Effect of nerve section on β-endorphin and α-melanotrophin immunoreactivity in motor nerves of normal and dystrophic mice. *Neurosci. Lett.*, **92**, 1–7.

Hughes, S. and Smith, M.E. (1989) Proopiomelanocortin-derived peptides in mice with motoneurone disease. *Neurosci. Lett.*, **103**, 169–73.

Hughes, S. and Smith, M.E. (1990) Opioid receptors in skeletal muscle of normal and dystrophic mice. *Neurosci. Lett.*, **116**, 29–33.

Hunt, S.P. (1983) Cytochemistry of the spinal cord, in *Chemical Neuroanatomy* (ed. P.C. Emson), Raven Press, New York, pp. 53–84.

Hunt, S.P., Allanson, J. and Mantyh, P.W. (1986) Radioimmunocytochemistry, in *Immunocytochemistry: Modern Methods and Applications* (eds J.M. Polak and S. Van Noorden), John Wright, Bristol, pp. 99–114.

Iwasaki, T., Kinoshita, M., Ikeda, K. *et al.* (1989) Trophic effects of cholecystokinin and calcitonin gene-related peptide on ventral spinal cord in culture. *Int. J. Neurosci.*, **48**, 285–9.

Iwasaki, Y., Kinoshita, M., Ikeda, K. *et al.* (1990) Trophic effects of enkephalin β-endorphine and dynorphine on ventral spinal cord in culture. *Int. J. Neurosci.*, **50**, 131–5.

Iwasaki, Y., Kimoshita, M., Ikeda, K. *et al.* (1991) Trophic effect of various neuropeptides on the cultured ventral spinal cord. *Neurosci. Lett.*, **48**, 285–9.

Iwata, M. and Hirano, A. (1979) On the problems in the pathology of amyotrophic lateral sclerosis, in *Progress in Neuropathology* (ed. H.M. Zimmerman), Raven Press, New York, pp. 277–98.

Jackson, I.M.D., Adelman, L.S., Munsat, T.L. *et al.* (1986) Amyotrophic lateral sclerosis; Thyrotropin-releasing hormone and histidyl proline diketopiperazine in the spinal cord and cerebrospinal fluid. *Neurology*, **36**, 1218–23.

Jacobsohn, L. (1908) Uber die Keine des menschlichen Ruckenmarks. *Abh. Konigl. Preuss Akad. Wiss. Phys. Math. Classe (1)*.

Jacobsohn-Lask, L. (1931) Uber den medialen Sympathikuskern des menschlichen Ruckenmarks. *Z. Ges. Neurol. Psychiat.*, **134**, 344–656.

Jamal, G.A., Weir, A.E., Hansen, S. *et al.* (1985) Sensory involvement in motor neuron disease: further evidence from automated thermal threshold determination. *J. Neurol. Neurosurg. Psychiat.*, **48**, 906–10.

Jennings, C.G.B. and Mudge, A.W. (1989) Chick myotubes in culture express high-affinity receptors for calcitonin gene-related peptide. *Brain Res.*, **504**, 199–205.

Jinnai, K., Chihara, K., Kanda, F. *et al.* (1989) Calcitonin gene-related peptide enhances spontaneous acetylcholine release from the rat motor nerve terminal. *Neurosci. Lett.*, **103**, 64–8.

Johansson, O., Hokfelt, T., Pernow, B. *et al.* (1981) Immunohistochemical support for three putative transmitters in one neuron: coexistence of 5-hydroxytryptamine, substance P-, thyrotrophin releasing hormone-like immunoreactivity medullary neurons projecting to the spinal cord. *Neuroscience*, **6**, 1857–81.

Jones, C.R., Hiley, C.R., Pelton, J.T. *et al.* (1989) Autoradiographic visualization of the binding sites for (^{125}I) endothelin in rat and human brain. *Neurosci. Lett.*, **97**, 276–9.

Juurlink, B.H.J., Munoz, D.G. and Devon, R.M. (1990) Calcitonin gene-related peptide identifies spinal motoneurones in vitro. *J. Neurosci. Res.*, **26**, 238–41.

Kar, S., Chabot, J.-G. and Quirion, R. (1991) Neuropeptide receptors in developing and adult rat spinal cord: an in vitro quantitative autoradiography study. *Soc. Neurosci. Abstr.*, **17**, 320.11.

Kar, S., Gibson, S.J. and Polak, J.M. (1990) Origins and projections of peptide-immunoreactive nerves in the male rat genitofemoral nerve. *Brain Res.*, **512**, 229–37.

Kar, S., Bretherton-Watt, D., Gibson, S.J. *et al.* (1989) Pancreastatin a novel neuropeptide: Occurrence and co-distribution with chromogranin A in porcine central nervous system. *J. Comp. Neurol.*, **288**, 627–39.

Kar, S., Gibson, S.J., Rees, R.G. *et al.* (1991) Increased calcitonin gene-related peptide (CGRP), substance P, and enkephalin immunoreactivities in dorsal spinal cord and loss of CGRP-immunoreactive motoneurones in arthritic rats depend on intact peripheral nerve supply. *J. Mol. Neurosci.*, **3**, 7–18.

Karanth, S.S., Springall, D.R., Kar, S. *et al.* (1991) Time-related decrease of substance P and CGRP in central and peripheral projections of sensory neurones in *Myobacterium leprae* infected nude mice: A model for lepromatous leprosy in man. *J. Pathol.*, **161**, 335–45.

Katagiri, T., Gibson, S.J., Su, H.C. *et al.* (1986) Composition and central projections of the pudendal nerve in the rat investigated by combined peptide immunocytochemistry and retrograde fluorescent labelling. *Brain Res.*, **372**, 313–22.

Katagiri, T., Kuzirai, T., Nihei, M. *et al.* (1988) Immunocytochemical study of Onuf's nucleus in amyotrophic lateral sclerosis. *J. Med.*, **27**, 23–8.

Kato, T., Hirano, A. and Manaka, H. (1991) Calcitonin gene-related peptide immunoreactivity in familial amyotrophic lateral sclerosis. *Neurosci. Lett.*, **133**, 163–7.

Kato, T., Katagiri, T., Hirano, A. *et al.* (1988) Sporadic motor neuron disease

Neuropeptides

with Lewy body-like inclusions: a new subgroup. *Acta Neuropathol.*, **76**, 208–11.

Kato, T., Katagiri, T., Hirano, A. *et al.* (1989) Lewy body-like hyaline inclusions in sporadic motor neuron disease are ubiquitinated. *Acta Neuropathol.*, **77**, 391–6.

Kato, T., Katagiri, T., Hirano, A. *et al.* (1991) Calcitonin gene-related peptide immunoreactivity in spinal spheroids in motor neuron disease. *Acta Neuropathol.*, **82**, 302–5.

Kinderman, N.B. and Jones, K.J. (1991) Testosterone effects on ribosomal RNA levels in injured peripheral motor neurons – a preliminary report. *Metabolic Brain Dis.*, **6**, 157–64.

Komuro, I., Kurihara, H., Sugiyama, T. *et al.* (1988) Endothelin stimulates c-fos and c-myc expression and proliferation of vascular smooth muscle cells. *FEBS Lett.*, **238**, 249.

Konno, H., Yamamoto, T., Iwasaki, Y. *et al.* (1986) Shy–Drager syndrome and amyotrophic lateral sclerosis. *J. Neurol. Sci.*, **73**, 193–204.

Kruger, L., Silverman, J.D., Mantyh, P.W. *et al.* (1989) Peripheral patterns of calcitonin-gene related peptide general somatic sensory innervation: cutaneous and deep terminations. *J. Comp. Neurol.*, **280**, 291–302.

Lackie, P.M., Cuttitta, F., Minna, J.D. *et al.* (1984) Localization of receptors using a dimeric ligand and electron immunocytochemistry. *Histochemistry*, **83**, 57–9.

Laufer, R. and Changeux, J.-P. (1987) Calcitonin gene-related peptide elevated cyclic AMP levels in chick skeletal muscle: possible neurotrophic role for a coexisting neuronal messenger. *EMBO J.*, **6**, 901–6.

Laurelle, L. (1937) La structure de la moelle epinere en coupes longitudinales. *Rev. Neurol.*, **67**, 695–725.

Lee, M.E., de la Monte, S.M., Ng, S.-C. *et al.* (1990) Expression of the potent vasoconstrictor endothelin in the human central nervous system. *J. Clin. Invest.*, **86**, 141–7.

Leigh, P.N., Anderton, B.H. and Dodson, A. (1988) Ubiquitin deposits in anterior horn cells in motor neuron disease. *Neurosci. Lett.*, **93**, 197–203.

Lewis, P.D. (1977) *Motor Neurone Disease* (ed. F.C. Rose), Grune & Stratton, New York, pp. 30–5.

Lowe, J., Lennox, G., Jefferson, D. *et al.* (1988) A filamentous inclusion body within anterior horn neurones in motor neurone disease defined by immunocytochemical localization of ubiquitin. *Neurosci. Lett.*, **94**, 203–10.

McBride, J.T., Springall, D.R., Winter, R.J.D. *et al.* (1990) Quantitative immunocytochemistry shows calcitonin gene-related peptide-like immunoreactivity in lung neuroendocrine cells is increased by chronic hypoxia in the rat. *Am. J. Respir. Cell Mol. Biol.*, **3**, 587–93.

McNeill, D.L., Carlton, S.M., Coggeshall, R.E. *et al.* (1990) Denervation-induced intraspinal synaptogenesis of calcitonin gene-related peptide-containing primary afferent terminals. *J. Comp. Neurol.*, **296**, 263–8.

Mallonga, R.L. and Ontell, M. (1991) Reinnervation of murine muscle following fetal sciatic nerve transection. *J. Neurobiol.*, **22**, 887–96.

Manaker, S., Shulman, L.H., Winokur, A. *et al.* (1985) Autoradiographic localization of thyrotrophin-releasing hormone receptors in amyotrophic lateral sclerosis spinal cord. *Neurology, 35,* 1650–53.

Manaker, S., Barack, S., Caine, P. *et al.* (1988) Alterations in receptors for thyrotrophin releasing hormone, serotonin and acetylcholine in amyotrophic lateral sclerosis

Mannen, T., Iwata, M., Toyokura, Y. *et al.* (1977) Preservation of a certain motoneuron group of the sacral cord in amyotrophic lateral sclerosis; its clinical significance. *J. Neurol. Neurosurg. Psychiatr., 40,* 464–9.

Mantyh, P.W. and Hunt, S.P. (1984) Evidence for cholecystokinin-like immunoreactive neurons in the rat medulla oblongata which project to the spinal cord. *Brain Res., 291,* 49–54.

Marti, E., Gibson, S.J., Polak, J.M. *et al.* (1987) Ontogeny of peptide- and amine-containing neurones in motor sensory and autonomic regions of rat and human spinal cord, dorsal root ganglia and skin. *J. Comp. Neurol., 226,* 322–59.

Matteoli, M., Haimann, C. and De Camilli, P. (1991) Substance P-like immunoreactivity at the frog neuromuscular junction. *Neuroscience, 37,* 271–5.

Matteoli, M., Haimann, C., Tori-Tarelli, F. *et al.* (1988) Differential effect of alphalatrotoxin on exocytosis from small synaptic vesicles and from large dense core vesicles containing calcitonin gene-related peptide at the frog neuromuscular junction. *Proc. Natl. Acad. Sci. USA, 85,* 7366–70.

Matteoli, M., Balbi, S., Sala, C. *et al.* (1990) Developmentally regulated expression of calcitonin gene-related peptide at mammalian neuromuscular junction. *J. Mol. Neurosci., 2,* 175–84.

Melki, J., Blondet, B., Pincon-Raymond, M. *et al.* (1991) Generalized molecular defects of the neuromuscular junction in skeletal muscle of the Wobbler mutant mouse. *Neurochem. Int., 18,* 425–33.

Merighi, A., Polak, J.M., Fumagalli, G. *et al.* (1989) Ultrastructural localisation of neuropeptides and GABA in the rat dorsal horn: a comparison of different immunogold labelling techniques. *J. Histochem. Cytochem., 37,* 529–40.

Millan, M.J., Millan, M.H., Czlonkowski, A. *et al.* (1984) Vasopressin and oxytocin in the rat spinal cord: distributions and origins in comparison to (Met) enkephalin, dynorphin and related opioids and their irresponsiveness to stimuli, modulating neurohypophyseal secretion. *Neuroscience, 13,* 179–88.

Mitsuma, T., Nagimori, T. and Adachi, K. (1984) Concentrations of immunoreactive thyrotrophin releasing hormone in spinal cord of patients with amyotrophic lateral sclerosis. *Am. J. Med. Sci., 287,* 34–6.

Mitsuma, T., Adachi, K., Mukoyama, M. *et al.* (1988) Concentrations of thyrotrophin-releasing hormone and substance P are increased in several areas of the central nervous system of shambling mutant mice. *Neurochem. Int., 13,* 261–4.

Mitsuma, T., Adachi, K., Mukoyama, N. *et al.* (1990) Pro-thyrotrophin-releasing hormone concentrations in the brain of ataxic mice. *J. Neurol. Sci., 98,* 163–7.

Neuropeptides

Mitsumoto, H. and Bradley, W.G. (1982) Murine motor neuron disease (the Wobbler mouse). Degeneration and regeneration of the lower motor neuron. *Brain*, **105**, 811–34.

Moore, R.Y. (1989) Cranial motor neurones contain either galanin or calcitonin gene-related peptide like immunoreactivity. *J. Comp. Neurol.*, **282**, 512–22.

Mora, M., Marchi, M., Gibson, S.J. *et al.* (1989) Calcitonin gene-related peptide immunoreactivity at the human neuromuscular junction. *Brain Res.*, **492**, 404–7.

Moser, P.C. and Pelton, J.T. (1991) Behavioral effects of central administration of endothelin in rat. *Br. J. Pharmacol.*, **10**, 124–6.

Moss, S.J., Harkness, P.C., Mason, I. *et al.* (1991) Evidence that CGRP and cAMP increase transcription of AChR α-subunit gene, but not of other subunit genes. *J. Mol. Neurosci.*, **3**, 101–8.

Murayama, S., Ookaura, Y. and Mori, H. (1989) Immunocytochemical and ultrastructural study of Lewy body-like hyaline inclusions in familial amyotrophic lateral sclerosis. *Acta Neuropathol.*, **78**, 143–52.

Nakano, K. (1969) On the autonomic nuclei in the dog spinal cord. *Mie. Med. J.*, **18**, 243–57.

New, H.V. and Mudge, A.W. (1986) Calcitonin gene-related peptide regulates muscle acetylcholine receptor synthesis. *Nature*, **323**, 809–11.

Nicoll, R.A. (1977) Excitatory action of TRH on spinal motoneurones. *Nature*, **265**, 242–3.

Nicoll, R.A. (1978) The action of thyrotrophin-releasing hormone, substance P and related peptides on frog spinal motoneurones. *J. Pharmacol. Exp. Therapeut.*, **207**, 817–24.

Nistri, A., Fisher, N.D. and Gurnell, M. (1990) Block by the neuropeptide TRH of an apparently novel K^+ conductance of rat motoneurones. *Neurosci. Lett.*, **120**, 25–30.

Ohhashi, T. and Jacobowitz, D.M. (1988) Effect of calcitonin gene-related peptide on neuromuscular transmission in the isolated rat diaphragm. *Peptides*, **9**, 613–17.

Ono, H. and Fukuda, H. (1982) Ventral root depolarization and spinal reflex augmentation by a TRH analog in rat spinal cord. *Neuropharmacology*, **21**, 39–44.

Onuf, B. (Onufrowicz) (1900) On the arrangement and formation of the cell groups of the sacral region of the spinal cord in man. *Arch. Neurol. Psychopathol.*, **3**, 387–412.

Oppenheim, R.W., Haverkamp, L.J. and Prevette, D. (1988) Reduction of naturally occurring motor neuron death in vivo by a target derived neurotrophic factor. *Science*, **240**, 919–22.

Otsuka, M., Kanazawa, I., Sugita, H. *et al.* (1978) Substance P in the spinal cord and serum in amyotrophic lateral sclerosis, in *Amyotrophic Lateral Sclerosis* (eds T.A. Toyokura and Y. Tsubaki), University Park Press, Baltimore, pp. 405–11.

Oyanagi, M., Makifuchi, T. and Ikuta, F. (1983) A topographic and quantitative

References

study of neurons in human spinal gray matter, with special reference to their changes in amyotrophic lateral sclerosis. *Biomed. Res.*, **4**, 211–24.

Palacios, J.M. and Dietl, M.M. (1989) Regulatory peptide receptors: visualisation by autoradiography, in *Regulatory Peptides* (ed. J.M. Polak), Birkhauser, Basle, pp. 70–97.

Palkovits, M. (1984) Distribution of neuropeptides in the central nervous system. *Prog. Neurobiol.*, **23**, 151–89.

Patten, B.M. and Croft, S. (1984) Spinal cord substance P in amyotrophic lateral sclerosis, in *Research Progress in Motor Neurone Disease: Progress in Neurology Series* (ed. F. Clifford Rose), Pitman, London, pp 283–9.

Piehl, F., Arvidsson, U., Johnson, H. *et al.* (1991) Calcitonin gene-related peptide (CGRP)-like immunoreactivity and CGRP messenger RNA in rat spinal cord motoneurones after different types of lesions. *Eur. J. Neurosci.*, **3**, 737–57.

Polak, J.M. (1989) *Regulatory Peptides*, Birkhauser, Basle.

Polak, J.M. and McGee, J.O. (eds) (1990) *In situ Hybridization: Principles and Practice*, Oxford University Press, Oxford.

Polak, J.M. and Van Noorden, S. (eds) (1986) *Immunocytochemistry: Modern Methods & Applications*, 2nd edn, John Wright, Bristol.

Polak, J.M., Gibson, S.J., Gentleman, S. *et al.* (1991) Galanin: distribution, ontogeny and expression following manipulation of the endocrine and nervous system, in *Galanin. Werner-Gren Center Int. Symposium Series* (eds T. Hokfelt, T. Bartfai, D. Jacobowitz and D. Ottoson), MacMillan Press, Basingstoke, pp. 117–34.

Pons-Tortella, E., Roca-de-Vinales, R. and Rodriguez-Arias, B. (1951) La collone fibrillaire de la moelle sacree: Sa morphologie, ses lesions dans la poliomyelite antereue aigue, sa valuer foncinnelle. *Rev. Neurol.*, **85**, 165–77.

Popper, P. and Micevych, P.E. (1989) Localization of calcitonin gene-related peptide and its receptors in a striated muscle. *Brain Res.*, **496**, 180–6.

Popper, P. and Micevych, P.E. (1990) Steroid regulation of calcitonin gene-related peptide mRNA expression in motoneurones of the nucleus of the bulbocavernous. *Mol. Brain Res.*, **8**, 159–66.

Popper, P., Ulibarri, C. and Micevych, P. (1992) The role of target muscles in the expression of calcitonin gene-related peptide messenger RNA in the spinal nucleus of the bulbocavernous. *Mol. Brain Res.*, **13**, 43–51.

Post, C., Freedman, J., Paulsson, I. *et al.* (1987) Antinociceptive effects in mice after intrathecal injection of a substance P receptor antagonist, spantide: lack of neurotoxic action. *Regul. Pept.*, **18**, 243–52.

Rethelyi, M., Metz, C.B. and Lund, P.K. (1989) Distribution of neurons expressing calcitonin gene-related peptide mRNA in the brain stem, spinal cord and dorsal root ganglia of rat and guinea-pig. *Neuroscience*, **29**, 225–39.

Rethelyi, M., Mohapatra, N.K., Metz, C.B. *et al.* (1991) Colchicine enhances mRNAs encoding the precursor of calcitonin gene-related peptide in brainstem motoneurons. *Neuroscience*, **42**, 531–9.

Rexed, B. (1954) A cytoarchitecture atlas of the spinal cord in the cat. *J. Comp. Neurol.*, **100**, 297–379.

Neuropeptides

Roa, M. and Changeux, J.-P. (1991) Characterization and developmental evolution of a high-affinity binding site for calcitonin gene-related peptide on chick skeletal muscle membrane. *Neuroscience*, **41**, 563–70.

Rodrigo, J., Polak, J.M., Terenghi, G. *et al.* (1985a) Calcitonin gene-related peptide immunoreactive sensory and motor nerves of the mammalian palate. *Histochemistry*, **82**, 67–74.

Rodrigo, J., Polak, J.M., Fernanez, L. *et al.* (1985b) Calcitonin gene-related peptide-immunoreactive sensory and motor nerves of the rat, cat and monkey oesophagus. *Gastroenterology*, **88**, 441–51.

Rosenfeld, M.G., Mermod, J.J., Amara, S.J. *et al.* (1983) Production of a novel neuropeptide encoded by the calcitonin gene via tissue-specific RNA processing. *Nature*, **304**, 129–35.

Rubanyi, G.M. (ed.) (1992) *Endothelin*, Oxford University Press, New York.

Ruda, M.A. (1988) Spinal dorsal horn circuitry involved in the brain stem control of nociception, in *Progress in Brain Research* (eds H.L. Fields and J.-M. Besson), Elsevier, Amsterdam, pp. 129–40.

Ruda, M.A., Bennett, G.J. and Dubner, R. (1986) Neurochemistry and neural circuitry in the dorsal horn, in *Progress in Brain Research* (eds P.C. Emson, M.N. Rosser and M. Tohyama), Elsevier, Amsterdam, pp. 219–67.

Rutishauser, U. and Jessell, T.M. (1988) Cell adhesion molecules in vertebrate neural development. *Physiol. Rev.*, **68**, 819–57.

Saint-Come, C. and Strand, F.L. (1988) ACTH 4–9 analogue (Org 2766) improves qualitative and quantitative aspects of motor nerve regeneration. *Peptides*, **8**, 215–21.

Saint-Come, C., Acker, G.R. and Strand, F.L. (1985) Development and regeneration of motor systems under the influence of ACTH peptides. *Psychoneuroendocrinology*, **10**, 445–95.

Salt, T.E. and Hill, R.G. (1983) Neurotransmitter candidates of somatosensory primary afferent fibres. *Neuroscience*, **10**, 1083–103.

Schiffmann, S.N., Tellgels, E., Halleux, P. *et al.* (1991) Cholecystokinin mRNA detection in rat spinal cord motoneurons but not in dorsal root ganglia. *Neurosci. Lett.*, 123–6.

Schmidt-Achert, K.M., Askanas, V. and Engel, W.K. (1984) Thyrotrophin-releasing hormone enhances choline acetyltransferase and creatine kinase in cultured spinal ventral horn neurons. *J. Neurochem.*, **43**, 586–9.

Schoenen, J. (1990) Anatomie biochimique des systemes peptidergiques spinaux. Etude de materiel normal et pathologique: plasticite des neuro-peptides du ganglion rachidien adulte. Symposium international de Pharmacologic Clinique, Marseille. Jan. *Therapie*, **45**, 243–9.

Schoenen, J., Lostra, F., Vierendeels, G. *et al.* (1985a) Substance P, enkephalins, somatostain, cholecystokinin, oxytocin and vasopressin in human spinal cord. *Neurology*, **35**, 881–90.

Schoenen, J., Reznik, M., Delwaide, P.J. *et al.* (1985b) Etude immunocytochimique de la distribution spinale de substance P, des enkephalins, de cholecysokinine et de serotonine dans la sclerose laterale amyotrophique. *C.R. Soc. Biol. Soc. Belge de Biol.*, **179**, 528–34.

Schroder, H.D. (1980) Organization of the motoneurones innervating the pelvic muscle of the male rat. *J. Comp. Neurol.*, **192**, 567–87.

Schroder, H.D. (1981) Onuf's nucleus X. A morphological study of a human spinal nucleus. *Anat. Embryol.*, **162**, 443–53.

Shinmi, O., Kimura, S., Yoshizawa, T. *et al.* (1989) Presence of endothelin-1 in porcine spinal cord: isolation and sequence determination. *Biochem. Biophys. Res. Commun.*, **162**, 340–6.

Simonson, M.S., Wann, S., Mene, P. *et al.* (1989) Endothelin stimulates phospholipase C, Na^+/H^+ exchange, c-fos expression, and mitogenesis in rat mesangial cells. *J. Clin. Invest.*, **83**, 708–12.

Springall, D.R., Steel, J.H., Gentleman, S. *et al.* (1992) *Immunocytochemistry and image analysis.* Submitted to *Symposium Biomedical Imaging in Diagnostic Pathology. A view of the 21st Century*, 81st Annual Meeting of US and Canadian Academy of Pathology, Atlanta, March 14–20 1992.

Sternberger, L.A. (1979) The unlabelled antibody enzyme peroxidase antiperoxidase (PAP) method, in *Immunocytochemistry* (ed. Sternberger, L.A.), John Wiley, New York, pp. 104–69.

Stober, T., Schimrigk, K., Pietzson, S. *et al.* (1985) Intrathecal thyrotropin-releasing hormone therapy of amyotrophic lateral sclerosis. *J. Neurol.*, **232**, 13–14.

Strand, F.L., Kung, T.T. and Saint-Carne, C. (1981) Regenerative ability of spinal motor systems is influenced by ACTHMSH peptides, in *Functional Recovery from Brain Damage. Developments in Neuroscience* (eds M.W. Hoff and G. Mohn), Elsevier, Amsterdam, pp. 369–409.

Strand, F.L., Rose, K.J., King, J.A. *et al.* (1989) ACTH modulation of nerve development and regeneration. *Prog. Neurobiol.*, **33**, 45–85.

Strand, F.L., Rose, K.J., Zuccarelli, L.A. *et al.* (1991) Neuropeptide hormones as neurotrophic factors. *Physiol. Rev.*, **71**, 1017–46.

Streit, W.J., Dumoulin, F.L., Raivich, G. *et al.* (1989) Calcitonin gene-related peptide increases in rat facial motoneurones after peripheral nerve transection. *Neurosci. Lett.*, **101**, 143–8.

Suburo, A.M., Gibson, S.J., Moscoso, G. *et al.* (1992) Transient expression of neuropeptide Y and its C-flanking peptide immunoreactivities in the spinal cord and ganglia of human embryos and fetuses. *Neuroscience*, **46**, 571–84.

Sung, J.H. (1979) Autonomic neurons affected by lipid storage in the sacral cord. *J. Neuropathol. Exp. Neurol.*, **38**, 87.

Sung, J.H. (1982) Autonomic neurons of the sacral spinal cord in amyotrophic lateral sclerosis, anterior poliomyelitis and neuronal intranuclear hyaline inclusion disease. Distribution of sacral autonomic neurons. *Acta Neuropathol.*, **56**, 233–7.

Tacke, R. and Martini, R. (1990) Changes in expression of mRNA specific for cell adhesion molecules (L1 and NCAM) in the transected peripheral nerve of the adult rat. *Neurosci. Lett.*, **120**, 227–30.

Takami, K., Kawai, Y., Shiosaka, S. *et al.* (1985a) Immunohistochemical evidence for the coexistence of calcitonin gene-related peptide and choline

Neuropeptides

acetyltransferase-like immunoreactivity in neurons of the rat hypoglossal, facial and ambiguus nuclei. *Brain Res.*, **328**, 386–9.

Takami, K., Kawai, Y., Uchida, S. *et al.* (1985b) Effect of calcitonin gene-related peptide on contraction of striated muscle in the mouse. *Neurosci. Lett.*, **60**, 217–30.

Takuwa, N., Takuwa, Y., Yangisawa, M. *et al.* (1989) A novel vasoactive peptide endothelin stimulates mitogenesis through inositol lipid turnover in Swiss 3T3 fibroblasts. *J. Biol. Chem.*, **264**, 7856–61.

Tang, F., Cheung, and Vacca-Galloway, L.L. (1990) Measurement of neuro-peptides in the brain and spinal cord of Wobbler mouse: a model for motoneuron disease. *Brain Res.*, **518**, 329–33.

Terenghi, G., Polak, J.M., Rodrigo, J. *et al.* (1986) Calcitonin gene-related-immunoreactive nerves in the tongue, epiglottis and pharynx of the rat: occurrence, distribution and origin. *Brain Res.*, **365**, 1–14.

Tschopp, F.A., Henke, H., Petermann, J.B. *et al.* (1985) Calcitonin gene-related peptide and its binding sites in the human central nervous system and pituitary. *Proc. Natl. Acad. Sci. USA*, **82**, 248–52.

Tsujimoto, T. and Kuno, M. (1988) Calcitonin gene-related peptide prevents disue-induced sprouting of rat motor nerves. *J. Neurosci.*, **8**, 3951–7.

Vacca-Galloway, L.L., Steinberger, C.C., Poole, E. *et al.* (1987) Substance P, thyrotrophin releasing hormone and serotonin neurons sprout in cervical spinal cord of Wobbler mouse, a model for motoneuron disease, in *Substance P and Neurokinins* (eds J.L. Henry, R. Couture, A.C. Cuello, C.R. Pelletier and R. Quirion), Springer, New York, pp. 359–62.

Vandenbergh, P., Octave, J.N. and Lechan, R.M. (1991) Muscle denervation increases thyrotrophin-releasing hormone (TRH) biosynthesis in the rat medullary raphe. *Brain Res.*, **566**, 219–24.

Varndell, I.M. and Polak, J.M. (eds) (1984) *Immunolabelling for Electron Microscopy*, Elsevier, Amsterdam.

Villar, M., Huchet, M., Hokfelt, T. *et al.* (1988) Existence and coexistence of calcitonin gene-related peptide, vasoactive intestinal polypeptide and somatostatin-like immunoreactivities in spinal cord motoneurones of developing embryos and post-hatch chicks. *Neurosci. Lett.*, **86**, 114–18.

Villar, M.J., Cortes, R., Theodorsson, E. *et al.* (1989) Neuropeptide expression in rat dorsal root ganglion cells and spinal cord after peripheral nerve injury with special reference to galanin. *Neuroscience*, **33**, 587–604.

Weill, C.L. (1991) Somatostatin (SRIF) prevents natural motoneuron cell death in embryonic chick spinal cord. *Dev. Neurosci.*, **13**, 377–81.

White, D.M. and Zimmerman, M. (1988) Changes in the content and release of substance P and calcitonin gene-related peptide in rat cutaneous nerve neuroma, in *Proceedings of the V. World Congress on Pain, Pain Research and Clinical Management* (eds R. Dubner, G.F. Gebhart and M.R. Bond), Elsevier, Amsterdam, pp. 109–13.

White, D.M., Leah, J.D. and Zimmerman, M. (1989) The localization and release of substance P and calcitonin gene-related peptide at nerve fibre ending in a rat cutaneous nerve neuroma. *Brain Res.*, **503**, 198–204.

Wiklund, N.P., Ohlen, A., Wiklund, C.U. *et al.* (1989) Neuromuscular actions of endothelin on smooth, cardiac and skeletal muscle from guinea pig, rat and rabbit. *Acta Physiol. Scand.*, **137**, 399–407.

Woolf, C. and Wiesenfeld-Hallin, Z. (1986) Substance P and calcitonin gene-related peptide synergistically modulate the gain of the nociception flexor withdrawal reflex in the rat. *Neurosci. Lett.*, **66**, 226–30.

Yamamoto, T., Satomi, H., Ise, H. *et al.* (1977) Sacral spinal innervations of the rectal and vesical smooth muscles and the sphincter muscles as demonstrated by the horseradish peroxidase method. *Neurosci. Lett.*, 741.

Yanagisawa, M., Kurihara, H., Kimura, S. *et al.* (1988) A novel potent vasoconstrictor peptide. *Nature*, **332**, 411–15.

Yoshizawa, I., Kimura, S., Kanazawa, I. *et al.* (1989) Endothelin localizes in the dorsal horn and acts on spinal neurones: Possible involvement of dihydropyridine-sensitive calcium channels and substance P release. *Neurosci. Lett.*, **102**, 179–84.

Young, W.S. and Kuhar, M.J. (1979) A new method for receptor autoradiography: (^{3}H) opioid receptors in rat brain. *Brain Res.*, **179**, 255–70.

Yung, K.K.L., Tang, R., Fielding, R. *et al.* (1990) Alterations of thyrotropin releasing hormone, substance P and enkephalins in the spinal cord, brainstem, hypothalamus and midbrain of the Wobbler mouse at different stages of the motoneuron disease. *Neurosci. Lett.*, Suppl. 40, S55.

Zhang, Y.Q. and Vacca-Galloway, L.L. (1992) Decreased immunoreactive (IR) calcitonin gene-related peptide correlates with sprouting of IR-peptidergic and serotonergic neuronal processes in spinal cord and brain nuclei from the Wobbler mouse during motoneuron disease. *Brain Res.*, **587**, 169–77.

Zoli, M., Fuxe, K., Agnati, L.F. *et al.* (1986) Computer-assisted morphometry of transmitter-identified neurons: new openings for the understanding of peptide-monoamine interactions in the mediobasal hypothalamus, in *Neurohistochemistry: Modern Methods and Applications* (eds P.P.H. Soinila and S. Panula), Alan R. Liss, New York, pp. 137–72.

29 *Animal models of motor neuron disease*

JOSEPH E. MAZURKIEWICZ

29.1 INTRODUCTION

Human motor neuron disease (HMND) is a progressive disorder characterized clinically by muscular wasting and weakness. The disease is neuronopathic, the muscle effects being secondary to anterior horn cell dysfunction and loss (Hughes, 1982; Hays, 1991). There are four major clinically defined forms of the disease:

1. amyotrophic lateral sclerosis;
2. spinal muscular atrophy;
3. progressive bulbar palsy; and
4. primary lateral sclerosis (Brooks *et al.*, 1989).

In most countries, these are generally grouped together under the name amyotrophic lateral sclerosis (ALS). In amyotrophic lateral sclerosis the entire motor system is involved pathologically, including the motor cortex, brainstem and spinal cord. Diagnosis of ALS requires lower motor neuron signs detected by clinical and electrophysiologic examination, upper motor neuron signs detected by clinical examination and progression of the disease, once identified.

The classic description of the pathology is based on autopsy material and represents the end stage of the disease. When autopsy specimens of ALS spinal cord are examined, large losses of motor neurons are evident. It has been estimated that because of compensatory reinnervation a loss of up to 50% of motor neurons can occur before clinical weakness develops (Hansen and Ballantyne, 1978).

The early pathologic changes that contribute to neuronal dysfunction and, eventually, lead to this loss are not known because it is not possible to study the biology of affected neurons during life. Thus, a number of experimentally induced and naturally occurring animal models have been investigated in attempts to understand the pathogenesis of these diseases. Thirty-eight of these animal models were discussed in a

659

comprehensive review by Smitt and de Jong (1989) that included literature up to 1988. Several naturally occurring, genetic animal models were being developed at that time, and Messer (1992) selectively updated the list (up to 1990) by including a discussion of the hereditary canine spinal muscular atrophy (HCSMA) disease in Brittany spaniels (Cork *et al.*, 1979) and the then newly described inherited diseases in the mouse: *Mnd* (motor neuron degeneration) (Messer and Flaherty, 1986; Messer, Strominger and Mazurkiewicz, 1987) and *wst* (wasted) (Lustep and Rodriguez, 1989). This chapter will focus primarily on work done on the hereditary models for motor neuron disease since that time: both published and newer studies of the *Mnd* (motor neuron degeneration) mutation in the mouse (Messer and Flaherty, 1986; Messer, Strominger and Mazurkiewicz, 1987); of hereditary canine spinal muscular atrophy (HCSMA) disease in the dog (Cork *et al.*, 1979); and of the progressive motor neuronopathy (*pmn*) mutant in the mouse (Schmalbruch *et al.*, 1991); however, a brief discussion of selected experimentally induced animal models is warranted by way of introduction.

29.2 EXPERIMENTALLY INDUCED ANIMAL MODELS

Several etiologies have been proposed for ALS, including biochemical or metabolic abnormalities, excitatory amino acid intoxication, toxicity from heavy metals and trace elements, immunologic abnormalities, viral induction and genetic defect(s). Despite the initial insult, however, the ultimate pathology appears to be the same: neuronal loss. In experimentally induced animal models, an agent with a known mechanism of action is chosen to mimic one of the proposed etiologies, thus permitting analysis of the pathogenic events leading to neuronal cell loss. There has been a resurgence of interest in experimental models that coincides with a resurgence of interest in two of the proposed etiologies for motor neuron disease: neuronal loss induced by viruses (Jubelt, 1991, 1992) and by autoimmune mechanisms (Appel *et al.*, 1991a).

Viruses can induce a variety of alterations and degenerations in neurons in selected regions of the nervous system that have a similar distribution to lesions that are found in human neurodegenerative diseases (Kristensen, 1992). One viral model that has received recent attention is the neurologic disease produced by Cas-Br-E MuLv, a murine retrovirus (Jolicoeur *et al.*, 1991) isolated from a population of wild mice with a naturally occurring viral neurologic disease (Gardner *et al.*, 1973). While the distribution of the lesions in this retrovirally induced disease in mice coincides with those in ALS, being found primarily in ventral horn cells of the lumbar spinal cord, in the brainstem and in deep cerebellar nuclei, the pathology differs from the human. In mice, the disease appears first as spongiform changes in non-neuronal cells (glial and endothelial cells), suggesting that the neuronal loss seen in this disease is indirect and not due to viral infection of the neurons (Kay et al., 1991). The model system, however, does permit the development of hypotheses for neuronal death that may be pertinent in understanding motor neuron disease. To explain the observations, a model has been developed that centers on gp170, the glycoprotein encoded by the env gene in Cas-Br-E MuLv that is responsible for viral recognition of the receptor on susceptible cells and, within its amino acid sequence, includes the primary determinant of the spongiform encephalopathy induced by this retrovirus. Because this protein binds to receptors, the disease is hypothesized to be receptor mediated, with the putative receptor located on neurons (Jolicoeur, 1991). The gp170 protein could interfere with the binding of a trophic factor that could act through this receptor or, having bound to the receptor, it could induce cell death by mechanisms such as inappropriate opening of ion channels.

Alternatively, the receptor could be localized on non-neuronal cells and, following binding of gp170 to these receptors, the non-neuronal cell could be stimulated to overproduce a substance that is toxic to neurons. Conversely, it could suppress the production of a substance that is necessary for neuronal maintenance. Granted, these are all suppositions; however, the concepts do mirror current research, such as that on excitatory amino acid toxicity, which may act secondarily through induction of an inappropriate increase of intracellular calcium concentration. The increased calcium levels could ultimately be responsible for neuronal death through stimulation of intracellular proteases, phospholipases or endonucleases (Choi, 1988). These hypotheses also mirror the growing interest in growth factor involvement in motor neuron disease now that ciliary neurotrophic factor has been demonstrated to prevent degeneration of motor neurons following axotomy (Sendtner, Kreutzberg and Thoenen, 1990).

Interest in an immune basis for motor neuron disease was revived after reports of a disproportionate incidence of paraproteinemia (abnormal monoclonal serum immunoglobulins) among patients with lower motor neuron disease (Shy et al., 1986; Younger et al., 1990). Interest in such an etiology was heightened when an IgM paraprotein from similar patients was found to react with the gangliosides GM1 and GD1b (Latov et al., 1988), and was further intensified with the finding of antibodies to gangliosides in patients with motor neuron disease but without serum paraproteins (Pestronk, Adams and Clawson, 1988; Pestronk et al., 1989). Gangliosides are present in high concentrations in neuronal cell membranes, especially at the nerve terminal (Ledeen et al.,

1976; Ledeen, 1978); thus an autoimmune pathogenesis of ALS could arguably be inferred from the presence of anti-ganglioside antibodies (Drachman and Kuncl, 1989).

In support of an autoimmune etiology for ALS, two immune-mediated animal models have been developed in guinea-pigs: experimental autoimmune motor neuron disease (EAMND) and experimental autoimmune gray matter disease (EAGMD). EAMND was induced by injections of purified bovine spinal cord motor neurons and resulted in a slowly developing disease with limb weakness and lower motor neuron destruction (Englehart, Appel and Killian, 1989). EAGMD, a more acute disease, was induced by injections of spinal cord ventral horn homogenates, resulting in destruction of both lower and upper motor neurons (Englehart, Appel and Killian, 1990). In both diseases, denervation was evidenced by electromyographic and morphologic criteria; IgG was found at neuromuscular junctions and in the cytoplasm of spinal cord motor neurons. When serum or immunoglobulins from EAMND and EAGMD animals, and from ALS patients, were injected into non-diseased mice, the recipient mice developed motor neuron dysfunction and were shown to have IgG in motor neurons and at the motor endplate (Appel et al., 1991b). The localization of EAMND, EAGMD and ALS immunoglobulins at the neuromuscular junction suggests a direct effect of immunoglobulins on the motor endplate. This could result in an increase in intracellular calcium concentration, leading to an increase in resting acetylcholine release, and the triggering of processes leading to cell death (Appel et al., 1991b). It should be noted that the many and divergent proposed etiologies for ALS appear to be converging to involve a common mechanism for neuronal death that involves abnormalities in intracellular calcium levels and the pathogenic pathways in which this ion participates.

29.3 NATURALLY OCCURRING ANIMAL MODELS

The ideal animal model would exactly replicate the neuropathologic changes seen in the human disease it represents and have pathogenic mechanisms in common. Experimentally induced models focus on pathogenic mechanisms because agents with predictable mechanisms of action are used to produce pathology that closely resembles the human disease. Hereditary, natural models, on the other hand, are selected because of their pathologic similarity to the human disease, in onset, clinical progression and outcome. Pathogenic mechanisms are, for the most part, unknown. Hereditary models, however, provide a source of animals with reproducible abnormalities that can be analyzed at many points in time: from initiation of cellular dysfunction to ultimate cell death. Additionally, these models, especially those with a late-onset disease, can be used for testing possible therapies. While the primary etiology in these models is genetic, cellular and molecular processes will most likely be similar to the human disease, be it familial or sporadic ALS.

Of the large number of naturally occurring, hereditary models (reviewed in Smitt and de Jong, 1989; Messer, 1992), three appear to be particularly promising models for motor neuron disease: *Mnd* in the mouse for ALS and *pmn* in the mouse and HCSMA in the dog for the spinal muscular atrophies.

29.3.1 The *Mnd* mutation in the mouse

Mnd was initially identified as a spontaneous, adult-onset, genetically dominant, neurologic disease with clinical involvement evident at ~ 6.0 months of age, progressing to total spastic paralysis with premature death at 10–12 months of age (Messer and Flaherty, 1986). For the past several years, the mice have been bred for a consistent age of onset in *Mnd/Mnd*, a result of which is a greatly reduced penetrance displayed by the heterozygote (Messer, 1992); Messer *et al.* (1992) now consider *Mnd* to be semidominant with variable penetrance, and work continues primarily using *Mnd/Mnd* (please see the addendum at the end of this chapter for new information on a change in the symbol for the motor neuron degeneration mutation). The *Mnd* disease has been categorized into four broad stages based on the clinical signs displayed: presymptomatic, mild (5.5–6.5 months of age), moderate and severe (>8.5 months of age) (Callahan *et al.*, 1991).

A routine histopathologic survey of the *Mnd* nervous system, using hematoxylin and eosin and Nissl stains, showed degeneration of neurons primarily in spinal cord motor neurons until late in the disease when pathology was observed in other neurons in the central nervous system, again primarily involving the motor system. Initially, the pathology was more severe in the lumbosacral cord, progressing with time to involve thoracic and cervical regions of the cord. In the later stages of the disease, cranial nuclei, mainly X and XII, and upper motor neurons of the red nucleus, reticular formation of the pons and medulla, and restricted areas of the cerebral cortex also were affected (Messer, Strominger and Mazurkiewicz, 1987). A statistically significant decrease in the number of lumbar (L4) ventral horn neurons in moderate-stage *Mnd/Mnd* compared with age-matched controls has been found (Callahan *et al.*, 1991). This loss in ventral horn neurons was reflected in a progressive atrophy of large myelinated axons in ventral roots (Mazurkiewicz and Lawrence, 1990).

Animal models of motor neuron disease

Pathology in neurons was demonstrated by distorted plasma membranes, eccentric nuclei, a mild central chromatolysis and numerous cytoplasmic inclusions. These cytoplasmic inclusion bodies increase in number and size with progression of the disease, and, as they become larger, other cytoplasmic elements, including the cytoskeleton, are displaced (Messer, Strominger and Mazurkiewicz, 1987; Callahan *et al.*, 1991). No such inclusions were detected in the age-matched control mice. Histochemical and immunocytochemical studies showed that the inclusions in spinal neurons, especially those in spinal lamina IX, stain intensely with luxol fast blue (LFB), contain immunoreactivity for ubiquitinated protein and display enzyme histochemical reactivity for several lysosomal hydrolases (β-glucuronidase, acid phosphatase and trimetaphosphatase) (Mazurkiewicz, 1991; Mazurkiewicz *et al.*, 1993). Some extraneuronal ubiquitin deposits were also detected in the neuropil (Mazurkiewicz *et al.*, 1993). Ubiquitin deposits and LFB staining were present in the majority of spinal neurons, with ubiquitin immunopositivity found in presymptomatic animals (Mazurkiewicz, 1991), and LFB stained inclusions found as early as 1 month of age. Abnormally accumulating autofluorescent material has also been detected in spinal cord and other tissues as early as the first month of age (Messer and Plummer, 1993). As with the aforementioned inclusion bodies, the autofluorescent material was also found in increasing numbers of cells and in increasing amounts within individual cells, as the animals age. While the clinical disease begins late in life and then follows a slowly progressing time course, the precipitating event, as manifested by these abnormal cytoplasmic accumulations, would appear to occur very early in the life of the animal.

Many neuronal cell bodies in *Mnd/Mnd* spinal cord contained phosphorylated neurofilaments (Callahan *et al.*, 1991); using a particular monoclonal antibody, TA51 (Sobue *et al.*, 1990), the number of such cells was greatly increased when compared with age-matched controls (unpublished observations from this laboratory). All neurofilament (NF) proteins were markedly redistributed within the cytoplasm, as exemplified by a margination of NF to the region just beneath the plasma membrane. This left a region in the cytoplasm that was unreactive with the battery of monoclonal antibodies to each of the NF subunits with different degrees of phosphorylation that were used. The number of cells containing the cytoplasmic NF-immunonegative regions and the size of the regions within individual cells increased with severity of the disease; however, none were detected prior to the onset of clinical symptoms. In presymptomatic *Mnd* spinal neurons, the NF cytoskeleton retains a relatively normal distribution, even though the cytoplasm contains inclusion bodies, and appears to become displaced only after the number and size of the inclusions exceeds a certain volume. Taken at face value, this would suggest that the cytoskeletal rearrangement might be secondary to inclusion body information; however, NF and ubiquitin show an immunocytochemical co-localization (Mazurkiewicz, 1991), and both pathologic abnormalities could be linked directly with ubiquitin-mediated cellular processes.

Since NFs are a major determinant of axonal caliber and axonal caliber is controlled by NF transport (Hoffman, Griffin and Price, 1984), any changes in axonal transport should have a direct effect on local axonal NF content with a concomitant effect on axonal caliber. A consequence of the abnormal accumulation of NF proteins in the *Mnd* spinal motor neuron cell bodies should be an alteration in axonal geometry in ventral roots. In presymptomatic *Mnd* animals, the frequency of distribution of caliber of myelinated axons was bimodal and not different from age-matched controls at all ages. However, beginning with the mild stage and progressing through the rest of the stages, this normal bimodal distribution was shifted, with an apparent increase in smaller diameter axons at the expense of the larger diameter fibers (Mazurkiewicz and Lawrence, 1990). Apparently, the myelinated axons in ventral roots develop normally and remain indistinguishable from roots in normal, age-matched controls until 5.5–6.0 months of age, a time that coincides with the onset of clinical symptoms. The progressive atrophy of large ventral root fibers then parallels the progressive motor dysfunction displayed in hindlimbs and forelimbs.

Figure 29.1 is a time line chart that summarizes and compares the histopathology found in HMND at post-mortem examination with histopathologic findings in *Mnd* at post-mortem examination and throughout the course of the disease. The data in the chart emphasize the progressive nature of the two diseases and highlight the utility of animal models in which the course can be examined at all stages of the clinical disease as well as prior to onset of clinical disease.

Excitatory amino acids have been suggested as a possible cause for loss of motor neurons in sporadic ALS (Plaitakis and Caroscio, 1987; Rothstein *et al.*, 1990), and it has been reported that glutamate transport is lowered in synaptosomes from the spinal cord and motor cortex of patients with ALS (Rothstein, Martin and Kuncl, 1992). This deficit in transport could lead to excitotoxic levels of glutamate in the extracellular space (Plaitakis, 1990). The uptake of glutamate by synaptosomes from spinal cord of *Mnd/Mnd* mice has been shown to be reduced by 26% in the mild stage of the disease, progressing to a 47% reduction in the more severe stages (Battaglioli *et al.*, 1993). Uptake in synaptosomes from presymptomatic *Mnd* mice was not different from the uptake in age-matched control mice. Glutamate uptake did not decline significantly in

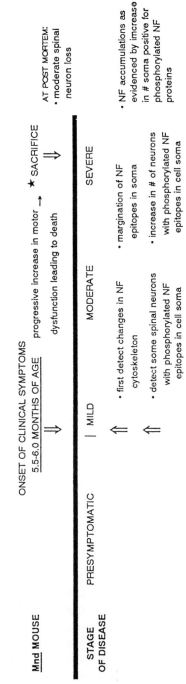

END STAGE DISEASE

HUMAN MOTOR NEURON DISEASE

ONSET OF CLINICAL SYMPTOMS
~40-50 YEARS OF AGE ⇒

progressive increase in motor → dysfunction leading to death

DEATH ⇒

¶ AT POST MORTEM:
spinal cord shows
• extreme neuronal loss
• NF accumulations
• increase # soma positive for phosphorylated NFs

• motoneurons contain abnormal inclusions that are: eosinophilic
• motoneurons contain ubiquitin deposits
• atrophy of ventral roots

dysfunction in axonal transport

Mnd MOUSE

ONSET OF CLINICAL SYMPTOMS
5.5-6.0 MONTHS OF AGE ⇒

progressive increase in motor → dysfunction leading to death

★ SACRIFICE ⇒

AT POST MORTEM:
• moderate spinal neuron loss

STAGE OF DISEASE   PRESYMPTOMATIC | MILD | MODERATE | SEVERE

• first detect changes in NF cytoskeleton
• detect some spinal neurons with phosphorylated NF epitopes in cell soma

• margination of NF epitopes in soma
• increase in # of neurons with phosphorylated NF epitopes in cell soma

• NF accumulations as evidenced by increase in # soma positive for phosphorylated NF proteins

3.5-4.0 months

1.0-1.5 months

• just able to detect autofluorescent inclusions

• Ubiquitin deposits in spinal neurons

• inclusions are clearly evident

progressive increase in size of Ubiquitin deposits and # of cells with such deposits → →

progressive increase in size of these inclusions → →

progressive increase in size of inclusions → →

• motoneurons contain ubiquitin deposits

• motoneurons contain autofluorescent inclusions

• motoneurons contain inclusion that are:
eosinophillic
PAS positive
Sudan Black Positive
stain with Luxol Fast Blue

• no difference in distribution of axon diameters in ventral roots between Mnd and control

• progressive atrophy of ventral root axons with change in bimodal distribution of axon diameters with severity of disease

• atrophy of ventral root axons with loss of large diameter axons

¶ In the human disease it is not known when and how these histopathologic changes develop since they can be analyzed only at post mortem.

★ Animals are usually sacrificed in early severe stage. At severe stage they can no longer assume an upright posture or adequately groom themselves.

⟹ and ⇑ arrows indicate time at which a certain event occurs.

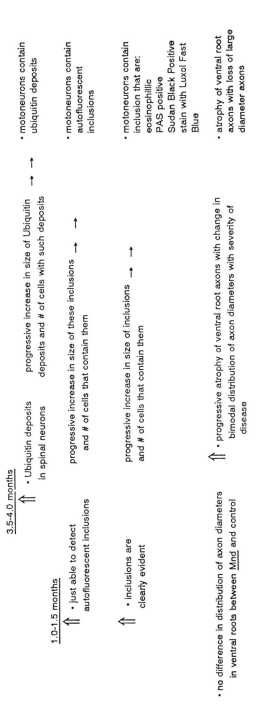

Figure 29.1 Time line comparison of histopathology of human motor neuron disease (ALS) and mouse *Mnd* disease.

corpus striatum, and GABA uptake did not change significantly in either spinal cord or corpus striatum in *Mnd* mice.

29.3.2 What can we learn about pathogenesis of motor neuron disease from *Mnd*?

Spinal motor neurons in *Mnd* and ALS have a number of histopathologic changes in common: abnormalities of the neurofilament cytoskeleton (Manetto *et al.*, 1988; Munoz *et al.*, 1988; Brooks *et al.*, 1989; Callahan *et al.*, 1991), ubiquitin-containing inclusion bodies (Leigh *et al.*, 1988; Lowe *et al.*, 1988a; Mazurkiewicz, 1991) and decreased synaptosomal uptake of glutamate (Rothstein, Martin and Kuncl, 1992; Battaglioli *et al.*, 1993). In the human, however, these observations were made at post-mortem and the origins of the abnormalities could only be speculated upon. In *Mnd* there was the opportunity to detect and follow these abnormalities from time of initial appearance in presymptomatic animals through onset of symptoms in adult animals onto the development of severe disease. Using the accumulated evidence to date, we can begin to describe a hypothetical sequence of events that results in cellular degeneration and dysfunction, leading eventually to neuronal cell death. Because basic cellular processes are shared by mammalian neurons, the sequence of events in the *Mnd* mouse might reflect the sequence in HMND.

The identity of the mutant gene product in *Mnd* is unknown. However, by 1 month of age the accumulation of substances in neuronal soma had already been triggered, mustering normal cytoplasmic degradative systems. Cells have two general pathways to deal with cytoplasmic accumulations: intralysosomal digestion and digestion via the ATP-dependent proteolytic system involving ubiquitin (Goldberg and St John, 1970; Hershko and Ciechanover, 1982); both systems are stimulated in *Mnd/Mnd* spinal neurons. The two systems would appear to intersect in the cytoplasmic accumulations or inclusion bodies: the inclusion bodies contain lysosomal hydrolases and are immunopositive for antibodies that recognize ubiquitin conjugates (Mazurkiewicz *et al.*, 1993).

The juxtaposition of several observations from the literature will amplify this connection and suggest that physiologic cell death in *Mnd* involves an autophagic mechanism. Originally believed to be involved only in non-lysosomal proteolysis, protein ubiquitination is now considered one of the signals for uptake of certain molecules into lysosomes (reviewed in Mayer *et al.*, 1991). It has been suggested that ubiquitin–protein deposits in hippocampal neurons in Alzheimer's disease might be present in autophagosomes (Lowe *et al.*, 1988b).

Autophagy has been implicated in the removal of abnormal cellular components that accumulate during cell toxicity or death (Dunn, 1990); in dying cells, one of the degradative mechanisms that is responsible for the destruction of the cytoplasm is autophagy (Clarke, 1990). Tying these points together are the observations that the stress-induced degradation of cellular proteins involves the autophagic–lysosomal pathway and is dependent on the presence of the ubiquitin-activating enzyme, E1 (Gropper et al., 1991), and that E1 is associated with the maturation of autophagocytic vacuoles (Lenk et al., 1992).

Preliminary results from electron microscopic analysis of neurons from 1-month-old Mnd/Mnd spinal cord have demonstrated the presence of inclusion bodies sequestered within a double membrane, and using an immunogold technique have shown an association of the ubiquitin-activating enzyme, E1, with the periphery of inclusion bodies (Mazurkiewicz, 1993). Thus, one of the first signs of cellular pathology is the formation of autophagosomes that contain material with the same morphology as the inclusion bodies that were observed throughout the course of the disease. The size and number of the inclusion bodies continue to increase until a point is reached at which normal cellular metabolism is compromised. Cytoskeletal rearrangements could follow, leading to a disruption of axonal transport and disruption of the maintenance of axonal integrity. Sequestration of NF protein in the cell body of the motor neuron would lead to atrophy of large myelinated axons, from which would follow muscle weakness and motor dysfunction. Ultimately, neuronal dysfunction and eventual death could proceed slowly by an autophagocytic mechanism.

However, the defect in glutamate uptake could play a role in the overall process of pathogenesis albeit late in the scheme: the extracellular concentration of glutamate could reach toxic levels and contribute to the loss of neurons seen in Mnd. Because frank histopathologic changes are evident long before the appearance of the decline in glutamate uptake, it would appear that this deficit in Mnd is a consequence rather than the primary cause of the disease. In the human disease, in contrast, it has not been possible to determine if the deficit in glutamate transport by synaptosomes from the spinal cord of patients with ALS precedes, accompanies or follows the onset of the disease.

This hypothetical scheme for the pathogenesis of Mnd disease was synthesized using the number of pathologic changes that were observed in severe-stage mice, which then, in a retrograde manner, were followed back in time to the point of initial appearance. Attribution of an abnormality to a primary or secondary cause was based solely on the relationship between the time of initial appearance and the clinical signs of the disease present at that time. When the identity of the *Mnd* gene product is known, this scheme could be further supported should the product be an abnormal protein that is made constitutively and simply clogs the normal cellular degradative pathways. Alternatively, the product itself could play a direct role in the dysregulation of these or other degradative pathways. Because all cells in the mouse are assumed to express the mutation, it remains to be explained why some cells degenerate and die while other cells function normally. Identity of the gene product is being pursued on two fronts: genetic and biochemical. In the first instance, the *Mnd* gene has been mapped to proximal chromosome 8 (Messer *et al.*, 1992), thus narrowing the scope of the search for the identification of the DNA sequence responsible for the mutation. Secondly, in preliminary work, a subcellular fraction that is enriched in inclusion bodies has been isolated from *Mnd* nervous tissue (Mazurkiewicz, 1992); refinements in the isolation protocol should furnish a cleaner fraction on which biochemical analyses can be performed. Knowledge of the content of the inclusion bodies might provide clues to the identity of the product of the mutation.

29.3.3 Hereditary canine spinal muscular atrophy

HCSMA is an autosomal dominantly inherited motor neuron disease in Brittany spaniels that shares clinical and pathologic features with HMND (Cork *et al.*, 1979, 1990). The disease produces progressive weakness and atrophy in muscle with a clinical progression in a caudal to rostral direction (Lorenz *et al.*, 1979). Three patterns of disease have been recognized: accelerated, intermediate and chronic. In the accelerated form, pups become weak by 6–8 weeks of age, progressing to complete tetrapareses by 13–16 weeks. Pups with accelerated disease are homozygous for the HCSMA trait. Pups with the intermediate and chronic form are heterozygous for the trait. Intermediate-form animals progress slowly to severe paresis over several years, while chronically affected dogs develop non-progressive weakness (Sack *et al.*, 1984). The principal neuropathologic changes are present in ventral horn of the spinal cord and in the brainstem; there appears to be no upper motor neuron involvement as the motor cortex or long motor tracts of the spinal cord are normal. Affected neurons display a pale chromatolysis and possess greatly distended axonal internodes with massive accumulations of maloriented neurofilaments (Cork *et al.*, 1982). A few motor neurons also contain increased numbers of NF, that are immunoreactive with antibodies directed against phosphorylated NF (Cork *et al.*, 1988). Axonal transport of the low molecular weight neurofilament peptide is significantly reduced in HCSMA and may contribute to the swellings of proximal axons (Griffin *et al.*, 1987). Rather than a loss of motor neurons in HCSMA, it appears that in accelerated and intermediate forms of HCSMA, neurons may never attain normal size and some may fail to undergo the normal period of cell death during development (Cork *et al.*, 1989a). Morphometric studies of ventral roots in animals with accelerated and intermediate forms of HCSMA mirror the above observations that suggest growth arrest; axons fail to achieve normal size during development and, subsequently, undergo atrophy (Cork *et al.*, 1989b). Preliminary data from pups in an early accelerated HCSMA suggested that levels of excitatory amino acids (including glutamate and aspartate) are decreased in spinal cord of affected dogs, but not in motor cortex (unpublished observations mentioned in Cork, 1991). HCSMA, like *Mnd* and ALS, appears to have a deficit in excitatory neurotransmitter transport, and this may play a role in the disease process.

HCSMA remains an important animal model for motor neuron disease because it provides an opportunity to analyze the biology of motor neurons and the properties that contribute to their vulnerability to disease at the clinical and the molecular level. The extended size of the HCSMA kindred may provide some advantage in a search for putative genetic markers for motor neuron disease; Cork (1991) reports that such studies are under way. However, genetic studies that can be done in dogs are limited. They are also large animals with a relatively long breeding cycle and are expensive to maintain.

29.3.4 Progressive motor neuronopathy (*pmn*)

Progressive motor neuronopathy, *pmn*, is an autosomal recessive mutant in the mouse (Schmalbruch *et al.*, 1991). In homozygotes, the pelvic girdle and hindlimb muscles atrophy and become paralytic during the third week of life; the forelimbs become affected soon thereafter, and the mice die by 7 weeks. Heterozygotes are normal. The brain of *pmn* mice is histologically normal and, within the first 5 weeks of life, motor neurons of the spinal cord and cranial nuclei appear normal. However, by 6–7 weeks, 40% of the facial motor neurons have degenerated, reflecting the rather precipitous nature of the degenerative process in *pmn* (Sendtner *et al.*, 1992a,b). In ventral roots, the numbers of fibers are normal, but the size of large fibers is somewhat reduced. By 4 weeks of age, the sciatic nerve and its branches, and the phrenic nerve show signs of axonal degeneration. This is most dramatic in the phrenic nerve, which at this time shows a 69% loss of myelinated axons. Motor endplates show signs of severe degeneration.

The disease causes a progressive degeneration of motor axons that is

671

manifested in a dying-back fashion, starting at the endplates and progressing in a cephalad direction. It would appear that the initial disease process, as it affects neuronal cell bodies up to 4–5 weeks of age, while rapid, is not as rapid as the process that follows in the remaining 2 weeks prior to death. In the seminal paper on *pmn*, the authors suggest that the absence of histopathology in motor neurons and the limited pathology in ventral roots might be because the animals die early (Schmalbruch *et al.*, 1991). However, by 6–7 weeks of age, a significant number of motor neurons in the facial nucleus is lost (Sendtner *et al.*, 1992). Presumably, if spinal cord had been examined at this later time, a concomitant loss in motor neurons would also have been found; however, this has not been determined. Death is suggested to result from the very rapid and extensive loss of fibers in the phrenic nerve, which innervates the diaphragm.

29.4 THERAPEUTIC TRIALS IN HEREDITARY ANIMAL MODELS

Mitsumoto, Hanson and Chad (1988) in reviewing pharmacologic trials in animal models, reported that such trials had been few and limited, and that each had been done using the wobbler mouse. Since the time of that review, however, the results from therapeutic trials in animal models have become very exciting. Trials involving the use of ciliary neurotrophic factor (CNTF) in the *pmn* (Sendtner *et al.*, 1992a) and the *Mnd* mouse (Helgren *et al.*, 1992) animal models have been reported. Ciliary neurotrophic factor is a small polypeptide isolated from chick ocular tissue and from rat and rabbit sciatic nerve. It can rescue avian motor neurons from cell death both *in vitro* and *in vivo* (Arakawa, Sendtner and Thoenen, 1990; Oppenheim *et al.*, 1991) and prevents the death of axotomized motor neurons in newborn rats (Sendtner, Kreutzberg and Thoenen, 1990). Based on these demonstrated biological properties of CNTF, both groups of researchers rationalized that this compound should be tested in an appropriate animal model of HMND.

In the study with *pmn* (Sendtner *et al.*, 1991a), the compound was delivered by intraperitoneal injection of a mouse cell line that had been transfected with a genomic construct that causes these cells to synthesize and release CNTF in high quantities. This treatment significantly prolonged the life of *pmn* mice; improved their motor performance; improved the survival time of facial motor neurons; and reduced the degeneration of myelinated axons in the phrenic nerve. Treatment began on post-natal day 21, at which time symptoms of paralysis may be evident and considerable axonal degeneration will have occurred. Strikingly, even at this advanced stage of the disease, CNTF was beneficial. Oppenheim (1992), in comments on the results of this trial, opined that despite the dramatic effect CNTF had in *pmn* mice several concerns needed to be addressed, among them being the need for a more systematic and quantitative analysis of the motor performance; a determination of how long beyond post-natal day 50 CNTF treatment is effective; and an examination of the effects of CNTF on muscle tissue, because CNTF receptors are expressed on skeletal muscle (Davis *et al.*, 1991), and the first manifestation of the *pmn* mutation is degeneration at the nerve–muscle interface.

The second trial of CNTF in an animal model involved the *Mnd* mutant (Helgren *et al.*, 1992). Five-month-old *Mnd* mice received subcutaneous injections of recombinant human CNTF three times a week for 8 weeks; the trial thus began just prior to onset of the clinical signs and continued into what would be considered the late moderate stage in the disease. This group of researchers used a systematic and quantitative analytical paradigm to assess the effect that the growth factor had on hindlimb performance. Three spatial parameters of goal-directed locomotion were determined: stride length (distance between ipsilateral footprints), intra-step distance (distance between the right and left hindlimb footprints within one step) and the base of support. The rate of decline of stride length and intra-step distance was significantly lower in the CNTF-treated group, suggesting that this treatment could retard the progression of motor dysfunction by 30–40% in the *Mnd* mouse. As with the study on *pmn*, the effect that CNTF has on skeletal muscle in *Mnd* also needs to be determined. While muscle degeneration is not a hallmark of the *Mnd* disease until very late, there is clear motor dysfunction leading to paralysis. As CNTF appears to spare the myelinated axons in peripheral nerve in *pmn*, perhaps CNTF is involved in the Schwann cell/axon interaction and retards the atrophy of the large myelinated fibers that had been observed in ventral roots in *Mnd*. Some objective measure of the effect of CNTF on the neuropathology in *Mnd* is warranted.

Clearly the reports of the ameliorative effects of CNTF on the progression of disease in these two animal models are of enormous significance and raise hopes that treatments for human motor neuron disease can indeed be developed.

29.5 CONCLUSIONS

This chapter has selectively reviewed some experimentally induced and naturally occurring animal models of HMND, focusing on three of the hereditary motor neuron diseases in the mouse and the dog. While the ideal model may not yet have been found, some possess enough clinical and pathologic characteristics in common with HMND to permit their

Animal models of motor neuron disease

use in testing hypotheses for the pathogenesis of motor neuron disease, in uncovering molecular and cellular processes involved in neuronal cell death and in testing possible therapies. Recent results have once again emphasized the utility of animal models in studies that are difficult or impossible to perform in HMND patients.

ACKNOWLEDGMENTS

I thank Drs Anne Messer, Linda Callahan, Norman Strominger and Esther Wylen and Ms Kaddee Lawrence for their contributions to various parts of this work. I thank Dr Gordon I. Kaye for his discussions and editorial skills. Experimental studies of *Mnd* in this laboratory were supported by funds from the National Institutes of Health (J.E.M.) and the ALS Association in conjunction with Anne Messer, and by a fellowship from the Fogarty International Center (J.E.M.).

ADDENDUM

Since completion of this chapter, the symbol for motor neuron degeneration has been changed from *Mnd* to *mnd* (Cook *et al.*, in press). The *mnd* mutation arose in a C57BL/6 H-2 recombinant congenic and has been maintained with sister × brother matings on this original background, both at Albany and at The Jackson Laboratory. The proper strain designation for the *mnd* strain is B6.KB1-*mnd*.

REFERENCES

Appel, S.H., Engelhardt, J.I., Garcia, J. and Stefani, E. (1991a) Autoimmunity and ALS: a comparison of animal models of immune-mediated motor neuron destruction and human ALS. *Adv. Neurol.*, **56**, 405–12.

Appel, S.H., Engelhardt, J.I., Garcia, J. and Stefani, E. (1991b) Immunoglobulins from animal models of motor neuron disease and from human amyotrophic lateral sclerosis patients passively transfer physiological abnormalities to the neuromuscular junction. *Proc. Natl. Acad. Sci. USA*, **88**, 647–51.

Arakawa, Y., Sendtner, M. and Thoenen, H. (1990) Survival effect of ciliary neurotrophic factor (CNTF) on chick embryonic motoneurons in culture: comparison with other neurotrophic factors and cytokines. *J. Neurosci.*, **10**, 3507–15.

Battaglioli, G., Martin, D.L., Plumer, J. and Messer, A. (1993) Synaptosomal glutamate uptake declines progressively in the spinal cord of a mutant mouse with motor neuron disease. *J. Neurochem.*, **60**, 1567–9.

Brooks, B.J., Sufit, R.L., DePaul, R. *et al.* (1989) Design of clinical therapeutic trials in amyotrophic lateral sclerosis. *Adv. Neurol.*, **56**, 521–46.

Callahan, L.M., Wylen, E.L., Messer, A. and Mazurkiewicz, J.E. (1991)

Neurofilament distribution is altered in the *Mnd* (Motor neuron degeneration) mouse. *J. Neuropathol. Exp. Neurol.*, **50**, 491–504.

Choi, D.W. (1988) Calcium-mediated neurotoxicity and diseases of the nervous system. *Neuron*, **1**, 623–34.

Clarke, P.G.H. (1990) Developmental cell death: morphological diversity and multiple mechanisms. *Anat. Embryol.*, **181**, 195–213.

Cook, S., Davisson, M., Bronson, R. and Messer, A. Symbol change. *Mouse Genome* (in press).

Cork, L.C. (1991) Hereditary canine spinal muscular atrophy: an animal model of neuron disease. *Can. J. Neurol. Sci.*, **18**, 432–4.

Cork, L.C., Griffin, J.W., Munnell, J.F. *et al.* (1979) Hereditary canine spinal muscular atrophy. *J. Neuropathol. Exp. Neurol.*, **38**, 209–21.

Cork, L.C., Griffin, J.W., Choy, C. *et al.* (1982) Pathology of motor neurons in accelerated hereditary canine spinal muscular atrophy. *Lab. Invest.*, **46**, 89–99.

Cork, L.C., Troncoso, J.C., Klavano, G.G. *et al.* (1988) Neurofilamentous abnormalities in motor neurons in spontaneously occurring animal disorders. *J. Neuropathol. Exp. Neurol.*, **47**, 420–31.

Cork, L.C., Altschuler, R.J., Bruha, P.J. *et al.* (1989a) Changes in neuronal size and neurotransmitter marker in hereditary canine spinal muscular atrophy. *Lab. Invest.*, **61**, 69–76.

Cork, L.C., Struble, R.G., Gold, B.G. *et al.* (1989b) Changes in size of motor axons in hereditary canine spinal muscular atrophy. *Lab. Invest.*, **61**, 333–42.

Cork, L.C., Price, D.L., Griffin, J.W. and Sack, G.H. (1990) Hereditary canine spinal muscular atrophy: canine motor neuron disease. *Can. J. Vet. Res.*, **54**, 77–82.

Davis, S., Aldrich, T.H., Valenzuela, D.M. *et al.* (1991) The receptor for ciliary neurotrophic factor. *Science*, **253**, 59–63.

Drachman, D.B. and Kuncl, R.W. (1989) Amyotrophic lateral sclerosis: an unconventional autoimmune disease? *Ann. Neurol.*, **26**, 269–74.

Dunn Jr, W.A. (1990) Studies on the mechanisms of autophagy: formation of the autophagocytic vacuole. *J. Cell Biol.*, **110**, 1923–33.

Engelhardt, J.I., Appel, S.H. and Killian, J.M. (1989) Experimental autoimmune motoneuron disease. *Ann. Neurol.*, **26**, 368–76.

Englehardt, J.I., Appel, S.H. and Killian, J.M. (1990) Motor neuron destruction in guinea pigs immunized with bovine spinal cord ventral horn homogenate: experimental autoimmune grey matter disease. *J. Neuroimmunol.*, **27**, 21–31.

Gardner, M.B., Henderson, B.E., Officer, J.E. *et al.* (1973) A spontaneous lower motor neuron disease apparently caused by indigenous type-C RNA virus in wild mice. *J. Natl. Cancer Inst.*, **51**, 1243–5.

Goldberg, A.L. and St John, A.C. (1976) Intracellular protein degradation in mammalian and bacterial cells: 2. *Annu. Rev. Biochem.*, **45**, 747–803.

Griffin, J.W., Cork, L.C., Adams, R.J. and Price, D.L. (1982) Axonal transport in hereditary canine spinal muscular atrophy (HCSMA). *J. Neuropathol. Exp. Neurol.*, **41**, 370.

Animal models of motor neuron disease

Gropper, R., Brandt, R.A., Mayer, A.M. *et al.* (1991) The ubiquitin-activating enzyme, E1, is required for stress-induced lysosomal degradation of cellular proteins. *J. Biol. Chem.*, **266**, 3602–10.

Hansen, S. and Ballantyne, J.P. (1978) A quantitative electrophysiological study of motor neurone disease. *J. Neurol. Neurosurg. Psychiatr.*, **41**, 773–83.

Hays, A.P. (1991) Separation of motor neuron diseases from pure motor neuropathies: pathology. *Adv. Neurol.*, **56**, 385–98.

Helgren, M.E., Wong, V., Kennedy, M. *et al.* (1992) Ciliary neurotrophic factor (CNTF) slows the progression of motor dysfunction in the Mnd mouse. *Neurology*, **42**, 1426–7.

Hershko, A. and Chiechanover, A. (1982) Mechanisms of intracellular protein breakdown. *Annu. Rev. Biochem.*, **51**, 335–64.

Hoffman, P.N., Griffin, J.W. and Price, D.L. (1984) Control of axonal caliber by neurofilament transport. *J. Cell Biol.*, **99**, 705–14.

Hughes, J.T. (1982) Pathology of amyotrophic lateral sclerosis, in *Human Motor Neuron Diseases* (ed. L.P. Rowland) Raven Press, New York, pp. 75–88.

Jolicoeur, P. (1991) Neuronal loss in a lower motor neuron disease induced by a murine retrovirus. *Can. J. Neurol. Sci.*, **18**, 411–13.

Jolicoeur, P., Rassart, E., DesGroseillers, L. *et al.* (1991) Retro-virus induced motor neuron disease of mice: molecular basis of neurotropism and paralysis. *Adv. Neurol.*, **56**, 481–93.

Jubelt, B. (1991) Viruses and motor neuron diseases. *Adv. Neurol.*, **56**, 463–472.

Jubelt, B. (1992) Motor neuron diseases and viruses: poliovirus, retroviruses and lymphomas. *Curr. Opin. Neurol. Neurosurg.*, **5**, 655–8.

Kay, D.G., Gravel, C., Robitaille, Y. and Jolicoeur, P. (1991) Retrovirus-induced spongiform myeloencephalopathy in mice: regional distribution of infected target cells and neuronal loss occurring in the absence of viral expression in neurons. *Proc. Natl. Acad. Sci. USA*, **88**, 1281–5.

Kristensen, K. (1992) Potential role of viruses in neurodegeneration. *Mol. Chem. Neuropathol.*, **16**, 45–58.

Latov, N., Hays, A.P., Donofrio, P.D. *et al.* (1988) Monoclonal IgM with unique specificity to gangliosides GM_1 and GD_{1b} and to lacto-N-tetrose associated with human motor neuron disease. *Neurology*, **38**, 763–8.

Ledeen, R.W. (1978) Ganglioside structures and distribution: are they localized at the nerve ending? *J. Supramolecular Structure*, **8**, 1–17.

Ledeen, R.W., Skrivanek, J.A., Tirri, L.J. *et al.* (1976) Gangliosides of the neuron: localization and origin. *Adv. Exp. Med. Biol.*, **71**, 83–103.

Leigh, P.N., Anderton, B.H., Dodson, A. *et al.* (1988) Ubiquitin deposits in anterior horn cells in motor neurone disease. *Neurosci. Lett.*, **93**, 197–203.

Lenk, S.E., Dunn, W.A., Trausch, J.S. *et al.* (1992), Ubiquitin-activating enzyme is associated with maturation of autophagocytic vacuoles. *J. Cell Biol.*, **118**, 301–8.

Lorenz, M.D., Cork, L.C., Griffin, J.W. *et al.* (1979) Hereditary spinal muscular atrophy in Brittany spaniels: clinical manifestations. *J. Am. Vet. Med. Assoc.*, **175**, 833–9.

Lowe, J., Lennox, G., Jefferson, D. *et al.* (1988a) A filamentous inclusion body within anterior horn neurones in motor neurone disease defined by immunocytochemical localisation of ubiquitin. *Neurosci. Lett.*, **94**, 203–10.

Lowe, J., Blanchard, A., Morrell, K. *et al.* (1988b) Ubiquitin is a common factor in intermediate filament inclusion bodies of diverse type in man, including those of Parkinson's disease, Pick's disease and Alzheimer's disease, as well as Rosenthal fibers in cerebellar astrocytomas, cytoplasmic bodies in muscle and Mallory bodies in alcoholic liver disease. *J. Pathol.*, **75**, 345–53.

Lustep, H.L. and Rodriguez, M. (1989) Ultrastructural, morphometric and immunocytochemical study of anterior horn cells in mice with 'wasted' mutation. *J. Neuropathol. Exp. Neurol.*, **48**, 519–33.

Manetto, V., Sternberger, N.H., Perry, G., Sternberger, L.A. and Gambetti, P. (1988) Phosphorylation of neurofilaments is altered in amyotrophic lateral sclerosis. *J. Neuropathol. Exp. Neurol.*, **47**, 642–53.

Mayer, R.J., Arnold, J., Laszlo, L. *et al.* (1991) Ubiquitin in health and disease. *Biochim. Biophys. Acta*, **1089**, 141–57.

Mazurkiewicz, J.E. (1991) Ubiquitin deposits are present in spinal motor neurons in all stages of the disease in the Motor neuron degeneration (*Mnd*) mutant of the mouse. *Neurosci. Lett.*, **128**, 182–6.

Mazurkiewicz, J.E. (1992) Inclusion bodies in motoneurons of the *Mnd* mouse share chemical and physical properties with lysosomes. *Mol. Biol. Cell*, **3**, 310a.

Mazurkiewicz, J.E. (1993) Intraneuronal inclusions in the motor neuron degeneration mouse (*mnd*) stem from an autophagocytic mechanism. *Soc. Neurosci. Abs.*, **19**, 635.

Mazurkiewicz, J.E. and Lawrence, K.A. (1990) A correlation may exist between abnormal neurofilament distribution and axonal size in the Motor neuron degeneration (*Mnd*) mouse. *J. Cell Biol.*, **111**, 42a.

Mazurkiewicz, J.E., Callahan, L.M., Swash, M. *et al.* (1993) Cytoplasmic inclusions in spinal neurons of the Motor neuron degeneration (*Mnd*) mouse. I. light microscopic analysis. *J. Neurol. Sci.*, **116**, 59–66.

Messer, A. (1992) Animal models of amyotrophic lateral sclerosis, in *Handbook of Amyotrophic Lateral Sclerosis* (ed. R. Smith), Marcel Decker, New York, pp. 433–51.

Messer, A. and Flaherty, L. (1986) Autosomal dominance in a late-onset motor neuron disease in the mouse. *J. Neurogenet.*, **3**, 345–55.

Messer, A. and Plummer, J. (1993) Accumulating autofluorescent material as a marker for early changes in the spinal cord of the *Mnd* mouse. *Neuromusc. Disord.*, **3**, 129–34.

Messer, A., Strominger, N.L. and Mazurkiewicz, J.E. (1987) Histopathology of the late-onset motor neuron degeneration (*Mnd*) mutant of the mouse. *J. Neurogenet.*, **4**, 201–13.

Messer, A., Plummer, J., Maskin, P., Coffin, J.M. and Frankel, W.N. (1992) Mapping of the Motor neuron degeneration (*Mnd*) gene. *Genomics*, **18**, 797–802.

Animal models of motor neuron disease

Mitsumoto, H., Hanson, M.R. and Chad, D.A. (1988) Amyotrophic lateral sclerosis. Recent advances in pathogenesis and therapeutic trials. *Arch. Neurol.*, **45**, 189–202.

Munoz, D.G., Greene, C., Perl, D.P. and Selkoe, D.J. (1988) Accumulation of phosphorylated neurofilaments in anterior horn motoneurons of amyotrophic lateral sclerosis patients. *J. Neuropathol. Exp. Neurol.*, **47**, 9–18.

Oppenheim, R.W. (1992) High hopes of a trophic factor. *Nature*, **358**, 451–2.

Oppenheim, R.W., Prevette, D., Quin-Wei, Y. *et al.* (1991) Control of embryonic motoneuron survival in vivo by ciliary neurotrophic factor. *Science*, **251**, 1616–18.

Pestronk, A., Adams, R.N. and Clawson, L. (1988) Serum antibodies to GM_1 ganglioside in amyotrophic lateral sclerosis. *Neurology*, **38**, 1457–61.

Pestronk, A., Adams, R.N., Cornbluth, D. *et al.* (1989) Patterns of serum antibodies to GM_1 and GD_{1a} gangliosides in ALS. *Ann. Neurol.*, **25**, 98–102.

Plaitakis, A. (1990) Glutamate dysfunction and selective motor degeneration in amyotrophic lateral sclerosis: an hypothesis. *Ann. Neurol.*, **28**, 3–8.

Plaitakis, A. and Caroscio, J.T. (1987) Abnormal glutamate metabolism in amyotrophic lateral sclerosis. *Ann. Neurol.*, **22**, 575–9.

Rothstein, J.D., Martin, L.J. and Kuncl, R. (1992) Decreased glutamate transport by the brain and spinal cord in amyotrophic lateral sclerosis. *New Engl. J. Med.*, **326**, 1464–68.

Rothstein, J.D., Tsai, G., Kuncl, R.W. *et al.* (1990) Abnormal excitatory amino acid metabolism in amyotrophic lateral sclerosis. *Ann. Neurol.*, **28**, 18–25.

Sack Jr, G.H., Cork, L.C., Morris, J.M. *et al.* (1984) Autosomal dominant inheritance of hereditary canine spinal muscular atrophy. *Ann. Neurol.*, **15**, 369–73.

Schmalbruch, H., Skovgaard Jensen, H.-J., Bjaerg, M. *et al.* (1991) A new mouse mutant with progressive motor neuronopathy. *J. Neuropathol. Exp. Neurol.*, **50**, 192–204.

Sendtner, M., Kreutzberg, G.W. and Thoenen, H. (1990) Ciliary neurotrophic factor prevents the degeneration of motor neurons following axotomy. *Nature*, **345**, 440–1.

Sendtner, M., Schmalbruch, H., Stökll, K.A. *et al.* (1992a) Ciliary neurotrophic factor prevents degeneration of motor neurons in mouse mutant progressive motor neuronopathy. *Nature*, **358**, 502–4.

Sendtner, M., Stökll, K.A., Carroll, P. *et al.* (1992b) More on motor neurons. *Nature*, **360**, 541–2.

30 *Cell culture of motor neurones*

SARAH HARPER and FRANK WALSH

The molecular pathology of diseases of the lower motor neurone is poorly understood. It is clear that in motor neurone disease (MND) there is selective death of motor neurones and the lesion affects the cell body with little evidence to support the idea that there is any dying back of the motor axon. However, a number of studies have reported changes in motor neurones that are similar to those seen after axotomy often after addition of serum to cell cultures containing motor neurones (Wolfgram and Myers, 1973; Roisen *et al.*, 1982). One of the major problems in MND is that despite many years of extensive research it is not clear if the disease is an autoimmune disease or is caused by a toxin, virus or other agent. Although progress has been slow it is likely that clearer answers to defined questions can be given now more than ever before. This is because there have been major developments in cell culture methods and our understanding of the trophic factor dependence of motor neurones and the molecular processes of axonal growth. Motor neurone cell culture allows the study of these cells in a controlled environment and specific experiments can be designed to test specific hypotheses. In this chapter we discuss some of the issues related to motor neurone cell culture and how these cells may be of value in deciphering the molecular pathology of MND.

30.1 NATURALLY OCCURRING NEURONE CELL DEATH

It has been known for many years that in early development more neurones are generated than are required. During a critical period neurones that do not make successful connections or have access to sufficient quantities of trophic factors will die. This form of developmental cell death led to the hypothesis that cells in a target field supply the innervating neurones with neurotrophic factors that support the selective survival of the neurones (Landmesser and Pilar, 1978). This has subsequently become known as the neurotrophic theory (reviewed in Thoenen and Barde, 1980; Davies, 1988a,b; Purves, Snider and Voyvodic, 1988; Barde, 1989; Oppenheim, 1989). A substantial amount of evidence for the neurotrophic theory has come from work on nerve growth factor (NGF), and more recently from work on neurotrophin 3 (NT-3) and brain-derived neurotrophic factor (BDNF).

Competition for limited amounts of target-derived trophic molecules is thought to control the number of innervating neurones that can ultimately survive. An alternative to this limited production hypothesis is that survival of a proportion of neurones in a population is controlled by limited access via axonal branches and synaptic sites to trophic factors (Dahm and Landmesser, 1988; Oppenheim, 1989). In this case sufficient amounts of neurotrophic factor would be produced to support virtually all neurones that are generated. The availability would be limited by the ability of neurones to branch and form sufficient numbers of target contacts, which provide the means for gaining access to trophic support (Oppenheim, 1989). Support for the access hypothesis has come from studies on pharmacologically paralysed chicken embryos, in which neurones that would normally die during cell death survive. Muscle extract from these animals is no more effective than that from normal animals at promoting motor neurone survival both *in vitro* (Tanaka, 1987) and *in vivo* (Houenou, Prevette and Oppenheim, 1989). This suggests that the level of neurotrophic factor synthesis is identical in normal and hyperinnervated muscle (Oppenheim, 1989).

Those neurones that do not gain access to a neurotrophic factor die during a period of cell death. This period of cell death begins shortly after the first neurones reach their targets and is thought to eliminate inappropriately connected neurones and adjust the number of neurones to the size of the target field (Cowan *et al.*, 1984). After the phase of neuronal cell death, the continued dependence of neurones on their targets is manifested by the ongoing adjustment of axonal branching and dendritic arborization with the changing size of the target as the animal grows (Purves, 1988; Purves, Snider and Voyvodic, 1988).

Although many other putative neurotrophic factors have been proposed to play a similar role to NGF, albeit on different populations of neurones (Berg, 1984; Walicke, 1989), NGF remains the only completely characterized molecule that satisfies virtually all the criteria for a neurotrophic factor in regulating the survival of discrete populations of developing neurones *in vivo*. The evidence for the neurotrophic theory based on the work on NGF is as follows.

Firstly, NGF promotes the survival of sympathetic and some sensory neurones in culture, and these neurones are also dependent on NGF *in vivo* (Levi-Montalcini and Angeletti, 1968; Johnson *et al.*, 1980;

Hamburger and Yip, 1984). Secondly, anti-NGF antibodies administered during the period of target field innervation eliminate NGF-dependent neurones, whereas exogenous NGF rescues them (Levi-Montalcini and Angeletti, 1968; Johnson *et al.*, 1980; Hamburger and Yip, 1984). Thirdly, NGF is present in the target field of NGF-responsive neurones during innervation and is transported back to the cell bodies (Davies *et al.*, 1987; Korsching and Thoenen, 1988). The receptor–ligand complex is conveyed by fast axonal transport to the cell body, where it exerts its survival effects (Korsching and Thoenen, 1983; Palmatier, Hartman and Johnson, 1984; Davies *et al.*, 1987). Disruption of axonal transport leads to the death of developing sympathetic neurones, which can be prevented by administration of NGF (Levi-Montalcini *et al.*, 1975; Hendry and Campbell, 1976; Menescini-Chen, Chen and Levi-Montalcini, 1977).

30.2 MOTOR NEURONE DEVELOPMENT

The spinal motor neurone is one of the best-studied cells of the adult nervous system. Spinal cord motor neurones appear at the germinal neuroepithelium, and migrate towards and congregate in the lateral aspect of the ventral neural tube to form the lateral motor column and extend axons outside the cord (Bennett, 1983).

Naturally occurring cell death and the role of the target have been clearly shown for the chick spinal motor neurones that depend on their peripheral target for survival. Motor neurone cell death in the chick begins at embryonic day (E) 5.5–6, a time when motor neurones have differentiated and assembled into the lateral motor columns with their axons projecting to their peripheral targets (Landmesser and Morris, 1975). Approximately 50% of motor neurones die over the next 5 days (Oppenheim, Chu-Wang and Maderedrut, 1978), and the extent of cell death can be modulated by removal or enlargement of the target tissue (Hollyday and Hamburger, 1976). Survival is also impaired by mutations affecting muscle. It has been proposed that embryonic motor neurones require muscle-derived trophic factors for survival (for reviews see Henderson, 1988; Oppenheim, 1989). As yet, however, no muscle-derived trophic molecule specific for motor neurones has been purified to homogeneity despite an enormous amount of effort.

30.3 CULTURE OF MOTOR NEURONES

The ability to culture pure populations of motor neurones is hampered by their location within the spinal cord, and therefore cultures obtained from the spinal cord contain a mixed population of neurones. The absence, until recently, of specific markers for motor neurones has made identification of these cells in culture very difficult. To date two approaches have been adopted. These are, firstly, identification of motor neurones in mixed populations and, secondly, enrichment of motor neurones prior to culture.

30.3.1 Identification of motor neurones in mixed neurone populations

Immunocytochemical methods have been used to identify motor neurones. This work is based on the observations that these cells synthesize unique gene products. One of these is the enzyme choline acetyltransferase (ChAT). Antibodies against ChAT have been used to identify cholinergic neurones in spinal cord cultures (Smith *et al.*, 1986). These antibodies are generally difficult to use with early neurones and have been found not to be completely specific as other cholinergic neurones appear in the neural tube. The low abundance of ChAT also is a major problem, as is the general lack of reactivity of antibodies across different species.

Antibodies against the SC1 antigen have also been of value. The antibody was originally obtained by immunizing mice with crude chicken embryo spinal cord membranes (Tanaka and Obata, 1984). Subsequent cloning of the SC1 antigen revealed that the protein shows sequence similarity to cell adhesion molecules that are members of the immunoglobulin superfamily (Burns *et al.*, 1991; Tanaka *et al.*, 1991). It is likely that the SC1 antigen functions as an important cell adhesion molecule, but this has not been shown formally yet. In the early spinal cord SC1 is expressed on the cell surface of motor neurones and floorplate cells. This selective expression of SC1 has led to its use as a marker for motor neurones both *in vitro* (Bloch-Gallego *et al.*, 1991) and *in vivo* (Yamada *et al.*, 1991). In cultures of total spinal cord antibodies against SC1 label two morphologically distinct cell types. These are, firstly, large multipolar motor neurones and, secondly, flat fibroblast-like floorplate cells. The total number of motor neurones in these cultures ranges from 10 to 30%, suggesting that SC1 antibody probably labels all motor neurones rather than a selected population. *In vivo* labelling occurs in all cells of the ventral horn at all rostral–caudal levels tested (Tanaka and Obata, 1984), whereas antibodies to another putative motor neurone marker called calcitonin gene-related peptide only label half the motor neurones present in this region (Fontaine *et al.*, 1986; New and Mudge, 1986). The 30% of labelled cells with SC1 antibody is considerably greater than previous reported numbers (14%) using retrograde labelling methods (Schaffner, St John and Barker, 1987; Henderson, 1988). Also the figure of 30% motor neurones in the spinal cord also corresponds to the number of neurones that extend processes in the presence of muscle-derived factors in mixed cell cultures.

Retrograde labelling has also been widely used and involves back-filling of neurones by retrograde transport of fluorescent or enzyme tracers. Labels such as horseradish peroxidase (HRP, Tanaka and Obata, 1983), fluorescein conjugates or diI (Honig and Hume, 1986) are injected into the primary muscle masses of the hindlimbs around E6 and subsequently transported along the axons of innervating motor neur-ones. The major disadvantage of this technique is that it can only be used to label neurones that have achieved sufficient outgrowth to reach their targets. Not all motor neurones will label with this technique and the tracer may be lost rapidly once the neurones are placed in culture. Additionally the dye may affect the development of the neurones. The major advantage of using fluorescent tracers is the ability to use the fluorescence-activated cell sorter (FACS) to enrich for motor neurones, but only a small proportion of these cells are recovered. The cell losses are high because of apparent harshness of the procedure and, as the FACS is not routinely available for sterile work, the procedure is not in widespread use.

30.3.2 Identification of motor neurones prior to culture

Enriched cultures of motor neurones can be obtained by dissection of the neural tube at very early stages prior to cell death when motor neurones are relatively abundant (Masuko, Kuromi and Shamida, 1979; Berg and Fishbach, 1978; Henderson, Huchet and Changeux, 1981, 1983; Longo, Manthorpe and Varon, 1982). Cell death begins at around E5.5, so this technique is useful for studying very early motor neurones. Alternatively, subdissection of the neural tube and culture of only the ventral region, where motor neurones are present, substantially increases the proportion of motor neurones present (Smith, McMana-man and Appel, 1985). This method is more suited for older spinal cords as subdissection of the spinal cord is difficult at early stages.

30.4 PANNING FOR MOTOR NEURONES WITH THE SC1 ANTIBODY

The recent technique of panning (Barres et al., 1988) offers a relatively simple method for purification of motor neurones using SC1 anti-bodies (Bloch-Gallego et al., 1991). Polystyrene Petri dishes are coated with secondary antibody followed by binding of the SC1 antibody.

Cell culture of motor neurones

After blocking to prevent non-specific binding, a suspension of spinal neurones is added to the panning dish, incubated for 1 h and then washed gently to remove any non-adherent cells. SC1-positive cells can then be eluted from the dish by competition with an excess of anti-SC1 and seeded on to polyornithine–laminin-coated culture dishes. All cells purified by this method are SC1 positive, and most of them develop the complex neuronal morphology associated with motor neurones. Floor-plate cells are present in these cultures, but their morphology is sufficiently different from that of motor neurones that they can be unambiguously identified.

30.5 METRIZAMIDE GRADIENT SEPARATION

Schnaar and Schaffner (1981) have described a centrifugation method utilizing metrizamide density gradients. Motor neurones separate from other cell types based on their lighter buoyant density. This method is only suitable for motor neurones from E6 embryos onwards since there is not a sufficient difference in size of motor neurones and other neurones in the spinal cord prior to this age. After dissociation of spinal cords in trypsin, cells are applied to iso-osmotic metrizamide density gradients. After a brief centrifugation three fractions of viable cells are obtained. Cholinergic cells migrate to lower densities than other spinal cord cells and can thus be separated. Using this method Schnaar and Schaffner (1981) reported that motor neurones purified in this way survive only in the presence of muscle conditioned medium and on a highly adhesive substratum. Additional studies by Flanigan, Dickson and Walsh (1985) confirmed the generality of the procedures.

30.6 TROPHIC FACTORS FOR CULTURED MOTOR NEURONES

All cells both *in vivo* and *in vitro* generally require trophic factors for their long-term survival and maintenance. Tissue culture of spinal motor neurones has been used extensively to study putative trophic factors for these cells. In general, tissue culture systems are based on either dissociated spinal cord or micro-explants from spinal cords. The advantages of dissociated cultures are that prelabelled motor neurones can be studied. The number of surviving motor neurones can be quantified, and also neurite extension from individual neurites can be assessed. The main disadvantage of this method is that neurones are being cultured under non-physiological conditions. The advantage of explant culture is that it more closely mimics the *in vivo* environment.

684

The disadvantages, however, are that in a more heterogeneous culture system it is impossible to determine whether any trophic action is achieved through direct action on motor neurones or action through neighbouring cells. For this reason most experiments are performed using motor neurones that have been purified free from other cells.

30.7 TROPHIC INFLUENCES ON CULTURED EMBRYONIC SPINAL MOTOR NEURONES

30.7.1 Skeletal muscle-derived factors

In vivo motor neurones depend on their target muscle for survival. Removal of a limb bud in the developing chick embryo leads to the death of all motor neurones destined to innervate the limb (Hamburger, 1934). Giller *et al.* (1973) were the first to demonstrate that ChAT activity increases in mouse spinal cord neurones after co-culture on muscle. Subsequently the same authors found that conditioned medium from muscle cells was sufficient to increase ChAT activity (Giller *et al.*, 1977). Muscle conditioned medium supports the survival of motor neurones purified by cell sorting, but the response is significantly smaller than that observed using only partially purified motor neurones. This suggests that other neurones in the culture, in co-operation with factors from muscle conditioned medium, contribute to survival *in vitro*.

Myotube-conditioned medium is reported to contain two activities that promote the survival of motor neurones in culture (Calof and Reichardt, 1984). The first is a neurite-promoting activity that acts by adsorbing to the culture substratum. This activity has subsequently been identified as laminin (Calof and Reichardt, 1985). The second action of myotube conditioned medium enhances survival of cultured motor neurones over longer periods and its identity is still unknown (Henderson, 1988). Henderson (1988) has recently reviewed the literature on his and other studies aimed at isolating motor neurone growth factors. The consensus is that despite many attempts by a variety of groups standard protein purification has not yielded any positive results. It is likely that alternative strategies such as expression cloning may be more productive.

30.7.2 ChAT development factor and cholinergic differentiation factor

One of the few molecules to be characterized as a motor neurone trophic factor is the ChAT development factor (McManaman *et al.*, 1990). A polypeptide of 22 kDa, it was purified over 5000-fold from rat skeletal muscle by conventional chromatography and sodium dodecyl sulphate (SDS) gel electrophoresis, and enhances the survival of motor neurones both *in vivo* and *in vitro*. *In vivo* ChAT development factor increases the number of surviving motor neurones and decreases the number of pyknotic cells with no effect on other neuronal cell types. In addition to increasing survival *in vitro*, the factor also increases ChAT activity in purified motor neurones in culture. Martinou *et al.* (1989a) showed that, in addition to the presence of the ChAT development factor in skeletal muscle conditioned media, there was a second distinct activity. This is believed to be the cholinergic differentiation factor (CDF), which was originally identified by Weber (1981). Subsequent studies showed that this was also involved in the choice of neurones to have a cholinergic or an adrenergic phenotype (Patterson and Chun, 1977). More recently the active factor was cloned and was found to correspond to a previously studied factor called leukaemia inhibitory factor (LIF). As LIF is available in an active recombinant form, it has now been possible to analyse its effect on rat motor neurones. Martinou, Martinou and Kato (1992) have now shown that LIF promotes the survival of E14 rat motor neurones. The motor neurones were retrogradely labelled with diI and then purified by FACS. Low concentrations of LIF in the nM region were sufficient to promote the survival of about 85% of the motor neurones in the culture. LIF was also able to induce ChAT activity in these pure cultures. Thus, LIF has quite dramatic effects on these neurones and is extremely active, whereas NGF and other factors are completely inactive in this model. It will be of great interest to extend studies on LIF to *in vivo* models of motor neurone cell death.

30.7.3 Ciliary neurotrophic factor (CNTF)

Ciliary neurotrophic factor (CNTF) was originally identified, purified and cloned based on its ability to support the survival of embryonic neurones of the ciliary ganglion (Adler *et al.*, 1979; Barbin, Manthorpe and Varon, 1984; Manthorpe *et al.*, 1986; Lin *et al.*, 1989; Stockli *et al.*, 1989). CNTF is now known to support sensory, sympathetic, retinal and spinal motor neurones in culture (Hoffman, 1988; Arakawa, Sendtner and Thoenen, 1990; Eckstein *et al.*, 1990) and treatment of chick embryos during the period of naturally occurring cell death rescues approximately 50% of those motor neurones that would normally die (Oppenheim *et al.*, 1991). Again, increased survival is manifest by a decrease in the number of pyknotic cells. *In vitro*, CNTF promotes the survival of 64% of lumbar spinal cord motor neurones (Arakawa, Sendtner and Thoenen, 1990). CNTF has also been shown to prevent the death of axotomized facial motor neurones and preganglionic sympathetic neurones *in vivo* (Sendtner, Kreutzberg and Thoenen, 1990; Blottner, Bruggemann and Unsicker, 1989), and promote cholinergic differentiation *in vitro* (Ernsberger, Sendtner and Rohrer, 1989). Recent studies (reviewed in Jessell and Melton, 1992) indicate that CNTF is a member of a large and diverse family of growth factors that includes growth hormone, prolactin, interleukins and a number of growth factors involved in haemopoiesis. These molecules show little primary sequence identity but have common structural features, including a characteristic helical core in the protein.

30.7.4 Fibroblast growth factor (FGF)

Fibroblast growth factor (FGF), a previously identified growth factor for fibroblasts and myoblasts (for review see Gospodarowicz, 1988), has been shown to support *in vitro* survival of embryonic neurones. Neurones that respond to FGF (acidic and basic) include those from the hippocampus (Walicke *et al.*, 1986), cerebral cortex (Morrison *et al.*, 1986; Walicke, 1988), striatum, septum and thalamus of E18 rats (Walicke, 1988), the early post-natal mouse cerebellum (Hatten *et al.*, 1988) and chick ciliary ganglion and spinal cord (Unsicker *et al.*, 1987). FGF can also induce fibre outgrowth from a variety of cells, including PC12 cells (Togari *et al.*, 1985; Neufield *et al.*, 1987; Rydal and Green, 1987), newborn rat adrenal chromaffin cells (Claude *et al.*, 1988; Stemple, Mahanthappa and Anderson, 1988) and post-natal retinal ganglion cells (Lipton *et al.*, 1988). Both FGF and CNTF differ from the neurotrophin family of trophic factors in that they are expressed at very high levels and their method of secretion is unknown as neither possesses a signal sequence. Thus, the mechanism of action of these neurotrophic factors may be very different from that of other target-derived neurotrophic factors. The fact that CNTF prevents lesion-mediated degeneration of motor neurones in newborn rats makes it a promising candidate for treatment of degenerative disorders of motor neurones. Both acidic and basic FGF promote survival of motor neurones in culture. Basic FGF is more effective, although the activity of acidic FGF can be increased by supplementing the cultures with heparin, which prevents its inactivation. Basic FGF supports the survival of 50% of lumbar spinal motor neurones, while acidic FGF with heparin is able to support only 35% (Arakawa, Sendtner and Thoenen, 1990).

The data published on the survival of motor neurones in the presence of both CNTF and FGF are somewhat ambiguous. Some authors report

Cell culture of motor neurones

that they are unable to achieve any significant survival responses with either of these molecules. Because the mechanism of secretion is unknown and neither is believed to be secreted, the likelihood of these molecules playing a role during the period of naturally occurring cell death is extremely small.

30.7.5 Transforming growth factor beta-1 (TGF-β_1)

TGF-β_1 was first identified as promoting anchorage-dependent growth of fibroblasts and has been purified from porcine and human platelets. This factor regulates the proliferation and differentiation of many cell types; for example, it blocks myogenesis and adipogenesis and promotes chondrogenesis and the differentiation of epithelial cells (for review see Massague, 1990). Martinou et al. (1990) report that purified E14 rat motor neurones respond to TGF-β_1 with increased survival in low-density cultures. The effect is not observed when motor neurones are grown in high-density cultures, raising the possibility that cell–cell contacts may have a beneficial effect on cell survival. However, other workers have not been able to achieve similar effects on motor neurone survival with TGF-β_1 (Bloch-Gallego et al., 1991).

30.7.6 Astroglial growth factors (AGFs)

AGFs (AGF-1 and AGF-2) have been reported to support the survival of lumbar spinal cord cells in vitro (Unsicker et al., 1987). AGF-1 and AGF-2 were purified from bovine brain (Pettman et al., 1985) but have subsequently been found to have significant homology to (and are believed to be) acidic and basic FGF respectively. Monoclonal antibodies against AGF-2 recognize both AGF-2 and bFGF. Interestingly, these workers find acidic and basic FGF to be equally potent at maintaining the survival of lumbar spinal cord cells in vitro.

30.8 THE ROLE OF THE SUBSTRATUM IN MOTOR NEURONE SURVIVAL

Laminin has been reported as being one of the crucial factors in muscle conditioned medium that supports neurite outgrowth and cholinergic development (Calof and Reichardt, 1985; Martinou et al., 1989b). The extrajunctional region of adult skeletal muscle is virtually devoid of neurite growth-promoting activity (Slack and Pockett, 1982). Increased neurite-promoting activity has been demonstrated in denervated muscle as compared with innervated muscle (Henderson, Huchet and Chan-geux, 1983; Hill and Bennet, 1983). These authors suggest that the

688

muscle fibre matrix may be important in promoting outgrowth. This idea has received support from Glicksman and Sanes (1983), who demonstrated that adult spinal motor axons regenerate to contact the basal lamina in the absence of myofibres.

30.9 NEURAL CELL ADHESION MOLECULES

An alternative to the production hypothesis of target-dependent cell death is the access hypothesis. According to this view, motor neurones compete for access to a target-derived neurotrophic factor by means of axonal terminals and synapses. In contrast to the production hypothesis, sufficient amounts of neurotrophic factor would normally be produced to support all motor neurones that are generated. In this case the limiting factor is axonal branches and synaptic sites needed to gain access to the trophic factor. Any perturbations that affect branching and synaptogenesis would therefore affect motor neurone survival. This hypothesis suggests that a major factor behind the competition for access for a trophic factor is the capacity of motor neurones to branch and form contacts.

The cell adhesion molecule N-CAM is expressed in muscle during the period of innervation and synaptogenesis (Grumet et al., 1982; Moore and Walsh, 1985) and N-CAM antibodies inhibit the binding of nerve to muscle in vitro (Rutishauser, Grumet and Edelman, 1983). These observations have led to the suggestion that N-CAM may play an important role in the process of synaptogenesis, and thus expression of cell adhesion molecules on muscle may determine access of neurones via axonal branching and synaptogenesis. N-CAM is expressed on muscle during the actual period of neuronal innervation but is downregulated as development proceeds.

Paralysis or denervation of adult skeletal muscle causes an increase in expression of N-CAM which disappears on reinnervation (Couvalt and Sanes, 1985; Moore and Walsh, 1986). Partial denervation, which occurs during the initial stages of neurodegenerative diseases, is accompanied by sprouting of the remaining motor axons to compensate for the loss. This could be mediated via cell adhesion molecules.

The importance of cell adhesion molecules in survival of neurones is clearly demonstrated in culture by the fact that neurones do not survive unless grown on an adhesive substrate. Laminin is the usual molecule of choice, but purified N-cadherin also promotes neurite outgrowth (Bixby and Zhang, 1990) and N-CAM, N-cadherin and L1 expressed on the surface of transfected fibroblasts also promote neurite outgrowth (Doherty et al., 1991; Williams et al., 1992). Thus, both trophic factors and cell adhesion molecules play important roles in promoting the survival of motor neurones.

30.10 CULTURE OF FACIAL MOTOR NEURONES

The cranial motor nerve nuclei are arranged segmentally within the hindbrain of the developing chicken embryo. The hindbrain is divided into segmental units or rhombomeres which appear between stage 9 and 12 (Hamburger and Hamilton, 1951) and remain visible until stage 25. The cranial motor nuclei lie within pairs of segments with their exit points in the anterior rhombomere of the pair. Facial motor neurones in rhombomere 4 extend axons directly towards their exit point, which is also in rhombomere 4. Facial motor neurones in rhombomere 5 first extend laterally and then turn anteriorly to reach the exit point in rhombomere 4. Subdissection of rhombomere 4 is possible as early as stage 12, permitting the culture of these neurones prior to their reaching their target muscles. The segmental arrangement of these motor neurones within the hindbrain and the use of motor neurone-specific antibody (SC1) means that it is now possible to look at the outgrowth of specifically facial motor neurones.

Using this method we have looked at the survival and outgrowth of these neurones cultured on laminin, collagen and fibronectin. These early motor neurones grow well on laminin in the absence of trophic factors from muscle for at least 48 h, but show limited outgrowth on either collagen or fibronectin. Neurones were also grown in co-culture with 3T3 cells and 3T3 cells transfected with the cell adhesion molecules N-CAM or N-cadherin. The results (shown in Figure 30.1) demonstrate that facial motor neurones grow longer neurites when cultured on the cell adhesion molecule substrate.

30.11 MOTOR NEURONE DISEASE AND CELL CULTURE OF MOTOR NEURONES

The availability of pure populations of motor neurones or the ability to identify these cells has allowed specific questions to be asked regarding cell death in MND. In recent years there has been continuing interest in the question of autoimmunity. While plasmapheresis does not have any great beneficial effect in altering the progress of the disease there has been a continuing interest in this topic. Certainly it has seemed possible that there is a specific autoimmune attack against a trophic factor or even a motor neurone cell-surface antigen. Until the identification of motor neurones in culture and the factors that alter their survival it has not been possible to address these questions. In addition to these more

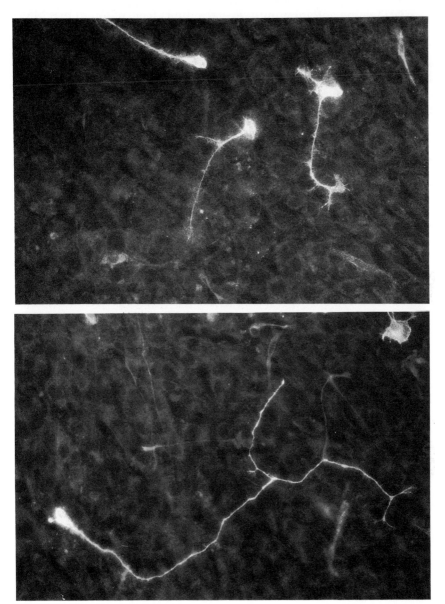

Figure 30.1 Examples of stage 15 chicken facial motor neurones cultured for 24 h on a monolayer of 3T3 fibroblasts expressing human N-CAM. Cells were cultured in Sato medium with 2% fetal calf serum added, fixed and stained with SC1 antibody. Both micrographs (A and B) show the extended multipolar morphology of motor neurones grown in contact with the N-CAM-expressing monolayer.

specific ideas on autoimmunity several authors have reported that MND serum contains a factor that is toxic to primary cultures (see Doherty *et al.*, 1986). With this as background we initiated some studies to address questions regarding toxic factors and also autoimmunity using sera from control and MND patients (Doherty *et al.*, 1986). We showed that levels of neurofilament protein (a marker of neuronal differentiation) in cultures maintained in the presence of MND serum were lower than in cultures maintained in the presence of control serum, suggesting a toxic component in sera. However, this was a general feature of MND and did not also portionate with the immunoglobin portion, showing that it was not an antibody. However, when these cultures were maintained under conditions that promote the survival of a muscle-dependent population of motor neurones, the magnitude of the inhibition did not increase, suggesting that the toxicity is not specifically directed at those neurones that respond to muscle derived factors. In agreement with this finding, Touzeau and Kato (1983) observed a small but consistent reduction in neuronal survival, ChAT activity and [^{3}H]-acetylcholine synthesis in primary cultures of embryonic chick ciliary ganglia on treatment with serum from MND patients. However, these effects were not statistically significant. Similarly, Gurney *et al.* (1984) have reported that botulinum toxin-induced sprouting of motor neurones is also inhibited by serum from MND patients. However, the validity of this study has seriously been called into question with the cloning of the so-called sprouting factor (Gurney *et al.*, 1986). It turned out to be the glycolytic enzyme, glucose-6-phosphate isomerase, which is clearly not a trophic factor (Faik *et al.*, 1988). These types of analytical studies, which were carried out a few years ago on spinal cord cell cultures and muscle extracts that contained trophic activities, provided evidence against the autoimmune hypothesis in MND. However, they do not obviously invalidate the hypothesis, and clearly any of the newly discovered trophic factors could be a target of immune attack or indeed the motor neurones themselves. Our studies used chicken neurones, which may have antigenic differences from rodent or human motor neurones. Also, the disease has a time course over a number of years, and any active immune component may be present at any one stage of the disease. As the sera used were not collected at any one time, this obviously limits the conclusions that can be derived from this type of negative study.

The developments in cell culture methods and the availability of trophic factors in recombinant forms should allow more defined questions to be addressed in the future. These systems also offer the opportunity for testing the role of other components that may be involved in causing motor neurone cell death. The results obtained in

692

tissue culture and *in vivo* experiments such as for the role of CNTF suggest that trophic factors may be useful agents for altering the course of the disease. The interplay of cell cultures and trophic factors with more complex model systems will be central to providing an intellectual framework for pharmacological intervention in MND.

REFERENCES

Adler, R., Landa, K.B., Manthorpe, M. and Varon, S. (1979) Cholinergic neurotrophic factors; intraocular distribution of trophic activity for ciliary neurons. *Science*, **204**, 1434–6.

Arakawa, Y., Sendtner, M. and Thoenen, H. (1990) Survival effect of ciliary neurotrophic factor (CNTF) on chick embryonic motoneurons in culture: comparisons with other neurotrophic factors and cytokines. *J. Neurosci.*, **10**, 3501–15.

Barbin, G., Manthorpe, M. and Varon, S. (1984) Purification of the chick eye ciliary neurotrophic factor. *J. Neurochem.*, **43**, 1468–78.

Barde, Y.A. (1989) Trophic factors and neuronal survival. *Neuron*, **2**, 1525–34.

Barres, B.A., Silverstein, B.E., Corey, D.P. and Chun, L.L.Y. (1988) Immunological, morphological, and electrophysiological variation among retinal ganglion cells purified by panning. *Neuron*, **1**, 791–803.

Bennett, M.R. (1983) Development of neuromuscular synapses. *Physiol. Rev.*, **83**, 915–1048.

Berg, D.K. (1984) New neuronal growth factors. *Annu. Rev. Neurosci.*, **7**, 149–70.

Berg, D.K. and Fishbach, G.D. (1978) Enrichment of spinal cord cell cultures with motoneurons. *J. Cell Biol.*, **77**, 83–98.

Bixby, J.L. and Zhang, R. (1990) Purified N-cadherin is a potent substrate for rapid induction of neurite outgrowth. *J. Cell Biol.*, **110**, 1253–60.

Bloch-Gallego, E., Huchet, M., El M'Hamdi, H. *et al.* (1991) Survival *in vitro* of motoneurons identified or purified by novel antibody-based methods is selectively enhanced by muscle-derived factors. *Development*, **111**, 221–32.

Blottner, D., Bruggemann, W. and Unsicker, K. (1989) Ciliary neurotrophic factor supports target derived preganglionic sympathetic spinal cord neurons. *Neurosci. Lett.*, **105**, 316–20.

Burns, F.R., Von Kannen, S., Guy, L. *et al.* (1991) DM-Grasp, a novel immunoglobulin superfamily axonal surface protein that supports neurite extension. *Neuron*, **7**, 209–20.

Calof, A.L. and Reichardt, L.F. (1984) Motoneurons purified by cell sorting respond to two distinct activities in myotube-conditioned medium. *Dev. Biol.*, **106**, 194–210.

Calof, A.L. and Reichardt, L.F. (1985) Response of purified chick motoneurons to myotube conditioned medium; laminin is essential for the substratum-binding, neurite outgrowth promoting activity. *Neurosci. Lett.*, **59**, 183–9.

Claude, P., Parade, I.M., Gordon, K.A. *et al.* (1988) Acidic fibroblast growth factor stimulates adrenal chromaffin cells to proliferate and to extend neurites but is not a long-term survival factor. *Neuron*, **1**, 783–90.

Couvalt, J. and Sanes, J. (1985) Neural cell adhesion molecule (NCAM) accumulates in denervated and paralysed muscles. *Proc. Natl. Acad. Sci. USA*, **82**, 4544–8.

Cowan, W.M., Fawcett, J.W., O'Leary, D.D.M. and Stanfield, B.I.B. (1984) Regressive events in neurogenesis. *Science*, **225**, 1258–65.

Dahm, L.M. and Landmesser, L. (1988) The regulation of intra-muscular nerve branching during normal development and following activity blockade. *Dev. Biol.*, **130**, 621–44.

Davies, A.M. (1988a) The emerging generality of the neurotrophic hypothesis. *Trends Neurosci.*, **11**, 24–5.

Davies, A.M. (1988b) Role of neurotrophic factors in development. *Trends Genetics*, **4**, 139–43.

Davies, A.M., Bandtlow, C., Heumann, R. *et al.* (1987) Timing and site of nerve growth factor synthesis in developing skin in relation to innervation and expression of the receptor. *Nature*, **326**, 353–8.

Doherty, P., Dickson, J.G., Flanigan, T.P. *et al.* (1986) Effects of amyotrophic lateral sclerosis serum on cultured chick spinal neurons. *Neurology*, **36**, 1330–4.

Doherty, P., Rowett, L.H., Moore, S.E. *et al.* (1991) Neurite outgrowth in response to transfected N-CAM and N-cadherin reveals fundamental differences in neuronal responsiveness to CAMs. *Neuron*, **5**, 209–19.

Eckstein, F.P., Esch, F., Holbert, T. *et al.* (1990) Purification and characterisation of a trophic factor for embryonic peripheral neurons: comparisons with fibroblast growth factors. *Neuron*, **4**, 623–31.

Ernsberger, U., Sendtner, M. and Rohrer, H. (1989) Proliferation and differentiation of embryonic chick sympathetic neurons; effects of ciliary neurotrophic factor. *Neuron*, **2**, 1275–84.

Faik, P., Walker, J.I.H., Redmill, A.A.M. and Morgan, M.J. (1988) Mouse glucose-6-phosphate isomerase and neuroleukin have identical 3' sequences. *Nature*, **332**, 454–5.

Flanigan, T.P., Dickson, J.G. and Walsh, F.S. (1985) Cell survival characteristics and choline acetyltransferase activity in motor neurone-enriched cultures from chick embryo spinal cord. *J. Neurochem.*, **45**, 1323–6.

Fontaine, B., Klarsfeld, A., Hokfelt, T. and Changeux, J.P. (1986) Calcitonin gene-related peptide, a peptide present in spinal cord motoneurons, increases the number of acetylcholine receptors in primary cultures of chick embryo myotubes. *Neurosci. Lett.*, **71**, 59–65.

Giller, E.L., Schrier, B.K., Shainberg, A. *et al.* (1973) Choline acetyl transferase activity is increased in combined cultures of spinal cord and muscle cells from mice. *Science*, **10**, 588–9.

Giller, E.L., Neale, J.H., Bullock, P.N. *et al.* (1977) Choline acetyl transferase activity of spinal cord cultures increased by co-culture of muscle and muscle-conditioned medium. *J. Cell Biol.*, **74**, 16–29.

Glicksman, M.A. and Sanes, J.R. (1983) Differentiation of motornerve terminals formed in the absence of muscle fibres. *J. Neurocytol.*, **12**, 661–71.

Gospodarowicz, D. (1988) Molecular and developmental biology aspects of fibroblast growth factor, in *Biology of Growth Factors*, Vol. 234 (eds J.E.

Kudlow, D.H. Maclennan, A. Bernstein and A.I. Gotlieb), Plenum Publishing, New York, pp. 23–39.

Grumet, M., Rutishauser, U. and Edelman, G.M. (1982) Neural cell adhesion molecule is an embryonic muscle cell and mediates adhesion to nerve cells *in vitro*. *Nature*, **295**, 693–5.

Gurney, M.E., Belton, A.G., Cashman, N. and Antel, J.P. (1984) Inhibition of terminal axon sprouting by serum from patients with amyotrophic lateral sclerosis. *New Engl. J. Med.*, **311**, 933–99.

Gurney, M.E., Heinrich, S.P., Lee, M.L. and Yin, H.-S. (1986) Molecular cloning and expression of neuroleukin, a neurotrophic factor for spinal and sensory neurons. *Science*, **234**, 566–74.

Hamburger, V. (1934) The effects of wind bud extirpation on the development of the central nervous system in the chick embryo. *J. Exp. Zool.*, **68**, 449–94.

Hamburger, V. and Hamilton, H.L. (1951) A series of normal stages in the development of the chick embryo. *J. Morphol.*, **88**, 49–92.

Hamburger, V. and Yip, J.W. (1984) Reduction of experimentally induced neuronal death in spinal ganglia of the chick embryo by nerve growth factor. *J. Neurosci.*, **4**, 767–74.

Hatten, M.E., Lynch, M., Rydel, R.E. *et al.* (1988) *In vitro* neurite extension by granule neurons is dependent upon astroglial-derived fibroblast growth factor. *Dev. Biol.*, **125**, 280–9.

Henderson, C.E. (1988) The role of muscle in the development and differentiation of spinal motoneurons: *in vitro* studies, in *Selective Neuronal Death. Ciba Foundation Symposia*, Vol. 126, pp. 65–81.

Henderson, C.E., Huchet, M. and Changeux, J.-P. (1981) Neurite outgrowth from embryonic chicken spinal neurons is promoted by media conditioned by muscle cells. *Proc. Natl. Acad. Sci. USA*, **78**, 2625–9.

Henderson, C.E., Huchet, M. and Changeaux, J.P. (1983) Denervation increases in neurite promoting activity in extracts of skeletal muscle. *Nature*, **302**, 609–11.

Hendry, I.A. and Campbell, J. (1976) Morphometric analysis of rat superior cervical ganglion after axotomy and nerve growth factor treatment. *J. Neurocytol.*, **5**, 351–60.

Hill, M.A. and Bennett, M.R. (1983) Cholinergic growth factor from skeletal muscle elevated following denervation. *Neurosci. Lett.*, **35**, 31–5.

Hoffman, H.-D. (1988) Ciliary neurotrophic factor stimulates choline acetyltransferase activity in cultured chicken retina neurons. *J. Neurochem.*, **51**, 109–13.

Hollyday, M. and Hamburger, V. (1976) Reduction of naturally occurring motor neuron cell loss by enlargement of the periphery. *J. Comp. Neurol.*, **170**, 311–20.

Honig, M.G. and Hume, R.I. (1986) Fluorescent carbocycine dyes allow living neurons of identified origin to be studied in long term cultures. *J. Cell Biol.*, **103**, 171–87.

Houenou, L., Prevette, D. and Oppenheim, R. (1989) Motoneuron survival *in vivo* following treatment with extracts from active and inactive muscle. *Soc. Neurosci. Abstr.*, **15**, 436.

Cell culture of motor neurones

Jessell, T.M. and Melton, D.A. (1992) Diffusible factors in vertebrate embryonic induction. *Cell*, **68**, 257–70.

Johnson, E.M., Gorin, P.D., Brandeis, L.D. and Pearson, J. (1980) Dorsal root ganglion neurons are destroyed by exposure in utero to maternal antibody to nerve growth factor. *Science*, **210**, 916–18.

Korsching, S. and Thoenen, H. (1983) Quantitative demonstration of the retrograde axonal transport of endogenous nerve growth factor. *Neurosci. Lett.*, **39**, 1–4.

Korsching, S. and Thoenen, H. (1988) Developmental changes of nerve growth factor levels in sympathetic ganglia and their target organs. *Dev. Biol.*, **126**, 40–6.

Landmesser, L. and Morris, D.G. (1975) The development of functional innervation in the hindlimb of the chick embryo. *J. Physiol.*, **248**, 301–26.

Landmesser, L. and Pilar, K.G. (1978) Interactions between neurons and their targets during *in vivo* synaptogenesis. *Fed Proc.*, **37**, 2016–22.

Levi-Montalcini, R. and Angeletti, P.V. (1968) Nerve growth factor. *Physiol. Rev.*, **48**, 534–69.

Levi-Montalcini, R., Aloe, L., Mugnaini, E. *et al.* (1975) Nerve growth factor induces volume increase and enhances tyrosine hydroxylase synthesis in chemically axotomised sympathetic ganglia of newborn rats. *Proc. Natl. Acad. Sci. USA*, **72**, 595–9.

Lin, L.H., Mismer, D., Lile, J.D. *et al.* (1989) Purification, cloning and expression of ciliary neurotrophic factor (CNTF). *Science*, **246**, 1023–5.

Lipton, S.A., Wagner, J.A., Madison, R.D. and D'Amore, P.A. (1988) Acidic fibroblast growth enhances regeneration of processes by postnatal mammalian retinal ganglion cells in culture. *Proc. Natl. Acad. Sci. USA*, **85**, 2388–92.

Longo, F.M., Manthorpe, M. and Varon, S. (1982) Spinal cord neurotrophic factors: bioassay of Schwannoma and other conditioned media. *Dev. Brain Res.*, **3**, 277–94.

McManaman, J.L., Oppenheim, R.W., Prevette, D. and Marchetti, D. (1990) Rescue of motoneurons from cell death by a purified skeletal muscle polypeptide: effects of the ChaT development factor, CDF. *Neuron*, **4**, 891–8.

Manthorpe, M., Skaper, S.D., Williams, L.R. and Varon, S. (1986) Purification of adult rat sciatic nerve ciliary neurotrophic factor. *Brain Res.*, **367**, 282–6.

Martinou, J.-C., Martinou, I. and Kato, A.C. (1992) Cholinergic differentiation factor (CDF/LIF) promotes survival of isolated rat embryonic motoneurons *in vitro*. *Neuron*, **8**, 737–44.

Martinou, J.-C., Le Van Thai, A., Cassar, G. *et al.* (1989a) Characterization of two factors enhancing choline acetyltransferase activity in cultures of purified rat motoneurons. *J. Neurosci.*, **9**, 3645–56.

Martinou, J.-C., Bierer, F., Le Van Thai, A. and Weber, M.J. (1989b) Influence of the culture substratum on the expression of choline acetyltransferase activity in purified motoneurons from rat embryos. *Dev. Brain Res.*, **47**, 251–62.

Martinou, J.-C., Le Van Thai, A., Valette, A. and Weber, M.J. (1990) Transforming growth factor β_1 is a potent survival factor for rat embryo motoneurons in culture. *Dev. Brain Res.*, **52**, 175–81.

696

Massaque, J. (1990) The transforming growth factor-β family. *Annu. Rev. Cell Biol.*, **6**, 597–641.

Masuko, S., Kuromi, H. and Shamida, V. (1979) Isolation and culture of motoneurons from embryonic chicken spinal cords. *Proc. Natl. Acad. Sci. USA*, **76**, 3536–41.

Menescini-Chen, M.G., Chen, J.S. and Levi-Montalcini, R. (1978) Sympathetic nerve fibres ingrowth in the central nervous system of neonatal rodents upon intracerebral NGF injections. *Arch. Ital. Biol.*, **116**, 53–84.

Moore, S.E. and Walsh, F.S. (1985) Specific regulation of N-CAM/D2-CAM cell adhesion molecule during skeletal muscle development. *EMBO J.*, **4**, 623–30.

Moore, S.E. and Walsh, F.S. (1986) Nerve dependent regulation of N-CAM expression in muscle. *Neuroscience*, **18**, 499–505.

Morrison, R.S., Kornblum, H.I., Leslie, F.M. and Bradshaw, R.A. (1986) Trophic simulation of cultured neurons from neonatal rat brain by epidermal growth factor. *Science*, **238**, 72–5.

Neufeld, G., Gospodarowicz, D., Dodge, L. and Fujii, D.K. (1987) Heparin modulation of the neurotrophic effects of acidic and basic fibroblast growth factors and nerve growth factor on PC12 cells. *J. Cell. Physiol.*, **131**, 131–40.

New, H.V. and Mudge, A.W. (1986) Calcitonin gene-related peptide regulates muscle acetylcholine receptor synthesis. *Nature*, **323**, 809–11.

Oppenheim, R.W. (1989) The neurotrophic theory and naturally occurring motoneuron death. *Trends Neurosci.*, **12**, 252–5.

Oppenheim, R.W. (1991) Cell death during development of the nervous system. *Annu. Rev. Neurosci.*, **14**, 453–501.

Oppenheim, R.W., Chu-Wang, I.W. and Maderedrut, J.L. (1978) Cell death of motoneurons in the chick embryo spinal cord. The differentiation of motoneurons prior to their induced degeneration following limb bud removal. *J. Comp. Neurol.*, **177**, 87–112.

Oppenheim, R.W., Prevette, D., Qin-Wei, Y. *et al.* (1991) Control of embryonic motoneuron survival *in vivo* by ciliary neurotrophic factor. *Science*, **251**, 1616–18.

Palmatier, M.A., Hartman, B.K. and Johnson, E.M. (1984) Demonstration of retrogradely transported endogenous nerve growth factor in axons of sympathetic neurons. *J. Neurosci.*, **4**, 751–6.

Patterson, P.H. and Chun, L.L.Y. (1977) The induction of acetylcholine synthesis in primary cultures of dissociated rat sympathetic neurons. Effects of conditioned medium. *Dev. Biol.*, **56**, 263–80.

Pettmann, B., Weibel, M., Sensenbrenner, M. and Labourdette, G. (1985) Purification of two astroglial growth factors from bovine brain. *FEBS Lett.*, **189**, 102–9.

Purves, D. (1988) *Body and Brain: A Trophic Theory of Neuronal Connections.* Harvard University Press, Cambridge, MA.

Purves, D., Snider, W.D. and Voyvodic, T. (1988) Trophic regulation of nerve cell morphology and innervation in the autonomic nervous system. *Nature*, **336**, 123–8.

Roisen, F.J., Bastfield, H., Donnenfield, H. and Baxter, J. (1982) Neuron specific

697

Cell culture of motor neurones

in vitro cytoxicity of sera from patients with amyotrophic lateral sclerosis. *Muscle Nerve*, **5**, 48–53.

Rutishauser, U., Grumet, M. and Edelman, G. (1983) N-CAM mediates initial interactions between spinal cord neurons and muscle cells in culture. *J. Cell Biol.*, **97**, 145–52.

Rydel, R.E. and Greene, L.A. (1987) Acidic and basic fibroblast growth factors promote stable neurite outgrowth and neuronal differentiation in cultures of PC12 cells. *J. Neurosci.*, **7**, 3639–53.

Schaffner, A.E., St John, P.A. and Barker, J.L. (1987) Fluorescence-activated cell sorting of embryonic mouse and rat motoneurons and their long term survival *in vitro*. *J. Neurosci.*, **7**, 3088–104.

Schnaar, R.L. and Schaffner, A.E. (1981) Separation of cell types from embryonic chicken and rat spinal cord: characterization of motoneuron-enriched fractions. *J. Neurosci.*, **1**, 204–17.

Sendtner, M., Kreutzberg, G.W. and Thoenen, H. (1990) Ciliary neurotrophic factor prevents the degeneration of motor neurons after axotomy. *Nature*, **345**, 440–1.

Slack, J.R. and Pockett, S. (1982) Motor neurotrophic factor in denervated adult skeletal muscle. *Brain Res.*, **247**, 138–40.

Smith, R.G., McManaman, J. and Appel, S.H. (1985) Trophic effects of skeletal muscle extracts on ventral spinal cord neurons in vitro: separation of a protein with morphologic activity from proteins with cholinergic activity. *J. Cell Biol.*, **101**, 1608–21.

Smith, R.G., Vaca, K., McManaman, J. and Appel, S.H. (1986) Selective effects of the skeletal muscle extracts fractions on motoneuron development *in vitro*. *J. Neurosci.*, **6**, 439–47.

Stemple, D.L., Mahanthappa, N.K. and Anderson, D.J. (1988) Basic FGF induces neuronal differentiation, cell division and NGF dependence in chromaffin cells: a sequence of events in sympathetic development. *Neuron*, **1**, 517–25.

Stockli, K.A., Lottspeich, F., Sendtner, M. *et al.* (1989) Molecular cloning, expression and regional distribution of rat ciliary neurotrophic factor. *Nature*, **342**, 920–3.

Tanaka, H. (1987) Chronic application of curare does not increase the level of motoneurone survival-promoting activity in limb muscle extracts during naturally occurring motoneurone cell death period. *Dev. Biol.*, **124**, 347–57.

Tanaka, H. and Obata, K. (1983) Survival of HRP labelled spinal motoneurons of chick embryo in tissue and cell cultures. *Dev. Brain Res.*, **9**, 390–5.

Tanaka, H. and Obata, K. (1984) Developmental changes in unique cell surface antigens of chick embryo spinal motoneurons and ganglion cells. *Dev. Biol.*, **106**, 26–37.

Tanaka, H., Matsui, T., Agata, A. *et al.* (1991) Molecular cloning and expression of a novel adhesion molecule, SC1. *Neuron*, **7**, 535–45.

Thoenen, H. and Barde, Y.A. (1980) Physiology of nerve growth factor. *Physiol. Rev.*, **60**, 1284–335.

Togari, A., Dickens, G., Kuzaya, H. and Guroff, G. (1985) The effect of fibroblast growth factor on PC12 cells. *J. Neurosci.*, **5**, 307–16.

Touzeau, G. and Kato, A.C. (1983) Effect of amyotrophic lateral sclerosis sera on cultured cholinergic neurons. *Neurology*, **33**, 317–22.

Unsicker, K., Reichert-Preibesch, H., Schmidt, R. *et al.* (1987) Astrological and fibroblast growth factors have neurotrophic functions for cultured peripheral and central nervous system neurons. *Proc. Natl. Acad. Sci. USA*, **84**, 5459–63.

Walicke, P.A. (1988) Basic and acidic fibroblast growth factors have trophic effects on neurons from multiple CNS regions. *J. Neurosci.*, **8**, 2616–27.

Walicke, P.A. (1989) Novel neurotrophic factors, receptors and oncogenes. *Annu. Rev. Neurosci.*, **12**, 103–26.

Walicke, P., Cowan, W.M., Ueno, N. *et al.* (1986) Fibroblast growth factor promotes the survival of dissociated hippocampal neurons and enhances neurite extension. *Proc. Natl. Acad. Sci. USA*, **83**, 3012–16.

Weber, M. (1981) A diffusible factor responsible for the determination of cholinergic functions in cultured sympathetic neurons. *J. Biol. Chem.*, **246**, 3447–53.

Williams, E.J., Doherty, P., Turner, G. *et al.* (1992) Calcium influx into neurons can solely account for calcium-dependent neurite outgrowth promoted by L1. *J. Cell Biol.*, **119**, 883–92.

Wolfgram, F. and Myers, L. (1973) Amyotrophic lateral sclerosis: the effect of serum on the anterior horn cells in tissue culture. *Science*, **179**, 579–80.

Yamada, T., Placzek, M., Tanaka, H. *et al.* (1991) Control of cell pattern in the developing nervous system: polarizing activity of the floor plate and notochord. *Cell*, **64**, 635–47.

31   *Clinical trials*

T.J. STEINER

31.1 INTRODUCTION

Motor neurone disease (MND) offers no prospect of simple-design clinical trials. Why this is so will be explained in this chapter.

There are medical conditions that do offer such a prospect. As an example, hypertension appears to be one: find patients, of whom there are many, with blood pressure levels above a clearly defined norm; divide randomly into two groups; treat one group for a short period with the test drug and the other with a control medication, all under double-blind conditions; measure the effect directly and parametrically in the members of each group and compare the groups with statistical tests of significance. Yet, lowered blood pressure is a surrogate end-point. What evidence comes from such a trial that illness is reduced, or health or well-being improved? When matters such as these become the trial objectives, a Pandora's box of difficulties is opened.

Back, therefore, to MND. This is a condition that presents extremely variably. It may exist in different forms, has its onset in an enormously wide age range, progresses largely unpredictably and, again, very variably, and offers no obvious manner of measurement. As far as the pathophysiology of MND is understood, reversal of the condition seems unattainable, arrest is the best effect ever likely to be achieved, and slowed rate of progression is the most realistic outcome presently to hope for.

In addition, MND is relatively uncommon when set against other major neurological degenerations such as cerebrovascular disease. Three unhelpful consequences follow. Firstly, adequate trials require multicentre, probably multinational, collaboration. Secondly, in the relatively young science of well-conducted clinical trials, experience in MND has yet to be obtained, whereas large multinational collaborative stroke trials, for example, are becoming so commonplace that we shall soon have learnt how to do them. Thirdly, commercial interest is lacking, favouring more common illnesses. Without commercial support it is extraordinarily difficult not only to set up and do large trials, but also to apply to them the sort of quality control now rightly demanded by drug regulatory authorities.

A further difficulty is the lack of putative therapies available in the past. Without a treatment of promise, developing the method for clinical trials has been seen as a sterile exercise. Yet, in the now necessary process of inventing the wheel for the MND cart, help is available from several sources: from an understanding of the general principles of clinical trials method; from solutions that have been developed to some of the specific problems arising in trials of those other conditions, such as stroke, from which extrapolation is possible; and from the one major collaborative multinational trial so far undertaken in MND (Steiner, 1991). In this, the SPECIALS trial of branched-chain amino acids (BCAA), the need to develop and test a method was seen as an aim of importance equal to that of evaluating the treatment, for which scientific support was rather lacking at the outset.

In the following discussion, the issues are principally those specific to MND. In identifying the issues, and in the occasional suggestion of solutions, there is heavy dependence upon what has been learnt within the SPECIALS collaboration (Steiner, 1991), although the BCAA trial is unfinished at the time of writing, and certainly unpublished. Issues specific to MND relate to the disease, the patients and the therapy. However, there are important general issues too, of science, ethics and judgements of cost–benefit. The extent to which these can produce special problems in MND trials is a matter of relevance here also, and they are briefly reviewed first.

31.2 SCIENTIFIC ISSUES

Scientific requirements in MND trials are the usual ones: adequate experimental design combined with valid assessments. The basic principles (see the simple hypertension trial above) are taken here for granted. In MND, adequate design and valid assessment obtain special significance because the nature of the illness makes both of these difficult to achieve. More detail follows in the discussions specific to the illness (section 31.5.1).

Control is particularly difficult; the problems brought by the variable symptoms and signs that present or develop in MND, the relentless but inconstant progression and the range of possible ways in which therapeutic intervention may occur are all compounded by ethical pitfalls (see below, sections 31.3 and 31.5.2).

Whereas clinical trials are usually discussed in the context of testing drug treatments, in MND potential treatments also, and importantly, include remedial (physical) therapy. This is a discipline in which objective research is problematic because of the nature of the intervention. The double-blind conditions of drug trials cannot be reproduced for a therapy that depends upon patient–therapist interaction. Nor can physical therapy be dispensed in fixed doses within a standard regimen, since standardization of therapy is a contradiction of the philosophy behind all forms of remedial therapy. If therapy is not standardized, can the assessments be? If these are not, what manner of comparative trial is possible? The tendency for investigators in this field to resort to limited-value single-case studies is easily understood.

The difficulties special to trials of physiotherapy are mentioned again in the discussion related to treatments (see section 31.5.3), but they have been described previously in some detail (Brooke and Steiner, 1990) in response to Basmajian's (1975) dispassionate comment:

> Almost all therapeutic procedures in rehabilitation departments must be regarded with suspicion; it is sound science to start on the premise that they may be either useless or harmful. The science behind them is not as strong as the faith.

This remark, today, probably does equally well for the whole MND therapeutic repertoire (leaving aside non-specific symptomatic treatments). There is no need to undertake trials comparing one drug treatment with another because no treatment standards exist. Placebo appears, scientifically, to be the best available, and that on which we need to improve. Trials must measure **efficacy** and **safety**, which are absolute qualities, not **usefulness**, which comes later when efficacy is proven and the place of one therapy in the context of others available is to be determined. In the terms of Schwartz and Lellouch (1967), trials should rather be explanatory (per protocol) than pragmatic (intention-to-treat). More is said of this later (section 31.5.2).

31.3 ETHICAL ISSUES

Ethical pitfalls are everywhere in the study of numbers of terminally ill patients, many of whom in desperation will try, even demand, any treatment available. The danger is that this frees investigators of many constraints more normally imposed by what patients will not allow to be done to them. Consent is too easily obtained. The same factor creates tensions over allocation of patients to untreated or placebo-treated comparative groups, even though it is in the nature of clinical trials that the treatment may be found to be ineffective, or even harmful.

Ethical issues have been discussed in detail by Robinson (1990), who wrote about risk-taking in relation to disease severity. The thinking of both investigator and patient is too easily distorted when the only apparent alternative to trial entry is progressive functional decline unremitting until death. To physicians, high risk for even limited promise of gain becomes acceptable; for patients, all hope is invested in the new treatment, and why would they accept a placebo?

Robinson's arguments are worth reading, although few answers are found to the problems he presents. I shall not reiterate this entire debate, but one issue he addressed is that of small (i.e. too small) trials. Cure of MND seems not to be a realistic goal, and total arrest of progression has not hitherto been thought of as a likely outcome of any treatment. Why, then, are trials done with statistical power to show only that (Munsat and Brooks, 1987)?

What Robinson did not consider is how large trials need to be. He could not have been aware of the clinical implications of the answer. If several hundred patients need to be recruited (section 31.5.1), it might be expected that several tens of centres need to participate over many months, necessarily from several countries. These figures reflect availability of resources in terms of interested investigators and adequately equipped centres (for trials as well as patient care). Actual numbers of patients may be less a limiting factor than the ability to locate them, a discovery, albeit not unexpected, made by the SPECIALS collaborators. The ethical implication is that a single major trial may substantially tie up most of the resources in an area as large as Western Europe. There is an imperative requirement to ensure, if this is so, that the trial that is done is the one that most needs doing, 'need' in this context representing the need of patients.

It is not clear that any force exists to bring this about, and more likely that commercial interests will determine the issue unless a pressure movement comes into being as patients' advocate. Even more detrimental to patients' interests would be a financially motivated abandonment of a half-completed trial, wasting the commitment of patients to it, to start another.

31.4 COST–BENEFIT

Judgements of cost–benefit ratio cannot be avoided, and rightly should not be. The need to put a price on benefit is a consequence of limited resources in health care provision. For clinical trialists the ethical issue is that resources may not be available for the treatment to continue even if found successful. Physical therapy, for example, is very expensive, and so are some drugs, especially those emerging from biotechnology programmes. Brooke and Steiner (1990) referred to:

> the almost unanswerable question of what cost society should bear to postpone death of an individual, or to improve quality of life until a foreseeable death, assuming either of those benefits is attainable. What cost should society bear for merely a reasonable prospect of such benefits?

Cost per patient may be high, but the disease is rare. Does that increase the obligation on society (lower cost), or make it lower priority (benefit to fewer)? Society, not trialists, makes these decisions, but it is the trialists' responsibility (since no-one else can) to put society in the position of being able to make an informed decision. In other words, if these questions are generated because of a trial outcome, that trial's additional duty is to provide the data to enable answers to be given. Otherwise a new ethical problem is created, and it is unfortunate in the extreme if the trial designers had failed to plan for this.

Cost containment in the treatment of a disease is an ethical requirement in itself because others, with other illnesses, supposedly will inherit the benefit of freed resources (opportunity gain). The 'value' of a treatment can therefore be measured in these terms: does it reduce other costs of treating MND, for example by maintaining mobility and independence, reducing the need for domiciliary services, residential care or hospital admissions? The equations are not easy: what weight is to be given to the unfortunate but recognizable truth that extending the life of an MND patient generally increases treatment costs?

Brooke and Steiner (1990) wrote also of the costs to be borne by the patient, or by other members of the family, rather than by society at large. The patient is clearly not the sole bearer, within the family, of the cost. If a group study of a treatment finds, say, marked benefit in 50%, moderate benefit in 25% and none in 25%, how, they asked, does the spouse of an affected parent estimate the probability of benefit to one individual and decide whether to continue the therapy at their own cost and at the price of taking their children out of private school (for example)?

The reason why this problem was especially relevant to their discussions of physiotherapy trials in MND is that disease and therapy seemed to allow matching of one to the other. The objectives of trials where this is so should not be limited to learning whether patients **as a group** can expect to gain from the treatment, but should ask also which patients have the greatest expectation, and how much of the therapy gives the best cost–benefit ratio. Clinical trialists are not used to posing such questions, or designing their protocols to answer them. It is an expertise they appear to have a duty to learn.

31.5 SPECIFIC ISSUES

31.5.1 Issues specific to the illness

DIAGNOSIS

No test is diagnostic for MND, but Mitsumoto, Kanson and Chad (1988) noted that diagnosis of the condition was made with 'surprising uniformity by physicians'. On the contrary, Li *et al.* (1991) found striking differences in diagnostic behaviour between three countries. Li *et al.* (1986) proposed a four-step diagnostic procedure based on clinical examination alone, claiming 86% specificity and therefore value in clinical research. On this criterion (14% false positives) it would not be. This paper merely illustrates that research brings extra considerations to those of routine management. Electromyography is generally believed to be a necessary part of diagnostic confirmation, essentially by contributing to the probability of being correct through the exclusion of other possibilities. Specific EMG criteria have been proposed (Denys *et al.*, 1989), but these are put forward as the 'minimum criteria needed to support the diagnosis of MND'.

How to make the diagnosis is not the subject of this chapter, although questions of diagnostic certainty are. Criteria to be adopted, therefore, may be considerably more strict in clinical trials than in conventional therapy, or may need supplementation to limit variability (Kuether, Struppler and Lipinski, 1986) (see below). But this is commonly so in other diseases too, as is the important consequence that the trial result may not be reliably extrapolated to the larger group more 'loosely' diagnosed. It would be quite undesirable if acceptance in a trial only of patients with unequivocal diagnoses led to exclusion of all except those with advanced disease (Kuether, Struppler and Lipinski, 1986). Apart from being unrepresentative, intuitively it seems that these are the least likely to gain from treatment.

The E1 Escorial criteria for diagnosis (Swash and Leigh, 1992) attempt at least to standardize the diagnostic process, compromising between specificity and selectivity. Until these, or a descendant of them, or an entirely newly generated set of criteria, become widely accepted, the SPECIALS approach to diagnosis may be the most realistic (Table 31.1).

Table 31.1 Diagnostic criteria employed by the SPECIALS collaboration in the branched-chain amino acids trial

---

Clinical diagnosis of primary ALS

The diagnosis of primary ALS requires involvement of upper **and** lower motor neurones and involvement of more than one limb or the tongue, confirmed by clinical examination by a fully trained neurologist.

This definition:

1. excludes progressive muscular atrophy (PMA) with **only** lower motor neurone signs, but includes all patients with unequivocal upper motor neurone involvement even if this is minimal and lower motor neurone signs strongly predominate;

2. excludes pure bulbar palsy (PBP) with **only** bulbar signs, but includes predominantly bulbar cases with even minimal limb involvement **provided that** both upper and lower motor neurone signs (bulbar or spinal) can be demonstrated.

(This implies that a patient with only lower motor neurone involvement when first seen may not be entered at that time, but could later become eligible if other signs appear within the first 24 months. Similarly, a patient with only bulbar involvement when first seen may not be entered at that time, but could later become eligible if spinal signs appear within the first 24 months.)

Second opinion

The confirmatory second opinion may be given by another fully trained neurologist, or by a senior trainee in a post recognized for neurological training.

EMG support

An EMG requires the following features to support a clinical diagnosis of ALS:

The EMG must in the opinion of the investigator

- support the diagnosis; **and**
- show evidence of chronic partial denervation in more than one site; **and**
- exclude peripheral neuropathy.

Essentially, whilst setting basic diagnostic rules, this approach accepts as MND whatever two independent neurologists agree is MND in any individual case. Thereby avoided are inflexible definitions that may become unintendedly exclusive. The truth is that there is no gold standard by which to judge this approach, right or wrong.

Clinical trials

The variable nature of MND has been referred to already, and of course is well known. The disease presents in many ways, with bulbar symptoms at onset or more commonly distal weakness of either upper or lower limbs. Respiratory problems can initiate medical referral (Miller et al., 1957).

These wide disparities in presentation, coupled with equal variations in the rate and pattern of disease progression that cannot be predicted, create enormous difficulties for studies of effects of intervention. Munsat, Andres and Taft (1988) found deterioration rates indicative of motor neurone loss to be remarkably linear. Andres et al. (1986), using their Tufts quantitative neuromuscular examination (TQNE), found an average deterioration of 4.5% per month. The rate of progression in such terms may be linear, but at critical times small decrements in muscle power cause major functional losses, and decline with heterogeneous patterns of disease.

Robinson (1990) referred to the need to ensure that severely affected patients are expected to survive to the end of the trial, perhaps on the basis of pulmonary function at entry, a criterion adopted by SPECIALS (Table 31.2). It is clear what he meant, even though the logic does not hold if the treatment aims to cure or arrest progression. Robinson observed that atypical cases of MND might be preferentially selected if follow-up is intended to be long term (relative to the ordinary course of MND).

Much depends on the end-point to be assessed (see below). Death is always one of the end-points in MND trials, and of course all patients enter trials alive. A more appropriate end-point might be loss of independence, however defined, but if so all patients entered must be independent. If that is the case, will benefit associated with treatment under trial conditions to this subgroup of patients extrapolate to those in routine management who are already dependent?

In the BCAA trial, SPECIALS took loss of independence as its principal end-point, but faced two major difficulties. First was that of defining independence, when some patients who could be independent were not because of indulgent carers, and some who really were not independent managed nevertheless to exist without day-to-day support through lack of provision or dogged insistence. As a way around this, SPECIALS attempted to measure what reasonably could be done, not what usually was done (Table 31.2), the opposite approach to that of the Barthel functional evaluation system (Mahoney and Barthel, 1965) used for outcome measurement.

708

Table 31.2 Entry criteria employed by the SPECIALS collaboration in the branched-chain amino acids trial

---

Inclusion critieria

1. Clinical diagnosis of primary ALS (see Table 31.1).
2. Second (confirmatory) opinion (see Table 31.1).
3. EMG supports clinical diagnosis (see Table 31.1).
4. Less than 2 years from onset.
5. History of progression over at least 3 months.
6. Forced vital capacity > 50% predicted.
7. Independence, defined as
   - feeding by mouth (i.e. not nasogastric tube or gastrostomy **and** swallowing score of 3 or 2 on Norris scale); **and**
   - self-feeding (score of 3 or 2 on Norris scale); **and**
   - ambulatory [walking 20 feet (6.5 m) unassisted, with aids; if needed assistance may be given to stand up].
8. Other medication optimized (especially anti-spasticity drugs).
9. Aged 25–80 years.
10. Informed consent.

Exclusion criteria

1. Familial ALS.
2. Known antecedent polio infection.
3. CSF protein > 100 mg/dl (if known).
4. Other neurological degenerative illness (including dementia).
5. Other severe physical disability.
   Other illness:
   - metabolic disorders (e.g. dysthyroid state) not controlled by treatment;
   - diabetes mellitus;
   - hepatic or renal disease with impaired function;
   - autoimmune disease;
   - known malignancy (affecting general health or life expectancy);
   - disabling cardiac disease (angina or heart failure).
6. Need for neuroleptics or steroid medication.
7. Therapeutic administration of BCAA in the past.

The second difficulty was that dependence might come about in several quite different ways, reflecting bulbar, upper limb, lower limb or respiratory involvement, yet adoption of such an end-point made these equal. At least they might be equivalent in a cost–benefit sense (see above, section 31.4). In any other sense, equivalence had meaning only in group comparisons, with numbers large enough that treatment groups were matched at entry (see below, section 31.5.1). High numbers, with randomization, are always the statistical solution to

Clinical trials

variability, scientifically better than measuring outcome in small non-representative groups. Very high numbers furthermore offer some hope of subgroup analysis to answer secondary questions about who, within the whole population of patients, seems most likely to gain from the tested treatment.

The Committee on Health Care Issues of the American Neurological Association (1987) noted a possible therapeutic window that might otherwise be missed: 'beneficial effects may not be seen . . . if the patient was examined too soon or too late'. As Robinson (1990) observed, 'there are grounds for believing that not all points in a trajectory of neurological deterioration are equally amenable to therapeutic attention'. Again the implications are that subgroup selection, within the overall diagnosis of MND, is on the one hand a possible prerequisite for seeing a treatment effect at all, and on the other a genuine danger in extrapolating from trial populations to those coming for routine management.

ENTRY CRITERIA: TIME FROM ONSET

Restrictive entry criteria underly Lasagna's law of clinical trials (Gorringe, 1970), which states that as soon as a clinical trial begins the supply of patients becomes one-tenth of what it was thought to be beforehand. Glasberg (1990) described a typical MND trial exemplifying Lasagna's law perfectly. In practice, Lasagna is almost invariably right, and if he is to be cheated there should be no exclusion criterion that is not based on sound argument.

Following the discussion of variability above, one issue that arises is duration of illness prior to entry, and with it the question of whether or not this matters to a treatment trial. The answer is affirmative if there is impact upon prognosis.

If time from onset is very short, a degree of diagnostic uncertainty is highly likely since a recognizable pattern of progression over time is an important contributor to diagnostic probability. Wrong diagnosis would certainly affect prognosis. (It would also alter treatment effect, if treatment is in any way specific to MND.) Progression over a minimum period should therefore be within the diagnostic criteria of a trial (Table 31.1). It will then automatically be within the entry criteria.

The same minimum time from onset will tend to exclude patients with very rapid progression, in whom it may seem that there is little opportunity for therapeutic salvation. This is more contentious, but intuitively right. In any event, specifying a minimum time from onset has both effects, and the remaining debate addresses only how long that period should be.

There is a problem also with very long times from onset. A patient who has had the illness already for 5 years demonstrates quite a slow progression. If the entry criteria specify that a patient must be independent at entry, and he still qualifies, two things are indicated. Firstly, it is a relatively unusual course, not fitting the ideal of a 'typical' patient. Secondly, and more importantly, if the slope of deterioration so far is maintained during the trial, the follow-up period will need to be very prolonged to observe a change at all, let alone a change altered by treatment.

The SPECIALS trial of amino acids set limits at 3 months and 2 years (Table 31.1). The latter limit was the single factor most responsible for loss of patients to the trial: the significance of this should not be overlooked.

ENTRY CRITERIA: RESPIRATORY FUNCTION

Poor respiratory function is the second buttress in MND trials to Lasagna's law of clinical trials (Gorringe, 1970). Its importance to trial recruitment lies in the potently adverse prognosis evidently attaching to impaired respiration. Commonly, respiratory function is measured as forced vital capacity (FVC). The measurement can be technically difficult in patients with poor bulbar function who cannot make a good mouth seal: masks are an unsatisfactory alternative, as anyone will testify who has tried the exercise with one. However, poor bulbar function of this sort is also associated with short life expectancy, so the prognostic value of FVC is not lost. Values below 60% of predicted are rarely compatible with long survival, a fact confirmed in interim safety analyses of the SPECIALS amino acids trial (unpublished data).

How this factor of respiratory impairment should be dealt with may depend rather on the anticipated or hoped for treatment effect. If a treatment may postpone death, it needs to be tested in those in whom death is expected in at least a substantial proportion. Such trials can achieve considerable statistical power with quite low numbers. Expectations tend, however, to be more modest, and the usual though not necessarily correct view is that patients 'predestined' to die should be left out. This theory is good in acute stroke trials, for example, where it might be truly said that patients unconscious early after cerebral infarction are destined to die. It is less convincing that the argument extends to MND patients who meet other reasonable entry criteria, even though their untreated life expectancy may be short.

More thought needs to be given to the usual practice of excluding such patients. I suggest instead, as it clearly is of major prognostic significance, that stratification for low FVC is a better alternative.

711

Clinical trials

The foregoing paragraphs indicate that non-entry rates will be high: 90% is predictable, but the exact figure will depend upon how inclusion/ exclusion criteria are formulated (see above). Such selectiveness, based or not upon sound reasoning, raises serious doubts about extrapolating from the select few to the many (see above and section 31.5.2).

There is no possibility of putting these doubts to rest if the entered sample cannot be related to those excluded because the characteristics of this latter group are unknown. Without some record, even the size of this group may not be known. Tiresome though it may be, diagnostic information, presentation details and basic demographic data must be kept as reference material for each patient known of but not entered (primary exclusions). The more of these there are, and therefore the more tiresome the procedure, the more important it can be seen to be.

NUMBERS

Not much can be said on requirements for group size, which are essentially statistically determined. There are few grounds for generalization since all depends on what is expected of the treatment upon what outcome measure. Numbers can be low, as in the example above, where a treatment potentially postpones death in a group selected for high expectation of death.

More modest expectations call for higher numbers. I will give one example. In a series of patients followed at Charing Cross Hospital between 1986 and 1989, outcome after 1 year can be summarized as follows: 50% still independent, 33% dependent or in institutional care, 17% dead. How these figures might extrapolate to other series defined by particular entry criteria is questionable, and this will be a problem whenever entry criteria select a subgroup not representative of the greater population from which they derive. However, if a similar outcome can be expected in those untreated, 80% power to see a treatment effect that increases those remaining independent by 25% (i.e. to 62.5%) requires 247 patients per group, testing at a significance level of 5%.

Two further points should be mentioned. The first is that larger numbers may be necessary to ensure group matching. What this means, in other words, is that a smaller sample is less likely adequately to represent the population from which it is drawn (see above). The second point is a reflection that, regardless of statistics, clinicians seem to have become desensitized to trials. Only those with grossly large numbers impress. In acute stroke, trials of 20 000 patients are being contemplated. In MND, there is still common sense, maintained by confronting patients who, untreated, get worse; in stroke, those who survive by and large get better.

ASSESSMENT OF OUTCOME

Valid and appropriate measurement of change in an illness, usually attempted by some measurement of the patient before and after intervention as well, perhaps, as during it, is at once a *sine qua non* of clinical trials and, in MND, an issue so difficult that no acceptable and widely accepted solution to it has yet been found. The disease affects the integrity of nerve cells, but manifests principally as loss of muscle power, and the patient complains of loss of a range of functional abilities. Assessment of outcome therefore implies measurement of some or all of these. Death of a patient is an outcome too, measurable in absolute terms or in terms of time until it happens. Such ultimate measures may be important, and should never be omitted, but are insensitive unless the impact of treatment is great and the stage of disease is advanced so that death is an expected outcome in at least a substantial proportion. Alternatively, follow-up may be very prolonged.

An issue relevant to death as an apparently unequivocal outcome, and to its use in illness measurement, is that of permanent artificial ventilation. This might be counted as a further separate end-point, or discounted altogether in favour of continuing neurological and functional measurements, together with time-to-death in non-survivors. The problem is that artificial ventilation is not everywhere available, and, where it is, not always offered. A pragmatic, though perhaps debatable, approach is to regard permanent artificial ventilation as the final ending of independent life, and not different for purposes of measuring treatment efficacy from death, which in any event would be the presumable consequence of withholding artificial ventilation.

For accurate and objective assessment of the neuromuscular system, especially the monitoring of muscle strength and tone, no definitive methods exist. The Medical Research Council (1976) clinical grading system for muscle power, scoring 0–5, was not developed for such purposes as this. It is limited by insensitivity, subjectivity and greatly unequal intervals between grades (Andres *et al.*, 1986) so that summation, although often practised, is meaningless. Dynamometry may yield more accurate and reproducible results – with correct use.

Isometric contractions produce muscle cramps in many MND patients, and results are invalidated where this happens. Isokinetic measures are useless in severe weakness. All measures of muscle power are altered where there is significant or, worse, variable spasticity. The measurement of spasticity, as resistance to passive movement in the limb, is always difficult, largely unhelped by technology. Clinical scores for spasticity exist too, notably the Ashworth (1964) scale of 0–4. This works quite well in upper motor neurone disease, but to judge how interaction occurs between these parameters of muscle functioning requires great clinical skill – not to mention self-confidence! Anyway, what is the 'true' measure of muscle power: with or without allowance for spasticity?

Muscle testing in MND patients is further hampered by muscle contractures and painful joints, fatigue, dyspnoea, communication difficulty and emotional lability. Muscle power in MND is also subject to fluctuations during the day, and from day to day. Muscle power may be unaltered yet functioning greatly changed through modification of muscle tone, body position and posture and emotional state. Standardization of medication taken to reduce spasticity is an issue to be considered separately, especially since there may be paradoxical consequences for function when loss of lower limb tone causes loss of posture, or support in gait.

Gait is fortunately objectively quantifiable in many ways, although good measures of quality of gait remain elusive. Timed measures of gait in any event destroy quality, and have little functional meaning. As they are also dangerous where gait is impaired, they are wisely avoided. Gait at least is an activity whose measurement is relevant to the illness, but it is soon lost in many patients, remains hardly impaired in a few, and in all cases other functional losses occur.

Scores of 'overall' function are available (e.g. Norris et al., 1974; Andres et al., 1986; Hillel et al., 1988), generally producing figures whose meaning is difficult to conceptualize. The Norris scale (Norris et al., 1974; Hillel et al., 1990), and modifications thereof, have gained popularity in a vacuum of alternatives. These scores are non-linear, and difficult to repeat accurately at home where function, according to common sense, is most appropriately measured. Many factors affecting functional assessment are subjective, and Robinson (1990) debated whether or not these assessments are valid contributors to group outcome measurement, arguing elsewhere (Robinson, 1987) that they may be.

The SPECIALS BCAA protocol has included a modification of the Barthel score (Mahoney and Barthel, 1965), devised by a physiotherapist for patients undergoing rehabilitation. The objective was more an attempt to assess its validity in ALS (see Louwerse, de Jong and Kuether, 1990) than actually to make use of it. But even a simplistic approach to functional measurement, with categorical assessments of 'can' or 'cannot', is beset with difficulties. Is a patient who can comfortably walk 20 feet unaided independent in that activity if he cannot get out of his chair? What is the real-life meaning of 'independence in feeding' if the food initially has to be brought to the patient?

The answer is that true functions, in the 'activities of daily living' sense, are not ideal measures because they are so subject to living conditions. A patient may one day lose the ability to clean his teeth because the last user of the toothpaste tube replaced the top too tightly. These things are not useful to measure, because they are not disease specific. Instead, we isolate facets of function, recognizing that they are artificial and may not relate to real-life function, but selecting them because they appear on the one hand to be important and on the other so affected by disease that change can be regarded as consequent upon disease (disease-specific). We might call these faculties, as opposed to functions. Because the course of MND runs differently in different individuals, unequally represented in bulbar symptoms and signs and those affecting upper and lower limbs and respiration, some faculty specific to each of these needs to be measured: hence swallowing, self-feeding (with food laid ready), walking (from standing) and respiration (as forced vital capacity), as adopted by SPECIALS (Table 31.2).

On a further note, it is as well to keep in mind the possibility that patient's views of benefit may differ from the physician's (Wynne, 1989). This **may** be because the physician's perception of what constitutes benefit is misjudged. Robinson (1990) introduced a note of caution possibly relevant to this. 'Fundamentally', he wrote, 'the issue is to what extent trials should be concerned with the precise measurement of motor neurone loss and possible regeneration, or be concerned with functional changes which may or may not be correlated with such loss or regeneration.'

Robinson saw this question reflecting the debate on whether trials should be concerned with therapeutic efficacy alone, or had a role also in exploring pathogenesis. (This raises a separate issue of patient's consent in terms of what they believe to be the **purpose** of what they consent to, which I will not go into.) The further issue Robinson perceived was of the whole status of objective measurements, whether fundamental or functional in emphasis, in relation to subjective indicators of improvement. Wynne's (1989) message, strongly expressed, was essentially the same. The ultimate response might be to abandon all indices of illness in favour of a single, necessarily subjective measure of quality of life.

Robinson's arguments can be read in his paper (Robinson, 1990). However these might be resolved, a separate question, to my mind important but often neglected, is that of who should do these

715

Clinical trials

assessments. Senior hospital specialists with a long-developed interest in MND or other neurological disabling illness may be highly skilled in assessment, but out of their element in patients' homes. Junior medical staff 'taken on' for the trial may be equally unfamiliar with home visiting, without having the advantage of assessment skills based on long experience and a deep understanding of the illness and patients who are its victims. Nurses, at least in the UK, in general have very limited training in clinical measurement, and little understanding of the scientific principles on which it is based.

Physiotherapists do have this training, and mostly are substantially more skilled at muscle, movement and functional assessments than recently qualified doctors. Furthermore, they are more used to notions of community-based medical care than most hospital doctors, and respond better and more flexibly to the idea of home assessment. They may be too individualistic in approach, failing to see the importance of measurement in terms relevant to groups, but this calls only for education.

Whoever does the assessments needs careful and repeated standardization training, and there is a lot to be said for some form of recurrent performance validation as a quality control measure. If this is done, the so-called 'ideal' of one assessor throughout the trial may lose importance. It may as well be admitted that this is anyway less practical in a prolonged study than is often claimed, and quite devalued in the context of multicentre, let alone multinational, studies.

PRACTICALITIES OF FOLLOW-UP

The central feature of MND is progressively increasing disability, eventually becoming severe in all cases. Greatly disabled patients cannot reasonably be expected to travel long distances for assessment, and if they do so it is at considerable cost to them. Rarely can they do so repeatedly. If hospital admission for this purpose is the result, it should be noted that the upset to the patient's routine during a stay of any length may be detrimental in its own way. Altered diet and enforced inactivity affect health and mobility. Aids to mobility, however thoughtfully provided, never replicate home, where a clutter of strategically placed pieces of furniture can be the key to a patient's movement about the house.

For the serial assessments that this progressive disease demands, patients whose disability is increasing will not return again and again to the hospital, even if they were able to initially. In any event, faced with continuing deterioration, patients may make their own judgements of treatment efficacy. The consequence in both cases is a loss to the trial of patients in whom worsening continues apace, a potential source of serious bias.

In my opinion, patients who enter MND trials with prolonged follow-up must be offered the option of reassessment at home if this bias is to be avoided, and to be fair to them. This is so notwithstanding the logistic problems for the investigator, and the fact that testing then does not take place under ideally standardized conditions. Assessments made in difficult circumstances are better than none at all, and if there is to be difficulty either way does the assessment gain from placing this on the patient rather than the investigator? Equally importantly, because it has a potential impact on assessment validity, is it not worthwhile to have the opportunity during home assessment for direct observation of what is provided in services, and of intrafamily relationships?

31.5.2 Issues specific to the patients

SELECTION BIAS

MND is an uncommon condition, and trials may need to recruit from a large geographical area. The resulting requirement to travel considerable distances may deter those with more advanced disease, and particular manifestations, from entering. Elderly patients on the one hand, and those with young dependants on the other, may be less inclined to take part. A sample will poorly represent those still working and unwilling to take time off work repeatedly. This may exclude from the trial those most highly motivated. Conversely, patients in whom the disease provokes depression, perhaps highly represented in a particular subgroup, will not be inclined to take part.

Thus there is no obvious means of access to a population of MND patients representative of all MND sufferers. To recognize this limitation in conclusions drawn from trial outcomes is one thing: to define or quantify its effect is quite another.

Agencies such as the Motor Neurone Disease Association, a patient-based UK charity in touch with many patients for purposes primarily of care-giving, not research, have a role to play in recruitment – if they wish to take it. Such a source may be relatively free of bias, although possibly unrepresentative of social class. Organizations of this nature do not exist in many other countries. But always left out will be those in whom the diagnosis has not been made, is incorrect or for some reason not imparted, and others who have not yet sought any help. Nobody knows how these factors bias entry to trials, or even if it matters whether they do. Still other patients do not wish to take part in research, whereas the opposite extreme – patients desperate to try anything, consenting to everything, however offered, and if possible all at once – is not uncommonly encountered.

CONTROLS

If the need for a controlled experiment is unarguable (and perhaps it is not, for it is questioned below), finding an untreated group of similar patients may not be easy because of the issues discussed above. Variability is one problem but, at least in theory, this can be overcome statistically, by randomization of large numbers. Yet matching for age, sex, disease subtype, stage of disease and rate of progression, areas affected, functional consequences, psychological adjustment and response and coping abilities, impossible in a small and heterogeneous population, makes heavy demands of randomization even in quite large groups. So recruitment targets get bigger and bigger, notwithstanding the difficulties noted above in finding large numbers.

Published experience here is zero: only SPECIALS so far has exceeded a target of 200 per treatment group. Matching at entry (*a priori*) by stratification reduces outcome variability in a smaller number so long as what is matched is what is important prognostically. The SPECIALS experience suggests that, with the exception of impaired respiratory function (as indicated by forced vital capacity reduced to < 50% of predicted), what we thought we knew of prognostic markers (age, duration of illness since onset, bulbar involvement) may be quite in error.

There are other very serious problems in generating a control group. It is ethically difficult to recruit patients without offering the therapy. The concept of equipoise makes no difference: patients envisage only a single chance for themselves. For patients with a life expectancy of a few months, that period on placebo treatment is a sacrifice of everything. The possibility that the treatment may be on trial for safety as well as efficacy has little real meaning in such a context.

Intention-to-treat trials (section 31.2) are particularly problematic, requiring the patient to remain under review, and without other trial treatments, for the originally envisaged follow-up period even if for some reason they do not continue the treatment. They are 'locked in without further hope'.

Intention-to-treat trials are not mandatory, and, in consequence of this issue alone, perhaps should be avoided. Intention-to-treat trials are intended to replicate current practice, to reflect the problems, inconsistencies and compliance failures of routine management of the disease. What meaning does this have when there is no current treatment? The one thing that is certain above all is that when a treatment is found, or appears to have been found, 'routine' management will change.

Is there a mandate for controlled trials in MND? This question is equally contentious in other diseases, and discussion generally begs the question of what is actually controlled. Self-deception is not unknown in trial design. What, for example, determines survival in a trial, if this is to be the measure of outcome?

According to Munsat, Andres and Taft (1988), longevity in MND is as dependent on 'external' health factors such as emphysema, smoking history, general medical care and respiratory support as on actual motor neurone loss. How well are these taken into account, and, if they are not, how good is the control? Other important 'external' factors are qualities of the carer, and of the home, availability of mobility aids, provision of services, and a variety of personality factors that determine ability to cope. Other treatments can also be 'external' to the trial (see below).

It is left only to argue that, against the background of chronic progressive incurable disease, patients perhaps can act as their own controls, and to question whether, in such a context, placebo effect has any lasting power that needs to be isolated and corrected for.

31.5.3 Issues specific to the therapy

Brooke and Steiner (1990) discussed the difficulties of putting physical therapy on trial. Many of these are specific to that type of therapy, and readers are referred to that paper.

Drug treatment protocols may seem to be free of many of these problems. Yet one point coming from that discussion is the need to be aware of other treatments the patient may be receiving. Drug trial protocols as a matter of course draw up lists of excluded concomitant medication. Do they always, however, consider the possible impact of a newly started course of hydrotherapy, for example, or the functional improvement suddenly achieved by provision of a much-needed aid?

The problem here, of course, is that these matters are highly patient specific: what can bring about profound change for one may have no impact whatsoever on another. In trial protocols it is difficult to legislate for all possibilities even if there were ethical freedom to do so.

COMPLIANCE

Cooperation with treatment programmes in MND trials is not usually a problem initially. Most patients are eager to help themselves, and participate to the full if the project is proposed to them in the spirit of being a collaborative venture against the disease. However, compliance with treatment is sooner or later influenced by three adverse factors.

Firstly, it may be affected by treatment side-effects. These of course are generally treatment specific. In SPECIALS they include difficulty in swallowing the large bulk of not very edible BCAA powders, and an equal problem with the placebo. This last point is important in preservation of blindness, which can all too easily be undone even by minor but consistently reported side-effects, as was discovered in many of the TRH trials (Brooke *et al.*, 1986; Caroscio *et al.*, 1986; Mitsumoto *et al.*, 1986).

Secondly, the start of a treatment programme for an incurable disease risks hopes being inappropriately raised with the proposition that therapy can help. Wynne (1989) showed that multiple sclerosis patients were not necessarily driven to unreasoning optimism, but unrealistically high expectations have led, in terminal cancer patients, for example, to later anger, frustration and disillusionment (Chatterton, 1988). All of these promote the growth of non-compliance, and artificially poor retest results after a while.

The opposite side of this coin is sometimes seen: patients who argue that 'more of a good thing must be better' and increase the dose of self-administered therapy. If the treatment has been correctly prescribed in the first place this can lead only to a raised incidence of side-effects without prospect of extra benefit, and ultimately may undo all good.

Thirdly, simple treatment failure, real or apparent, with disease progression even in the absence of unrealistic expectation, can dull the motivation of anyone. There is a danger here not only of non-random drop-out, referred to earlier, but also of non-random non-compliance. Reduction of this risk is seen as a compelling argument for intention-to-treat analyses, but this does not solve this problem. It may reduce the risk of overestimating efficacy, but in this disease to miss identifying real benefit by diluting it with the non-response of non-compliers may be the greater of the two evils.

These several circumstances establish the importance of compliance monitoring, both to promote compliance (a concept foreign to intention-to-treat trial design) and to be aware of compliance failures. A secondary but important reason for wishing the second of these is that compliance failure may not be whimsical but covertly reflect adverse side-effects of the treatment. The mainstay procedure for compliance monitoring in drug trials is pill counting, which has never been shown to be a valid method. Alternatives such as occasional and anticipated blood level monitoring have little claim to greater validity. Methods that do, such as electronic event monitors in the form of pill containers, are expensive and need, in this disease, to be shown to be necessary. Motivation is usually accompanied by honesty, and in most cases there is a carer to ask as well as the patient.

DURATION OF FOLLOW-UP

The dilemma here results from a multiple conflict. Firstly, consideration for patients brings awareness that longer follow-up makes greater demands, and possibly consigns them to a useless therapy for the remainder of their lifetime. Secondly, concern for the trial is that longer follow-up results in more drop-outs and falling compliance. Thirdly, to obtain the trial result in as short a time as possible is a wish for the benefit of all future patients, as well as those involved in it presently. Fourthly, the duration of therapy might be chosen so that it is most likely to reveal benefit, but there is awareness too that perhaps it is life-long treatment that will subsequently be offered and that should, therefore, be tested.

Of course the resolution of this complex conundrum is again dependent on the nature of the treatment, and the hoped-for effect. But throughout I have assumed that the purpose is to modify the disease progression. In that case, a short follow-up time (say 3 months) is likely to identify only a fairly remarkable change in the natural history. Even if such occurred, it would still be of rather major importance to know whether such an effect was maintained – and that means more prolonged follow-up. Periods of a year, or longer, seem to be an inescapable minimum.

STOPPING RULES AND MONITORING COMMITTEES

The question of when, and in what circumstances, a trial should be prematurely halted is by and large a general issue (Zelen, 1974, 1979; Pocock, 1983, 1992). Robinson (1990) found it particularly apposite to MND trials, but perhaps this is only because MND patients tend to vote with their feet if doubts about continuing arise: they look at once for another trial, because they are short of time.

I will not discuss what the rules should be: essentially they are determined statistically upon a statement of what risks the investigators are prepared to accept on their patients' behalf (section 31.3). The risks here are of continuing a relatively or actually harmful treatment in one group versus that of throwing away the trial and the resources, including patient commitment, that the trial has already consumed. It should be remembered that, in the present state of the MND treatment art, actual harm from the active treatment is as likely as relative harm (from withholding treatment) on placebo. These are very difficult issues

Clinical trials

to explain to patients but, if this is not done, it might be thought that they are not issues for the investigators instead to determine. If they do determine them, it might be thought that they should be subject to external review in the process.

This is the place of the monitoring committee, **which every large multicentre trial should have**, without exception. And until we know better, it should be set up in a way that follows the spirit of guidelines for the constitution of research ethics committees generally: with a mixture of experts, non-experts and lay. SPECIALS included a statistician and a lawyer: this may be a good model!

REFERENCES

Andres, P.L., Hedlund, W., Finison, L. *et al.* (1986) Quantitative motor assessment in amyotrophic lateral sclerosis. *Neurology*, **36**, 937–41.

Ashworth, B. (1964) Preliminary trial of carisoprodol in multiple sclerosis. *Practitioner*, **192**, 540–2.

Basmajian, J.V. (1975) Research and retrench. *Physical Therapy*, **55**, 607–8.

Brooke, A.S. and Steiner, T.J. (1990) Special problems of physiotherapy trials in motor neuron disease, in *Amyotrophic Lateral Sclerosis* (ed. F. Clifford Rose), Demos, New York, pp. 181–93.

Brooke, M.H., Florence, J.M., Heller, S.L. *et al.* (1986) Controlled trial of thyrotropin releasing hormone in amyotrophic lateral sclerosis. *Neurology*, **36**, 146–51.

Caroscio, J.T., Cohen, J.A., Zawodniak, J. *et al.* (1986) A double-blind, placebo-controlled trial of TRH in amyotrophic lateral sclerosis. *Neurology*, **36**, 141–5.

Chatterton, P. (1988) Physiotherapy for the terminally ill. *Physiotherapy*, **74**, 42–6.

Committee on Health Care Issues of the American Neurological Association (1987) Current status of thyrotropin-releasing hormone therapy in amyotrophic lateral sclerosis. *Ann. Neurol.*, **22**, 541–3.

Denys, E.H., Guiloff, R.J., Kelly, J.J. *et al.* (1989) The role of EMG in ALS treatment trials: Committee Report. *Internat. ALS.MND Update*, **3Q89**, 10–12.

Glasberg, M.R. (1990) Selection of patients in therapeutic trials, in *Amyotrophic Lateral Sclerosis* (ed. F. Clifford Rose), Demos, New York, pp. 33–8.

Gorringe, J.A.L. (1970) Initial preparation for clinical trials, in *The Principles and Practice of Clinical Trials* (eds E.L. Harris and J.D. Fitzgerald), Livingstone, Edinburgh, pp. 41–6.

Hillel, A.D., Miller, R.M., McDonald, E. *et al.* (1988) Amyotrophic lateral sclerosis severity scale, in *Amyotrophic Lateral Sclerosis: Recent Advances in Research and Treatment* (eds T. Tsubaki and Y. Yase), Excerpta Medica, Amsterdam, pp. 247–52.

Hillel, A.D., Miller, R.M., Yorkston, K. *et al.* (1990) Amyotrophic lateral sclerosis severity scale, in *Amyotrophic Lateral Sclerosis* (ed. F. Clifford Rose), Demos, New York, pp. 93–7.

Kuether, G., Struppler, A. and Lipinski, H.G. (1986) Therapeutic trials in ALS –

the design of a protocol, in *Amyotrophic Lateral Sclerosis* (eds V. Cosi, A.C. Kato, W. Parlette, P. Pinelli and M. Poloni), Plenum, New York, pp. 265–76.

Li, T.M., Day, S.J., Alberman, E. and Swash, M. (1986) Differential diagnosis of motoneurone disease from other neurological conditions. *Lancet*, **ii**, 731–3.

Li, T.M., Swash, M., Alberman, E. and Day, S.J. (1991) Diagnosis of motor neuron disease in three countries. *J. Neurol. Neurosurg. Psychiatr.*, **54**, 980–3.

Louwerse, E.S., de Jong, J.M.B.V. and Kuether, G. (1990) Critique of assessment methodology in amyotrophic lateral sclerosis, in *Amyotrophic Lateral Sclerosis* (ed. F. Clifford Rose), Demos, New York, pp. 151–79.

Mahoney, F.I. and Barthel, D.W. (1965) Functional evaluation: the Barthel index. *Maryland State Med. J.*, **14**, 61–5.

Medical Research Council (1976) Aids to the examination of the peripheral nervous system. *Memorandum No. 45*. HMSO, London, pp. 1–2.

Miller, R.D., Mulder, D.W., Fowler, W.S. and Olsen, A.M. (1957) Exertional dyspnoea: a primary complaint in unusual cases of progressive muscular atrophy and amyotrophic lateral sclerosis. *Ann. Int. Med.*, **46**, 119–22.

Mitsumoto, H., Hanson, M.R. and Chad, D.A. (1988) Amyotrophic lateral sclerosis: recent advances in pathogenesis and clinical trials. *Arch. Neurol.*, **45**, 189–202.

Mitsumoto, H., Salgado, E.D., Negroski, D. *et al.* (1986) Amyotrophic lateral sclerosis: effects of acute intravenous and chronic subcutaneous administration of thyrotropin-releasing hormone in controlled trials. *Neurology*, **36**, 152–9.

Munsat, T.L. and Brooks, B.R. (1987) Don't throw the baby out with the bathwater (letter). *Neurology*, **37**, 544–5.

Munsat, T.L., Andres, P. and Taft, J. (1988) The nature of clinical change in amyotrophic lateral sclerosis, in *Amyotrophic Lateral Sclerosis: Recent Advances in Research and Treatment* (eds T. Tsubaki and Y. Yase), Excerpta Medica, Amsterdam, pp. 203–6.

Norris, F.H., Calanchini, P.R., Fallat, R.J. *et al.* (1974) The administration of guanidine in amyotrophic lateral sclerosis. *Neurology*, **24**, 721–8.

Pocock, S.J. (1983) *Clinical Trials: A Practical Approach*. Wiley, London.

Pocock, S.J. (1992) When to stop a clinical trial. *Br. Med. J.*, **305**, 235–40.

Robinson, I. (1987) Analysing the structure of 23 clinical trials in multiple sclerosis. *Neuroepidemiology*, **6**, 46–76.

Robinson, I. (1990) Ethical issues and methodological problems in the conduct of clinical trials in amyotrophic lateral sclerosis, in *Amyotrophic Lateral Sclerosis* (ed. F. Clifford Rose), Demos, New York, pp. 195–213.

Schwartz, D. and Lellouch, J. (1967) Explanatory and pragmatic attitudes in therapeutic trials. *J. Chron. Dis.*, **20**, 637–48.

Steiner, T.J. (1991) Branched-chain amino-acids in ALS: the European trial, in *New Evidence in MND/ALS Research* (ed. F. Clifford Rose), Smith-Gordon, London, pp. 315–16.

Swash, M. and Leigh, N. (1992) Criteria for diagnosis of familial amyotrophic lateral sclerosis (workshop report). *Neuromusc. Disord.*, **2**, 7–9.

723

Clinical trials

Wynne, A. (1989) Is it any good? The evaluation of therapy by participants in a clinical trial. *Soc. Sci. Med.*, **29**, 1289–97.

Zelen, M. (1974) The randomisation and stratification of patients to clinical trials. *J. Chron. Dis.*, **27**, 365–75.

Zelen, M. (1979) A new design for randomised clinical trials. *New Engl. Med. J.*, **300**, 1242–5.

POSTSCRIPT

Laughter in Hell

GEORGE MACBETH

I'm a baby
Growing backwards. Every day
    A little bit less. Can't walk
    So many yards. Harder to pour the tea.
Phlegm in the throat. I have a bath
With qualms. Approach bumpy ground
    Leaning on someone's arm. Type
    With a lot of difficulty. Writing a cheque
When it's cold can take a long time. Why cold?
I don't know. There's a lot they don't know
    About life. But I'll tell you one thing.
    It's a lethal, progressive, incurable
Disease. Like mine.

Thus the man on splints, gritting his teeth
    As he fell on the terrace.
    But they came soon,
Bearing toast, a fur hippopotamus,
The new *Poetry Review*, anything.
    Anything at all
To block the bones in his hands,
The skeleton below the skin
Sneering at them. Old friends were worst
    With their frightening sympathy
Instead of news. What's the prognosis?
He's walking slower
Than last year. It must be terrible for you.

So make a joke,
Maybe take him away for a while. I can read
    The tea-leaves for myself.

Laughter in Hell

Some days he's fine, yes. I don't know, no.
I don't know what I'll do
    If he gets worse. I mean when, yes.
One fucker was even crying. I'll do the crying,
Sonny boy, you stand and listen. Give
    Me a break. Friends!
I'd rather have enemies,
They make me try harder. What's that?
    There's no pain.
He just gets very tired. He can hardly stand sometimes

Imagine buttons
That won't go into their holes. Shoelaces
    You can't untie. Fancy going to bed
    In your brogues? And a zip
You need two hands for. A scenario.
The man stumps into a lavatory
    On his dog-headed stick. Leans the stick
In a corner. Leans on the wall
With one hand, and fumbles. Meanwhile, the piss,
    Growing tired of waiting, comes
With a gush. Over the seat,
Over the whole world
    It sometimes seems. And he has to wipe it up.
There are nights
When I think of euthanasia. Nights.
    When I watch television, dreaming
    Of running for a bus again. Nights
When it all seems just like yesterday, except
    For the stiffness in my joints. Roll on,
    Cataclysm. Let someone else have it.
Lung cancer, blow up in Armagh, lose his daughter
In a car crash. Join the club.
    I'm sick of being alone
    In the wheel-chair dream.
The brakes fail. You can't get away
    From the mugger. I have to stand or choke.

It dissolves, though. There are mornings
When I wake fairly cheerful. I rise
    And manage to shave. Not so bad.
I look out and it's raining. The cows
Don't look so good either. I get downstairs,
    Eat some breakfast. I read a book

Or the papers. Maybe they'll find a cure. Pigs
    Might fly. Ironic laughter
    Can make you choke on a blood pressure pill.
It's a joke. There's no pain,
So you can't be ill. I laugh, I go
    On laughing. Remember, you laugh
And the world laughs with you. Laughter in paradise.
                        Laughter in hell.

Index

The following abbreviations are used throughout the index:
ALS   amyotrophic lateral sclerosis
MND   motor neuron disease
SMA   spinal muscular atrophies

731

Index

Index

Index

Index

Index

Index

Index

Index

Index

Index

Index